Child and Adolescent Communication Disorders

Organic and Neurogenic Bases

Child and Adolescent Communication Disorders

Organic and Neurogenic Bases

Marie R. Kerins, EdD, CCC-SLP

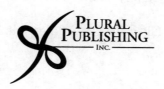

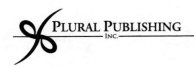

5521 Ruffin Road
San Diego, CA 92123

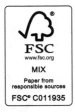

e-mail: info@pluralpublishing.com
Website: http://www.pluralpublishing.com

Typeset in 10.5/13 Palatino by Flanagan's Publishing Services, Inc.
Printed in the United States of America by McNaughton and Gunn, Inc.

Library of Congress Cataloging-in-Publication Data

Child and adolescent communication disorders : organic and neurogenic bases / [edited by] Marie R. Kerins.
     p. ; cm.
Includes bibliographical references and index.
ISBN 978-1-59756-656-8 (alk. paper)—ISBN 1-59756-656-X (alk. paper)
I. Kerins, Marie R., editor.
[DNLM: 1. Communication Disorders. 2. Adolescent. 3. Child. WL 340.2]
RC423
616.85'5—dc23
                                                        2014034175

Contents

v

Preface

One hundred years of practice, one thousand hours of assessment and treatment —that is what this collaborative text represents across the contributing authors. I am pleased and proud to present this textbook that was written by speech-language pathology and audiology faculty at Loyola University in Maryland. *Child and Adolescent Communication Disorders: Organic and Neurogenic Bases* is a textbook of disorders that we as clinicians have encountered in our own practice over the many years of working with children and adolescents. Each contributing author has had involvement and often extensive experience in both the practice and research in their respective chapter contribution. Participation in professional listservs has confirmed the need for such a text with a range of disorders from cleft palate to communication disorders concomitant with emotional and behavioral disorders.

It was important for us to include a representative sample of disorders. Organizing the content by disorder aides in text organization but also limits the reader to think beyond the restriction of the chapter's boundaries. Many of these disorders overlap and co-occur with one another. You will find this as you read through the respective chapters where there are often references to other communication disorders or other chapters. We were pleased to be able to include the new DSM-5 diagnostic criteria that serve as a common language among many health care providers. The following section will describe the text organization.

Text Organization

The intent of this book is to introduce the reader to disorders that a speech-language pathologist will likely encounter on his or her caseload. The range of disorders varies from those that affect the client physically or organically such as cleft palate and cerebral palsy to disorders that have a more neurogenic origin such as traumatic brain injury to disorders in between that may have aspects of both organic and neurogenic origin. As research evolves, identifying the etiology of the disorders becomes more specific and objective and less behavioral. Brain studies and genetic studies further illuminate our understanding of the disorders. Each chapter begins with chapter objectives followed by definitions, information on etiology, and characteristics of the disorder.

Next, information on assessment and treatment are presented as a general introduction to these disorders giving the reader a sense of direction in both choosing assessment measures and providing intervention. As the evidence base in the profession grows, SLPs can treat clients with more scientific support. However, there is still much room for growth in developing an evidence base for many of the disorders presented. The authors have tried to bring in evidence-based approaches but will also indicate approaches that are largely theoretical and/or need further replication due to conclusions from less rigorous research designs.

It is also critical that despite the most rigorous research designs clients are individuals who are complex. There are many factors that contribute to the outcomes of treatment and at the end of the day the savvy clinician will use not only the written research but his or her own expertise and the influence of the client's individual needs.

The text is divided into six parts, all of which have been written to include and be consistent with the new DSM-5 diagnostic categories. Part I includes *Developmental Disorders* of the brain with both neurogenic and organic bases. Chapter 1 *Autism Spectrum Disorders*, Chapter 2 *Language Learning Disabilities*, and Chapter 3 *Intellectual Limitations*. Part II *Organic Bases* includes more traditionally defined organic disorders. Chapter 4 *Cerebral Palsy* and Chapter 5 *Cleft Lip and Palate* are described. Part III *Neurogenic Disorders* includes Chapter 6, *Traumatic Brain Injuries,* which affect the nervous system. Part IV *Disorders Secondary to Environmental Factors* includes a disorder that can be argued to have both organic and neurogenic bases; however, I felt it best to include this under the heading *Fetal Alcohol Spectrum Disorders*, Chapter 7. Part V, *Emotional and Behavioral Disorders,* includes a chapter entitled *Communication Disorders Concomitant with Communication Disorders;* many of these have neurogenic implications. Finally, Part VI *Central Auditory Processing Disorders* includes an overview of the implications the central auditory nervous system has on processing language. This is the last chapter, Chapter 9, *Central Auditory Processing Disorders.*

Cover Design

As the editor, I was drawn to the cover picture illustrated by my nephew, William Reilly, for this text. Although the image of the chicken is somewhat an odd choice for a text on communication disorders it represents many thoughts and feelings that encapsulate the struggles and gifts of the children and adolescents we work with. Our students, so unique and talented in their contributions, are frequently at odds in their ability to adequately communicate their thoughts and needs whereas some also struggle to understand the essence of communication when spoken to. If asked to draw a picture of communication, a child draws an animal representing how they see themselves as a communicator—poorly understood. When asked to draw a chicken, the adolescent on the autism spectrum deliberates on which of the five breeds of chickens he/she should draw, yet fails to be able to forge friendships with his or her classmates.

Finally, the old adage of the chicken and egg comes to mind. As communication skills develop, the reciprocity between social-emotional development and skilled communication is intertwined. Communication skills develop in tandem with a rich language and literacy environment. One is dependent upon the other demonstrating that the causal relationship is not linear but reciprocal, with environmental factors contributing to language development and language development impacting how one communicates with the environment. Although difficult to disentangle, understanding their connection assists in the intervention process.

Acknowledgments

As editor and contributing author of the text I recognize the commitment and work it takes to publish a textbook. First, I would like to thank each of the contributing authors who made this possible. They were responsive, quick to turn their edits around, and remained cheerful in the process! There were also many others who made significant contributions by tirelessly checking references, proofing text, and designing tables among other tasks. These individuals include Elizabeth Watson, Diana Dautzenberg, Annmarie Langlois, Bernie Kremer, Lacey Cohen, Monique Bujold, Taylor Moore, Kathryn Hughes, and Natasha Sutton. I also want to thank the wonderfully supportive staff from Plural Publishing. Valerie Johns believed in the project and saw this through from beginning to end. Gem Rabanera and Taylor Eaton worked on the details of keeping me on a timeline, reminding me what needed to happen and creating action items for me to complete. Thank you all.

Finally, I want to thank my nephew William for his artistic contribution to the cover, and my husband, Mike, children Michael, Kaitlin, and Brendan, and daughter-in-law Lauren for their confidence, encouragement, and support.

Acknowledgements

Contributors

Libby Kumin, PhD, CCC-SLP
Professor
Department of Speech-Language
  Pathology and Audiology
Loyola University Maryland
Baltimore, Maryland
Chapter 3

Angela Strauch Lane, MS, CCC-SLP
Director of Assistive Technology
Unified Community Connections, Inc.
Affiliate Faculty
Department of Speech-Language
  Pathology and Audiology
Loyola University Maryland
Baltimore, Maryland
Chapter 4

Marie R. Kerins, EdD, CCC-SLP
Department Chair
Department of Speech-Language
  Pathology and Audiology
Loyola University Maryland
Baltimore, Maryland
Chapter 8

Donna L. Pitts, AuD, CCC-A
Assistant Professor
Department of Speech-Language
  Pathology and Audiology
Loyola University Maryland
Baltimore, Maryland
Chapter 9

Janet Preis, EdD, CCC-SLP
Associate Professor
Department of Speech-Language
  Pathology and Audiology
Loyola University Maryland
Baltimore, Maryland
Chapter 1

Brianne Higgins Roos, MS, CCC-SLP
Affiliate Faculty
Department of Speech-Language
  Pathology and Audiology
Loyola University Maryland
Baltimore, Maryland
Chapter 7

Lisa Schoenbrodt, EdD, CCC-SLP
Professor
Department of Speech-Language
  Pathology and Audiology
Loyola University Maryland
Baltimore, Maryland
Chapters 2 and 6

Kathleen Siren, PhD, CCC-SLP
Assistant Professor
Department of Speech-Language
  Pathology and Audiology
Loyola University Maryland
Baltimore, Maryland
Chapter 5

Kara Tignor, MS, CCC-SLP
Division Director
Speech-Language and Hearing Clinic
Loyola Clinical Centers
Loyola University Maryland
Baltimore, Maryland
Chapter 2

This book is dedicated to my brother Paul and sister Kathleen who taught me not to take anything for granted, to appreciate what we have, and that complaining is often not productive. And to all the children and adolescents whom I have worked with over the last 30 years; each individual is unique and there is always something we can learn from one another.

PART I

Developmental Brain Differences

CHAPTER 1

Autism Spectrum Disorders

Janet Preis

Chapter Objectives

Upon completing this chapter, the reader should be able to:

1. Define autism according to DSM-5 (and differentiate from DSM-IV)
2. Describe the characteristics of ASD across domains of socialization, language, and behavior
3. Describe the role of the speech-language pathologist as it relates to screening, diagnosis, and assessment
4. Explain appropriate means and content of communication assessment across life span of students with ASD
5. Describe overview of intervention for social communication
6. Delineate communication interventions according to levels of evidence

Introduction

Autism spectrum disorders (ASDs) have become one of the most prominent and challenging disabilities for children and their families. Recent statistical information (Centers for Disease Control [CDC], 2014) indicates that one child in every 68 is classified as having an ASD. These remarkable statistics have led the CDC to encourage the health professions to consider ASD as a critical and urgent public health concern (CDC). Although many professionals work with and are responsible for assessment and intervention of people with ASD, speech-language pathologists (SLPs) play a critical role. Two of the core components of an ASD are significant impairments in communication and socialization. Although these were divided into separate "entities" in the previous diagnostic criteria (see DSM-IV-TR, American Psychiatric Association [APA] 2000), it is most appropriate (as reflected in the 2013 DSM-5 criteria) to consider these deficits as one central impairment, that of *social communication*. Therefore, due to their knowledge base and scope of practice, SLPs are on the forefront of assessment and service provision for people with ASD. This chapter examines autism spectrum disorder (referred to interchangeably as ASD and autism) as it relates to the SLP, including the diagnostic criteria, particularly the characteristics of social communication and behavior, and their influence on assessment and service provision.

In 1943, Leo Kanner first proposed the diagnosis of infantile autism. Based on the observation of 11 children, Kanner outlined both social and communicative deficits, which, despite even the most recent diagnostic changes and research findings, are remarkably consistent with the definition currently in use more than 70 years later. Kanner used the term *autistic* to describe "the outstanding, 'pathognomonic,' fundamental disorder [that] is the children's inability to relate themselves in the ordinary way to people and situations from the beginning of life" (Kanner, p. 242), calling them "disturbances of affective contact." Until recently, autistic disorder was considered one of five conditions classified as a pervasive developmental disorder in the *Diagnostic and Statistical Manual of Mental Disorders-Text Revised* (DSM-IV-TR), along with Asperger's disorder, childhood disintegrative disorder, pervasive developmental disorder not otherwise specified, and Rett's syndrome (APA, 2000) (Table 1–1). For a diagnosis of autism, significant impairments were noted across three separate but related categories: communication, socialization, and behavior. In order for a person to qualify for a diagnosis of autism, he had to exhibit at least 6 of the 12 noted behaviors across these three categories.

Most recently, the American Psychiatric Association updated the diagnostic criteria for autism in its fifth edition of the *Diagnostic and Statistical Manual of Mental Disorders* (APA, 2013). These changes are the outcome of intensive research and analysis resulting in a new category: *autism spectrum disorder* (ASD). The primary catalyst for most of the change was the lack of specificity of the previous diagnostic categories with research finding that, although the global deficit of pervasive developmental disorder (PDD) was accurate, determining *which* PDD it was among the five was not (APA, 2012).

The new DSM-5 criteria meld the previously separate diagnoses of autistic disorder, pervasive developmental disorder not otherwise specified (PDD-NOS), childhood disintegrative disorder, and Asperger's disorder (a.k.a., Asperger's syndrome) into one diagnosis now entitled autism spectrum disorder (ASD), as the authors contend that they function more as a continuum of one disorder rather than four distinct entities. Rett's disorder is no longer considered a mental disorder due to its known genetic and medical origin. In addition, the categories of communication and socialization have been combined into *social communication*, requiring an exhibition of three deficits, along with two in the category of restrictive and repetitive behavior. In summary, the DSM-5 definition of ASD includes a range of severity as well as a description of overall developmental status, specific to social communication and patterns of behavior, interests, or activities.

The DSM-5 describes ASD as a lifelong, early-onset disorder characterized by marked impairments in social communication, in the presence of restricted, repetitive, and stereotypic behavior. It is a disorder that substantially impacts everyday function. Specifically, the DSM-5 definition includes the following criteria for the diagnosis of autistic disorder: "Persistent impairment in reciprocal social communication and social interaction (Criterion A), and restricted, repetitive patterns of behavior, interests, or activities (Criterion B). These symptoms are present from early childhood and limit or impair everyday functioning (Criteria C and D)" (APA, 2013, p. 53). As cited previously, current prevalence estimates yield rates of one per 68 (CDC, 2014), a significant increase from estimates less than 20 years ago of one per 1,000 (Wing,

Table 1–1. Progression of DSM

DSM (year)	Parent Category	Specific Disorders
DSM-I (1952)	None	N/A
DSM-II (1968)	None	N/A
DSM-III (1980)	Pervasive Developmental Disorders (PDD)	Childhood Onset PDD Infantile Autism Atypical Autism
DSM-III-R (1987)	Pervasive Developmental Disorders (PDD)	PDD-NOS Autistic Disorder
DSM-IV (1994)	Pervasive Developmental Disorders (PDD)	PDD-NOS Autistic Disorder Asperger Disorder Childhood Disintegrative Disorder Rett syndrome
DSM-IV-TR (2000)	Pervasive Developmental Disorders (PDD)	Autistic Disorder Asperger Disorder Childhood Disintegrative Disorder Rett syndrome Same diagnoses as DSM-IV, text correction for PDD-NOS
DSM-5 (2013)	Autism Spectrum Disorders	No disorders, but provide the following specifiers: • Associated medical or genetic condition (e.g., fragile X) or environmental factor (e.g., intrauterine exposure) • Verbal abilities • Cognitive abilities • Severity of symptoms

1993). The male to female ratio is almost 5:1 with little difference across racial and ethnic groups (Frombonne, 2003); non-Hispanic white children, however, are the most likely group to be identified with an ASD (CDC). Cultural factors contribute to inconsistent and even inaccurate classification and diagnosis of ASD as well as influence whether services are obtained once a diagnosis has been made (Wilder, Dyches, Obiaker, & Algozzine, 2004). Cultural differences include overall views on disabilities (e.g., acceptance, shame) and the specific perceptions on what is considered an area of need (e.g., differences in eye contact expectations across cultures).

Epidemiology

In the 70-plus years since Kanner's original description, research has produced a myriad of products reflecting a constant search for cause, cure, and treatment. ASD by definition is a lifelong condition, and although not considered to be curable, significant progress has been made in recent years regarding potential factors influencing its presence. Although there is no single cause that can account for all cases of ASD, researchers appear to agree that both genetics and the environment play important roles (National Institute of Mental Health [NIMH], 2011). Direct examination of the brains of individuals with ASD through neuroimaging and neuropathology has found differences from those without ASD, specifically for brain growth and development, cortical connections, and neuronal organization (Grafodatskaya, Chung, Szatmari, & Weksberg, 2010). In addition, research has identified more than 100 autism risk genes (Liu et al., 2014) and in approximately 15% of the cases, a specific genetic cause of a person's ASD can be identified (Geschwind, 2011).

Some of the genetic causes are passed down in families, and others are spontaneous mutations that occur in either the egg or the sperm or very early in embryo development.

A number of studies examining the incidence of ASD in twins have provided strong support for its genetic basis (Bailey, Raspa, Olmsted, & Holiday, 1995; Folstein & Rutter, 1977; Steffenburg et al., 1989). These studies calculated a measure of genetic influence known as a *heritability index*, comparing the influence of genetics to that of the environment, each determining that this index was high. Accord-

ing to the NIMH, the genetic influence can be noted in identical twins who, by definition, have identical genetic makeup; both will have autism on almost 9 out of 10 occasions (2011). In addition, NIMH noted that in families with similar, but not identical genetic systems, a sibling of a person with ASD is 35 times more likely to have the disorder. Even if an ASD does not manifest itself, first-degree relatives are reported to have a greater incidence of lesser, but similar, forms of the behavioral or social language difficulties found in the disorder (Losh et al., 2009). There is also a significant association of ASD with genetic disorders such as fragile X, tuberous sclerosis, Prader-Willi, and Angelman syndromes. For example, approximately 30% and 50% to 61% of people with fragile X and tuberous sclerosis, respectively, also show traits of ASD (Sek et al., 2014; NIMH; Rutter, 2011). And the incidence of this co-occurrence, specifically for FXS, was reported to be as high as 67% for males with FXS who met "at least of one of the AD/ASD criteria on one test [ADI or ADOS], providing support to the claim that autistic behaviour is a major component of the fragile X phenotype" (p. 743, Clifford et al., 2007). However, as noted by Zafeiriou, Ververi, and Vargiami in 2007, although there is a strong correlation between autism and various genetic factors, the exact genetic background of the disorder remains unclear.

Research is not implying, however, that a genetic risk indicates automatic onset; nor does it imply that genetics is the sole cause of autism. Most recently following an extensive study of twins, researchers Hallmayer et al. (2011) concluded that the genetic influence may have been overestimated (estimated by the researchers to be a *moderate influence* [i.e., 37%] as opposed to the previously reported 90% influence) causing the focus of research to be less on environmental triggers or causes. Their 2011 study concluded that the shared environment of twins is a critical influence on the development of ASD. The environment is considered to be a substantial "contributor" to the prevalence of ASD as, although a specific genetic cause can be identified in around 15% of cases, most cases appear to involve both the genetic risk and environmental factors that influence early brain development (Grafodatskaya et al., 2010).

The influence of multiple factors as a cause of ASD is supported by the National Institutes of Environmental Health Sciences (2012), who report that autism may be caused by an interaction between genetic and environmental factors, hypothesizing it may be triggered during early fetal development, with environmental exposures during pregnancy contributing to its cause. Some of the environmental contributors currently under examination are maternal and paternal age, illness during pregnancy, and oxygen deprivation during birth. None of these, however, have been found to be a definitive cause of ASD.

until later) and impact everyday functioning (APA). In addition, the DSM-5 breaks down ASD into three levels of severity for the domains of social communication and behavior ranging from requiring support to requiring very substantial support (see DSM-5, p. 52, *Levels of Support*).

The designated levels of support (i.e., "requiring support, requiring substantial support, requiring very substantial support," APA, 2013, p. 52) illustrate the heterogeneity across the population of ASD. Even within the same diagnosis, a great range of functioning can occur, all causing lifelong impairment. There are, however, common characteristics and challenges central to the development of social communication skills. For the SLP it is critical to recognize and understand these core features, as they are the focus of ongoing assessment and appropriate therapeutic intervention. As we know, a diagnosis is not synonymous with an intervention plan; therefore, therapeutic approaches can both differ and overlap within the spectrum of the disorder. However, in order to most appropriately provide intervention, it is necessary first to understand how having an ASD specifically affects all aspects of communication, the realm of the SLP.

Diagnostic Criteria

Diagnostically, ASD is a complex neurological disorder, referred to as a spectrum due to its wide range of symptoms and manifestations. In the updated DSM-5 (APA, 2013), the key components of ASD are significant impairments in social communication, and restricted and repetitive behaviors, which must be present in early childhood (although may not be noted

Areas of Impairment

As noted previously, the central challenge in ASD is impaired social communication. This is a broad reaching term, encompassing the true purpose of communication where components of language and socialization merge to allow for social, human interaction. The American Speech-Language-Hearing Association (ASHA) delineated these core characteristics in the 2006 document, *Guidelines for Speech-Language Pathologists in Diagnosis, Assessment, and Treatment of Autism Spectrum Disorders across the Life Span* as follows:

> . . . social communication including aspects of joint attention (e.g., social orienting, establishing shared attention, monitoring emotional states, and considering another's intentions), social reciprocity (e.g., initiating bids for interaction, maintaining interactions by taking turns, and providing contingent responses to bids for interaction initiated by others), language and related cognitive skills (e.g., understanding and using nonverbal and verbal communication, symbolic play, literacy skills, and executive functioning—the ability to problem solve and self-monitor future, goal-directed, behavior), and behavior and emotional regulation (e.g., effectively regulating one's emotional state and behavior while focusing attention on salient aspects of the environment and engaging in social interaction) (p. 2).

It is important to examine each of the entities of social communication remembering that these areas are affected simultaneously. In order to understand the implications of these deficits, it is necessary to explain the overall social development and distinction of children and adolescents with autism. Descriptively these delays remain throughout development, although changes typically occur over time.

Social Communication

Social Orienting

For children with ASD, impairments in joint attention and social orienting are found to most strongly distinguish them from other disorders as young children. As noted by Dawson et al. (2004), one of the earliest noted impairments in ASD is also its most basic: a lack of orientation to social stimuli that likely contributes to the social communication needs noted later in life. Specifically, in their 2004 study comparing 3 to 4-year-old children with autism spectrum disorder to developmentally delayed and typically developing children, Dawson et al. found that the children with autism were significantly below the other groups in all domains for measures of social orienting, joint attention, and attention to another's distress.

Research (e.g., Bryant, 1991; Mundy & Neal, 2001; Symons, Hains, & Muir, 1998) has established that in typical development, infants orient to social stimuli by focusing on a caregiver's eyes (including the direction of gaze), facial expressions, voice, and gestures. These skills support the later development of social language use where a child learns to consider the knowledge of a communication partner specific to experiences, and begin to be most relevant when communicating (Baron-Cohen, 1988; Carpenter & Tomasello, 2000). Being able to recognize and interpret a communication partner's eye gaze, facial expressions, intonation, and gestures also allows typically developing children to understand and predict the emotional states of others. These skills are necessary for a child to infer how actions and emotional responses are interrelated. Developmentally, a child begins by attending to the emotional state of others to determine how a novel experience should be perceived. As a child progresses, intentional communication and language may be used to obtain specific emotional responses such as comfort, social games, and praise. Even later developing skills that involve self-monitoring require the ability to recognize and understand how personal behaviors and interactions affect the emotional state of others (ASHA, 2006b).

Joint Attention

Although the individual element of joint attention is not specifically noted in the DSM-5, it is commonly recognized as the foundation of social skills and language development, and considered to be a necessary precursor to effective communication. Research has consistently found that social orienting is significantly impaired in children with autism, initially noted through their restricted ability to notice others or respond to a caregiver's voice (Dawson, Meltzoff, Osterling, Rinaldi, & Brown, 1998; Klin, 1991, 1992; Lord, 1995), often giving an initial impression of impaired sensory function (i.e., appearing to be deaf). In addition, impairments of joint attention are noted in autism, which include difficulty following another's visual or gestural focus of attention, as well as reduced skills shifting gaze between people and objects (Dawson, Hill, Spencer, Galpert, & Watson, 1990; Mundy & Neal, 2001; Wetherby, Prizant, & Hutchinson, 1998). The absence or impairment of these language precursors substantially interferes with the ability to comment, request information, and share experiences (ASHA, 2006b). Although joint attention is often considered "the realm" of early childhood (meaning, it is often only addressed with young children), these deficits continue across the life span in autism, contributing to ongoing challenges in social language. For example, research conducted by Klin, Jones, Schultz, Volkmar, and Cohen (2002) using

eye-tracking technology found that individuals with ASD attend less frequently to a speaker's eyes and more frequently to their mouths. In addition, Vivanti, Nadig, Ozonoff, and Rogers (2008) found that children with high-functioning autism were similar to typical developing peers when attending to a demonstrated action but were notably different in their decreased attention to the demonstrator's face. The inability to notice and interpret these nonverbal cues, particularly those found in facial expressions, interferes with social communication, well beyond the early childhood years.

Monitoring Emotional States and Shared Intentions

One of the primary features in very young children with autism that often differentiate them from children without disabilities are the lack of reciprocal eye contact and a social smile (meaning in response or along with another). Even though minor environmental changes may be easily detected by the child with ASD, human faces and social interaction are not of great interest, resulting in significantly reduced eye contact. This absence of reciprocal gaze between child and caregiver severely interrupts early interpersonal patterns central to communication such as turn taking, as well as sharing of affective states and construction of shared emotional meaning. Research has found that people with autism both attend less to others' emotions, particularly distress or discomfort (Dawson et al., 2004; Sigman, Kasari, Kwon, & Yirmiya, 1992), and display positive affect in a shared interaction less frequently (Dawson et al., 1990; Wetherby et al., 1998) than typical developing peers. As noted previously, in typical development intentional communication is often used to obtain specific emotional responses such as comfort, social games, and praise; in ASD this is usually restricted or later to develop. Even in the presence of being able to identify emotions when presented statically such as in photographs, identifying these emotions in ongoing social interactions is an area of need (Klin, 2000; Klin et al., 2002; Yirmiya, Sigman, Kasari, & Mundy, 1992). Some of these needs are related to the deficits in social orientation, as (according to Klin et al., 2002) people with ASD focus primarily on a communicative partner's mouth rather than the eyes, missing critical social cues including a partner's emotional state. These restricted skills in social orientation may contribute to the lessened ability to identify, and subsequently address, the cause of emotions in others.

Social Reciprocity

According to the DSM-5, a deficit in social-emotional reciprocity is described as ranging from an abnormal social approach and failure of normal back and forth conversation through reduced sharing of interests, emotions, and affect and response to total lack of initiation of social interaction (APA, 2013). Along with, and possibly because of, deficits in joint attention, children with ASD have difficulty initiating, maintaining, and responding appropriately during social interactions. These skills are necessary for the development of social language, and contribute to the acquisition of more sophisticated use (ASHA, 2006a, 2006b). Social-emotional reciprocity is at the core of conversational skills, and individuals with autism typically have difficulty initiating communication spontaneously (Wetherby et al., 1998) and are often lim-

ited to conversations that are structured and predictable. Even when very young, children with ASD initiate less often than typical peers, and engage in fewer turn-taking events between themselves and a partner. As language develops, the needs in social reciprocity become more evident particularly the skills necessary for social conversation such as providing adequate background information to a listener, making appropriate and relevant comments, and keeping the conversation going through expansion and questions (Lord & Paul, 1997). Even once comments and questions have been acquired, social exchanges continue to be notable for their lack of relevance and interest to all conversational partners, as people with ASD are often noted to dominate the conversation with their particular, but possibly not shared, areas of interest (Klin & Volkmar, 1997).

Language Skills

Communication, by definition, is a system of shared meanings ranging from gestures, single words, word combinations, rote phrases, and sentences, culminating in complex fluid, conversations. Language is the medium, according to ASHA, 2006b, that allows us to share our own experiences, learn about another's perspective, and engage in goal-directed, problem-solving behavior. Early development of social skills is often correlated with a child's use of nonverbal modes of communication (e.g., gestures, gaze), and atypical language patterns are often central to an appropriate differential diagnosis of autism versus other disabilities.

For families, although characteristics of impaired socialization have been present, a deficit in language is often one of the first warning signs that a child has a disability. Language skills have been cited as a predictor of later social-communication outcomes, specifically the presence of expressive language by age 5 (Rutter, 1970, 2011). According to Rutter's 2011 summative review of research from 2007 to 2010, "Very few children who have not developed some useful communicative speech by the age of 5 to 6 years have a positive outcome" (p. 398).

Language skills include both comprehension and use, and both are affected in ASD, interfering with the ability to communicate and understand the intent of others. Expressive language, however, tends to improve more readily and rapidly than receptive language (Paul & Cohen, 1984), possibly leaving the impression that comprehension is more intact than it is. Even for the children with ASD who develop verbal, symbolic language as a means of communication, needs for language are evident for both understanding and independent, functional use. The following sections describe the language characteristics of children with ASD in the areas of speech development, grammatical complexity, semantics, and pragmatic language use.

Speech

Generally children with autism speak at a later age and develop speech at a slower rate than children without autism (LeCouteur et al., 1989), with approximately 15% having a speech disorder (Shriberg, Paul, Black, & van Santen, 2011). Approximately 25% of children with autism have been described as having words (at around 12 to 18 months) and losing them. Recent research indicates that as many as 30% of children with ASD are considered to be nonverbal, explained as using few or no

words consistently by the age of 9 (Anderson et al., 2007). This statistic was even higher in earlier studies with up to 50% of children with ASD reported as nonverbal possibly due to inconsistent definitions of functional speech. Despite the inconsistent findings, verbal expression for many children with autism is (and will continue to be) an area of significant need. In the area of expressive phonology, children who are verbal are unremarkable when compared to other disabled populations, with a similar pattern of the less frequently a phoneme occurs in language the greater the incidence of error. For children considered to be nonverbal, motor planning deficits appear to interfere with the complex productions required for articulation of speech, and imitation of specific oral movements are difficult (Bryson, 1997; Lord & Paul, 1997; National Research Council [NRC], 2001). It is critical to note that the acquisition of verbal expression is substantially compromised by the deficits in social communication, particularly that of joint attention, and that nonverbal social and cognitive skills are central to the development of speech (Wodka, Mathy, & Kalb, 2013).

Finally, the paralinguistic features of speech are another area of difference when compared to the patterns noted for typical developing children and adolescents. Research (see Diehl, Watson, Bennetto, McDonough, & Gunlogson, 2009) has noted differences in rate, rhythm, volume, and intonation, as well as an inability to appropriately change language register dependent on the setting. Although prosodic differences were noted in the original description of autism by Kanner (1943), they have been described as being both monotonous and exaggerated, probably due to great heterogeneity of the population (Nadig & Shaw, 2012). Although often neglected in intervention, these differences can impact a communication partner's perception of the person with autism, as unintended and often negative impressions may occur (Paul et al., 2005).

Grammar

In the expressive arenas, sentence length and complexity, both functions of syntax and morphology, can be variable in children with autism. One study (Bartolucci, Pierce, & Streiner, 1980) found that children with autism produced the 14 grammatical morphemes (e.g., articles, present progressive -*ing*, plural *s*) less frequently than their cognitively matched, nondisabled peers, with most errors noted for the use of articles (i.e., *a*, *the*, *an*) and verb tenses. Development of syntax and the use of varying sentence forms appear to be similar to that of peers of equal cognition, with a relation to a developmental rather than age level. Some children with autism treat language as gestalt chunks and expressively produce phrases and sentences in such a manner. In these instances sentence length and grammatical complexity are not indicators of language development and increased complexity, but of an atypical style in language production. Pronoun reversal is also a commonly discussed error of expressive morphology noted in children with autism. Though this is an error in grammatical form, some researchers believe it is born of the deficits in joint attention and understanding another's perspective (Hobson, Lee, & Hobson, 2009). Even when grammatical and syntactic structure appear to be intact, more sophisticated syntax is often lacking, such as establishing relationships between sentences when engaged in conversation (Volkmar, Klin, Schultz, Rubin, & Bronen, 2000).

Receptively, less is known about the processing skills of children with autism in the areas of morphology and syntax. Syntactically, errors noted in early development tend to stabilize, although some needs continue when relating personal events (Losh, 2003). Although overall research (see Vulchanova, Talcott, Vulchanov, Stankova, & Eshuis, 2012) has found strengths in structural language tasks as compared to pragmatic skills and language comprehension, little research has been done to analyze general patterns in receptive language form in autism.

Semantics

Semantics, otherwise known as language content, is the area of language and communication involving the comprehension and use of vocabulary and concepts. As noted previously, the acquisition of language is substantially affected by the needs in joint attention, interfering with the typical process of learning and using words and phrases. Children with autism often remain in the first phase of lexical development, where words are learned slowly and only for significant people, things, and events (Carpenter & Tomasello, 2000). Generalization of these words to other uses is reduced, and the method for learning is not systematic. Even when there is a loss of previously acquired words, this occurs before children have a vocabulary burst, a time when vocabulary is acquired quickly and widely generalized. The second phase of typical development follows a vocabulary spurt in which words are learned rapidly, often with little exposure, and are generalized to new situations. This process, known as "fast mapping," is a skill children with ASD have difficulty with due to their needs in joint attention (Baron-Cohen, Baldwin, &

Crowson, 1997; Priessler & Carey, 2005). Children with autism may fail to reach the level of language learning that is not strictly associative, resulting in a limited or atypical repertoire of words and phrases. Parent report has indicated that preschool-aged children with ASD have vocabularies that are significantly smaller than same-aged children with developmental delays (Coonrod & Stone, 2004).

Semantically, children with autism appear to demonstrate a separation of language function and language form. Though they may understand basic concepts and vocabulary, the appropriate use of these words in multiple and varied communicative situations is impaired. That is, the words may be recalled and retrieved, but the shared commonalities may not be extracted resulting in impaired category formation (Minshew, Meyer, & Goldstein, 2002).

This may be the reason that some words, as originally noted by Volden and Lord (1991), take on unusual meanings possibly associated with events or intents unfamiliar to most listeners. Some words may be modifications of the intended one, resulting in odd but understandable language (e.g., "cuts and blusers" for cuts and bruises). Other modifications include the use of neologisms in which the source of the word or phrase was not easily evident (e.g., "poomba" for hairdryer), possibly related to a similar event (Volden & Lord). Although vocabulary may be noted as a relative strength for verbal children with ASD (Landa, 2007), difficulty is often reported for the understanding of abstract words (Tager-Flusberg & Caronna, 2007). Even for individuals previously diagnosed as having Asperger's syndrome where receptive and expressive vocabulary has been found to be generally commensurate with typical developing peers, higher-order language processing such as reading comprehension or the detection of verbal absurdities is more impaired than vocabulary (Kjelgaard & Tager-Flusberg, 2001; Williams, Goldstein, & Minshew, 2006).

One of the most notable characteristics of children with autism who develop verbal speech is the presence of echolalia. Children with autism may be slow to shift from preverbal communication to symbolic language, with patterns that are "idiosyncratic, less readable, and more context-bound than linguistic communication" (Prizant, Schuler, Wetherby, & Rydell, 1997, p. 573). Additionally, children with autism may engage in unconventional verbal behaviors (UVBs), including echolalia, perseverative speech, and language with private meaning, making communication with a less familiar partner difficult or impossible. Though these forms of verbal expression are aberrant, they are not meaningless. Research (McEvoy, Loveland, & Landry, 1988; Prizant & Duchan, 1981) has found that both immediate and delayed echolalia may serve a purpose in the conversation of a child with autism. Some of the functions of echolalia may be turn taking, rehearsal, affirmative answers (i.e., "yes"), declaration of information, and making a request. Echolalia is generally viewed as a communicative strategy in the absence of consistent, spontaneous verbal expression, which typically reduces as more language is acquired (Loveland & Tunali-Kotoski, 1997).

Pragmatics

The area of language found to be the most significantly impaired in children with autism is pragmatics, or the social use of language. For young children, or children at the emerging stage of language development, acquisition of "communicative intentionality" (Prizant et al., 1997) is the major task. Once children use language, the challenge is to expand the range of communicative functions. Expressing these communicative functions in comprehensible and appropriate ways as well as across differing contexts becomes the primary pragmatic goal.

Communicative intent is typically very restricted, with regulation of another's behavior, as demonstrated through requests and protests, noted to exist more frequently than socially driven communication (e.g., sharing feelings, commenting, requesting permission) (Stone & Caro-Martinez, 1990). Even in the presence of symbolic language, use is typically much less flexible across multiple environments. Typically, language forms and usage are context-driven, concrete, and cue-dependent. Communicative abilities can also be greatly influenced by a child's emotional state as well as variables in communicative environments, resulting again in great variability in skills dependent on setting (Klin & Volkmar, 2005). Additionally, children with autism have difficulties understanding verbal information as well as nonverbal signals. This difficulty will limit the reciprocity of a conversational exchange, as a child with autism is often unaware of what a listener is expecting of him or her. As children develop in their language skills, these needs translate into difficulties making conversational repairs and reading the emotional state of others (Wetherby, Prizant, & Schuler, 2000).

Individuals with ASD and higher verbal skills are typically verbose, engaging in incessant talking (not necessarily conversation) about a favorite topic, regardless of a listener's level of interest or comprehension (de Villiers, Fine, Ginsberg, Vaccarella, & Szatmari, 2007; Paul, Orlovski, Marcinko, & Volkmar, 2009). Con-

versations are typically monologues that often appear to exist without a clear point or conclusion (Nadig, Lee, Singh, Bosshart, & Ozonoff, 2010). Their expressive language may be confusing to a listener, as individuals with ASD often fail to provide appropriate background information on a subject or clearly mark a change in topic. Conversation may also include internal thoughts seemingly inappropriate in an exchange, making a two-way conversation difficult to impossible (Paul et al.).

Overall, children with autism differ from children without autism in their rate of communicative initiation, with most attempts directed at regulation rather than social interaction. The presence of perseverative comments or questions is reported, as well as reduced incidence of appropriate responses to a partner's comment in conversation. This deficit, as well as previously noted difficulties regarding taking the perspective of a listener, contributes to poor conversational skills. From reduced use of communicative intents at the prelinguistic level to breakdowns in conversational interactions at a more advanced social language level, children with autism manifest significant needs in the area of pragmatic language use.

Nonverbal Behavior

The DSM-5 specifies deficits in nonverbal communicative behaviors used for social interaction; ranging from poorly integrated verbal and nonverbal communication, through abnormalities in eye contact and body language, or deficits in understanding and use of nonverbal communication, to total lack of facial expression or gestures (APA, 2013). Differences in nonverbal communication are evident in early development, with one of the hallmark features being the absence of gestures (Wetherby et al., 2004). Although presymbolic gestures may be noted, such as pulling a person to a desired object, conventional gestures such as waving goodbye are either delayed or absent. So it is not unusual to find a child with autism who can act out an event by using actions or even words, but who cannot use gestures where the action is symbolic in nature, such as shaking the head for no, or pointing a finger to indicate something of interest in the distance (Stone & Caro-Martinez, 1990; Wetherby et al., 1998). Research has indicated that the lack of gesture development contributes to the creation of and reliance on problem behaviors such as unusual vocalizations and running away (Fox, Dunlap, & Buschbacher, 2000).

Children with autism are remarkable for their limited facial expressions, particularly joy, notable for a lack of coordination of expression with eye-gaze (Wetherby et al., 2004). Deficits in nonverbal communication are not limited to expressive use, as comprehension is also impaired. Differences have been reported for facial recognition, a fundamental skill in socialization for children, adolescents, and adults with autism (Klin et al., 1999). Research has posited that some of the needs in facial recognition and comprehension of emotional expressions may be more a function of psychological and neural factors rather than solely a deficit in social function (Behrmann, Thomas, & Humphreys, 2006).

Play Skills

Previously in the DSM-IV-TR, the absence of make-believe and functional play was part of the diagnostic criteria (APA, 2000).

In the updated DSM-5, symbolic play is integrated into "Deficits in developing, maintaining, and understanding relationships" (APA, 2013, p. 50). Although no longer its "own section," play continues to be an area of need for children with autism, and continues across the lifespan as it influences relationships and the ability to make and keep friends.

As noted across most areas of development, the previously identified needs in the area of joint attention and social orientation have a substantial impact on the development of play. In particular, children with autism have fewer shared social experiences in which to imitate the actions of others, a primary means of interaction in play. In early development, according to Libby, Powell, Messer, and Jordan (1998), children with autism engage in less functional play and more sensorimotor play (e.g., oral exploration, spinning). In addition, when functional play develops it tends to be qualitatively different as children are only being able to use objects as function denotes. Finally, symbolic play is often reduced or absent with an inability to engage in object substitution (i.e., pretend a car is a plane), or attribution of false properties (i.e., pretend the doll is hungry). Overall, play appears to be rigid, with difficulty noted for changing routines or materials. It can be especially difficult for children with autism to integrate the ideas or themes of a play partner into their own play. Even simple games such as "tag" or "hide and go seek" may be difficult, as although these appear to have "rigid" rules and routines, they require an awareness of a play partner and the expectation of others. Overall, the impairments in play are affected by the needs previously noted in social communication and social reciprocity. These needs, although typically attributed to young children, affect interactions across the life span, and even, as noted by ASHA (2006b) "compromises the ability to enact social sequences in a representational manner, a capacity that allows individuals to visualize an event before it takes place and even prepare for unfamiliar or potentially distressful situations" (p. 11).

Literacy Skills

According to ASHA, 2006b, "The printed word is a modality of communication that is central to social and communicative competence, as both reading and writing play a primary role in the ability to function effectively in academic and vocational settings and participate in social cultural rituals and routines (e.g., reading books and writing letters/e-mails) that contribute to social membership" (p. 12). This is an area of recent interest and research for people with autism, often marked by irregular development, consistent with those noted previously for language. Specifically, students with autism are often noted to have relative strengths for decoding printed words allowing for a sight word vocabulary that is disproportionate to their reading comprehension. Overall, high-functioning students with ASDs have decoding skills that are "generally adequate, but that can be below, equal to, or above chronological age norms" (O'Connor & Klein, 2004, p. 116). As language skills progress, reading comprehension also improves, however the central needs noted for language form, content, and use remain. Specifically, students with autism demonstrate more syntactic errors and fewer referents (Norbury & Bishop, 2003), as well as have shorter stories with fewer causal relationships noted, specifi-

cally regarding the feelings and thoughts of the characters (Tager-Flusberg, 1995). In addition, comprehension of narratives is affected by difficulty with inferential and indirect language and intent. Beyond fictional narratives, students with autism are less likely to convey recent events through a personal narrative, showing relatively stronger skills for retelling a fictional story, also reflective of areas of need in social communication, organization, and understanding listener perspective. Overall, narratives skills appear to be related to all areas of functioning including language, cognition, and social-emotional functioning (Losh, 2003).

Cognitive Skills

The cognitive, social, and linguistic development of children with autism, though often examined as separate entities, are interrelated, with each area affecting the other (Wetherby & Prutting, 1984). Kanner (1943) originally maintained that persons with autism had normal intellectual functioning. This fact, however, has been repeatedly challenged (Lockyer & Rutter, 1969; Volkmar, Hoder, & Cohen, 1985; Volkmar, Klin, & Cohen, 1997), with previous research finding that 70% to 80% of people with autism obtained IQ scores in the range of intellectual impairment, primarily falling into the moderate to severe categories (DeMeyer et al., 1972; Wing & Gould, 1979). However, recent research (CDC, 2012) indicates that the majority of children with ASD did not have intellectual disability (i.e., IQ less than or equal to 70). According to Sigman, Dissanayake, Arbelle, and Ruskin (1997), children with ASD are not delayed or deviant in spatial knowledge, perceptual organization, or short-term memory skills. Rather, primary difficulties are noted for the derivation of abstract information "necessary for sequencing material and in transforming this information into symbolic representations" (p. 259). These deficits, in turn, significantly impact both social and communicative functioning, as representational thinking is necessary to extract knowledge of other people, their language, and the environment.

One particular area of cognitive functioning found to be impaired in ASD is executive functioning, or the mental ability to solve problems and monitor behavior. Executive functioning involves skills in organization, attention, and planning. The greatest areas of need, even when compared to children with other disabilities (i.e., ADHD), were cognitive flexibility and planning (Geurts et al., 2004) particularly in novel settings and when having to manage complex information. Needs in executive functioning contribute to the perseverative behavior and impaired social skills noted in the diagnosis, as although "rules" of socialization may be learned appropriately, the ability to modify these "rules" to a specific situation is often difficult.

Theory of mind is another cognitive process that affects the social communication and behavior of people with autism (Baron-Cohen, 2001). Theory of mind is the ability to infer a range of mental states of others including emotions, beliefs, and intentions, all of which are the cause of an action; its lack sometimes is referred to as "mind blindness." Having theory of mind allows us to think about what we are thinking and feeling as well as what others are thinking and feeling and allows us to understand emotions, take on another's perspective, predict behavior or emotional state, and overall, understand that behavior impacts how others think or

feel. The implications of these needs are great for the person with autism, as it is necessary to be aware of and regulate our behavior based on another's thoughts and reactions. Theory of mind is needed for understanding unwritten social rules, sarcasm, "white lies," and figures of speech; it is a critical component of effective social communication.

Behavior and Emotional Regulation

Restricted, repetitive patterns of behavior, interests, or activities is a critical diagnostic component of autism, possibly manifested through stereotypes, insistence on routines and rituals, fixated interest, and unusual sensory reactions. Some, if not all, of these behaviors may be due to the substantial needs in emotional regulation. As noted by the NRC (2001), the developmental trajectory in emotional regulation significantly impacts a person's with autism ability to be socially engaged, attend to the most salient aspects of an interaction, and to appropriately regulate emotions and behavior, all of which directly affect social communication. The challenges in social orienting, joint attention, social reciprocity, language, and cognition all contribute to the restricted, repetitive patterns of behavior.

Many patterns of behavior noted in autism appear to be similar to those noted in typical early development for emotional regulation, such as mouthing and rocking. Other behaviors are idiosyncratic, such as needing an unusual "transition object" or wandering, that also appear to serve to support emotional regulation. Some repetitive language may also be a form of emotional regulation, often connected to events that are not immediately evident to caregivers and peers. For example, a child with autism may use the phrase "want milk" each time he hears a sound of distress indicating that if you give a baby milk, he will stop crying. In addition, more pronounced behaviors may be present when emotional regulation is more critically disrupted such as tantrums or "bolting," all of which may be a form of communication. The impairment in social communication to convey wants and needs as well as understand the expectations of others may exacerbate the patterns of behavior, often misunderstood by family, peers, and educators, contributing further to the child's distress.

One of the additions noted to the DSM-5 is "hyper- or hyporeactivity to sensory input or unusual interest in sensory aspects of environment" (2013, p. 50). Although all children with ASD do not need to exhibit these characteristics, many will manifest an observable difference in how they manage sensory input. These sensory differences combined with the needs in social communication often lead to unusual, rigid, and routinized behavior. Recent research found that children with autism differed from children with language impairments and developmental disabilities in both frequency and manifestation of sensory impairments (Leekam, Nieto, Libby, Wing, & Gould, 2007), with only 6% of the ASD group *not* affected. In addition, abnormalities were reported across multiple domains, with specific needs reported in vision and smell/taste.

Feeding issues have recently been reported as a pervasive need for children with ASD, primarily for food selectivity (Twachtman-Reilly, Amaral, & Zebrowski, 2008). Although issues with "picky eating" are often analyzed (and subsequently treated) from a strictly behavioral view, physiological elements must also be considered; particularly sensory processing issues and gastrointestinal (GI) issues. Specifically, considerations of sensory issues related to taste processing (i.e., accuracy in identifying tastes) as well as sensory overload in an eating environment (e.g., school cafeteria) have been reported to be key elements (Twachtman-Reilly et al.). Although research found that children with ASD had similar incidence of GI disorders when compared to typical peers (Black, Kaye, & Jick, 2002), its impact differed specific to appetite. That is, children with ASD with concomitant GI problems were reported to have a poor appetite more frequently than their counterparts without GI problems.

Assessment

Adequate and ongoing assessment of individuals with autism spectrum disorder is the foundation of any intervention program and, given the critical importance of social communication, speech-language pathologists play an important role. Typically, SLPs work in conjunction and collaboration with other professionals, including psychologists, neurologists, pediatricians, and educators, as well as other service providers such as audiologists and occupational therapists allowing for an optimal, interdisciplinary assessment. It is critical that all professionals involved in the diagnosis of ASD, according to Filipek et al., are conversant and proficient with guidelines presented in the DSM as well as diagnostic assessment tools (1999). This includes competence with screening, which involves the recognition of the early symptoms of ASD and knowledge of available screeners.

Screening

Screening for ASD has improved over time, as researchers have found that symptoms of ASD are observable by 12 months of age (Wetherby et al., 2004), and an accurate diagnosis can be made by the age of 24 months (Filipek et al., 1999). Screeners can be broadband or specific to autism, and the SLP must be knowledgeable of ones that are valid and reliable in order to most accurately identify children at risk for ASD. There are a number of broadband screeners that are psychometrically sound, such as the Ages and Stages Questionnaire, Third Edition (ASQ-3; Squires, Twombly, Bricker, & Potter, 2009), the Parents' Evaluation of Developmental Status (PEDS; Glascoe, 2012), and the Communication and Symbolic Behavior Scales Developmental Profile (CSBSDP) Infant Toddler Checklist (ITC; Wetherby & Prizant, 2002). All are effective in identifying children with disabilities (i.e., at least 80% effective) with the ITC receiving the highest rating from ASHA (2006a). Screeners that are "autism specific" have received less validation from research involving the general population, as most have been examined only with children already identified to be at risk or with already established developmental delays (ASHA, 2006a). It is critical for the SLP to examine a screener for its reported sensitivity and specificity; in other words screeners that "truly" rule in (i.e., true positives) or rule out (i.e., true negatives) should be used. At present, the Modified Screening Test for Autism in Toddlers, Revised with Follow-up (M-CHAT-R/F; Robins, Fein, & Barton, 2009), the Pervasive Developmental Disorders Screening Test-II (PDDST-II; Siegel, 2004), the Screening Test for Autism in Two-Year-Olds (STAT; Stone, Coonrod, & Ousley, 2000; Stone, Coonrod, Turner, &

Pozdol, 2004), and Systematic Observation of Red Flags (SORF; Wetherby et al., 2004) all have strong (i.e., >85%) sensitivity and specificity for identification of young children with autism.

According to Wetherby et al., (2004), the "red flags" for ASD in young children are as follows: (a) lack of appropriate gaze; (b) lack of warm, joyful expressions with gaze; (c) lack of sharing enjoyment or interest; (d) lack of response to name; (e) lack of coordination of gaze, facial expression, gesture, and sound; (f) lack of showing; (g) unusual prosody; (h) repetitive movements or posturing of body, arms, hands, or fingers; and (i) repetitive movements with objects. In addition, the following four "red flags" further differentiated children with ASD and those with developmental delay from children who were typically developing: (a) lack of response to contextual cues; (b) lack of pointing; (c) lack of vocalizations with consonants; and (d) lack of playing with a variety of toys conventionally.

Beyond the warning signs for young children, ASD may be suspected but not yet diagnosed in school age children as well as adolescents. As noted in the DSM-5 (2013):

> Symptoms are present from early childhood and limit or impair everyday functioning (Criteria C and D). The stage at which functional impairment becomes obvious will vary according to characteristics of the individual and his or her environment. Core diagnostic features are evident in the developmental period, but intervention, compensation and current supports may mask difficulties in at least some contexts. Manifestations of the disorder also vary greatly depending on the severity of the autistic condition, developmental level, and chronological age; hence the term spectrum. (p. 53)

In addition, a loss of language at any age is grounds for assessment. According to the Scottish Intercollegiate Guidelines Network (SIGN; 2007) there are warning signs in communication, socialization, and behavior that warrant screening and possible assessment, often creating an unusual profile of strengths and needs. For communication these include: (a) atypical language development including muteness; (b) unusual prosody; (c) persistent echolalia; (d) difficulty with proper pronoun use, particularly "I" and "me"; (e) atypical vocabulary for level of development; and (f) limited language use and/or limited topic focus. Warning signs for socialization include: (a) inappropriate attempts at or inability to join in peer play; (b) lack of awareness of social "rules"; (c) atypical relationships with adults (e.g., too intense/no relationship); and (d) escalated responses to stimulus (e.g., personal space; being hurried). Finally, restricted, repetitive interests or behaviors may include: (a) lack of flexibility as noted in play; (b) difficulty in unstructured spaces (e.g., playground, hallways); (c) marked resistance to change in routine or unstructured activities; and (d) unusual behaviors in response to sensory input.

Finally, adolescents may also demonstrate symptoms that are notable and specific to ASD (see SIGN, 2007). Some of these may appear as subtle, or practitioners may not consider particularly notable if the young person is successful in school academically. However, it is critical to examine the difference between academic and social competence and level of independence in social situations. It is also important to note the effect of context and environment as social communication and behavior difficulties are noted most frequently during transitions, unstructured social situations, and inter-

actions that require a dynamic back and forth (e.g., casual conversation). Overall, an adolescent suspected of ASD may appear socially naïve and have difficulty with same age peers, although can often interact well with adults. The needs noted previously for vocabulary, perseverative areas of interest, vocal affect, rigid behavior, and sensory responsiveness are also evident. In summary, it is incumbent that the SLP, in conjunction with other professionals, monitor young children for these characteristics, and refer for further evaluation if ASD is suspected.

Diagnosis

According to ASHA (2006a),

> The SLP who has been trained in the clinical criteria for ASD, as well as in the use of reliable and valid diagnostic and assessment tools for individuals with ASD, and who is experienced in diagnosis of developmental disorders, may be qualified to diagnose these disorders as an independent professional. (p. 8)

However, it is still considered ideal for the SLP to serve as critical member of an interdisciplinary team supporting and contributing to the collective expertise. In a diagnostic evaluation of children at risk for ASD, it is necessary to gather the following information: (a) relevant background information; (b) health, developmental, and behavioral history of the child and health history of the family; and (c) direct behavior observation. In addition, the American Academy of Pediatrics recommends that a medical evaluation should be completed (American Academy of Pediatrics, 2001). Obtaining relevant background information from the caregiver will help drive the evaluation and support the appropriate selection of a diagnostic tool. The child's history for health, development, and behavior offers critical insights for the evaluation team to determine the patterns of development as they relate to ASD. In particular, SIGN (2007) recommends using ASD-specific history-taking instruments such as the Autism Diagnostic Interview-Revised (ADI-R; Rutter, Le Couteur, & Lord, 2003) as they improve the reliability of an ASD diagnosis. A family history, in particular for genetic conditions occasionally associated with ASD (e.g., fragile X) or cognitive impairments. Finally, direct behavior observation must be conducted including interaction with the person suspected of an ASD, in order to compare present behaviors in social communication and restricted repetitive behaviors (RRBs) such as those noted in the DSM-5.

Typically, a diagnostic evaluation requires extensive time and may not be completed in one session in order to accurately obtain a reliable picture of performance. In addition, observation across a variety of contexts and people at varying levels of structure is needed to fully assess social communication. ASD-specific diagnostic instruments such as the Autism Diagnostic Observation Schedule, Second Edition (ADOS-2; Lord et al., 2012) are recommended to supplement the process of a clinical observation, as they systematically address the behaviors central to an ASD diagnosis such as communication, reciprocal social interaction, play, stereotypic behavior, restricted interests, and other abnormal behaviors. Although there are other autism-specific diagnostic instruments currently available (i.e., Childhood Autism Rating Scale [CARS-2], Schopler, Van Bourgondien, Wellman, & Love, 2010; Gilliam Autism Rating Scale

[GARS], Gilliam, 2006), none has achieved the high levels of specificity, sensitivity, and interrater reliability of the ADOS (ASHA, 2006b).

Assessment

For an assessment to be adequate it must be comprehensive and, according to researchers, involve "evaluating multiple areas of functioning that are relevant to the child's adaptation, taking the developmental aspects of each of these areas into consideration, and analyzing interrelationships between domains" (Klin et al., 1997, p. 412). In particular, Klin et al. (1997) describe six principles that should drive the assessment of children with autism: (a) assess multiple areas of functioning; (b) adopt a developmental perspective; (c) profile any variability in skills; (d) analyze variability in performance across settings; (e) evaluate the impact on everyday life and functional adjustment; and (f) document both delays and differences. Assessment methods must consider the quality of measures used and the information obtained, with specific consideration given to a child's variability in performance over time and across settings, as well as any possible impacting environmental factors.

Assessment also requires continuous contact, tracking progress from the diagnostic phase to the phase of intervention to ensure the information obtained is adequately and appropriately translated into functional goals. To most adequately achieve this end, assessment should focus on multiple areas of performance, including current level of functioning, behavioral components, and functional abilities. Delineation of strengths and needs is critical, as variability across differing skills is common and a general "score" or single result gives little information regarding such variability. Variability across settings, including people and structure, is also common. Information regarding optimal environments and less optimal settings is valuable. Relating and interpreting assessment information into everyday settings has a multilayered benefit; that is, it considers what a child does in "real life," relates the assessment immediately to intervention, and correlates social/emotional functioning to both assessment and intervention.

Lastly, both delays and differences need to be considered. Though a standardized instrument can often easily measure delays, deviance from the norm cannot be as easily measured. This does not mean, however, that the deviancies are irrelevant, but that alternative methods must be employed to obtain the information. Parents and service providers from multiple disciplines need to be involved to create a cohesive picture of strengths and needs in academic as well as social, communicative, and behavioral performance.

Regardless of the area assessed (e.g., communication, cognition, socialization, behavior) some guidelines need to be followed. In general, assessment should be dynamic, meaning that support is provided systematically in order to determine what factors affect and augment task completion. It is important to know what supports and what detracts from success, especially for tasks that may be too difficult for independent completion. Dynamic assessment helps identify the skills that are intact, but also helps determine those that may be emerging and what supports are needed for optimal functioning. In addition, the testing environment should be considered in terms of simplicity, use of effective reinforcers, pacing of tasks, and structure. The level and intensity of the social demands involved in the testing should also be monitored. Typically as the level of social demands increases, the performance level on a task decreases for individuals with ASD. The component of impaired social interaction impedes the assessment process as issues of motivation are often questioned in relation to a child's test performance. As noted previously, parents/caregivers should be involved to the maximum extent possible. Parent and caregiver input is crucial regarding the testing environment and its impact on their child, including the "typicalness" of the child's performance. In addition, caregivers are a critical source of information about specific strengths and needs noted in assessment. An even more critical reason for parent involvement may be a family's ability to associate assessment results and intervention recommendations immediately to specific observable behaviors during testing. When the assessment is complete, whenever possible, multiple examiners should combine their results into a single report, one that is cohesive rather than solely chronological. Discussion of findings should be integrated with each other; for example the communication results should be interpreted in light of the psychological and educational findings and vice versa. Finally, assessments, by nature, should be ongoing and geared toward the development of goals and objectives. Overall, the primary goal of assessment is to determine the current profile of social communication skills, to identify and prioritize functional, natural communication objectives, and to evaluate the role of the environment, including communication partners, on overall social communicative competence (ASHA, 2006a).

Communication Assessment

Marked impairment in social communication is the central characteristic in the diagnosis of autism spectrum disorders. Given the impact an individual's communication skills have on the ability to function in a primarily language-based society, thorough understanding of what a child can and cannot do is crucial. Comprehensive and ongoing assessment is key to designing appropriate interventions to address the individual needs in the domain of communication. Typically, a communication evaluation addresses speech production as well as receptive and expressive functioning in the areas of form (morphology, syntax), content (semantics), and use (pragmatics). In addition, according to ASHA (2006) it is especially important when working with children with ASD to determine the communicative intent of prelinguistic, preverbal, and verbal behavior, as well as unconventional verbal output. A functional communication assessment, including interview, direct observation, and experiment, is also suggested to determine the purpose of an atypical or unusual behavior and its correlation to communicative intent (Carr et al., 1994).

Information about a student's communicative functioning, as mentioned previously, must be considered in light of the whole student functioning in multiple environments. Standardized tests are one part of an assessment, but it is necessary to understand that the results of formal testing often do not capture all, or sometimes many, of a child's strengths and needs.

Typically, pragmatic and social functioning cannot be assessed through formal testing, particularly in the area of communicative intent and social competence.

When approaching assessment it is crucial to remember what we know about the profile of language and communication; that is, that language form is often more intact than language content which in turn is typically stronger than language use. In addition, language comprehension is generally more impaired than expressive language, with greater needs noted as the language becomes more complex, subtle, and abstract. Therefore, a communication assessment must be comprehensive in many aspects, allowing comparison between the broad areas of language form, content, and use. In addition, it is important to compare receptive and expressive capabilities for both discrete skills (e.g., grammatical recognition and use) and complex tasks (e.g., story retelling and explanation). Social communication needs are pervasive and may not be evident solely through standardized testing of formal language skills. The examination of all of a student's performance is needed in order to initiate an effective program of intervention, with particular focus on those "that affect social adaptive functioning within the ever-changing social contexts of an individual's natural routines" (ASHA, 2006a, p. 27).

Speech

Though many students with autism do not differ markedly from nondisabled peers in articulatory development (Lord & Paul, 1997), a notable percentage of the population are nonverbal. Due to the variation in speech production among children with ASD, the terminology of language as "expressive" must be considered beyond the scope of speech. Comprehension and use of augmentative and alternative communication systems should be evaluated as well as the role and impact of visual stimulus (e.g., pictures, words, photographs). For individuals who are verbal, assessment of their phonemic repertoire is beneficial to determine the ability to form and produce sounds in the language. In addition, the paralinguistic aspects of speech are often atypical, warranting an informal assessment of voice quality (e.g., hoarse; hypernasal), loudness, prosody (e.g., monotonous; singsong), and rate of speech.

Oral motor issues, especially those related to motor planning and eating, should be considered, as intervention may vary greatly depending on the type of speech disorder present. The presence of limb and/or verbal dyspraxia has significant implications for the protocol of treatment. The inability to motor-plan limb and oral movements will negatively affect a child's ability to gesture, imitate sounds, and use phonemes in connected speech. Along with the specific motor functions associated with speech, oral functions necessary for feeding should also be examined if this is an area of concern. These motor-planning and praxis issues need to be considered when evaluating nonverbal motor movements and oral functioning.

Language

The most critical areas of language assessment are those that derive from the core needs in ASD. Many of these, such as joint attention, turn taking, and imitation, can be assessed across a number of formal and informal procedures. Later developing language skills, such as those necessary for effective and efficient social interac-

tion (e.g., conversation; comprehension of complex information) can be assessed through formal and informal means as well. As noted previously, all of the behaviors observed during assessment are valuable, not just those noted during administration of formal tests.

The specific tools selected for assessment will depend on an individual's age and level of functioning, and should include a combination of standardized assessments, teacher/parent reports, interviews, simulated functional tasks, natural observation, and dynamic assessment (ASHA, 2014). For all children with ASD, particularly those in the prelinguistic and developing language stages, all aspects of communication should be assessed, not just that which is considered conventional. In particular, for children who are developmentally young, it is important to assess the communicative, symbolic, and social-affective abilities by measuring communicative functions, gestural and vocal communicative means, reciprocity, and social-affective signaling or behavior. In addition, nonverbal symbolic behavior typically noted in play should be examined along with the "traditional" areas of receptive and expressive verbal symbolic behavior. Results of such an assessment for young children with ASD should lead, according to ASHA, to the development of specific intervention approaches.

Once language emerges, battery type tests can be used that comprehensively assess receptive and expressive language domains. As language develops, it is helpful to implement assessments specifically designed to identify higher-level language skills such as ambiguous sentences, inferences, speech acts, and figurative language. Tests and assessments that consider the contextual and situational demands of conversation along with the discrete semantic and syntactic abilities will provide important information for the intervention plan. Overall, a language assessment should include (a) the core elements of social communication, (b) learning readiness, style, and potential, and (c) receptive and expressive competencies (NIASA & Le Couteur, 2003).

Other means of language assessment may be achieved through either the collection of a language sample or a narrative assessment. Although neither of these procedures is standardized, they can each provide valuable information on expressive language skills (i.e., sentence length; syntactical complexity; vocabulary; communicative intent) across contexts. In particular, a narrative assessment can provide the SLP with information for tasks that most closely resemble those expected in an academic environment. Narrative assessments can provide valuable information as it is an assessment tool that is both structured enough to allow for comparison between children and naturalistic enough to collect individual language and conversational styles (Botting, 2002). Competence with story retelling may be compared to story generation; in particular for stories where the student is provided with a wordless picture book such as, "Frog, where are you?" (Mayer, 1969). This 24-picture storybook without words allows for spontaneous generation of a story, and has been researched extensively in typical developing children and children with language impairments (see Botting). The narrative produced can be evaluated for microstructure (e.g., length, grammatical complexity) and macrostructure (e.g., cohesion, narrative devices) as well as comprehension of abstract events and outcomes depicted in the story.

As noted repeatedly, needs with social communication are central to the diagnosis of ASD, therefore information on current level of functioning for language use or pragmatic language is necessary for intervention planning. By definition, pragmatic skills need to be examined across a number of social situations with varying communication partners, not just in one-on-one formal testing sessions. Caregiver and teacher interviews and questionnaires can also be a valuable source of information in addition to measures of competence in natural conversational exchanges. A number of resources are available to support pragmatic assessments, including checklists in comprehensive test batteries (e.g., CELF-5, Semel, Wiig, & Secord, 2013; Test of Language Competence, Wiig & Secord, 1989) and stand-alone assessments (e.g., Children's Communication Checklist, Bishop, 1998, 2001; Language Use Inventory, O'Neill, 2009; Pragmatic Rating Scale, Landa et al., 1992). (See Table 1–2 for a list of tests appropriate to assess the social communication and language use of individuals with ASD.)

A final responsibility of the SLP in an assessment is to determine the link between behavior and communication by analyzing problem behaviors. By determining the antecedent and consequence of problem behaviors across environments, the SLP can play a critical role in determining the communicative intent (e.g., attention, escape, frustration, requesting, sensory). This assessment is necessary to implement functional communication training where teaching the communicative equivalence for the purpose of a challenging behavior will reduce that problem behavior, an approach solidly grounded in research (see Carr et al., 1999; Horner, Albin, Sprague, & Todd, 2000).

Table 1-2. Assessments of Language Use and Social Communication

Test	Author (year); Publisher	Publisher	Age Range (years; months)	Administration Time	Description
Children's Communication Checklist-2 (CCC-2)	D. V. M. Bishop (2006)	Pearson	4;0–16;11	15–30 minutes	A caregiver rating scale designed to assess communication skills in the areas of pragmatics, syntax, morphology, semantics, and speech.
Clinical Evaluation of Language Fundamentals-Fifth Edition (CELF-5) • Pragmatics Profile • Pragmatics Activities Checklist	Eleanor Semel, Elisabeth H. Wiig, and Wayne A. Secord (2013)	Harcourt Assessment	5;0–21;0	Not stated	-Pragmatics Profile: A checklist on verbal rituals, expression of intentions, and nonverbal communication completed by the examiner with input from teacher, caregiver, and informants. • Pragmatic Activities Checklist: Report of direct observation of student's functional communication skills during authentic interactions.
Comprehensive Assessment of Spoken Language (CASL) • Inference subtest • Pragmatic Judgment	Elizabeth Carrow-Woolfolk (1999)	Pearson	3;0–21;0	15 minutes	-Inference subtest: For 7;0-17;11 designed to assess the ability to use world knowledge to determine the meaning of inferences through direct questioning • Pragmatic Knowledge: For ages 3;0-21;0 designed to assess language use through situational examples where the examinee is asked for the appropriate thing to say or do in the situation. (Not normed on ASD but recommended by Reichow, Salamack, Paul, Volkmar, & Klin, 2008.)

Test	Author (year); Publisher	Publisher	Age Range (years; months)	Administration Time	Description
Evaluating Acquired Skills in Communication Third Edition (EASIC-3)	Anita Marcott (2009)	Pro-Ed	0;3–6;0	15–30 minutes	An inventory of prelinguistic skills, semantics, syntax, morphology, and pragmatics developed for children with ASD, DD, cognitive impairment, language disorders.
Functional Communication Profile Revised (FCP-R)	Larry Kleiman (2003)	LinguiSystems	PreK–Adult	45 minutes to 1½ hours	An inventory for individuals developmental (including ASD) and acquired delays of overall communication abilities, mode of communication (e.g., verbal, sign, nonverbal, augmentative), and degree of independence obtained through direct observation, teacher and caregiver reports, and one-on-one testing.
Language Use Inventory (LUI)	Daniella K. O'Neill (2009)	Knowledge in Development, Inc.	1;6–3;11	20 minutes	A standardized parent-report questionnaire assessing pragmatic language development in a wide range of settings functions; has been recommended for ASD (see Tager-Flusberg et al., 2009).
Pragmatic Communication Skills Protocol	Academic Communication Associates (1989)	Academic Communication Associates	3;0–11;0	20 minutes	Records observations of the effectiveness of children's pragmatic communication behaviors in natural contexts (e.g., describing events, expressing feelings, requesting information, maintaining conversational topics); no scores given.

continues

Table 1–2. *continued*

Test	Author (year); Publisher	Publisher	Age Range (years; months)	Administration Time	Description
Pragmatic Language Skills Inventory (PLSI)	James A. Gilliam and Lynda Miller (2006)	Pro-Ed	5;0–12;11	5–10 minutes	Rating scale (45 items) designed to assess pragmatic language abilities in personal (e.g., initiating conversation, asking for help), social (e.g., taking turns in conversations), and classroom (e.g., writing stories, using slang) interactions; normed on ASD.
Pragmatic Protocol	Carol Prutting and Diane Kirchner (1987)	Prutting, C.A., & Kirchner, D.M. (1987). A clinical appraisal of the pragmatic aspects of language. Journal of Speech and Hearing Disorders, 52(2), 105–119.	5;0–adult	15 minutes	The descriptive protocol consists of 30 pragmatic parameters of language across verbal, paralinguistic, and nonverbal aspects, reported as appropriate, inappropriate, or no opportunity to observe.
Pragmatic Rating Scale	Rebecca Landa (2011)	Unpublished material Kennedy Kreiger Institute, Baltimore, MD (contact author for copy)	4;0–adult	40–60 minutes	A rating scale (using 0 to 2, with higher indicative of greater severity) according to operational definitions of 34 features related to pragmatic language (e.g., verbosity, scripting, social appropriateness, redundancy, eye contact, communicative gestures) producing a total score.

Test	Author (year); Publisher	Publisher	Age Range (years; months)	Administration Time	Description
Social Communication Profile (previously known as the Perspective Taking Spectrum)	Michelle Garcia Winner, Pamela Crooke, and Stephanie Madrigal (2011)	Unpublished material, go to http://www.socialthinking.com for article. (Not yet scientifically validated)	School–age to adult	Not stated	Descriptive profile designed to show abilities and issues across disabilities; has six descriptive categories (2 with subcategories): (a) Significantly Challenged Social Communicator (SCSC) (b) Challenged Social Communicator (CSC) (c) Emerging Social Communicator (ESC) (d) Nuance Challenged Social Communicator (NCSC) (e) Neurotypical Social Communicator (NSC) (f) Resistant Social Communicator (RSC)
Social Emotional Evaluation (SEE)	Elisabeth Wiig (2008)	Super Duper Publications	6;0–12;0	20–25	Standardized, norm-referenced assessment of social skills and higher level language through the presentation of typical social situations and emotional reactions that elementary and middle school students encounter frequently. The 5 subtests (i.e., Recalling Facial Expressions; Identifying Common Emotions; Recognizing Emotional Reactions; Understanding Social Gaffes; Understanding Conflicting Messages) are designed for students with ASD, language delays/disorders, learning disabilities, or other executive functioning disorders.

continues

29

Table 1–2. *continued*

Test	Author (year); Publisher	Publisher	Age Range (years; months)	Admin-istration Time	Description
Social Language Development Test Adolescent	Linda Bowers, Rosemary Huisingh, and Carolyn LoGiudice (2010)	LinguiSystems	12;0–17;11	45 minutes	Standardized assessment for adolescents' social language skills with subtests on perspective taking, social interpretation, interpreting visual cues, and social interaction. Measures age-appropriate skills such as response to sarcasm, sensitive information, and rumors.
Social Language Development Test Elementary	Linda Bowers, Rosemary Huisingh, and Carolyn LoGiudice (2008)	LinguiSystems	6.0–11.11	45 minutes	Standardized assessment for school-aged children that evaluates social language and differentiates typically developing children from those with autism and language learning disorders. Includes subtests on making inferences, interpersonal negotiation, multiple interpretations, and supporting peers.
Social Responsiveness Scale-2	John Constantino (2012)	Western Psychological Services	2;6–adult	15–20 minutes	Standardized assessment that rates social behaviors on a 4-point scale (not true, sometimes true, often true, almost always true) to identify the presence and severity of ASD across 5 subscales (Social Awareness, Social Cognition, Social Communication, Social Motivation, Restricted Interests and Repetitive Behavior). Allows for parent, teacher, and self-report (adult), and different forms for male and female.

Test	Author (year); Publisher	Publisher	Age Range (years; months)	Administration Time	Description
Social Skills Improvement System Rating Scales (previously Social Skills Rating Scale)	Frank Gresham and Steven N. Elliott (2008)	Pearson	5;0–21;0	10–25 minutes	Standardized teacher, parent, and student rating scale of social skills (i.e., cooperation, assertion, responsibility, empathy, self-control) Problem behaviors (i.e., externalizing, internalizing, hyperactivity), and academic competence (i.e., reading and math competence, motivation to learn) using norms and an importance scale to facilitate intervention planning. Includes *Communication, Engagement, Bullying,* and *Autism Spectrum* subscales.
Test of Pragmatic Language-2 (TOPL-2)	Diana Phelps-Terasaki and Trisha Phelps (2007)	Pro-Ed	6;0–18;11	45–60 minutes	Standardized, norm-referenced direct assessment of the ability to use pragmatic language effectively in 6 areas (i.e., physical setting, audience, topic, purpose/speech acts, visual-gestural cues, abstraction). Reported by Young et al. (2005) as a helpful tool to document the pragmatic needs of students with ASD relative to typical development.

continues

Table 1–2. *continued*

Test	Author (year); Publisher	Publisher	Age Range (years; months)	Administration Time	Description
Test of Problem Solving-2 Adolescent (TOPS-2)	Linda Bowers, Rosemary Huisingh, and Carolyn LoGiudice (2007)	LinguiSystems	12;0–17;0	40 minutes	Standardized, direct assessment of how adolescents use language to think, reason, and solve problems. Includes questions related to 18 situations that focus on critical thinking skills such as clarifying, analyzing, generating solutions, evaluating, and affective thinking. (Students with IEPs for special services were included in the normative sample.)
Test of Problem Solving-3 Elementary (TOPS-3)	Linda Bowers, Rosemary Huisingh, and Carolyn LoGiudice (2005)	LinguiSystems	6;0–12;0	35 minutes	Standardized, direct assessment composed of 18 situations that examine six thinking tasks (i.e., inferences, sequencing, negative questions, problem solving, predicting, determining causes) that are relevant to most students and cultures. Recommended by the authors to not be used as a test of pragmatic or social language but to be part of a battery to assess pragmatic competence.

Test	Author (year); Publisher	Publisher	Age Range (years; months)	Administration Time	Description
Vineland Adaptive Behavior Scales, Second Edition (Vineland II)	Sara S. Sparrow, Domenic V. Cicchetti, and David A. Balla (2005)	AGS Publishing/ Pearson Assessments	Survey Interview Form, Parent/ Caregiver Rating Form, Expanded Interview Form: Birth–90 Teacher Rating Form: 3;0-21;11	20–60 minutes	Standardized interview and rating scales that assess social and personal skills needed for daily living; assists in diagnosing and classifying developmental disabilities including ASD by examining the domains of communication, daily living, socialization, motor, and behavior.
Vineland Social-Emotional Early Childhood Scales (SEEC)	Sara S. Sparrow, David A. Balla, and Domenic V. Ciccetti (1998)	Pearson Assessments	Birth–5;11	15–25 minutes	Standardized rating scale that measures social-emotional development using 3 scales (i.e., Interpersonal Relationships, Play and Leisure Time, Coping Skills) in individuals with disabilities, and gauges how the disabilities affect their daily functioning.

Correlation of Assessment with Intervention

For students with ASD, as with all communicatively impaired children, functionality should drive intervention. Remembering this, goals for intervention at all stages of development should be able to answer the question of, "So what?" For example, when developing expressive and receptive vocabulary goals focus should be on "power words," or words that facilitate a response in the environment, rather than the presentation of predictable vocabulary units. Specifically, teaching the vocabulary for individual items and events with which a child comes in contact such as names of family and peers, labels for routine events, and language for desired items and routines is far more effective and meaningful than teaching standard vocabulary units of "farm animals, clothing, household items," and the like. Assessment results will be especially helpful in answering this question, as a student's inability to be successful in many domains is often correlated with the needs in communication. The goals for language intervention should, therefore, be presented similarly to any other functional goals, following the sequence of acquisition, demonstration across environments, and spontaneous initiation. Spontaneous communication is the desired outcome, in the absence of adult intervention to the greatest degree possible.

Finally, ASHA guides us to focus our intervention on the core deficits noted in autism: communication, socialization, cognition, behavior. We are directed as SLPs to "prioritize assessment and intervention approaches that are related to improvements in social communicative competence, that is, the ability to form relationships, function effectively, and actively participate in natural routines and settings" (2006b, p. 22).

Intervention

The goal of intervention for all students, including those with ASD, is the development and application of functional skills necessary to live as independently as possible within a community. Autism spectrum disorders are lifelong disorders that begin early in life, with changes occurring across the life span for the manifestation of symptoms as well as for an individual's personal and social needs. ASD is by definition a descriptive disorder, with variations noted across individuals in cognition, language, level of socialization, behavior, and concomitant disorders. These individual differences make the goal of intervention a significant and often daunting challenge. Each person with autism has unique strengths and needs, many of which were identified during initial assessment, which must be taken into account when designing a treatment plan. Along with variations in ability, chronological age and developmental functioning must be considered when designing an effective intervention program. Development of skills is central, but adaptive functioning must be held as equally important. The constant and critical focus of any intervention program, therefore, must be the development of skills that allow a person to participate ultimately at the highest level possible in his or her family, with peers, and in the community.

As SLPs, it is incumbent that we keep the core deficits of ASD in mind while developing, implementing, and revising our treatment goals and intervention plans. As previously noted, assessment must continue across intervention for all goals as well as for the specific procedures of implementation. This assures us that the outcomes are functional, achievable, and designed to achieve spontaneous social communication. It is critical that as SLPs, we remain current with the principles of best practice and the evidence supporting our intervention. In addition, we must work as part of a team, which not only includes but is focused on the person with autism and the family, to create and implement treatment plans that meet the social communication needs of our clients with ASD. Finally, our plans must be individualized and include baseline and follow-up assessments to measure changes over time (Maglione, Gans, Das, Timbie, & Kasari, 2012).

Over the past 10 years, there has been remarkable work from researchers around the world examining a variety of intervention approaches. In addition, there have been a number of researchers who have examined and analyzed a multitude of studies to determine which strategies are empirically supported for individuals with ASD. Examining the evidence is critical to best practice and as ASHA (2006a) reminds us, as new research evidence becomes available, recommended practices will change. At present, there is solid evidence for choosing particular approaches, as well as information on emerging treatments and those that are not based on evidence. Overall, the findings indicate that there are a variety of approaches that are deemed effective ranging on a continuum from behavioral to developmental. In addition, the research has not yet shown which specific approaches or strategies are most

effective for particular profiles of ASD. In summary, the research continues to support what was noted by the NRC in 2001, that "no one approach is equally effective for all individuals with ASD" (p. 64). However, even in light of these differences, the NRC concluded and ASHA (2006a) agreed that there are several critical features to any effective intervention program, including "repeated, planned teaching opportunities" (ASHA) focused on the following six priorities:

(a) functional, spontaneous communication; (b) social instruction in various settings throughout the day; (c) play skills with a focus on play with peers and peer interaction; (d) new skill acquisition and generalization and maintenance in natural contexts; (e) functional assessment and positive behavior support to address problem behaviors; and (f) functional academic skills when appropriate. (p. 17)

ASHA's recommendations are supported by the Ministries of Health and Education who compiled a 2008 systematic review urging practitioners to focus on increases in spontaneous initiation of communication, increased participation in functional activities, generalization of skills, including communication, across partners, environments, functional activities, and an increase in conventional means of communication. In addition, these researchers found strong evidence in their systematic review to indicate that "Communication should be seen as a high-priority learning area, and communication goals should be included in individual plans for all children and young people with ASD" with "spontaneous communication, socialization and play goals" a priority (p. 22).

Recently, two substantial reviews of current treatment methods for individuals with ASD were conducted: in 2009 by the National Autism Center (NAC) and in 2010 by Young, Corea, Kimani, and Mandell. Both reviews inform service providers of the efficacy of various interventions that currently exist for children, transitioning youth, and adults with ASD, providing critical data on which interventions are effective, which are emerging, and which should not be implemented. (The NAC evaluated 775 research studies; Young et al. reviewed 271.) After implementing a rigorous review process, studies were rated and specific interventions were categorized according to a "strength of evidence rating," which "reflect the quality, quantity, and consistency of research findings that have been applied specifically to individuals with ASD" (NAC, p. 31). The resulting categories were *Established* or *Evidence-Based Interventions* (i.e., sufficient evidence to confidently determine there are beneficial treatment effects for ASD), *Emerging Interventions* (i.e., one or more studies suggest beneficial treatment effects for ASD, but more research needed), *Unestablished Interventions* (i.e., little or no evidence to establish treatment effectiveness for ASD), and *Ineffective/Harmful Interventions* (i.e., sufficient evidence to determine that it is ineffective or harmful for ASD). (There were no interventions ranked in the latter category.) Although all ratings were not identical between the two reviews, most interventions yielded similar rankings. Regardless of differences, both the NAC and Young et al. implore clinicians to choose treatments that are deemed to be solidly established as evidence based as the first consideration for intervention.

Established Evidence-Based Interventions

Both NAC and Young et al. determined that the following interventions rated as *Established* (NAC) or *Evidence Based* (Young et al.); all were beneficial for both communication and socialization: (a) antecedent package, (b) behavioral package, (c) comprehensive behavioral treatment for young children, (d) joint attention, (e) naturalistic teaching strategies, (f) peer training, and (g) story based. In addition, the NAC found modeling, pivotal response treatment, and self-management to be ranked as *Established*. Each treatment will be briefly explained reflective of the NAC's findings.

Antecedent

The NAC reviewed 99 peer-reviewed studies and found that antecedent interventions improved skills in the areas of communication and socialization, as well as in learning readiness, personal responsibility, play, and social responsiveness across the individuals with ASD aged 3 to 18 years. Antecedent interventions are ones that modify the "situational events" that occur prior to a target behavior, and are designed to either increase or decrease its occurrence. Some examples of antecedent interventions are positive behavior supports, behavioral momentum, choice, errorless learning, inclusion of special interests or rituals into task, priming, prompting, and time delay

Behavioral Approach

The NAC separated studies into a "package approach" ($N = 231$) and "comprehensive treatment" ($N = 22$; pp. 58–59).

A package approach was defined as interventions that teach alternative behaviors or skills to reduce problem behavior, "through the application of basic principles of behavior change" (p. 58); these include using the concepts of applied behavior analysis including verbal operants. The review of 231 studies indicated positive findings for all areas of development (i.e., academics, communication, socialization, learning readiness, personal responsibility, play, and self-regulation) for all ages (0 to 21 years). Comprehensive treatments were from programs that combined various ABA procedures such as discrete trial training and incidental teaching; these were across environments but all were intensive programs with a low student-teacher ratio, following prescribed procedures. This approach was successful for ages 0 to 9 years and improvement was noted for communication and socialization as well as cognition, motor skills, personal responsibility, and play.

Modeling

The NAC evaluated 50 studies and found that interventions that used modeling for simple and complex behaviors (often in conjunction with other strategies such as prompting and reinforcement) were effective. Positive effects were noted for communication and socialization as well as improved cognition, personal responsibility, and play, and spanned the ages of 3 to 18 for individuals with ASD. These findings included studies for both live modeling and video modeling.

Natural Teaching Approach

A natural teaching approach, also known as, incidental teaching, milieu teaching, and responsive education, teach func-tional skills in a child's natural environment and rely primarily on child-directed interactions. The 32 studies reviewed by the NAC showed positive outcomes for children with ASD ages birth to 9 years for communication and socialization as well as learning readiness and play. Typically these approaches encourage interaction and communication with peers, and provide natural choices and reinforcement in a motivating environment.

Peer Training

Although studies involving peer training spanned a variety of treatment packages, research found that the interventions were effective to improve communication, socialization, and play for children ages 3 to 14 years of age. This approach teaches typically developing peers and siblings how to facilitate interactions with children with autism.

Pivotal Response Training (PRT)

PRT is an intervention that targets the "pivotal" skills of motivation and responsivity to multiple cues. (The review of 14 studies included Natural Language Paradigm due to its similarity to PRT.) PRT's goal is integrated growth across a wide variety of skill areas, including social communication, self-initiation, and self-management, in a child's natural environment. It was found to be most effective for children ages 3 to 9, in the areas of communication, interpersonal, and play.

Story Based

Story-based interventions are effective for ages 6 to 14, and typically describe a situation and the expected behaviors associated with it. The most familiar story-based intervention is Social Stories™, and is typically supported with other interventions such as prompting and reinforcement. The 21 studies reviewed indicated that story-based interventions are effective for improved communication, socialization, and self-regulation.

Beyond the approaches noted above, the NAC found that interventions with a particular focus were effective, specifically *joint attention* (N = 6) and *self-management* (N = 21). Joint attention intervention focuses on this foundational skill by teaching the child to "respond to the nonverbal social bids of others or to initiate joint attention interactions" (p. 47). These were effective to improve communication and socialization for children with ASD ages 0 to 5 years. Self-management intervention was effective for ages 3 to 18 years of age, and yielded improvements in communication and socialization, as well as self-regulation. Promoting independence was the focus of these interventions (e.g., checklists, tokens, visual prompts) with the goal to teach individuals with ASD to motor and regulate their own behavior, and to seek and provide their own reinforcement.

Finally, although improvements were not noted in communication or socialization, implementation of *schedules* yielded improved skills in the area of self-regulation for individuals ages 3 to 14 years (N = 12). This intervention provides a visual list of what is needed to complete a specific activity (including a task or a day) and included words and pictures.

Emerging Interventions

Besides the previously noted established interventions, the NAC (2009) also determined a number of interventions to be *Emerging*, defined as ones that the research suggests "favorable outcomes," but more evidence is needed. Specifically, the NAC noted, "Based on the available evidence, we are not yet in a position to rule out the possibility that *Emerging Treatments* are, in fact, not effective" (p. 57).

The NAC does not recommend beginning with *Emerging Treatments*, but they should be considered as "promising" and can be seriously considered if the previously noted *Established Treatments* are found to be inappropriate. The NAC determined that the following interventions rated as *Emerging*, showing promise for both communication and socialization: (a) developmental relationship-based treatment, (b) picture exchange communication system, (c) social communication intervention, (d) structured teaching, and (e) technology-based treatment. In addition, the following *Emerging Interventions* were found to increase communication skills alone: (a) augmentative and alternative communication, (b) language training, and (c) sign instruction. Finally, (a) imitation training, (b) peer mediated structural arrangement, and (c) scripting yielded improvements in the area of socialization not specific to communication. (Most of these findings are consistent with the review conducted by Young et al. in 2010; however, the authors in the 2010 review rated the interventions of (a) multicomponent packages, (b) picture exchange communication system, (c) structured teaching, and (d) technology-based treatment as *Evidence Based* for children.)

Augmentative and Alternative Communication (AAC)

AAC interventions incorporate both high and low technological devices to facilitate and support communication, such as picture symbols, communication books, and electronic devices. The 14 studies found these interventions to be effective for children ages 3 to 9.

Developmental Relationship-Based Treatment

These treatments are grounded in a developmental theory and focus on creating and improving social relationships. All use a developmental approach, following a child's interest, with a strong emphasis on parent training and involvement, but can be implemented across teaching environments. Some specific examples noted were the Denver Model, DIR (Developmental, Individual Differences, Relationship-based)/Floortime, Relationship Development Intervention (RDI), and Responsive Teaching; improvements were found for children ages birth to 5.

Imitation Training

Treatments that focused on the adults imitating a child with ASD typically in the context of play (ages birth to 14 years) were ranked as emerging based on 6 studies.

Initiations

Seven studies showed emerging evidence for interventions that directly teach individuals with ASD ages 6 to 14 to initiate peer interactions.

Language Training (Production)

Thirteen studies found that language training specifically focused on the production of speech was an emerging treatment for children ages 3 to 9 years. Some examples noted were echo relevant word training, oral verbal communication training, structured discourse, simultaneous communication, and individualized language remediation.

Language Training (Production and Understanding)

Seven studies found that interventions that target speech production and comprehension of language combined (such as total communication training) were effective for children ages 3 to 9.

Peer-Mediated Structural Arrangement

These interventions are often known as peer tutoring where the same-age peer supports learning. These were considered emerging for 6 to 9 year olds (based on 11 studies).

Picture Exchange Communication System (PECS)

PECS is a treatment that follows a behavioral approach to teach children with ASD how to communicate by manually exchanging symbols with communication partners. The approach implements six phases of instruction: (a) physical exchange of a symbol for a desired object; (b) expanding the use of symbols across people, places, and things, including retrieving them from a distance; (c) requests using the phrase "I want"; (d) discrimination training to discern the meaning of symbols; (e) responding to questions; and (f) commenting using simple phrases (e.g., "I see"). The summative research ($N = 13$) found that PECS is an emerging treatment for children ages birth to 9 years of age; some evidence of ancillary speech development is reported (although this is not a focus of the intervention).

Scripting

This treatment relies on a verbal or written script as a model to rehearse prior to entering specific contexts, for children with ASD. Six studies were reviewed; it was ranked as an emerging intervention for 6 to 14 year olds.

Sign Instruction

Interventions that directly taught the use of sign language to communicate with others was an emerging treatment for 3 to 9 year olds, based on 11 studies.

Social Communication Intervention

These interventions are often called social pragmatic interventions and target pragmatic communication. The five studies reviewed indicated this approach is emerging for ages 0 to 5, and also supports motor development and personal responsibility.

Structured Teaching

These programs are designed to support the learning styles of people with ASD by adapting the learning environment to their specific needs. Structured teaching interventions are typically known as TEACCH (Treatment and Education of Autistic and related Communication-handicapped CHildren) and focus primarily on the physical organization of the environment, implementation of schedules, and individualized teaching methods. The four studies reviewed found improvements in communication and socialization as well as cognition, learning readiness, motor, and personal responsibility across all ages until 18 years of age.

Technology-Based Treatment

These treatments varied in their theoretical base, but all 19 studies relied on computers or related technology to present instructional materials (e.g., Alpha Program, the Emotion Trainer Computer Program, Personal Digital Assistant). These were most effective for individuals with ASD ages 6 to 18, improving communication and academics, personal responsibility, and self-regulation.

Unestablished Interventions

According to the NAC (2009) there are five interventions, due to their poor quality of research and inconsistency of outcome results specific to ASD, that are ranked as *Unestablished* Interventions. These are as follows: (a) academic interventions (i.e., use of traditional teaching methods to improve academics); (b) auditory integration training (AIT; i.e., presentation of sounds in a headphone for the purpose of retraining the auditory system); (c) facilitated communication; (d) gluten- and casein-free diet; and (e) sensory integrative package (i.e., using all of the senses to assist with environmental stimulation). (Young et al. rated academic interventions to be *Emerging* for children; was in agreement about AIT; and did not review the last three.) This does not, however, mean that all unnamed interventions fall into the previous categories of *Established* or *Emerging*, as there are many practices for which research has not been conducted or published in peer-reviewed journals.

In sum, for SLPs working with individuals with ASD it is incumbent to understand and follow the guidelines of effective service provision, to stay current with evidence, and to investigate treatment approaches before implementation. Intervention must keep social communication at its core and, as ASHA's Position Statement (2006c) states, "honor and adapt to differences in families, cultures, languages, and resources." Regardless of the specific approach, communication intervention must focus on and enhance functional, spontaneous communication across people, settings, and functions, including comprehension and production of verbal and nonverbal means. SLPs must work in collaboration with others, including the person with autism, the family, other professionals, and all invested partners. Finally, SLPs must continue in their professional development both as trainers and trainees to continue in their growth of knowledge and skills on how to provide functional, meaningful service for individuals with ASD (ASHA, 2006c).

Case Study 1: Young Child with Autism Initial Evaluation

Jessie is a 4-year-old girl presenting with limited to absent verbal communication, atypical social interactions, occasional outbursts of hitting herself and others, and some repetitive behaviors. Her parents initially became concerned about her lack of expressive communication, believing that "she understood all of what others said to her." She appeared, according to parental report, to be very independent, easily entertained by certain toys (especially dolls), and to experience frustration primarily due to her inability to communicate with others. When questioned how Jessie had her needs met, her parents reported she usually obtained items on her own (e.g., pushing a chair to a counter to open a cabinet containing food; acti-

vating DVDs and iPad independently), or led them by the hand to desired items and events. Both parents reported they were anxious to "rule out the diagnosis of autism" based on the consistently "good eye contact" observed at home with members in and outside of the family as well as her demonstration of affection.

Talk Aloud

It will be important to see what she understands in verbal and nonverbal communication as comprehension is often the most impaired area of language for children with ASD. It is also important to consider any means of communication in which she engages, as even though she isn't talking, she probably attempts communication in some less than traditional ways. Her interest in toys seems to be a good place to "get in" with her, as this may allow her to engage with me and I can observe joint attention, joint reference, and imitation skills. The ADOS and the CSBS will be excellent for observing her social communication skills and finding what she can do, rather than just a list of what she cannot.

Diagnostic testing was conducted over a period of 2 weeks, consisting of a psychological evaluation to determine her level of cognitive functioning, a speech-language evaluation to determine her current level of communicative functioning, an educational evaluation to assess present levels of preacademic skills, and an occupational therapy evaluation to determine the level of self-help skills and sensory functioning. A combination of parent interview, direct observation, and standardized testing was conducted. The Psychoeducational Profile-Revised (PEP-R) was administered to identify characteristic uneven learning patterns exhibited by children with autism or related developmental disorders. The scores are distributed among seven Developmental Scales and four Behavioral Scales. The Developmental Scales are norm-referenced and indicate where a child is functioning relative to peers. Jessie's overall Developmental Score was 20 months, well below her chronological age. Her strengths were in the areas of fine and gross motor and eye hand coordination. Her weakest areas were cognitive performance and cognitive verbal, as she had not yet mastered some of the early skills necessary for preschool learning, such as matching pictures to objects, recognizing shapes and letters, and labeling colors. Limited attention to task also affected her performance. Encouragement to continue to work was met with resistance when the task was not preferred. Alternately, she had difficulty transitioning from preferred tasks and made attempts to escape from less desirable ones by whining and arching her back as a form of resistance.

The Vineland Social Maturity Scales, an instrument using parent report to measure functional skills and adaptive behaviors not readily observed in an assessment session, was administered. Jessie's overall Adaptive Behavior Composite score fell in the range of moderate deficit with all areas of adaptive behavior affected (i.e., communication, daily living skills, socialization, and motor). Her strength was in the motor domain, with overall functioning similar to that of a child 18 months old. However, when Jessie's skills were compared with the special population of children with autism under age 10 who are nonverbal, her adaptive behavior skills were considered to be average, with the exception of daily living skills.

The Autism Diagnostic Observation Schedule (ADOS) was also administered. This is semistructured standardized assessment of play, reciprocal social-interaction, and a social communication skill that allowed the examiner to observe and score the occurrence or nonoccurrence of behaviors that are associated with a diagnosis of an autism spectrum disorder (ASD). The activities incorporated toys and other motivating materials in a variety of tasks such as construction, make-believe, joint interaction, picture description, and storytelling. Following the assessment of (a) language and communication, (b) reciprocal social interaction, (c) play, and (d) stereotyped behaviors and restricted interests, Jessie met the criteria for an autism spectrum disorder.

In the communicative assessment, Jessie was evaluated using the Communication and Symbolic Behavior Scales (CSBS) in the areas of (a) communicative functions, (b) gestural communicative means, (c) vocal communicative means, (d) reciprocity, (e) social-affective signaling, (f) verbal symbolic behavior, and (g) nonverbal symbolic play. Results of the assessment revealed the primary function of Jessie's communication to be requesting desired items or events, with occasional episodes of protesting. Jessie communicated for behavioral regulation but did not communicate for the purpose of calling, showing off, or commenting. The function of joint attention was limited, as she had difficulty attending to both objects and people, clearly focusing most frequently on only the objects. During the evaluation, Jessie communicated primarily through the conventional gesture of giving with no distal gestures observed. She often manipulated the hand of the examiner or her mother to request assistance or request items that were difficult to obtain independently. Occasionally, vocalizations were observed during these requests, primarily in the form of a single vowel sound with rising intonation. Repair strategies were attempted through the repetition of behaviors to request items or events, with few gaze shifts observed. Positive affect (i.e., facial expressions of pleasure or excitement with or without vocalization) was limited, with two instances of negative affect (i.e., vocal expressions of distress or frustration).

Talk Aloud

It will be important to evaluate Jessie's verbal communication specific to speech to determine what phonemes she produces spontaneously as well as what are noted in imitation. More information is needed on her receptive language skills to determine if she understands social phrases, directions, and vocabulary with and without visual supports like gestures and pictures. This will help us in our intervention planning to know how she learns and areas of strength.

A limited number of vowels and consonants was observed in Jessie's spontaneous phonemic repertoire, including four vowels (i.e., *ah, ih, uh, eh*) and five consonants (i.e., *b, d, k, m, n*), primarily during solitary play. These sounds were observed in isolation and occasional consonant-vowel combinations (e.g., *buh, kuh, dih*). No expressive language forms were heard. Impaired language comprehension was illustrated through Jessie's inconsistent response to verbal requests when accompanied by gestural cues. She did, however, point to a variety of pictures on demand, given up to a field of three choices. Jessie engaged in play with dolls, appearing to have them kiss and walk. She did not respond to the play of the exam-

iner and had difficulty relinquishing these items when presented with alternate toys. Other areas evaluated included imitation of gestures and oral movements. Jessie attempted to imitate a variety of gestural movements, including signs for "more, done, stop, go, and eat." Oral movements appeared more difficult, though she imitated mouth opening and closing, lip presses, and lip rounding when given assistance with oral positioning. Attempts to imitate the vowels within her repertoire were unsuccessful with the exception of *ah*. No consonants were imitated.

Talk Aloud

It appears to be most important to provide Jessie with an immediate means to communicate her wants and needs in a more socially appropriate and understandable way. She likes to look at pictures and appears to want to get her ideas and wants across to others; she may benefit from a copresentation of picture symbols and/or gestures with "phonemically accessible" utterances (e.g., CV & VC structures). Her aggressive behavior appears to be most related to her inability to have her needs met; therefore, assessing her "top 10 to 20" needs will be important as the initial focus of expressive vocabulary and communication intervention. Finally, Jessie appears to be an excellent candidate for direct teaching for sounds, signs, and pictures (possible discrete trial for massed practice for a high level of success and then moving into less directive approach) as she enjoys a structured teaching environment. She also appears to be an excellent candidate for an incidental teaching approach to support her in her preschool environment to use the communication skills. Finally, the elements of pivotal response training, using her high interest events (eating a snack; choosing a video) as the motivating elements upon which to focus her functional communication, joint attention, and play.

Based on the evaluation, communication intervention for Jessie will focus on: (a) the expansion of communicative functions (i.e., behavioral regulation, social interaction, joint attention); (b) imitation of gestural, vocal, and verbal behavior; (c) improved comprehension of gestural and verbal language; and (d) development of action play schemes used with familiar and novel objects. These goals will be addressed through the use of instructional routines to help develop anticipatory and intentional behaviors, replacing idiosyncratic communicative means (e.g., hitting, pushing away) with more conventional means (e.g., verbalizing "no"; head shake), and developing multiple means of communication. Jessie shows an interest in and a level of comprehension for pictures that will be used to establish a communication system for both receptive and expressive language development. Additionally, gestures and signs will be presented along with simple vocalizations for familiar and high-frequency intents. Speech sound production will be specifically directed toward the imitation of sounds and the correlation of sounds to meaningful utterances. Finally, play and communication will be simultaneously addressed thorough imitation of novel play schemes with a peer and/ or an adult, including turn taking, cooperative behavior, and tolerance of shared materials.

Review Questions

1. Are Jessie's parents "typical" regarding their concern about her lack of expressive communication? Why would

they believe that "she understood all of what others said to her?"

2. How would you address (and support) the parents' report of "good eye contact" and demonstration of affection when reporting the results of the diagnostic assessment?

3. What areas of overlap were noted in the testing? How relevant are each examiner's results to the speech/language intervention?

4. Is it appropriate to primarily address Jessie's expressive language needs and assume that the receptive skills will follow? Why or why not?

5. Why is it important to directly teach Jessie gestures and signs to go along with simple vocalizations for familiar and high-frequency intents?

Case Study 2: School Aged Student with Autism: Progress Summary

Charlie is a 10-year, 9-month-old boy currently enrolled in a 5th grade class at a public elementary school. Charlie was initially evaluated when he was 3 years old, and was diagnosed with Pervasive Developmental Disorder-Not Otherwise Specified (PDD-NOS). At the age of 6, Charlie received medical intervention to address his anxiety and attention problems which continues to date. A review of Charlie's progress and recent educational and communication testing revealed notable quantitative and qualitative gains, particularly over the last 3 years with the greatest gains noted in his language skills and his ability to interact with same age peers. He continues to demonstrate attention skills which are highly variable, most notably in his inability to remain seated in a chair for more than 10 minutes at a time. He can, however, complete tasks and responds well to redirection. Charlie's speech and language services have primarily focused on his social communication comprehension and specific verbal expression, particularly in his interactions with peers. The following is a progress report for his areas of language.

Language Form (Grammatical and Syntactic Complexity)

Overall, Charlie has made remarkable progress with his grammatical (word level) and syntactical (sentence level) complexity as he uses age appropriate endings, verb tenses, and pronouns. In addition since last report Charlie has improved in his verbal syntactical complexity. He does, however, continue to have needs for written syntax as written language is a substantial area of need for him (similar to the needs previously noted for verbal expression).

Language Content (Semantics)

Semantics is the "what" of language, typically assessed and addressed through teaching vocabulary and concepts. Charlie, however, no longer has difficulty with these aspects of language; rather his difficulty is closely connected to his pragmatic skills and tendency to evaluate the world as "black and white." At present, Charlie's semantic skills in need of intervention are figures of speech in everyday life and their intended meaning; social nuances such as "lying" (white lie vs. gray lie, etc.), and inferential thinking. The latter is especially necessary when reading lit-erature as Charlie must understand what is happening as well as what it "means" to the bigger picture of the story.

Language Use (Pragmatics)

Pragmatics is the "language part" of social skills; hence Charlie's core deficits with social communication become evident for both comprehension and use. This has been one of the primary areas of intervention for specific social skills, conversational skills, and specific verbal expression. Charlie continues to make substantial progress across all of these areas, with some areas improving exponentially. Charlie does, however, continue to exhibit the following behaviors (from the Pragmatic Language Scale): (a) Overly talkative, (b) Inappropriate/irrelevant detail, (c) Out of sync content, (d) Unannounced topic shifts, (e) Confusing accounts, (f) Topic preoccupation, (g) Unresponsive to examiner's cues (for interest and comprehension), (h) Insufficient background information, and (i) Inadequate background information.

In addition, Charlie has made substantial progress in coping skills, recognizing emotions of other, and dealing with his own emotions. Charlie has made solid and steady improvements identifying the overt emotions of others in pictures and in stories; however recognizing emotions 10 in vivo continues to be more difficult, particularly for those at a higher level (and expected by the age of 9) such as annoyance, boredom, and unfriendly or manipulative (i.e., bullying) behavior. In addition, when Charlie is in his own emotional struggle he is unable to recognize the response of another. The focus of intervention has recently been on "behavior maps" where Charlie can track the effects of his feeling, actions, and reactions of others. Although his "fuse" has certainly improved, Charlie continues to need support identifying the "size and solution" for a problem. Academically, Charlie continues to struggle with frustration, particularly when presented with written language tasks.

Summary

It is the recommendation of this clinician that Charlie continue to receive direct services to address his areas of need outlined in this report. Although the scores on his standardized testing indicate some areas of language to be "within normal limits," it is critical that all areas of Charlie's performance be examined. The following recommendations are made:

1. Written language: Charlie will explain and identify the stages of writing (brainstorm, outline, write, edit) and implement them across a variety of academic tasks for narrative and expository writing.
2. Semantics: Charlie will recognize, explain, and use figures of speech found in everyday life and literature, and identify the rationale for their use.
3. Pragmatics:
   a. Charlie will independently complete behavior maps and "social autopsies" for real life events, identifying and explaining antecedent and consequential events surrounding his and others' interaction.
   b. Charlie will develop strategies, and evaluate his performance with compromising with others, particularly for play and social interaction.
4. Executive functioning: Charlie will identify, plan, and implement a variety of strategies for organization of difficult or complex tasks, including breaking down the tasks into manageable chunks, persisting when tasks are difficult, and strategies of memorization.

Review Questions

1. What strategies could the SLP present to the classroom teacher to support Charlie with his anxiety and attention problems?

2. Charlie has recently made gains in his language skills and his ability to interact with same age peers. Since he is in the 5th grade now, doesn't this "justify" a reduction in service with the SLP? Why or why not?

3. Charlie has reported needs in his written language; how would these needs manifest themselves as they relate to his 5th grade curriculum? Should the SLP or the classroom teacher address Charlie's need with written syntax?

4. How can the SLP "combine" Charlie's needs in semantics with his needs in pragmatics during intervention?

Case Study 3: Adolescent With ASD: Continued Needs for Service

Louis is a 16-year-old presenting with a long history of academic and social difficulties first evident in his early childhood. He initially received services at age 2 through the infants and toddlers program. He subsequently received special education services from age 3 until the present, including education services, occupational and physical therapies, speech and language therapy, and psychological services. Presently Louis receives instructional support in the areas of English, science, and social studies. Although he currently participates in a social skills group co-led by the SLP and the school psychologist, he receives no other services by the SLP. Louis's current disabling condition is autism.

An original diagnosis of PDD-NOS was determined when Louis was 6 years of age by a psychiatrist not affiliated with the public school system. The medical report indicated uneven patterns of cognitive development and deficits in executive functioning leading to difficulties in attention, tendencies toward obsessiveness/perseveration, and poor impulse control. At the age of 10 years, Louis was diagnosed with severe anxiety with obsessive-compulsive disorder, separation anxiety, and poor self-esteem. Louis received multiple psychological evaluations in his academic history. His most recent results indicate his overall cognitive abilities are in the borderline range of functioning. Strengths noted in testing, falling in the average range, were visual-spatial reasoning, short-term auditory memory, and fund of factual knowledge. Significant weakness was revealed in the areas of mental mathematical reasoning, social reasoning, and visual-motor speed. Due to the continued concerns with social communication and Louis' strong negative view of himself, a request for additional services with the SLP was requested by the 13 parents, resulting in an updated assessment.

The communication assessment, conducted across four sessions, revealed significant needs in the areas of language content, auditory processing, and prag-matic language use. Articulation testing revealed no errors in single words or during a storytelling task. Informally, Louis's conversational speech is often less intelligible, with imprecise articulation and a rapid rate of speech. The Clinical Evaluation of Language Fundamentals-5th edition (CELF-5) was administered as a standardized assessment of language content, language structure, oral and written language, and pragmatics. Louis revealed age-appropriate skills for his language structure and memory (i.e., sentence comprehension, word structure, formulated sentences, recalling sentences, sentence assembly, and following directions). The greatest areas of needs were found in pragmatics (i.e., rituals and conversational skills; asking for, giving, and responding to information; and nonverbal communication skills) and oral and written language (i.e., understanding spoken paragraphs, reading comprehension, and writing).

The standardized test results were supported through informal measures, including a narrative assessment and observation across environments. During a narrative assessment, needs were noted for accurate and varied use of cohesive devices, clear use of referents, overall organization, and story length. A review of written academic tasks indicated that these needs are present in Louis' written language as well, with the teacher and Louis reporting he doesn't know where to start with an assignment. Observations and direct interaction with Louis revealed significant needs for social communication. Difficulties were noted and reported for staying on topic, continuing a topic not of his own initiation, social problem solving, body orientation and movement, and appropriate use and comprehension of facial expressions and gestures. Louis appeared to be impulsive regarding his verbalizations, often making negative comments about an 14 activity and about himself. He often became frustrated when a task was difficult and adopted a depressed and negative affect, occasionally hitting himself on the head when he interpreted a response as incorrect. Louis was also impulsive behaviorally, often grabbing for materials that belonged to the examiner, getting out of his seat to look out the window, and rocking in his chair. He was generally responsive to a verbal cue and appeared to have little awareness of his behavior, although he frequently said, "I'm sorry!" immediately following a verbal notice. Parent and teacher report indicated that Louis continues to present with poor impulse control and often blurts out ideas that are not related to the environment, limited social judgment, and obsessive/perseverative thought patterns.

Based on the evaluations, particularly the negative impact Louis' communication challenges are having on his self-perception, speech-language services are recommended to address the following areas of language and communication as recommended by ASHA (2006b):

(a) understanding and using more sophisticated syntax to show relationships between sentences in conversational discourse and academic tasks; (b) determining causal factors for emotional states of self and others; (c) understanding and using nonverbal gestures, facial expressions, and gaze to express and follow subtle intentions (e.g., sarcasm and other nonliteral meanings); (d) initiating and maintaining conversations that are sensitive to the social context and the interests of others; (e) perceiving one's actions within social events and predicting social behavior in others in order to self-monitor; and (f) understanding figurative language, multiple meaning words, and perspective taking in narratives and social interactions.

It is strongly recommended that the SLP work directly with Louis to teach him the skills needed for improved social communication, and with Louis' teacher, psychologist, and other service providers in order to ensure that all members on the team are working cohesively. His 15 goals will be addressed through direct instruction, clinician and student identification of areas of need, role-play, and "real-time" implementation of strategies. Specifically, direct instruction will be used to teach reading comprehension strategies, including "visualize/verbalize" to understand the "big picture." Narrative language skills and written language will also involve direct instruction on cohesive devices, identifying anaphoric devices, organization of thought, and increasing length and complexity. Language comprehension will be correlated to social communication, connecting figurative language and inferencing to contents of narratives and "real life." Pragmatic language skills will be addressed through self-identification of social skills critical for successful peer and adult interactions using behavior mapping, video analysis, video modeling, and "real time" implementation and assessment. An ecological assessment will be conducted by Louis to determine specific factors or "triggers" for target behaviors though social autopsies and role-play to practice more appropriate strategies. Finally, strategies will be implemented across a variety of settings with varying conversational partners, allowing Louis to self-evaluate and self-monitor his level of success and need.

Review Questions

1. Louis currently participates in a social skills group co-led by the SLP and the school psychologist; what is the "evidence" behind this intervention?

2. Why do you think the SLP chose The Clinical Evaluation of Language Fundamentals-5th edition (CELF-5) as a primary means of assessment for Louis? Why, then, did the SLP conduct a narrative assessment and observations of Louis in his environment?

3. How could Louis' impulsive verbalizations be addressed? Is this important for him as a 16-year-old young man? Why?

4. Is it important for Louis to learn how to self-evaluate and self-monitor his level of success and need? What characteristics of ASD "interfere" with him knowing this instinctively?

References

American Academy of Pediatrics. (2001). The pediatrician's role in the diagnosis and management of autism spectrum disorder in children. Committee on children with disabilities. *Pediatrics, 107,* 1221–1226. doi:10.1542/peds.107.5.1221

American Psychiatric Association. (2000). *Diagnostic and statistical manual* (4th ed., Text rev.). Washington, DC: Author.

American Psychiatric Association. (2012). *DSM-5 proposed criteria for autism spectrum disorder designed to provide more accurate diagnosis and treatment* [Press release]. Retrieved from http://www.dsm5.org/Documents/12-03%20Autism%20Spectrum%20Disorders%20-%20DSM5.pdf

American Psychiatric Association. (2013). *Diagnostic and statistical manual* (5th ed.). Washington, DC: Author.

American Speech-Language-Hearing Association. (2006a). *Guidelines for speech-language pathologists in diagnosis, assessment, and treatment of autism spectrum disorders across the life span* [Guidelines]. Retrieved from http://dx.doi.org/10.1044/policy.GL2006-00049

American Speech-Language-Hearing Association. (2006b). *Principles for speech-language pathologists in diagnosis, assessment, and treatment of autism spectrum disorders across the life span* [Technical report]. Retrieved from http://dx.doi.org/10.1044/policy. TR2006-001-43

American Speech-Language-Hearing Association. (2006c). *Roles and responsibilities of speech-language pathologists in diagnosis, assessment, and treatment of autism spectrum disorders across the life span* [Position statement]. Retrieved from http://dx.doi.org/10.1044/policy.PS 2006-00105

Anderson, D. K., Lord, C., Risi, S., DiLavore, P. S., Shulman, C., Thurm, A., . . . Pickles, A. (2007). Patterns of growth in verbal abilities among children with autism spectrum disorder. *Journal of Consulting and Clinical Psychology, 75*(4), 594–604. doi:10.1037/0022-006X.75.4.594

Bailey, A., Le Couteur, A., Gottesman, I., Bolton, P., Simonoff, E., Yuzda, E., . . . Rutter, M. (1995). Autism as a strongly genetic disorder: Evidence from a British twin study. *Psychological Medicine, 25*(1), 63–77.

Bailey, D. B., Raspa, M., Olmsted, M., & Holiday, D. B. (2008). Co-occurring conditions associated with *FMR1* gene variations: Findings from a national parent survey. *American Journal of Medical Genetics Part A, 146A*(16), 2060–2069. doi:10.1002/ajmg.a.32439

Baron-Cohen, S. (1988). Social and pragmatic deficits in autism: Cognitive or affective? *Journal of Autism and Developmental Disorders, 18,* 379–402. doi:10.1007/BF02212194

Baron-Cohen, S. (2001). Theory of mind in normal development and autism. *Prisme, 34,* 174–183.

Baron-Cohen, S., Baldwin, D. A., & Crowson, M. (1988). Do children with autism use the speaker's direction of gaze strategy to crack the code of language? *Child Development, 68*(1), 48–57.

Bartolucci, G., Pierce, S., & Streiner, D. (1980). Cross-sectional studies of grammatical morphemes in autistic and mentally retarded children. *Journal of Autism and Developmental Disorders, 10,* 39–50. doi:10.1007/BF02408431

Behrmann, M., Thomas, C., & Humphreys, K. (2006). Seeing it differently: Visual processing in autism. *Trends in Cognitive Sciences, 10,* 258–264. doi:10.1016/j.tics.2006.05.001

Bishop, D. V. M. (1998). Development of the Children's Communication Checklist (CCC): A method for assessing qualitative aspects of communication impairment in children. *Journal of Child Psychology and Psychiatry, 29,* 879–891. doi:10.1017/S0021963098002832

Bishop, D. V. M. (2001). Parent and teacher report of pragmatic aspects of communication: Use of the Children's Communication Checklist in a clinical setting. *Developmental Medicine and Child Neurology, 43,* 809–818. doi:10.1017/S0012162201001475

Black, C., Kaye, J. A., & Jick, H. (2002). Relation of childhood gastrointestinal disorders to autism: Nested case-control study using data from the UK General Practice Research Database. *British Medical Journal, 325,* 419–421. doi:10.1136/bmj.325.7361.419

Botting, N. (2002). Narrative as a tool for the assessment of linguistic and pragmatic impairments. *Child Language Teaching and Therapy, 18,* 1–21. doi:10.1191/0265659002ct224oa

Bryant, P. E. (1991). Face to face with babies. *Nature, 354,* 19. doi:10.1038/354019a0

Bryson, S. (1997). Epidemiology of autism: Overview and issues outstanding. In D. J. Cohen & F. R. Volkmar (Eds.), *Handbook of autism and pervasive developmental disorders* (2nd ed., pp. 41–46). New York, NY: Wiley.

Carpenter, M., & Tomasello, M. (2000). Joint attention, cultural learning, and language acquisition: Implication for children with autism. In A. M. Wetherby & B. M. Prizant (Eds.), *Communication and language issues in autism and pervasive developmental disorder: A transactional developmental perspective* (pp. 31–54). Baltimore, MD: Brookes.

Carr, E. G., Levin, L., McConnachie, G., Carlson, J. I., Kemp, D. C., & Smith, C. E. (1994). *Communication based intervention for problem behavior: A user's guide for producing positive behavior change.* Baltimore, MD: Brookes.

Centers for Disease Control. (2012). *Autism spectrum disorders (ASDs): Facts and statistics.* Retrieved from http://oceanresourcenet.org/linkservid/9EB95E4C-CEB7-95D1-948D034C1313DC2F/showMeta/0/

Centers for Disease Control. (2014). Prevalence of autism spectrum disorder among children aged 8 years: Autism and Developmental Disabilities Monitoring Network, 11 sites, United States, 2010. *MMWR, 63*(2), 1–22. Retrieved from http://www.cdc.gov/mmwr/pdf/ss/ss6302.pdf

Clifford, S., Dissanayake, C., Bui, Q. M., Huggins, R., Taylor, A. K., & Loesch, D. Z. (2007). Autism spectrum phenotype in males and females with fragile X full mutation and premutation. *Journal of Autism and Developmental Disorders, 37*(4), 738–747. doi:10.1007/s10803-006-0205-z

Coonrod, E., & Stone, W. (2004). Early concerns of parents of children with autistic and non-autistic disorders. *Infants and Young Children, 17,* 258–268.

Damico, J. S. (1985). Clinical discourse analysis: A functional approach to language assessment. In C. S. Simon (Ed.), *Communication skills and classroom success: Assessment of language-learning disabled students* (pp. 165–204). San Diego, CA: College-Hill Press.

Dawson, G., Hill, D., Spencer, A., Galpert, L., & Watson, L. (1990). Affective exchanges between young autistic children and their mothers. *Journal of Abnormal Child Psychology, 18,* 335–345. doi:10.1007/BF00916569

Dawson, G., Meltzoff, A., Osterling, J., Rinaldi, J., & Brown, E. (1998). Children with autism fail to orient to naturally occurring social stimuli. *Journal of Autism and Developmental Disorders, 28,* 479–485. doi:10.1023/A:1026043926488

Dawson, G., Toth, K., Abbott, R., Osterling, J., Munson, J., Estes, A., . . . Liaw, J. (2004). Early social attention impairments in autism: Social orienting, joint attention, and attention to distress. *Developmental Psychology, 40,* 271–283. doi:10.1037/0012-1649.40.2.271

DeMeyer, M. K., Alpern, G. D., Barton, S., DeMeyer, W. E., Churchill, D. W., Hingtgen, J. N., . . . Kimberlin, C. (1972). Imitation in autistic, early schizophrenic and nonpsychotic subnormal children. *Journal of Autism and Childhood Schizophrenia, 2,* 264–287. doi:10.1007/BF01537618

Diehl, J. J., Watson, D., Bennetto, L., McDonough, J., & Gunlogson, C. (2009). An acoustic analysis of prosody in high-functioning autism. *Applied Psycholinguistics, 30,* 385–404. doi:10.1017/S0142716409090201

Filipek, P. A., Accardo, P. J., Baranek, G. T., Cook, E. H., Dawson, G., Gordon, B., . . . Volkmar, F. R. (1999). The screening and diagnosis of autism spectrum disorders. *Journal of Autism and Developmental Disorders, 29,* 439–484. doi:10.1023/A:1021943802493

Folstein, S., & Rutter, M. (1977). Infantile autism: A genetic study of 21 twin pairs. *Journal of Child Psychology and Psychiatry, 18*(4), 297–321.

Fox, L., Dunlap, G., & Buschbacher, P. (2000). Understanding and intervening with young children's problem behavior: A comprehensive approach. In A. M. Wetherby & B. M. Prizant (Eds.), *Communication and language issues in autism and pervasive developmental disorder: A transactional developmental perspective* (pp. 307–332). Baltimore, MD: Brookes.

Frombonne, E. (2003). Epidemiological surveys of autism and other pervasive developmental disorders: An update. *Journal of Autism and Developmental Disorders, 33*, 365–382. doi:01 62-3257/03/0800-0365/0

Geschwind, D. H. (2011). Genetics of autism spectrum disorders. *Trends in Cognitive Sciences, 15*(9). doi:10.1016/j.tics.2011.07.003

Geurts, H. M., Verte, S., Oosterlaan, J., Roeryers, H., Hartman, C. A., Mulder, E. J., . . . Sergeant, J. A. (2004). Can the Children's Communication Checklist differentiate between children with autism, children with ADHD, and normal controls? *Journal of Child Psychology and Psychiatry, 45*, 1437–1453. doi:10 .1111/j.1469-7610.2004.00326.x

Glascoe, F. P. (2012). *Parents' Evaluation of Developmental Status: A method for detecting and addressing developmental and behavioral problems in children, 2nd edition.* Nashville, TN: Ellsworth & Vandermeer Press.

Grafodatskaya, D., Chung, B., Szatmari, P., & Weksberg, R. (2010). Autism spectrum disorders and epigenetics. *Journal of the American Academy of Child & Adolescent Psychiatry, 49*(8), 794–809.

Hallmayer, J., Cleveland, S., Torres, A., Phillips, J., Cohen, B., Torigoe, T., . . . Lotspeich, L. (2011). Genetic heritability and shared environmental factors among twin pairs with autism. *Archives of General Psychiatry, 68*(11), 1095–1102. doi:10.1001/archgenpsychiatry.2011.76

Hobson, P. R., Lee, A., & Hobson, J. A. (2010). Personal pronouns and communicative engagement in autism. *Journal of Autism and Developmental Disorders, 40*, 653–664. doi:10.1007/s10803-009-0910-5

Horner, R., Albin, R., Sprague, J., & Todd, A. (2000). Positive behavior support for students with severe disabilities. In M. Snell & F. Brown (Eds.), *Instruction of students with severe disabilities* (5th ed., pp. 207–243). Upper Saddle River, NJ: Prentice Hall.

Kanner, L. (1943). Autistic disturbances of affective contact. *Nervous Child, 2*, 217–250. Retrieved from http://simonsfoundation.s3 .amazonaws.com/share/071207-leo-kanner-autistic-affective-contact.pdf

Kjelgaard, M. M., & Tager-Flusberg, H. (2001). An investigation of language impairment in autism: Implications for genetic subgroups. *Language and Cognitive Processes, 16*, 287–308.

Klin, A. (1992). Listening preferences in regard to speech in four children with developmental disabilities. *Journal of Child Psychology and Psychiatry, 33*, 763–769. doi:10.1111/j.1469-7610.1992.tb00911.x

Klin, A. (1991). Young autistic children's listening preferences in regard to speech: A possible characterization of the symptom of social withdrawal. *Journal of Autism and Developmental Disorders, 21*, 29–42. doi:10.1007/BF0 2206995

Klin, A., Jones, W., Schultz, R. T., Volkmar, F., & Cohen, D. J. (2002). Visual fixation patterns during viewing of naturalistic social situations as predictors of social competence in individuals with autism. *Archives of General Psychiatry, 59*, 809–816. doi:10.1001/archpsyc.59.9.809

Klin, A., Sparrow, S. S., de Bildt, A., Ciochetti, D. V., Cohen, D. J., & Volkmar, F. R. (1999). A normed study of face recognition in autism and related disorders. *Journal of Autism Development and Disorders, 29*, 499–508. doi:10.1023/A:1022299920240

Klin, A., & Volkmar, F. (1997). Asperger's syndrome. In D. J. Cohen & F. R. Volkmar (Eds.), *Handbook of autism and pervasive developmental disorders* (2nd ed., pp. 94–122). New York, NY: Wiley.

Landa, R. (2007). Early communication development and intervention for children with autism. *Mental Retardation and Developmental Disabilities Research Reviews, 13*, 16–25.

Landa, R., Piven, J., Wzorek, M., Gayle, J., Chase, G., & Folstein, S. E. (1992). Social language use in parents of autistic individuals. *Psychological Medicine, 22*, 246–254. doi:10.1017/S0033291700032918

Le Couteur, A., Rutter, M., Lord, C., Rios, P., Robertson, S., Holdgrafer, M., . . . McLennan, J. D. (1989). Autism diagnostic interview: A standardized investigator-based instrument. *Journal of Autism and Developmental Disorders, 19*, 363–387. doi:10.1007/BF02212936

Leekam, S. R., Nieto, C., Libby, S. J., Wing, L., & Gould, J. (2007). Describing the sensory abnormalities of children and adults with autism. *Journal of Autism and Developmental Disorders, 37*, 894–910. doi:10.1007/s10803-006-0218-7

Libby, S., Powell, S., Messer, D., & Jordan, R. (1998). Spontaneous play in children with autism: A reappraisal. *Journal of Autism and Developmental Disorders, 28*, 487–497. doi:10.1023/A:1026095910558

Liu, L., Lei, J., Sanders, S., Willsey, A. J., Yan K., Cicek, A. E., . . . Roeder, K. (2014). DAWN: A framework to identify autism genes and subnetworks using gene expression and genetics. *Molecular Autism, 5*(1), 1–35. doi:10.1186/2040-2392-5-22

Lockyer, L., & Rutter, M. (1969). A five- to fifteen-year follow-up study of infantile psychosis: III. Psychological aspects. *British Journal of Psychiatry, 115*, 865–882. doi:10.1192/bjp.115.525.865

Lord, C. (1995). Follow-up of two-year-olds referred for possible autism. *Journal of Child Psychology and Psychiatry, 36*, 1365–1382. doi:10.1111/j.1469-7610.1995.tb01669.x

Lord, C., & Paul, R. (1997). Language and communication in autism. In D. J. Cohen & F. R. Volkmar (Eds.), *Handbook of autism and pervasive developmental disorders* (2nd ed., pp. 195–225). New York, NY: Wiley.

Lord, C., Rutter, M., DiLavore, P. C., Risi, S., Gotham, K., & Bishop, S. L. (2012). *Autism diagnostic observation schedule, second edition*. Los Angeles, CA: Western Psychological Services.

Losh, M. (2003). Narrative ability in autism: Strengths, weaknesses, and links to social understanding. *California Speech-Language-Hearing Association Magazine*. Retrieved from http://autism.justinecassell.com/autism08/wiki/images/0/07/Losh2003_NarrativeAbilityInAutism.pdf

Losh, M., Adolphs, R., Poe, M. D., Couture, S., Penn, D., Baranek, G. T., . . . Piven, J. (2009). Neuropsychological profile of autism and the broad autism phenotype. *Archives of General Psychiatry, 66*, 518–526.

Loveland, K., & Tunali-Kotoski, B. (1997). The school-age child with autism. In D. J. Cohen & F. R. Volkmar (Eds.), *Handbook of autism and pervasive developmental disorders* (2nd ed., pp. 283–308). New York, NY: Wiley.

Maglione, M. A., Gans, D., Das, L., Timbie, J., & Kasari, C. (2012). Nonmedical interventions for children with ASD: Recommended guidelines and further research needs. *Pediatrics, 130*(Suppl. 2), S169–178. doi:10.1542/peds.2012-0900O

Mayer, M. (1969). *Frog, where are you?* New York, NY: Dial Press.

McEvoy, R., Loveland, K., & Landry, S. (1988). Functions of immediate echolalia in autistic children: A developmental perspective. *Journal of Autism and Developmental Disorders, 18*, 657–688. doi:10.1007/BF02211883

Ministry of Health. (2008). *New Zealand autism spectrum disorder guideline*. Wellington, New Zealand: Ministry of Health.

Minshew, N. J., Meyer, J., & Goldstein, G. (2002). Abstract reasoning in autism: A dissociation between concept formation and concept identification *Neuropsychology, 16*(3), 327–334. doi:10.1037//0894-4105.16.3.327

Mundy, P., & Neal, R. (2001). Neural plasticity, joint attention and a transactional social-orienting model of autism. *International Review of Mental Retardation, 23*,139–168. doi:10.1016/S0074-7750(00)80009-9

Nadig, A., Lee, I., Singh, L., Bosshart, K., & Ozonoff, S. (2010). How does the topic of conversation affect verbal exchange and eye gaze? A comparison between typical development and high-functioning autism. *Neuropsychologia, 48*, 2730–2739. doi:10.1016/j.neuropsychologia.2010.05.020

The National Autism Center. (2009). *National standards report*. Retrieved from http://www.nationalautismcenter.org/pdf/NAC%20Standards%20Report.pdf

National Initiative for Autism: Screening and Assessment (NIASA) & Le Couteur, A. (2003). *National Autism Plan for Children (NAPC): Plan for the identification, assessment, diagnosis and access to early interventions for pre-school to primary school aged children with autism spectrum disorders (ASD)*. Retrieved from The National Autistic Society http://ncepmaps.org/_gl/_115/

National Institute of Environmental Health Science. (2012). *Autism*. Retrieved from http://www.niehs.nih.gov/health/topics/conditions/autism/

National Institute of Mental Health. (2011). *A parent's guide to autism spectrum disorder*. (NIH Publication No. 11-5511). Retrieved from http://www.nimh.nih.gov/health/publications/a-parents-guide-to-autism-spectrum-disorder/parent-guide-to-autism.pdf

National Research Council. (2001). *Educating children with autism.* Washington, DC: National Academies Press.

Norbury, C. F., & Bishop, D. V. (2003). Narrative skills of children with communication impairments. *International Journal of Language & Communication Disorders, 38,* 287–313. doi:10.1080/136820310000108133

O'Connor, I. M., & Klein, P. D. (2004). Exploration of strategies for facilitating the reading comprehension of high-functioning children with autism spectrum disorders. *Journal of Autism and Developmental Disorders, 34,* 115–127. doi:10.1023/B:JADD.0000022603.44077.6b

Paul, R., & Cohen, D. J. (1984). Outcomes of severe disorders of language acquisition. *Journal of Autism and Developmental Disorders, 14,* 405–421. doi:10.1007/BF02409831

Paul, R., Orlovski, S. M., Marcinko, H. C., & Volkmar, F. (2009). Conversational behaviors in youth with high-functioning ASD and Asperger syndrome. *Journal of Autism and Developmental Disorders, 39,* 115–125. doi:10.1007/s10803-008-0607-1

Paul, R., Shriberg, L. D., McSweeny, J. L., Cicchetti, D., Klin, A., & Volkmar, F. (2005). Brief report: Relations between prosodic performance and communication and socialization ratings in high functioning speakers with autism spectrum disorders. *Journal of Autism and Developmental Disorders, 35*(6), 861–869. doi:10.1007/s10803-005-0031-8

Priessler, M., & Carey, S. (2005). The role of inferences about referential intent in word learning: Evidence from autism. *Cognition, 97,* B13–B23.

Prizant, B., & Duchan, J. (1981). The functions of immediate echolalia in autistic children. *Journal of Speech and Hearing Disorders, 46,* 241–249. Retrieved from http://jshd.asha.org/

Prizant, B., Schuler, A., Wetherby, A., & Rydell, P. (1997). Enhancing language and communication development: Language approaches. In D. J. Cohen & F. R. Volkmar (Eds.), *Handbook of autism and pervasive developmental disorders* (2nd ed., pp. 572–605). New York, NY: Wiley.

Reichow, B., Salamack, S., Paul, R., Volkmar, F. R., & Klin, A. (2008). Pragmatic assessment in autism spectrum disorders: A comparison of a standard measure with parent report. *Communication Disorders Quarterly, 29*(3), 169–176. doi:10.1177/1525740108318697

Robins, D., Fein, D., & Barton, M. (2009). *The Modified Checklist for Autism in Toddlers, Revised with Follow-Up (M-CHAT-R/F),* Retrieved from http://www2.gsu.edu/~psydlr/M-CHAT/Official_M-CHAT_Website_files/M-CHAT-R_F_1.pdf

Rutter, M. (1970). Autistic children: Infancy to adulthood. *Seminars in Psychiatry, 2,* 435–450.

Rutter, M. (2011). Progress in understanding autism: 2007–2010. *Journal of Autism and Developmental Disorder, 41,* 395–404. doi:10.1007/s10803-011-1184-2

Rutter, M., Le Couteur, A., & Lord, C. (2003). *Manual for the Autism Diagnostic Interview Revised, WPS Edition.* Los Angeles, CA: Western Psychological Services.

Schopler, E., Van Bourgondien, M. E., Wellman, G. J., & Love, S. R. (2010). *The Childhood Autism Rating Scale, Second Edition.* Los Angeles, CA: Western Psychological Services.

Scottish Intercollegiate Guidelines Network. (2007). *Assessment, diagnosis and clinical interventions for children and young people with autism spectrum disorders: A national clinical guideline.* Retrieved from http://www.sign.ac.uk/pdf/sign98.pdf

Sek, W. K., Sahin, M., Collins, C. D., Wertz, M. H., Campbell, M. G., Leech, J. D., . . . Kohane, I. S. (2014). Divergent dysregulation of gene expression in murine models of fragile X syndrome and tuberous sclerosis. *Molecular Autism, 5*(16), 1–24. doi:10.1186/2040-2392-5-16

Semel, E., Wiig, E. H., & Secord, W. A. (2004). *Clinical Evaluation of Language Fundamentals-Preschool, Second Edition.* San Antonio, TX: The Psychological Corporation.

Semel, E., Wiig, E. H., & Secord, W. A. (2013). *Clinical Evaluation of Language Fundamentals, Fifth Edition.* San Antonio, TX: The Psychological Corporation.

Shriberg, L. D., Paul, R., Black, L. M., & van Santen, J. P. (2011). The hypothesis of apraxia of speech in children with autism spectrum disorder. *Journal of Autism and Developmental Disorders, 41,* 405–426. doi:10.1007/s10803-010-1117-5

Siegel, B. (2004). *Pervasive Developmental Disorders Screening Test-II (PDDST-II).* San Antonio, TX: Pearson.

Sigman, M. D., Dissanayake, C., Arbelle, S., & Ruskin, E. (1997). Cognition and emotion in children and adolescents with autism. In D. J. Cohen & F. R. Volkmar (Eds.), *Handbook of autism and pervasive developmental disorders* (2nd ed., pp. 248–265). New York, NY: Wiley.

Sigman, M. D., Kasari, C., Kwon, J. H., & Yirmiya, N. (1992). Responses to the negative emotions of others by autistic, mentally retarded, and normal children. *Child Development, 63*, 796–807. doi:10.2307/1131234

Sparrow, S. S., Cicchetti, D. V., & Balla, D. A. (2005). *Vineland Adaptive Behavior Scales, Second Edition*. San Antonio, TX: The Psychological Corporation.

Squires, J., Twombly, E., Bricker, D., & Potter, L. (2009). *ASQ-3 user's guide*. Baltimore, MD: Brookes.

Steffenburg, S., Gillberg, C., Hellgren, L., Andersson, L., Gillberg, I. C., Jakobsson, G., . . . Bohman, M. (1989). A twin study of autism in Denmark, Finland, Iceland, Norway and Sweden. *Journal of Child Psychology and Psychiatry, 30*(3), 405–416.

Stone, W. L., & Caro-Martinez, L. M. (1990). Naturalistic observations of spontaneous communication in autistic children. *Journal of Autism and Developmental Disorders, 20*, 437–453. doi:10.1007/BF02216051

Stone, W. L., Coonrod, E. E., & Ousley, O. Y. (2000). Brief report—screening tool for autism in two-year-olds (STAT): Development and preliminary data. *Journal of Autism and Developmental Disorders, 30*, 607–612. doi:10.1023/A:1005647629002

Stone, W. L., Coonrod, E. E., Turner, L. M., & Pozdol, S. L. (2004). Psychometric properties of the STAT for early autism screening. *Journal of Autism and Developmental Disorders, 34*, 691–701. doi:10.1007/s10803-004-5289-8

Symons, L. A., Hains, S. M. J., & Muir, D. W. (1998). Look at me: Five-month-old infants' sensitivity to very small deviations in eye-gaze during social interactions. *Infants Behavior and Development, 21*, 531–536. doi:10.1016/S0163-6383(98)90026-1

Tager-Flusberg, H. (1995). 'Once upon a ribbit': Stories narrated by autistic children. *British Journal of Developmental Psychology, 13*, 45–59. doi:10.1111/j.2044-835X.1995.tb00663.x

Tager-Flusberg, H. (1997). Perspectives on language and communication in autism. In D. J. Cohen & F. R. Volkmar (Eds.), *Handbook of autism and pervasive developmental disorders* (pp. 894–900). New York, NY: Wiley.

Tager-Flusberg, H., & Caronna, E. (2007). Language disorders: Autism and other pervasive developmental disorders. *Pediatric Clinics of North America, 54*, 469–481.

Tager-Flusberg, H., Rogers, S., Cooper, J., Landa, R., Lord, C., Paul, R., Rice, M., . . . Yoder, P. (2009). Defining spoken language benchmarks and selecting measures of expressive language development for young children with autism spectrum disorders. *Journal of Speech, Language, and Hearing Research, 52*, 643–652. doi:1092-4388/09/5203-0643

Twachtman-Reilly, S. C., Amaral, P., & Zebrowski, P. (2008) Addressing feeding disorders in children on the autism spectrum in school-based settings: Physiological and behavioral issues. *Language, Speech, and Hearing Services in Schools, 39*, 261–272. doi:10.1044/0161-1461(2008/025)

de Villiers, J., Fine, J., Ginsberg, G., Vaccarella, L., & Szatmari, P. (2007). Brief report: A scale for rating conversational impairment in autism spectrum disorder. *Journal of Autism and Developmental Disorders, 37*(7), 1375–1380.

Vivanti, G., Nadig, A., Ozonoff, S., & Rogers, S. (2008). What do children with autism attend to during imitation tasks? *Journal of Experimental Child Psychology, 101*, 186–205. doi:10.1016/j.jecp.2008

Volden, J., & Lord, C. (1991). Neologisms and idiosyncratic language in autistic speakers. *Journal of Autism and Developmental Disorders, 21*(2), 109–130. doi:10.1007/BF02284755

Volden, J., Smith, I. M., Szatmari, P., Bryson, S., Fombonne, E., Mirenda, P., . . . Thompson, A. (2011). Using the *Preschool Language Scale, Fourth Edition* to characterize language in preschoolers with autism spectrum disorders. *American Journal of Speech-Language Pathology, 20*, 200–208. doi:10.1044/1058-0360(2011/10-0035)

Volkmar, F., Hoder, L., & Cohen, D. (1985). Compliance, "negativism" and the effects of treatment and structure in autism: A naturalistic behavior study. *Journal of Child Psychology and Psychiatry, 26*, 865–877. doi:10.1111/j.1469-7610.1985.tb00603.x

Volkmar, F., Klin, A., & Cohen, D. J. (1997). Diagnosis and classification of autism and related conditions: Consensus and issues. In D. J. Cohen & F. R. Volkmar (Eds.), *Handbook of autism and pervasive developmental disorders* (2nd ed., pp. 5–40). New York, NY: Wiley.

Volkmar, F. R., Klin, A., Schultz, R. T., Rubin, E., & Bronen, R. (2000). Asperger's disorder. *American Journal of Psychiatry, 157*, 262–267. doi:10.1176/appi.ajp.157.2.262

Vulchanova, M., Talcott, J. B., Vulchanov, V., Stankova, M., & Eshuis, H. (2013). Morphology in autism spectrum disorders: Local processing bias and language. *Cognitive Neuropsychology, 29*, 584–600. doi:10.1080/02643294.2012.762350

Wetherby, A. M., & Prizant, B. M. (2002). *Communication and Symbolic Behavior Scales Developmental Profile, First Normed Edition.* Baltimore, MD: Brookes.

Wetherby, A. M., Prizant, B. M., & Hutchinson, T. (1998). Communicative, social-affective, and symbolic profiles of young children with autism and pervasive developmental disorder. *American Journal of Speech-Language Pathology, 7*, 79–91. Retrieved from http://ajslp.asha.org/

Wetherby, A. M., Prizant, B. M., & Schuler, A. L. (2000). Understanding the nature of communication and language impairments. In A. M. Wetherby & B. M. Prizant (Eds.), *Autism spectrum disorders: A transactional developmental perspective* (pp. 109–141). Baltimore, MD: Brookes.

Wetherby, A. M., & Prutting, C. (1984). Profiles of communicative and cognitive-social abilities in autistic children. *Journal of Speech and Hearing Research, 27*, 364–377. Retrieved from http://jslhr.asha.org/

Wetherby, A. M., Woods, J., Allen, L., Cleary, J., Dickinson, H., & Lord, C. (2004). Early indicators of autism spectrum disorders in the second year of life. *Journal of Autism and Developmental Disorders, 34*, 473–493. doi:10.1007/s10803-004-2544-y

Wiig, E. H., & Secord, W. (1989). *Test of Language Competence—Expanded Edition.* San Antonio, TX: The Psychological Corporation.

Wilder, L. K., Dyches, T. T., Obiaker, F. E., & Algozzine, B. (2004). Multicultural perspectives on teaching students with autism. *Focus on Autism and Other Developmental Disabilities, 19*(2), 105–113.

Williams, D. L., Goldstein, G., & Minshew, N. J. (2006). Neuropsychologic functioning in children with autism: Further evidence for disordered complex information-processing. *Child Neuropsychology, 12*(4/5), 279–298.

Wing, L. (1993). The definition and prevalence of autism: A review. *European Child and Adolescent Psychiatry, 2*, 61–74. doi:10.1007/BF02098832

Wing, L., & Gould, J. (1979). Severe impairments of social interaction and associated abnormalities in children: Epidemiology and classification. *Journal of Autism and Developmental Disorders, 9*, 11–29. doi:10.1007/BF01531288

Wodka, E. L., Mathy, P., & Kalb, L. (2013). Predictors of phrase and fluent speech in children with autism and severe language delay. *Pediatrics, 131*(e1128), 128–134. doi:10.1542/peds.2012-2221 Retrieved from http://pediatrics.aappublications.org/content/131/4/e1128.full.pdf+html

Yirmiya, N., Sigman, M. D., Kasari, C., & Mundy, P. (1992). Empathy and cognition in high-functioning children with autism. *Child Development, 63*, 150–160. doi:10.2307/1130909

Young, J., Corea, C., Kimani, J., & Mandell, D. (2010). *Autism spectrum disorders (ASDs) services: Final report on environmental scan.* Retrieved from http://www.impaqint.com/files/4-content/1-6-publications/1-6-2-project-reports/finalasdreport.pdf

Young, E. C., Diehl, J. J., Morris, D., Hyman, S. L., & Bennetto, L. (2005). The use of two language tests to identify pragmatic language problems in children with autism spectrum disorders. *Language, Speech, and Hearing Services in the Schools, 36*(1), 62–72.

Zafeiriou, D. I., Ververi, A., & Vargiami, E. (2007). Childhood autism and associated comorbidities. *Brain and Development, 29*, 257–272. doi:10.1016/j.braindev.2006.09.003

CHAPTER 2

Language Learning Disabilities

Kara Tignor and Lisa Schoenbrodt

Chapter Objectives

Upon completion of this chapter, the reader should be able to:

1. Have a clear concept of the exclusive nature of learning disabilities (LD) and how this term came to acquire its various definitions
2. Understand the environmental and genetic factors linked to LD
3. Be aware of the variety of characteristics that can signal a LD
4. Have a clear concept of what constitutes an LLD and understand the difference between isolated LD and LLD
5. Understand the connections between spoken and written language, as well as the evolutionary stages for both, especially in regard to the needs of a student with a LD or LLD
6. Understand the nature of and need for norm-referenced and naturalistic assessments and techniques for both
7. Have a grasp of the range of techniques available for intervention,

including *Response to Intervention* as an approach outlined in IDEA 2004

Introduction

For many years, researchers in the area of learning disabilities have debated numerous definitions. Even at the time of this writing, although there is a generally accepted definition, many other definitions still exist depending on the website, support group, or literature you may consult. The definitions all support the fact that language, (reading, writing, speaking, and listening) coexists frequently as part of the learning disability spectrum. Language disorders are frequently diagnosed during the preschool years, around 4 to 5 years of age, and may change to learning disabilities as children engage in more academic tasks when entering grade school (Watson, 2012). Speech-language pathologists (SLPs) and those in training need to be aware of the organic bases, historical context, characteristics, and definitions of the disorder. This chapter provides that information as well as methods for successful assessment and intervention with this population.

Definition

Practitioners in the field of LD have struggled to identify a common definition for the disorder, due perhaps to the field's youth. This difficulty in pinning down a definition may also be related to the fact that LD theories have arisen from a wide range of individuals of various backgrounds and representing different organizations. This continual struggle has led to the development of many different definitions, some of which are presented within this chapter.

The debate surrounding the definition of a LD resulted in the growth of many professional and advocacy organizations, including the Council for LD and the LD Association of America (LDA). These associations gave way to the development of the Division for LD and the National Joint Committee on LD (NJCLD), founded in 1975. This committee, comprised of 12 organizations with over 350,000 members, is committed to the education and welfare of individuals with learning disabilities (Table 2–1).

In 1990 the NJCLD revised its previous 1981 definition of a learning disability to the following one which is accepted by all of its member organizations:

LD is a general term that refers to a heterogeneous group of disorders manifested by significant difficulties

Table 2–1. Member Organizations of the National Joint Committee on Learning Disabilities Founded in 1975

Member Organizations of the NJCLD
• American Speech-Language-Hearing Association (ASHA)
• Association of Educational Therapists (AET)
• Association on Higher Education and Disability (AHEAD)
• Council for Learning Disabilities (CLD)
• Division for Communicative Disabilities and Deafness (DCDD)
• Division for Learning Disabilities (DLD)
• International Dyslexia Association (IDA)
• International Reading Association (IRA)
• Learning Disabilities Association of America (LDA)
• National Association of School Psychologists (NASP)
• National Center for Learning Disabilities (NCLD)

Note. The National Joint Committee on LD (NJCLD) was founded in 1975. This committee, comprised of 12 organizations with over 350,000 members, is committed to the education and welfare of individuals with learning disabilities.

in the acquisition and use of listening, speaking, reading, writing, resonating, or mathematical abilities. These disorders are intrinsic to the individual, presumed to be due to central nervous system dysfunction, and may occur across the life span. Problems in self-regulatory behaviors, social perception, and social interaction may exist with LD but do not by themselves constitute a LD. Although LD may occur concomitantly with other handicapping conditions (e.g., sensory impairment, mental retardation, serious emotional disturbance), or with extrinsic influences (such as cultural differences, insufficient or inappropriate instruction), they are not the result of those conditions or influences. (NJCLD, 1991 p. 20)

While the Learning Disabilities Association of America (LDA) initially disagreed with the definition originally proposed by the NJCLD in 1986 as they excluded the reading, writing and listening qualifications, their most recent definitions include these characteristics. "A LD is a neurological condition that interferes with a person's ability to store, process, or produce information. LD can affect one's ability to read, write, speak, spell, compute math, reason and also affect a person's attention memory, coordination, social skills, and emotional maturity" (http://ldaamerica .org/support/new-to-ld/).

Although the aforementioned 1991 NJCLD definition was widely used in the United States, there remained controversy regarding explicit conceptualization as to what constitutes a LD and what does not. As a result, the NJCLD (2011a) published a paper discussing both the points of general agreement regarding LD, as well as the common misconceptions related to these disabilities which have direct impli-

cations on the development of future policy. The NJCLD (2011a) states as the points of agreement the following:

1. *Individuals with LD may experience significant difficulties in one or a combination of areas of educational performance.*
2. *LD may coexist with other disorders, including but not limited to social-emotional, behavioral or attentional difficulties.*
3. *LD exists across cultures, races, and languages, but they may differ from one culture or language to another.*
4. *Individuals identified as intellectually gifted may also have LD.*
5. *Most students with LD have an uneven patter of strengths and weaknesses that affect learning.*
6. *Diverse disciplines—including education, psychology, speech-language pathology, and medicine, among others—have broadened understanding of the neurobiological and neuropsychological aspects of LD.* (pp. 237–238)

The NJCLD (2011a) warns of the dangers that the following misperceptions about LD can have not only on the well-being of the individuals with LD, but also on the development of policies and practices that serve these individuals.

1. *The first misperception is that LDs are mild impairments.* Although some individuals with LD may not struggle as much as others with this disability, this is by no means indicative of a "mild" degree of this disability.
2. *The second misperception is that high-quality instruction in the general education classroom or in supplementary intervention programs can prevent or eliminate LD.* There is consensus that early intervention may lessen the

effects of LD, but individuals with LD will likely need specialized instruction and accommodations throughout their lifespan.

3. *The third misperception is that LDs are synonymous with a reading disability.* Although the majority of students with LD have reading difficulties, there are also individuals diagnosed with LD who have difficulties in areas such as listening, speaking, mathematics, written expression, social-emotional, and executive functions.

4. *The fourth misperception relates to the term LD being used as a generic term for individuals with other disabilities.* These others disabilities may include intellectual impairment, developmental disabilities, hearing impairments, and autism. (p. 238)

Historical Perspective

LD did not achieve official recognition until the 1960s when Samuel Kirk first used the term learning disability to describe:

A retardation, disorder, or delayed development in one or more of the processes of speech, language, reading, writing, arithmetic, or other school subject resulting from a psychological handicap caused by a possible cerebral dysfunction and/or emotional or behavioral disturbances. It is not the result of mental retardation, sensory deprivation, or cultural and instructional factors. (Danforth, 2011; Kirk, as cited in Nelson, 2010, p. 137)

Prior to this recognition, children with LD were diagnosed with minimal brain dysfunction (MBD). As the field of research involving LD advanced, several aspects of Kirk's original definition remained intact, including the use of both inclusionary and exclusionary conditions. These characteristics developed over the course of several decades. Smith, Dowdy, Polloway, and Blalock (1999) identified several phases in the LD movement, including the foundations phase, the early years of the LD movement, and the modern phase. During the foundations phase a variety of theories regarding LD abounded. Franz Gall's early investigations in the 1800s led him to propose the existence of specific localization of brain function that differentiated mental retardation and language impairment (Supple & Söderpalm, 2010). Following Gall, Broca described motor aphasia in an individual and identified the defect's location in the brain. Pierre Paul Broca's research resulted in the discovery that alterations in the left side of the brain could result in speech and language problems. Another researcher, Carl Wernicke, made further contributions to the field of LD, leading to the location of the auditory speech area in the left side of the brain. According to this research, a lesion in or damage to this area, leads to difficulties in comprehending speech, reading, and writing. Disorders in reading and writing began to be linked to the same problems that were associated with aphasia. In 1887, an ophthalmologist named Rudolf Berlin used the term dyslexia to describe persons who have difficulty reading in the absence of visual problems. In the early 1900s, a neuropathologist named Samuel Orton asserted that listening, speaking, reading, and writing are all related functions. He stated that problems with any of these functions could be related to deficits in neurological functioning and identified several syndromes, including developmental aphasia, auditory aphasia, agraphia, motor speech deficits, and stuttering (Smith et al., 1999), each of which deal with some aspect of listening, speaking, reading, or writing.

Smith et al.'s second proposed phase covers the early years of the LD movement, beginning with Samuel D. Kirk's use of the term *LD*. Many legislative changes and modifications in educational services provided to children with LD also occurred during this phase. Major legislative changes included PL 89-10, the Elementary and Secondary Education Act of 1965; the Rehabilitation Act of 1973, specifically Section 504; PL 94-142, the Education for All Handicapped Children Act of 1974; the Individuals with Disabilities Education Act (IDEA) in 1990; PL 101-336, the Americans with Disabilities Act (ADA), and the Individuals with Disabilities Education Improvement Act in 2004. Due to these legislative changes, children with LD can now receive better educational and support services.

The final phase discussed by Smith et al. (1999) is the modern phase. From the 1990s to the present, service delivery models have continued to evolve. In the past, services were more categorical in nature, in that children with LD were educated in self-contained classrooms with other children with LD. During the 1990s a shift occurred in favor of the inclusion model, which calls for more fully incorporating children with disabilities in general education classrooms. This movement, which Madeline Will termed the Regular Education Initiative, called for a blending of special and general education services for children with disabilities. Children with LD would therefore be educated in the least restrictive environment (LRE) possi-

ble through methods such as mainstreaming. Other issues that continue to emerge during this phase include: (a) resolution of the definition of LD; (b) more efficient methods of identifying individuals with LD; (c) new methods for intervention, including more effective early intervention (EI) techniques; and (d) better teacher training in the areas of mild to moderate disabilities as well as research into outcomes of these training techniques.

IQ-Achievement Discrepancy

Samuel Kirk's 1962 definition was the first to indicate that LD involves psychological process disorders, and other more recent ones hold that stance as well. Kirk also noted the influence of processing problems on academic performance, and the existence of central nervous system dysfunction. Kirk's definition served as the foundation for the development of later definitions.

Barbara Bateman offered another early definition in 1965 that described the frequently present discrepancy between a student's intellectual potential and his or her current performance in a learning environment. Bateman's definition was the first to cite underachievement as a necessary component of LD, identifying its relationship to learning. Although her definition is also the first to discuss discrepancy (often referred to as IQ [Intellectual Quotient]-achievement discrepancy or aptitude-achievement discrepancy), Bateman does not indicate the level of discrepancy required or the best way to measure intellectual potential. Although her definition was not widely accepted, the idea of significant discrepancy was utilized in many of the criteria for identifying LD prior to the reauthorization of IDEA 2004 (Büttner & Shamir, 2011; Kavale & Forness, 2000; NJCLD, 2011b; NJCLD, 2005).

Moving forward into the 1970s, regulatory and legislative definitions began to appear. The first such definition emerged from the United States Office of Education (USOE, 1976):

A specific LD may be found if a child has a severe discrepancy between achievement and intellectual ability in one or more of several areas: oral expression, written expression, listening comprehension or reading comprehension, basic reading skills, mathematics calculation, mathematics reasoning, or spelling. A "severe discrepancy" is defined to exist when achievement in one or more areas falls at or below 50% of the child's expected achievement level, when age and previous educational experiences are taken into consideration (p. 52405).

A large debate ensued following this publication over the idea of employing a mathematical formula to identify children with LD. Due to the high volume of criticism received, the USOE published another definition in 1977, which removed the discrepancy criteria and instead focused on the manifestation of "an imperfect ability to listen, speak, read, write, spell, or to do mathematical calculations," (U.S. Office of Education, 1977, 65083, as cited in Nelson, 2010, p. 137). As with Kirk's original definition, this one also included the inclusionary and exclusionary nature of LD.

In 1993 Hammill reviewed the various definitions published in many LD textbooks and found they generally shared several important elements. First the definitions referred to the notion that underachievement is necessary for identification of a LD. Second, the definitions described underachievement using the concepts of discrepancy between ability or achievement (Gregg & Scott, 2000). Although both of these components continue to play a role in the identification process, additional data from a student's responsiveness to instruction was eventually added as a key component.

Response to Intervention

With the implementation of the *Individuals with Disabilities Education Improvement Act (IDEA)* in 2004, an emerging method of identification and intervention for students with a suspected LD was cultivated. Although variations of this identification practice were used prior to this reauthorization, the inclusion of the term response to intervention (RTI) in the federal law solidified the practice as a method for both identification of LD as well as a form of intervention (Fuchs & Vaughn, 2012; Ikeda, 2012; USDOE, 2006). Fuchs and Vaughn (2012) add that RTI is currently a method of identification of LD in all 50 states, and that this multitiered approach is a driving force in the areas of research and future legislation and policy development across many disciplines. In addition, RTI programs are said to not only reduce the number of students referred for special education, but can also lessen the degree to which a disability impacts a child's academic performance (Denton, 2012). As outlined by NJCLD 2005, the three (3) core concepts of RTI are:

1. Application of scientific, research-based interventions in general education;

2. Measurement of student's response to these interventions;
3. Use of the RTI data to inform instruction.

Although not universal, the RTI approach is often depicted in a three-tiered pyramidal diagram, with the following commonalities:

Tier 1 (i.e., primary prevention): High quality instruction and behavioral supports are provided for all students in general education. Universal screening is implemented to identify students who are at risk for learning difficulties.

Tier 2 (i.e., secondary intervention/ prevention): Students whose performance and rate of progress lag behind those of their classroom, school, or district peers based on the universal screeings in Tier 1 receive more specialized prevention or remediation within general education.

Tier 3 (i.e., tertiary intervention/ prevention): Comprehensive evaluation is conducted by an interdisciplinary team to determine eligibility for special education and related services. If warranted, more intensive services are provided. (Denton, 2012; NJCLD, 2005)

In addition to these three tiers of prevention and intervention, the implementation of ongoing professional development for teachers is essential in order to ensure the use of high-quality instruction at all levels (Denton, 2012; NJCLD, 2008).

There is general consensus that RTI's greatest achievement to date is the implementation of universal screenings at Tier 1

to help identify students who are at risk for potential reading and mathematical difficulties (Graves, Brandon, Duesbery, McIntosh, & Pyle, 2011). Based on those identified as being at risk, the theory is that if given quality instruction and remedial services as part of the general education, those *without* an LD will progress appropriately (NJCLD, 2005). This process seemingly separates learners who may be struggling from factors such as poor prior instruction or lack of education opportunity, linguistic diversity, poverty, or emotional interferences from those students with a LD who need more concentrated and specialized instruction (NJCLD, 2005; NJCLD, 2011b). However it is represented, the NJCLD (2005) states that:

RTI is a critical component of a multi-tiered service delivery system. The goal of such a system is to ensure that quality instruction, good teaching practices, differentiated instruction, and remedial opportunities are available in general education, and that special education is provided for students with disabilities who require more specialized services than what can be provided in general education (p. 4).

Etiology

Defining LD continues to be a difficult task given the fact that these disorders do not share a common cause; however, the most prevalent consensus is that individuals with LD have biologically based cognitive deficits (Büttner & Hasselhorn, 2011). Within this understanding, LD falls into several categories based on the associated etiological factors. These categories include both environmental and genetic factors.

Environmental Factors

There are many prenatal, perinatal, and postnatal environmental factors that may be related to brain development and that could be considered causes of LD. These factors may directly produce the overall LD or may contribute to the disorder.

During prenatal development, deficits in maternal nutrition may affect brain development (Owens, 2010). Various organs and systems go through critical developmental stages during this period and are sensitive to teratogens, a variety of chemicals that alter many aspects of fetal development (Nelson, 2010). The central nervous system (CNS) is most sensitive during the third and sixth weeks of embryonic development, when the brain begins to develop. Substance abuse during the prenatal period is particularly detrimental. Fetal alcohol spectrum disorder (FASD), fetal cocaine exposure (FCE), and maternal smoking are three major causes of deficits in fetal development.

Fetal Alcohol Spectrum Disorder

The effects of alcohol abuse during pregnancy were first documented as a specific syndrome in the 1970s. During this decade, researchers began to note a pattern of congenital malformations and developmental disabilities in children of alcoholic mothers (fetal alcohol syndrome [FAS]) that includes central nervous system (CNS) dysfunction, cognitive impairments, growth retardation, facial malformations, learning problems, behavioral problems, socioemotional deficits, and symptoms of attention deficit disorder (distractibility, short attention span, hyperactivity) and executive dysfunction (Owens, 2010). Fetal alcohol effect (FAE) is a less severe form of FAS and is similar to FAS except that the child may display some but not all of the clinical features associated with FAS. More recent terms that relate to this less severe diagnosis include alcohol-related neurodevelopmental disorder (ARND) and alcohol-related birth defect. Current statistics regarding the prevalence of FASD, FAE, ARND and ARBD estimate that approximately 10 out of every 1,000 births (1%) have one of these diagnoses. A majority of children diagnosed on this spectrum will be diagnosed with having an LD and/or ADHD (Nelson, 2010; Owens, 2010).

Fetal Cocaine Exposure

It is estimated that 11% to 35% of expectant mothers consume one or more illegal drugs, crossing all boundaries of "race, ethnicity, age, socioeconomic status, and geographic location," (Owens, 2010, p. 40). Prenatal exposure to cocaine may lead to several complications, including intrauterine growth retardation (IUGR), which occurs when an unborn baby is at or below the 10th weight percentile for his or her age [in weeks], premature birth, microcephaly (small head circumference), and low birth weight. In addition, a pattern of intellectual and cognitive deficits exists, as do sensory deficits in hearing and sight, a compromised nervous system, and difficulties in school performance. In addition, the infant mortality rate with consumption of crack cocaine is double the rate when compared to other noncocaine drug-dependent pregnant women (Owens, 2010).

Maternal Smoking

In 1993, the National Institute of Mental Health (NIMH) documented that maternal smoking during pregnancy produces infants who have a lower birth weight, which may increase the risk of developmental disabilities such as LD. In addition, studies show that there is an increased risk for hyperactivity, impulsivity, and reduced attention span (Sowan & Stember, 2000).

Perinatal Factors

Perinatal factors are those that occur during the time of birth. Several studies showed that birth histories that include hard labor, prolonged labor, or a combination of the two, fetal distress, and/or anoxia may lead to problems in neurobehavioral development. In addition, Owens (2010) reported a higher rate of birth complications among children with LD in comparison with "typically developing" (TD) children.

Postnatal Factors

Postnatal causes of LD include head injuries, lead exposure, and diet. Head injuries, or traumatic brain injury as discussed in Chapter 6, produce deficits in learning that parallel the profile of an individual who has a LD. There are differences between the two disabilities, but certainly the trauma to the brain causes changes that affect learning, emotional, and behavioral characteristics and outcomes.

Children who are exposed to significant levels of lead may display a variety of clinical signs, including retardation, seizures, irritability, hyperactivity, LD, and gastrointestinal problems. Lead poisoning is caused by the ingestion of lead-based paint, which is generally found in older homes (1950 and older). The Centers for Disease Control (2014) estimates that approximately 4 million households in the

United States have children in them being exposed to lead. Studies evaluated the deciduous teeth shed by children exposed to lead, finding that higher levels of lead concentration in children produced clinical signs. More research is under way in order to document the effects of low-level lead exposure in children.

Other environmental factors that may contribute to impaired neurological development generally involve the home environment and childrearing practices, a lack of structure and/or organization at home, a lack of parenting preparation or readiness (as is the case in teen pregnancy), cognitive limitations of parents, limited mother-child bonding, and lack of stimulation (Nelson, 2010; Owens, 2010). It is difficult to isolate the effects of these factors, which can work in combination with a biological predisposition to LD. Nevertheless, these factors are critical to development and should not be ignored.

Genetic Factors

Currently there are many research studies that strongly support the basis for genetic factors in some forms of LD (e.g., deficits in reading, spelling, and writing), including family studies, twin studies, and multiple regression studies using twins. Each investigation showed that reading disabilities run in families and are inherited at a rate of 50% (Owens, 2010).

Severe reading disability, or dyslexia, is characterized by an inability to identify words due to deficits in phonological skills in individuals who have no clear neurological, emotional, or intellectual problems. Recent studies show evidence of a biological basis of dyslexia through complex brain imaging, a promising indicator for future diagnosis and intervention with this population. Most recently, the DCDC2 gene has been isolated as a possible link to dyslexia; however, it is unlikely that one gene accounts solely for dyslexia, but rather several chromosomes contributing to this disorder (Nelson, 2010; Owens, 2010). More research continues to be conducted in order to isolate the component processes of reading.

In addition to a genetic predisposition to LD, many chromosomal disorders are associated with learning deficits, including Turner syndrome, Klinefelter syndrome, and fragile X syndrome (particularly in females, who carry the gene for this condition). Single-gene disorders associated with LD include neurofibromatosis, achondroplasia, and phenylketonuria.

Characteristics of LD

Numerous problems can be related to the lack of basic skills necessary for successful academic achievement in students with LD, including:

1. Phonological awareness of sounds
2. Memorization of sound-symbol association
3. Speed of pronouncing words for reading
4. Comprehension of sentences and paragraphs
5. Memory for reading
6. Summarization of information that was read
7. Spelling difficulties related to remembering letters and sounds
8. Visualization of words for spelling
9. Application of spelling rules consistently for words and in written narratives
10. Fine motor coordination for handwriting
11. Writing mechanics (punctuation, spelling, grammar)
12. Organization of written narratives
13. Conceptual knowledge of math
14. Memory for operations and order of operations for math
15. Comprehension of the "language" of mathematics
16. Utilization of problem-solving skills
17. Translation of mathematical concepts into word problems
18. Practical application of mathematical knowledge to the real world

The psychological processes involved in LD can be auditory-verbal, visual-motor, and/or perceptual. Auditory-verbal process deficits result in reading disorders and other language-based LD. Visual-motor and perceptual process deficits may result in reading problems, but more than likely will affect handwriting and mathematics (Goldstein & Reynolds, 1999).

Children whose difficulties relate primarily to visual-motor skills but that are independent of a reading disability (e.g., a nonlanguage-based LD) are identified in neuropsychology as having a "nonverbal LD" (NLD) (Rourke, 1989, as cited in Volden, 2004). Several descriptions of this disorder state that it is a right-hemisphere disorder, possibly due to damage, disorder, or destruction of white matter in this hemisphere (Casey, 2012; Rissman, 2010). As cited in Volden (2004), these children have problems with "(a) visual and tactile perception, (b) complex psychomotor skills, and (c) dealing with novel material" (p. 128). Deficits are seen in processing complex tactile information, gross and fine motor coordination, nonverbal problem-solving, understanding the more complex aspects of verbal material, using social skills, spatial organization, mathematics, handwriting, memory for facts, attention to detail, and judgment and reasoning. In addition, these students are more likely to have problems related to depression and anxiety (Casey, 2012).

Children who have difficulty in a variety of language areas, including reading, have a language-based LD. Although the term language learning disability is not universally accepted, the number of students demonstrating a LD concomitantly with communication disorders is on the rise (Paul & Norbury, 2012; Washburn et al., 2012).

Language Learning Disability

The boundaries of communication disorders and LD often overlap, making it difficult to determine the individual effects of each disorder versus their combined impact. Many researchers report that language impairments and LD are one and the same problem observed at different times throughout the life cycle. The diagnosis of LD can be made during a child's preschool experience; however, it is one that is predominantly diagnosed during the school-aged years when children begin to struggle with academic tasks (Nelson, 2010). There are some children who have a documented history of early language difficulties, both receptive and expressive; however, this does not apply to every person diagnosed with an LD. As stated by Paul and Norbury (2012), "not all LDs are language-based. A child could have a specific learning problem in, say, mathematics or graphomotor skills that might not be based on a language

weakness," (p. 399). As a result, the term language-learning disability (LLD) refers to those individuals whose primary LD affect both spoken and written language, including reading, writing, and spelling, with the majority of these students experiencing deficits in reading (Denton, 2012; Nelson, 2010; Owens, 2010; Paul & Norbury, 2012).

The influence that language development has on future learning is significant. In younger children, parents or family members quickly realize there are language-based problems when children have difficulty expressing their wants and needs. As the children age and go to school, academic needs become the main issue. According to some researchers (Carrow-Woolfolk & Lynch, 1982; Watson Gable, Gear, & Hughes, 2012), once the child enters school, language-based problems will affect performance in the school setting and will consequently be recognized as an LD. The use of terminology such as LLD often suggests the existence of one specific disability rather than two distinctly different disorders that coexist. This confusion in terminology reflects the earlier difficulty in defining LD and language disorders. Nevertheless, the "accepted" definitions for both terms clearly reflect the similarities and differences between the two. Paul and Norbury (2012) state that of the students diagnosed with LD, approximately 75% of them have deficits in reading, a skill that pulls on the "strong foundation of oral language abilities" (p. 399).

The 1991 NJCLD definition stated that LD is manifested by significant difficulties in listening, speaking, reading, writing, reasoning, mathematics, or social skills. There is obvious overlap in the area of language, as listening, speaking, reading, and writing comprise language as a whole. In addition, social skills fall under the realm of pragmatic language. Language also has a role to play in mathematics.

In 1990, the American Speech-Language-Hearing Association (ASHA) published the following definition:

> Specific LD means a disorder in one or more of the basic psychological processes involved in understanding or in using language, spoken or written, which may manifest itself in an imperfect ability to listen, think, speak, read, write, spell, or to do mathematical calculations. The term includes such conditions as perceptual handicaps, brain injury, minimal brain dysfunction, dyslexia, and developmental aphasia. The term does not include children who have learning problems that are primarily the result of visual, hearing or motor handicaps, of mental retardation, or emotional disturbance, or of environmental, cultural or economic disadvantage. (pp. 55–56).

In addition to this definition, which strongly parallels that of the NJCLD, ASHA (1993) stated that a language disorder is characterized by diminished understanding and/or use of spoken, written and/or other symbol systems. It is difficult to determine the exact prevalence rates of LD because, as Owens (2010) states, "they are associated with varied views on the identification and diagnosis of LD and are limited by the state of current scientific evidence" (p. 137). Despite these unknowns, current estimates from the National Center for Education Statistics (NCES) state that of the 13% of all school-aged children receiving special education (more than 2.5 to 2.8 million children), approximately 50% of them fall within the classification of LD, and

80% of them receive services for reading (Owens, 2010; Washburn et al., 2011). Estimates of co-occurrence between the LD and a language disorder range from 35% to 60%, with language disorder syndrome as the primary presenting syndrome among children and adolescents with LD. A recent study by Foster and Miller (2007) found a direct correlation in their school district from 2000 to 2003 in that of all of the students during this time period diagnosed with a LD, 52% of them had a previous diagnosis of a speech-language impairment. A review of individual state definitions of LD revealed that 48 of the states incorporate language disorders into their definitions of learning disabilities and into their criteria for service delivery (Mercer, King-Sears, & Mercer, 1990; nichcy.org).

Wallach and Butler (1994) offer additional research to support the overlap. The authors undertook a study of adolescents with LD and identified three major patterns in language and learning disorders: (a) significant language disorders exist at an early age; (b) the teen has a history of academic difficulty; and (c) language-related academic problems did not appear until adolescence. In 1984, Wiig and Semel concluded that language disorders change over time and during the school years frequently manifest as learning problems in reading, writing, and spelling. Despite all the reported overlap, not all students with LD have language disorders because this group is highly heterogeneous (Schoenbrodt, Kumin, & Sloan, 1997).

Characteristics

In 1978, Bloom and Lahey described language as a code whereby ideas about the world are represented through a conventional system of arbitrary symbols used for communication. This model included three major components: (a) form, which includes phonology, morphology, and syntax; (b) content, also known as semantics; and (c) use, also known as pragmatics.

Many researchers have described numerous characteristics of this population. In general, investigators note difficulties in basic vocabulary and information processing, as well as problems in cognition, comprehension and production of linguistic features, narrative and conversational discourse, nonverbal communication, and survival language. In addition, Paul and Norbury (2012) state that the majority of students identified as having a LLD have "underlying weaknesses in their oral language bases . . . and often have histories of delayed speech and/or language development" (p. 399). When a child's reading abilities are impacted, there are often reports of delayed acquisition of phonological skills, including difficulties with perception and production of complex phonemic configurations, and difficulty in phonological awareness (Nelson, 2010; Paul & Norbury, 2012).

According to a Technical Report by the NJCLD (2007), the characteristics of younger children with language disorders often include the following: (a) limited receptive and expressive vocabulary, often described as "late talkers;" (b) difficulty understanding simple directions; (c) monotone or other unusual prosodic features of speech; (d) reduced intelligibility; (e) infrequent or inappropriate spontaneous communication; and (f) immature syntax. Moyle, Stokes, and Klee (2011) divide a child's language development into three subgroups: phonology/articulation, semantics/syntax, and pragmatics, adding that a prominent indication of language impairment is the late onset of talking which is present in 10% to 20% of children. Sawyer (1985) reported the following characteristics in school-age children with LLD: word-finding difficulties, limited spontaneous speech, use of immature grammatical forms, difficulty untangling relationships in complex sentences, and trouble remembering and repeating information presented orally. In academic tasks, children demonstrated difficulty with spelling and decoding as well as comprehension in reading in the early grades. The characteristics noted 29 years ago still hold true today. Newer research has noted that school-age children with LLD have difficulty transitioning from the basic language skills including vocabulary development, sentence structure and use of language, to the more complex, higher levels of language expectations. As a result, these students struggle with the language demands necessary to be successful in academic settings. Both the younger child and the school-age child with LLD demonstrate greater difficulty with communication tasks associated with daily living activities. These children frequently have problems with pragmatic and social skills, which may become more apparent during school years (Paul & Norbury, 2012).

The characteristics of adolescents with LLD revolve around the social demands of language, as well as the increasing curricular demands and teacher expectations. At this level, students are in what Paul and Norbury (2012) refer to as the *advanced language developmental stage*. If diagnosed with LLD, these adolescents may experience difficulty processing and using complex language, elaborating the meanings of familiar words, processing and recalling critical information, retrieving words, making inferences, and comprehending basic classroom vocabulary and concepts.

In addition, they demonstrated a reduced ability to organize their thoughts prior to oral output and to engage in flexible thinking. The researchers also reported impairments in auditory memory, comprehension, and attention (Srivastava & Gray, 2012).

Teachers report that in the classroom, students with LLD have more difficulty interacting appropriately with their peers, particularly with comprehending and participating in adolescent banter (Gerber & Bryan, 1981; Mathinos, 1988; Rice, Sell, & Hadley, 1990; Watson et al., 2012). Watson et al. (2012) went on to conclude that when students with LLD are less adept at conversational skills, opportunities for social communicative interactions are lessened, which decreases the opportunity for practice and often leads to these students being rejected by their peers and socially isolated. This, in turn, creates problems with fitting in and acceptance, the quest for which is the hallmark of the adolescent years.

The connections between spoken and written language are clear. The 2001 Position Statement from the American Speech-Language-Hearing Association regarding the roles and responsibilities of speech-language pathologists with respect to reading and writing in children and adolescents supports this connection. According to this Position Statement, the connections between spoken and written language are well established in that (a) spoken language provides the foundation for the development of reading and writing; (b) spoken and written language have a reciprocal relationship, such that each builds on the other to result in general language and literacy competence, starting early and continuing through childhood into adulthood; (c) children with spoken language problems frequently have difficulty learning to read and write, and children with reading and writing problems frequently have difficulty with spoken language; and d) instruction in spoken language can result in growth in written language, and instruction in written language can result in growth in spoken language (Position Statement, Guidelines, p. 17).

Four conclusions emerge from the literature on literacy in nondisabled children: (a) the process of learning to read and write is a continuum that begins at birth; (b) reading, writing, speaking, and listening develop concurrently and interrelatedly and not sequentially; (c) the functions of literacy are as integral to literacy learning as the forms (i.e., phonology, morphology and syntax); and (d) children learn written language through active engagement in their world. With the clear connection between language development and literacy achievement, SLPs are playing a more active role in the development of literacy acquisition.

The above statement defines reading as the processes one uses to construct meaning from printed symbols. Reading can be divided into two areas: decoding and comprehension. Decoding incorporates word recognition processes that transform print into words. Comprehension involves the processes for understanding and interpreting language, where the development of meaning can occur at the word, sentence, and discourse levels. According to Allen, Ukrainetz, and Carswell (2012), a reciprocal relationship exists between decoding and comprehension. In other words, decoding without comprehension is not reading, and comprehension without decoding is not reading. In order for the reader to recognize written words, the reader uses lexical knowledge acquired during early language development. The National Research Council stated that children learn to read successfully when the following conditions occur (Snow, Burns, & Griffin, 1998, as cited in Washburn et al., 2011):

- Have normal or above average language skills;
- Have had experience in childhood that fostered motivation and provided exposure to literacy in use;
- Are given information about the nature of print via opportunities to learn letters and to recognize the sublexical structure of spoken words (i.e., phonology and morphology), as well as about the contrasting nature of spoken and written language; and
- Attend schools that provide coherent reading instruction and opportunities to practice (p. 165).

Difficulty learning to read and write may involve many of the components of language, including phonology, morphology, syntax, semantics, and pragmatics. In fact, the comprehension of spoken language provides the core for the development of reading comprehension and plays an essential role in academic success. Paul and Norbury (2012) use Chall's Stages of Reading Development to illustrate the progression (p. 412), which can be found in Table 2–2.

Chall's Stage 0 refers to "literacy socialization" or emergent literacy when children, through experience and exposure to literacy activities, learn that speech is a connection of individual sounds and that words often share some of these sounds, as in rhyming. During Chall's Stage 1 the focus is on phonics skills development where children are required to connect the sounds to printed letters and begin decoding (i.e., letter–sound identification, phoneme–grapheme identification). As a child progresses into Stage 2, his or her fluency and automaticity increase. Children learn to recognize words by sight,

Table 2–2. Jeanne Chall's Stages of Reading Development

Stage	Grade Level	Achievements
Stage 0: Prereading	Pre-K	Literacy socialization
Stage 1: Decoding	1–2	Phonological analysis and segmentation/synthesis in single words
Stage 2: Automaticity	2–4	Fluent reading; greater resources for comprehension available
Stage 3: Reading to Learn	4–8	More complex comprehension, increased rate
Stage 4: Reading for Ideas	8–12	Recognition of differing points of view, use of inferencing
Stage 5: Critical Reading	College	Synthesis of new knowledge, critical thinking

Source: "Language Disorders from Infancy through Adolescence," Rhea Paul, page 449, Copyright Elsevier 2007. Reprinted with permission.

which alleviates the need to decode familiar and reoccurring words. As a result of the decreased efforts needed for decoding, the emphasis on comprehension increases (Foster & Miller, 2007). As stated by Paul and Norbury (2012), "Stage 3 . . . marks a major change in the child's reading ability. Now instead of learning to read, the child is reading to learn" (p. 413). The effects of literacy learning problems at any age, therefore, are negative and long-lasting. Children who experience problems in literacy in early years may remain poor readers and writers throughout their school years, often reading slowly and/or inaccurately and lagging behind their peers. Of students who show reading difficulties in third grade, 74% of them will continue to display them in sixth grade, and if left untreated, can persist into adolescence and beyond (Graves et al., 2011; Seifert & Espin, 2012; Wankoff, 2011). In addition, these children are less likely to be accepted by their peers in school, and may be limited in vocational options as they get older (Foster & Miller, 2007; Washburn et al., 2011; Watson et al., 2012).

As indicated in the above discussion, children learn to read by progressing through a series of developmental stages. Frith's (1985) five-stage model illustrates this progression in a similar manner to Chall's, but with different labels. The first stage is referred to as the logographic stage, in which children associate spoken words with visual stimuli such as the first letter of each word. In the second stage, known as the transition stage, children use some letter-sound cues in order to recognize words. It is during this stage that children begin to develop sight-word vocabulary for frequently used words. During the alphabetic stage, children learn to use letter-sound relationships in order to decode words. Children next

begin to analyze words into units without phonological conversion, known as the orthographic stage. By the final stage, automatic word recognition, children have mastered the earlier stages in order to read words. Children who have difficulty in acquiring accurate and fluent word-identification skills may have the central deficit in a specific reading disability known as dyslexia. Based on the above stages, reading requires a foundation in "the language processes of holding phonological representations in memory, separating and manipulating phonemes, and retrieving the meaning attached to a phonological representation" (Adams, 1990, as cited in Allen, Ukrainetz, & Carswell, 2012, 206).

Reading comprehension also involves a developmental process rooted in listening comprehension and a wide range of other language skills that begins in preschool and progresses throughout the life span. As preschoolers, children are exposed to narrative and expository texts and learn to identify relevant and irrelevant information. They must then combine the identified words together to delineate meaning (Allen et al., 2012; Watson et al., 2012). It has been defined as "the process that excerpts and, at the same time, creates meaning by having the student interact and be involved with written language," (Shanahan et al., 2010, as cited in Watson et al., 2012, p. 79). With reading comprehension, students learn to question and respond to information that is read to them at home and at school.

During the elementary school grades, children refine their self-monitoring skills as they expand their knowledge for different types of text structures. They begin to develop skills for reading higher-level texts in a variety of styles and genres that are more linguistically complex. From the upper elementary grades through adolescence and into early adulthood, students are expected to read lengthy material as part of the curriculum. Much of this material contains abstract and unfamiliar language. The skilled reader needs to self-monitor comprehension and rely on metacognitive skills in order to develop strategies to facilitate comprehension. Watson et al. (2012) stated that the essential skills for reading comprehension are as follows: (1) working memory capacity and other executive processes; (2) prior knowledge; (3) motivation; (4) vocabulary; (5) text coherence; and (6) text structure (p. 80).

Like reading, writing is a developmental process that starts when children realize that they are "drawing" speech when representing objects, places, and ideas. These two processes, reading and writing, rely on an alphabetic code where a symbol has a somewhat direct correlation with a phoneme. The ability to both decode (break down) and encode (spell) words therefore relies heavily on an individual's phonological awareness skills, or the ability to understand and manipulate the various sound structures in words (Paul & Norbury, 2012; Vandewalle, Boets, Ghesquière, & Zink, 2012).

In the early elementary years, children write sentences that mimic the length of their own utterances. Early writing is ungrammatical and contains numerous spelling errors. By the time children reach the later elementary grades, their sentences exceed their spoken utterances and have become more grammatically correct. The writing process is complex, requiring the mastery of a variety of skills, including generation of ideas, planning and organization (executive function skills), editing and revising, and self-feedback (Owens, 2010, 2012). In addi-

tion, Koutsoftas and Gray (2012) state that typically developing writers show competence in the following areas: productivity, lexical diversity, grammaticality, sentence complexity, spelling accuracy, and story grammar (content). The process of revising drafts and proofreading the product continues to develop and is further refined during the secondary and postsecondary years.

In order to be a good writer, the child needs to be fluent in spelling. Owens (2012) states that young spellers practice what is often referred to as "invented spelling" where the names of letters are used when spelling, (e.g., writing "*SKP*" for *escape,* or "*LFT*" for *elephant*), similar to Frith's second developmental stage of reading. This method transitions into Frith's third developmental stage or phonemic spelling, where children have a stronger awareness of the phoneme-grapheme relationship (Owens, 2012).

In addition to phonological awareness, students also develop morphological awareness, the ability to recognize and break words down into individual morphemes, both bound and free (affixes, roots, base words, and derivatives). As stated by Kirk and Gillon (2009), "recent findings suggest that by 10 years of age, knowledge about the structure of words is a better predictor of decoding ability than is phonological awareness" (p. 341). Results from previous studies indicate that a student's performance on a measure of morphological awareness is a significant predictor of literacy acquisition and has an essential role in both word decoding and reading comprehension (Apel, Diehm, & Apel, 2013; Kirby et al., 2012). Strong morphological awareness skills expand on basic phonics skills and aid in both decoding and comprehension, as students are able to see the relationship between *rereading* and *read*, and *uncompli-cated* and *complicate* (Washburn et al., 2011).

Given the information concerning literacy, it is evident that spelling problems in this area can be related to spoken-language difficulties. Therefore, young children who demonstrate specific language impairments (SLI), "a language impairment in the absence of significant sensory, psychiatric, neurological, or intellectual impairment/disorder," may encounter difficulties in the development of literacy as well (Moyle et al., 2011, p. 160). Many longitudinal studies support this notion. Vandewalle et al. (2012), Kamhi and Catts (1989), and Wagner and Torgesen (1987) reported that reading disabilities are language-based disorders that can be identified long before children begin reading. Moyle et al. (2011) suggest that an SLI may be evident much earlier than the age is it typically diagnosed, around 4 to 5 years of age. Several symptomatic problems may appear, including expressive morphology, syntax, understanding words and sentences, and understanding what is read. In addition, written language is "highly decontextualized and its comprehension relies heavily on a well-developed vocabulary and clear understanding of the structural components and rules of language" (Kamhi & Catts, 1989, p. 86).

Although some LD children may not exhibit the above difficulties, they may have trouble with phonological processing, such as a lack of awareness of speech sounds in words, difficulty with word retrieval, verbal short-term memory, and speech production (Badian, McAnulty, Duffy, & Als, 1990; Torgesen, 1986; Vandewalle et al., 2012). Research has documented a relationship between phonological awareness and reading: phonological awareness develops prior to and influ-ences reading acquisition. Deficits in this area are highly associated with reading deficits and, in turn, intervention focusing on phonological awareness improves decoding skills (Paul & Norbury, 2012).

Based on the definitions and characteristics presented, there is an obvious overlap between language disorders and LD. This is not to say that all children with LD will evidence language disorders, or that all students with language disorders will eventually be defined as learning disabled. The child diagnosed with LD alone is likely to encounter difficulty in academic settings, whereas the child with both a language disorder and LD will struggle in social situations as well. Because both disabilities can be present in the same individual, assessment and intervention must imperatively surpass the traditional boundaries. Documenting both disorders requires multiple models for assessment and intervention, as well as collaboration with an interdisciplinary team.

Assessment

There are general assessment guidelines regardless of age. The first one is to understand that assessment is a process that includes more than simply administration of a test. For the students with a suspected LLD, it is essential to complete a dynamic assessment in which an examiner uses time to determine both strengths and weaknesses in the student, along with strategies that may help improve the student's performance. The type of information gained from this assessment will be the driving force in planning a course of intervention, if needed. Another guideline is that assessment should be naturalistic, a component discussed in the following sections. An additional guideline is that assessment should be interdisciplinary. In order to identify cognitive strengths and weaknesses and establish baseline behavior, the student with a suspected language disorder and LD should undergo an in-depth interdisciplinary evaluation. The assessment team should consist of in-dividuals with the skills, training, and qualifications to use the diagnostic tools. At the minimum, the speech-language pathologist (SLP), special and general education teachers, and the psychologist should be involved as part of the diagnostic team. Other specialists, such as the occupational therapist, may be called in for evaluation if the child demonstrates a specific problem in a particular area (e.g., speed and formation of letters for handwriting). Parents also play an important role on the assessment team, as they can provide critical information regarding the student's functioning in the home and community environments. Eligibility for educational services depends on the outcome of norm-referenced assessments and naturalistic assessments and on the student's ability to use language function appropriately in the academic setting (NJCLD, 2007).

Historically, professionals relied on a student's IQ-achievement (or ability-achievement) discrepancy as a basis for diagnosing a LD. Although this measure is still used for both research and diagnostic purposes, the debate regarding both the validity and reliability of its use continues (Maehler & Schuchardt, 2011). Sparks and Lovett (2009) summarize reports that criticize the sole use of IQ-achievement discrepancy scores stating several limitations to the use of these. They explain that (1) the discrepancy scores obtained are often less reliable than the tests used; (2) the IQ-achievement

discrepancy displayed by poor readers is not predictive of their responsiveness to remediation; (3) cognitive skills profiles suggest common etiologic factors and show no qualitative differences; and (4) cognitive deficits often found in LD may actually lower scores from a standard IQ test. Although IQ scores remain a component of the criteria needed to diagnose this disorder, the NJCLD (2007) determined that it should not be the *sole* basis for a diagnosis. Cahan, Fono, and Nirel (2012) add that relying heavily on this "regression-based discrepancy" often results in "overidentification of learning disabilities among individuals with high IQ scores and underidentification of learning disabilities among individuals with low IQ scores" (p. 170). Under the Individuals with Disabilities Act (2006), local education agencies (LEAs) are now able to use response to intervention as an essential component in the identification of students with a LD (Allen, Ukrainetz, & Carswell, 2012; Graves et al., 2011; Sparks & Lovett, 2009). Similarly, a diagnosis of LLD should be assigned with more than discrepancy testing. In order to determine eligibility for school-based services, standardized testing is necessary in most states.

Norm-Referenced Assessments

When discrepancy scores are used to determine eligibility for services for the student with both a language disorder and a LD, there are three common eligibility criteria: cutoff scores; a discrepancy criterion; and a clinical diagnostic model (Gregg & Scott, 2000). The sole use of discrepancy criteria to identify students with language disabilities and LD excludes many students who have difficulty with pragmatics, auditory processing, and executive function (problem-solving/ organizational abilities) and therefore should not be the sole basis for diagnosis (Allen et al., 2012; NJCLD, 2011b; Sparks & Lovett, 2009).

Standardized or formal evaluation is necessary to document comparable scores and eligibility for educational and support services for the student with both language disorders and LD. In addition to having good reliability and validity, a formal assessment battery should evaluate functioning in the following areas: intelligence, problem solving, attention, concentration, memory, receptive and expressive vocabulary, listening comprehension, auditory processing, and academic ability, including performance using language (speaking, listening, reading, and writing).

Equally as important as choosing the assessment tool is determining the appropriate derived score to be reported. The most frequently reported derived scores are age-equivalent scores, percentile ranks, and standard scores. Standard scores are considered the most accurate of the three as well as the most meaningful way to compare the score of the test taker to that obtained by a normative sample (Anastasiow, 1986; Haynes & Pindzola, 2012). The best method of reporting performance uses the standard error of measurement (SEM), which provides a confidence range of performance within which the true score falls, instead of assigning one specific value to test performance. Unfortunately, not all assessment manuals report the standard error of measurement.

In terms of assessment, the examiner should evaluate the student not only for his or her best performance, but also for performance as compared to peers when placed under the pressure of envi-

ronmental constraints, such as a timed test (Haynes & Pindzola, 2012; Lahey & Bloom, 1994). In any event, some modifications to the testing may be necessary in order to obtain important information about the student's level of language functioning. While the examiner must adhere to the instructions and time constraints outlined in the standardized assessment to ensure reliability, validity, and performance under stress, information obtained with modifications is invaluable. The student's abilities may be misinterpreted or, worse, missed altogether, if some modifications cannot be made.

Naturalistic Assessment

Norm-referenced tests are often necessary in order to determine eligibility for services and often provide important data regarding overall language performance. However, there are many reasons for not relying completely on this type of assessment alone. According to Launer (1994), norm-referenced tests (a) do not reflect actual communicative abilities, including pragmatics or language usage; (b) tap very specific skills with very specific methods; (c) produce anxiety and do not elicit realistic or optimal performance; (d) are not interactive, in that the student is in a position only to respond and not to initiate; (e) do not usually allow for creativity of response or flexibility in scoring and interpretation; (f) do not reflect language and communication in the classroom; and (g) are frequently culturally biased and do not reflect the diversity of cultures in the clinical population.

In order to counter these deficiencies, an in-depth assessment, which should also include an informal or naturalistic assessment, can provide important information regarding the language functioning of a student with language learning disability —information that may not be tapped by the norm-referenced assessment. Naturalistic assessments can take many forms, such as observation of performance through interviews, questionnaires, performance rating scales, behavioral observations, task analyses (in the form of narrative analysis or language samples), curriculum-based assessment (CBA), and ethnographic assessment (Haynes & Pindzola, 2012; Paul & Norbury, 2012). The student should be observed in a variety of settings and contexts that sample the type of environmental factors that exist in the natural setting, including the gymnasium, cafeteria, playground, classroom, and home. An observation of the student in the cafeteria, for example, may yield information regarding his or her ability to process information in a noisy environment, communicative competence with peers, ability to communicate under time constraints, word-finding difficulties, problem-solving abilities, and so forth. This type of invaluable information is not captured by a norm-referenced assessment. An informal evaluation can be descriptive, as it allows for a description of the student's communication patterns. Some informal assessment tools include:

1. Task analysis: According to Sohlberg and Mateer (1989), task analysis relies on four basic principles: (a) identification of the task parameters before the student completes the task; (b) evaluation of environmental factors, including the actual environment, and people, including teachers, peers, parents, and so on; (c) identification of the measurement criteria in a qualitative and quantitative manner; and (d) identification of the levels of cueing and compensatory strategies needed to complete the task.

2. Narrative assessment: A minimum of four samples should be collected from the student in the following areas: a personal-experience narrative, a television or movie program narrative, a book summary narrative, and a fictional story narrative. The samples should then be analyzed for style and story grammar development. Story grammar analysis determines if the narrative is a focused chain or a true narrative and answers questions such as: Is a setting given? Are the characters described? Is a goal presented? Narrative assessment evaluates true narrative by answering questions such as: Is the narrative grammatical? Is one topic presented? Is the vocabulary precise? and so forth (Hutson-Nechkash, 1990; Nelson, 2010; Westby, 1984).

3. Curriculum-based language assessment (CBLA): CBLA starts with the identification of curricular contexts in which language-related problems exist, and uses those contexts to develop assessments and interventions. CBLA assesses the types of language skills and strategies the student with a LD employs to process the language of the curriculum, the types of resources he or she uses to meet the demands of the curriculum, the additional abilities and strategies the student might need to make processing more effective and efficient, and the changes that could be made in the curriculum or its presentation to make it more accessible to the student (Nelson, 2010). In the CBLA process, the following should occur: (a) schoolwork

should be reviewed as a final product; (b) the student should be observed over several contexts or situations at various times of the day; and (c) once problem areas are identified, the student should be interviewed to obtain samples of expository and narrative discourse.

4. Portfolio assessment: This assessment approach involves collecting and retaining nonrandom samples of information over a period of time. The content of these samples should be identified so as to provide assessment data related to the goals of intervention. Examples of items to include are: narrative discourse samples, writing samples, student comments regarding assignments, samples of tests (essay writing), and observations of student behavior in terms of processing information (Paul & Norbury, 2012).

Naturalistic assessments provide the most functional information and depict the student's communicative abilities in the school environment. In terms of intervention, it makes sense to assess the areas in the school setting that are the most troublesome to the student with language LD. The information obtained from the entire assessment should be used not only to determine eligibility of services, but also to provide a basis for the formulation of functional and meaningful goals and objectives for the student (Schoenbrodt, Kumin, & Sloan, 1997).

Assessment in Young Children

Following the RTI framework, a significant emphasis with this population is the identification of young children (birth–3 years of age) who may be at risk for language and learning difficulties following Bloom and Lahey's content, form and use structure. As stated in Paul and Roth (2011), a young child's early language development, particularly receptive language development, continues to be a strong predictor of later language development. In other words, young children who struggle with language development continue to struggle, while those who meet language developmental milestones within normal limits continue progress without interferences. It is still difficult to delineate children who will "outgrow" their developmental delays versus those whose problems will persist throughout their life span. Because of this, the NJCLD (2007) developed a list of risk indicators and protective factors that need to be a considered with this population. Following is a comprehensive list of these essential components. Although one instance from the following list does not automatically correlate with a delay or disorder, the combination and/or existence of several risk factors requires SLPs and other professionals to monitor the child's development over time. Paul and Roth (2011) state that "In general, the greater the number of risk factors, the greater the developmental risk to the child" (p. 332). In addition, the presence of protective factors does not indicate that a disability is not/cannot be present.

Risk Indicators

- Perinatal conditions
  - Low Apgar scores
  - Low birth weight and/or preterm birth
  - Hospitalization for longer than 24 hours in a neonatal intensive care unit (NICU)

- Difficulty with sucking, sucking, and swallowing
- Chronic otitis media that may result in intermittent hearing loss
- Genetic or environmental conditions
  - Family history of LD
  - Adopted child status
  - Family history of spoken and/or written language problems
  - Exposure to environmental toxins or other harmful substances
  - Limiting language exposure in home, childcare, and other settings
  - Poverty
- Developmental milestones
  - Delay in cognitive skills
    - Not demonstrating object permanence
    - Limited understanding of means-ends relationship (e.g., using a stool to reach a cooking jar
    - Lack of symbolic play behavior
  - Delay in comprehension and/or expression of spoken language
  - Limited receptive vocabulary
  - Reduced expressive vocabulary
  - Difficulty understanding simple directions (e.g., one-step)
  - Monotone or other unusual prosodic features of speech
  - Reduced intelligibility
  - Infrequent or inappropriate spontaneous communication (vocal, verbal, or nonverbal)
  - Immature syntax
- Delay in emergent literacy skills
  - Slow speed for naming objects and colors
  - Limited phonological awareness (e.g., rhyming, syllable blending)
  - Minimal interest in print

- Limited print awareness (e.g., book handling, recognizing environmental print)
- Delay in perceptual-motor skills
  - Problems in gross or fine motor coordination (e.g., hopping, dressing, cutting, stringing beads)
  - Difficulty coloring, copying, and drawing
- Attention and behavior
  - Distractibility
  - Impulsivity
  - Hyperactivity
  - Difficulty changing activities or handling disruptions to routines
  - Perseveration (i.e., constant repetition of an idea)

Protective Factors

- Access to quality pre-, peri-, and postnatal care
- Maternal education
- High-quality learning opportunities
  - Exposure to rich and varied vocabulary, syntax, and discourse patterns
  - Responsive learning environments sensitive to all cultural and linguistic backgrounds
  - Access to printed materials
  - Involvement in structured and unstructured individual/group play interactions and conversations
  - Engagement in gross and fine motor activities
- Multiple supports
  - Assistance adapted to the child's responsiveness to instruction or intervention
  - Access to adaptive and assistive technology (AT) services

■ Transition planning between early intervention (EI) services (birth to age 3 years) and preschool programs (ages 3–5 years), and between preschool and elementary school
■ Service coordination

When the above elements are present in a young child's development, SLPs, in conjunction with other professionals (e.g., special educators, social workers, psychologists, occupational and physical therapists), need to complete the following:

■ Screening
■ Examination for the presence of risk indicators and protective factors
■ Systematic observations
■ Naturalistic
■ Thorough case history, including birth and developmental information
■ Language sample; MLU analysis
■ Comprehensive evaluation, if needed

Assessment in School-Aged Students
(Haynes & Pindzola, 2012; NJCLD, 2008; Paul & Norbury, 2012)

As with the young child population, the goal of assessment with the school-age population is to develop a comprehensive representation of a student's strengths and weaknesses, as well as a variety of strategies and supports available to address language, learning, and behavioral difficulties. At all developmental levels, assessments should be "individualized to address questions of concern related to the student's cognitive, academic, social, behavioral, motivational, and/or emo-

tional needs" (NJCLD, 2008, p. 9). Components of the assessment include the following:

■ Screening of speech and language skills
■ Screening of literacy development, including phonological awareness skills
■ Thorough case history; early developmental information
■ Examination of early risk factors and protective factors
■ CBLA
■ Portfolio assessment
■ Observations in multiple settings
■ Narrative and discourse analysis
■ Comprehensive evaluation, if needed
■ Academic progression
■ Interviews with teachers
■ Spelling/written language sample
■ Pragmatic language analysis

Assessment With Older Students
(Haynes & Pindzola, 2012; NJCLD, 2008; Paul & Norbury, 2012)

■ Student-centered assessment tied directly to educational planning
■ Thorough case history; early developmental information
■ CBLA
■ Portfolio
■ Observation
■ Narrative and discourse analysis
■ Comprehensive evaluation, if needed
■ Academic information/progression
■ Written language sample
■ Higher-level language skills
  ■ Inferencing, idioms, figurative language
■ Pragmatic language analysis

Intervention

As with assessment of students suspected of having an LLD, intervention with this population has several guiding principles. Regardless of age, intervention should employ naturalistic techniques that reflect experiences individualized for each student. It is essential that services be provided in inclusive and natural environments whenever possible to maximize the results. For school-aged students, intervention should be curriculum-based as well, using classroom content (e.g., vocabulary words, spelling lists, subject-specific reading and writing tasks) as the basis for intervention. Another key component with intervention is the introduction, modeling, and teaching of evidence-based compensatory strategies aimed at improving a student's overall performance. As stated by Watson et al. (2012) and Foster and Miller (2007), intervention strategies should be explicitly taught. As this process progresses throughout a student's academic career, there needs to be an emphasis on increasing a student's independence with learning, tapping into his or her metacognitive skills and self-advocacy so that he or she is able to better manage the demands and/or challenges presented (Srivastava & Gray, 2012; Watson et al., 2012).

Differentiated Intervention

There are skills that are often targeted with each age group. Although these lists are not all inclusive, they highlight the key skills addressed. Following the list is a more detailed description of several of these intervention approaches and techniques.

Intervention With Young Children
(ASHA/NJCLD; Snowling & Hulme, 2012; Watson et al., 2012)

- Improving language environment by modeling
- Parent/caregiver education
- Emergent literacy tasks, including phonological awareness (e.g., rhyming, syllabication, segmenting, and blending) and training in letter-sound knowledge
- Oral language development—narrative and discourse intervention
- Vocabulary development, both receptive and expressive
- Pragmatic language skills

Intervention With School-Age Students
(NJCLD, 2008; Paul & Norbury, 2012; Seifert & Espin, 2012; Snowling & Hulme, 2012; Watson et al., 2012)

- Curriculum-based language intervention
  - Content reading comprehension, including increasing prior knowledge, using text enhancements (e.g., text illustrations) and teaching strategies to help identify main ideas, identify text structure, and predict and summarize information
- Vocabulary development, both receptive and expressive
  - Content vocabulary
- Literacy skills, including phonological awareness, morphological awareness, oral and reading comprehension
- Narrative and discourse intervention

- Emerging writing skills
  - Planning, organization, revising
- Visual format strategies/graphic organizers
- Pragmatic language skills

Intervention With Older Students
(NJCLD, 2008; Paul & Norbury, 2012; Srivastava & Gray, 2012; Watson et al., 2012)

- Curriculum-based language intervention
- Higher-order language skills, both receptive and expressive
  - Inferencing, idioms, figurative language
  - Semantic flexibility—understanding multiple meanings of words, use of synonyms and antonyms
- Visual format strategies/graphic organizers
- Writing skills
  - Executive function skills needed for writing (e.g., planning, organization, self-evaluation, revising/editing)
  - Increasing semantic and syntactical skills in writing
  - Expository writing intervention and practice
- Transition to high school and possibly secondary school or vocational tract
- Technology—computer-based applications
- Compensatory strategies for identified weaknesses
- Metacognitive approach
- Narrative and discourse intervention
- Pragmatic language skills

Once the student with a language learning disability has been evaluated, a profile of his or her strengths and weak-nesses is developed. Students with language learning disability exhibit oral language deficits that affect both language comprehension and production. The type of intervention strategies provided to the student with language learning disability depends upon the results of the comprehensive assessment. In addition, there are many types of intervention strategies reported in the literature—far too many to outline here. The remainder of this chapter presents some intervention strategies that are particularly effective for students with language impairments and LD. For any intervention to be effective, however, it is important to present methods for enhancing these students' language environments. Additionally, collaboration between general and special education teachers, as well as specialists, is necessary for defining the problem, planning and providing services, and evaluating the outcomes of interventions. Critical elements in this process include interaction, communication skills, and assessment of consultation outcomes (Coufal, 1993; NJCLD, 2008; West & Cannon, 1988).

Enhancing the Language Environment

It is imperative that the education of students with LLD combine collaborative planning, problem solving, effective teaching methods, and learning strategies. The most effective language learning environments provide opportunities for frequent interaction: students encounter many opportunities to talk and hear talk used for various purposes and in a variety of settings. Based on the causal relationship between problems with language development and subsequent difficulties with learning, literacy in particular, Snowling and Hulme (2011) conclude that the "early implementation of programmes that foster oral language development in children with such difficulties" is essential (p. 32). The application of such a program should include activities that promote speaking and listening, vocabulary training, and narrative work.

ASHA's 2000 *Roles and Responsibilities* guidelines for SLPs with respect to reading and writing in children and adolescents further outlines the relationship between spoken language and the development of reading and writing, citing that "as many as half of all poor readers have an early history of spoken language disorders" (p. 9). These guidelines define an SLP's role in the early identification of language-based difficulties, stressing the mandate for identification and intervention as outlined in IDEA 1997 (reauthorized in 2004). As part of IDEA, ASHA reiterates that intervention for students needs to be related to the demands already present with the general education curriculum, and needs to be provided using what ASHA refers to as "best practice attributes, among them intervention practices that are research-based" (ASHA, 2000, p. 29). It is therefore essential that SLPs working with this population refer to these guidelines prior to and during their work with individuals and other professionals.

Targeting Classroom Vocabulary

Within the classroom environment, teachers need to target their instructional language, in addition to textbook language, identifying vocabulary words that are relevant, functional, and individualized for each student (Bashir & Scavuzzo, 1992; Snowling & Hulme, 2011; Watson et al., 2012). Watson et al. (2012) state that a stu-

dent's understanding of vocabulary is not only essential for their comprehension of narrative texts, but also for understanding "expository texts in various academic disciplines (e.g., science and math)" (p. 81). In other words, deficits in vocabulary knowledge will likely impact a student's performance in almost all academic subjects. Therefore, targeted words should be chosen from the academic curriculum, various literature forms, classroom units, or functional "survival" words.

For older students who are taking vocational courses or working, teachers should target vocabulary that is meaningful, functional, and appropriate for the student's level of functioning in that environment. This type of approach integrates language instruction across the curriculum, providing a more naturalistic and unified approach to intervention.

Content Enhancement Strategies

Content enhancement strategies involve the use of semantic information and discussion for organizing information in class, a technique more commonly known as a semantic organizer. These strategies are excellent in that they not only extend oral language production but also facilitate reading comprehension and writing production for students with LLD.

Visual format strategies are types of semantic organizers that help students to learn the meanings of and relationships among new words, recognize words they already know, and identify relationships among new and familiar words (Hamersky, 1993, 2000; Watson et al., 2012). There are five visual format strategies:

1. Attribute webs: In this format, the key word is written in the center of

the web. The students generate different attributes of the word, which are then written on extensions of the web. These characteristics are generated in a brainstorming session in which all responses are recorded on the web. A second web is then generated after students discuss similarities among the recorded characteristics.

2. Venn diagram: This strategy is used to help students visualize, understand, compare, and contrast the meanings and characteristics of two concepts. The ideas are written on an appropriate circle and similarities between concepts are written in the overlapping portion of the circle.

3. Multiple-meaning trees: A multiple-meaning tree can be used to help students visualize various meanings for content words. The concept is written in a rectangle (depicting the center of the tree) with various meanings of the word then written on branches that extend from the tree. Once the tree is completed, students should generate sentences for each meaning.

4. Semantic continuum: This strategy can be used to help students understand that groups of related words can be ranked according to changes in their meaning. Students must have an understanding of the specific attribute that is changing between the words. A key word or concept is identified, and students then generate words that relate to the key word. The concept and related words are then placed on a continuum.

5. Associated words format: This format targets the interrelationships among word meanings. Students apply the target concept to each of nine categories: (a) similar meaning, (b) part/whole relationships, (c) class name, (d) class member, (e) opposite meaning, (f) where something exists, (g) when something occurs, (h) function, and (i) rhyming (Hamersky, 1993, 2000).

Narrative Discourse

Another type of intervention strategy that concentrates on the development of syntax (structure) and semantics (content) involves narration. According to Nelson (2010), the discourse, or narrative, level requires the use of both syntax and semantics and the overall "organization of sentences into larger cohesive communication units" (p. 46). This type of language is what is used in the school environment and text information. Specifically, in narrative discourse, teachers present information by lecturing, reading stories aloud, and relating personal events. In response, students present reports or related events and also engage in the use of narratives at the conversational level. Given the fact that narrative discourse is used extensively in the school environment, students need to understand and use this form of discourse (Kaderavek & Sulzby, 2000; Nelson, 2010; Roth, Spekman, & Fye, 1995).

Discourse can take the form of conversational skills (to be discussed in the following section) or narrative skills, which are similar in that they require a sense of purpose, the selection of relevant information, a method for exchanging the information, the ability to assume the listener's perspective, and the ability to make any needed repairs. Differences in these forms are apparent, however. According to Paul and Norbury (2012), the generation of narratives requires the production of extended units of text. In addition, narratives should contain an introduction and a series of organized events that lead to a logical conclusion.

Narratives also require that the speaker produce a monologue, during which the listener maintains a passive role and is responsible for obtaining clarification if something is unclear. In narrative discourse, words take primary responsibility for carrying the overall meaning.

Conversational Discourse

Conversational discourse involves an interaction between two individuals in which the speaker/listener roles and topics change frequently (Paul & Norbury, 2012; Westby, 1984). Conversation is a complex event that is governed by certain rules regarding negotiation in turn-taking, the ability to maintain a discourse topic, and the ability to use repair techniques to recover from breakdowns in conversation (Brinton & Fujiki, 1989). These rules are further complicated by the influence of context and pragmatic conventions, which provide the background for the way in which language is to be used (Nelson, 2010). Context is determined by the number of participants in the conversation, the nature of their relationship, their shared experiences, the subject matter discussed, and the physical surroundings. In addition, speakers must be able to make assumptions about what their listeners know, otherwise known as presuppositional skills (Brinton & Fujiki, 1989; Paul & Norbury, 2012; Roth & Spekman, 1989).

Some students with language impairments may have difficulty with the use of language because they demonstrate poor syntactic and semantic skills (Leonard, 1986; Nelson, 2010). Others may have specific difficulty understanding the social uses of language (McTear, 1985; Paul & Norbury, 2012). These deficits may change in nature as the student gets older. Evidence suggests that students with LLD do not grow out of their deficits in comprehending and using syntactic and semantic structures. As the student gets older, these deficits may impair the learning of slang and idiomatic expressions, which in turn may interfere with the interpretation of jokes and sarcastic remarks, as well as interfere with the student's ability to use advanced discourse intentions, including persuasion and negotiation (Donahue & Bryan, 1984; Hall & Tomblin, 1978; Paul & Norbury, 2012).

Expository Text Intervention

In addition to discourse intervention, it is essential that SLPs, in collaboration with classroom teachers, target expository text, or the "language of the curriculum" (Ward-Lonergan & Duthie, 2013, p. 44). A majority of a student's time in school is spent both reading and listening to factual and informational content from a variety of sources including textbooks, classroom lectures, and other supplemental readings. These types of expository discourse are requirements in academic, social, and vocational settings and present unique challenges due to the unfamiliar vocabulary as well as the manner in which the text is organized. As a result, students with language disorders struggle with both comprehending and producing expository text (Nippold, Mansfield, Billow & Tomblin, 2008; Ward-Lonergan & Duthie, 2013). In addition, "the demand for adolescents to read expository materials such as textbooks, essays, lab reports, and newspaper articles dramatically increases from what was required of them during their elementary school years" (Ward-Lonergan & Duthie, 2013, p. 49).

SLPs are in a unique position to address the difficulties that students have with expository text. As Ward-Lonergan and Duthie (2013) note and as noted previously regarding intervention, it is important to use explicit instruction both in the classroom and in language treatment, adding that SLPs should not assume that this type of instruction is provided in the classroom. These authors outline detailed strategies from a variety of sources to address the difficulties in this area including ones to address reading comprehension and written expression of expository discourse. Many of these strategies, (e.g., *SQ3R* [Survey, Question, Read, Recite, Review], *POSSE* [Predict, Organize, Search, Summarize, Evaluation], and *RAP* [Read a paragraph, Ask about main ideas and details, Put main ideas and details into your own words]), are ones that are frequently used in classrooms but should also be targeted as part of individual or group language treatment. Graphic organizers also help address difficulties in this area (Ward-Lonergan & Duthie, 2013). In addition, SLPs have both the knowledge and skills to directly address the syntactic deficits with this population. As noted by Nippold et al. (2008), students with LLD show "poorer syntactic development in expository text" (p. 357) than the normal language development group, producing simple sentences with fewer subordinate clauses. Intervention needs to examine these deficits carefully and address them as needed.

Pragmatic Intervention

Students with LLD also have difficulty perceiving and interpreting social cues and frequently violate classroom rules by talking out and being off-task. These deficits may further inhibit the student's ability to gain social acceptance into the peer group (Conderman, 1995). For intervention to be effective, strategies such as those listed below, including direct and indirect instruction and incidental teaching in social and communicative skills, must take place and the environment should be enhanced to provide increased opportunities for learning to take place (Duchan, Hewitt, & Sonenmeier, 1994; Paul & Norbury, 2012).

- Direct pragmatic intervention: The primary goal of this approach is not just to teach behaviors such as turn taking, topic manipulation, and repair strategies, but also to facilitate these skills so that communication is enhanced in a variety of settings. This instruction is accomplished through the use of scaffolding techniques and representational play and story enactments, which include a theme of the script that is individualized for each student.
- Indirect instruction: This strategy structures the environment so that communication can occur in a naturalistic way. It is important that the student's peers be included in social interactions. Group activities in both academic and social settings, for example, offer a context for communication. This type of interaction provides a more natural way for students to gain information about slang terms and other expressions common to the peer group. Indirect instruction should also enhance the generalization of these skills across people and settings.
- Incidental teaching: In this method of intervention first introduced by Hart and Risley (1975), the clinician manipulates the physical environment to ensure that desired items and activities are visible

but not readily accessible. The clinician then waits for some type of topic initiation either through verbal or nonverbal means, and then uses that initiation to provide intervention through the form of questioning, prompting, and modeling (Paul & Norbury, 2012).

The interventions presented thus far are just a few of many that are used in the remediation of language problems in students with LLD. Although each intervention can be used to facilitate the development of form, content, and use, they are also complementary, sharing similar principles and based on the premise that intervention must be evidence-based, individualized, functional and meaningful to the student with LLD.

Conclusion

An LD can be a disorder either in isolation or in coexistence with other disorders, such as a language disability. A great deal of controversy surrounds the definition of an LD and this chapter presented an overview of the many methods of assessment and intervention for students with language LD. Research in assessment and intervention will continue to identify methods for the identification and remediation of language learning disability.

Case Study 1: Elena's Case History

This case study is designed as a Think Aloud to facilitate understanding of how a clinician might think through a case. The clinician's thoughts are shown in italics.

Elena, currently 7 years old, was diagnosed with a language disorder at age 4 when her preschool teacher noticed that she consistently had difficulty following directions that were presented orally. She also noticed that Elena had some difficulty interacting with her peers appropriately. Her teacher commented that Elena tends to "stand on the outside and wait for her peers to ask her to join." Once she does join the activity, she either makes comments that are off-topic or delayed in response to the question. Elena was evaluated for speech and language difficulties by an SLP at the local school system. The SLP ruled out hearing loss, but noted that receptive and expressive vocabulary skills were delayed. Speech-language therapy was recommended and continued while Elena entered kindergarten and first grade.

There doesn't seem to be specific information regarding Elena's early speech and language development. It would be beneficial to have a thorough case history including prenatal, perinatal, and postnatal development to determine any etiological factors that may be present. In addition, it is important to have family history information to determine if there is a reported history for language and/ or learning difficulties. With regard to her speech-language intervention, what were the goals and objectives? It seems pragmatic language skills should be addressed, but what about emergent literacy skills such as phonological awareness? With the inclusion of RTI's universal screening for all kindergarten students, what were those results? What are Elena's narrative skills like?

Once Elena entered public school, her teachers continued to note the same language issues but began to notice that Elena's academics were beginning to slip. Elena had a great deal of difficulty with sight word recognition for reading and seemed frustrated and distracted with activities related to reading. By the end of first grade, the school assessment team recommended a complete interdisciplinary evaluation. Elena's parents were supportive of the team and were eager to help in any way possible.

Initial Evaluation Results

A full psychoeducational assessment using the *Weschler Intelligence Scale for Children–Fourth Edition* (WISC-IV) was conducted by the school psychologist, which revealed a high average (SS = 113) Perceptual Reasoning Index, an average (SS = 103) Processing Speed Index, and below average scores for both Working Memory Index (SS = 81) and Verbal Comprehension Index (SS = 78).

Based on the above index scores, Elena's nonverbal functioning is her strength. When spoken and/or written language is removed from tasks, she performs better. Her weaknesses continue to be in the verbal domains including vocabulary and comprehension. In addition, under time constraints, she seems to struggle somewhat, as evidence from her Working Memory Index score.

In order to conduct a thorough language evaluation that will document the difficulties Elena is having with both receptive and expressive language tasks, the *Clinical Evaluation of Language Fundamentals-Fifth Edition* (CELF-5) was administered over two evaluation sessions to document Elena's strengths and weaknesses in a variety of language areas. Results were as follows in Table 2–3 and Table 2–4.

Following assessment, the team documented that a LD did exist and support services for reading and continued speech-language therapy were recommended. It

Table 2–3. Results for the CELF-5

Subtest	Raw Score	Scaled Score Mean = 10; SD = 3	%ile Rank	Age Equivalency
Sentence Comprehension	20	6	9th	6;0
Linguistic Concepts	21	8	25th	6;3
Word Structure	18	5	5th	4;7
Word Classes	18	9	37th	6;11
Following Directions	7	5	5th	5;2
Formulated Sentences	8	4	2nd	5;0
Recalling Sentences	36	10	50th	7;4
Understanding Spoken Paragraphs	9	7	16th	
Pragmatics Profile	161	8	25th	5;0

Table 2–4. Core Language and Index Scores of the CELF-5

Core Language & Index Scores	Sum of Scaled Scores	Standard Score Mean = 100; SD = 15	%ile Rank
Core Language Score	25	79	8th
Receptive Language Index	20	80	9th
Expressive Language Index	19	80	9th
Language Content Index	22	84	14th
Language Structure Index	25	79	8th

was also recommended that Elena participate in social skills groups and support groups to build self-esteem with the guidance counselor. She currently is excelling in these programs and her parents are pleased with the services offered by the school.

Understanding that speech-language intervention will continue, the goals and objectives need to be modified to address Elena's difficulties with receptive language, both at the sentence and paragraph level. Elena struggled significantly producing syntactically and semantically intact sentences, as evidenced by her performance on the "Formulated Sentences" subtest of the CELF-V. What is her conversational discourse performance? It is important to obtain narrative and conversational discourse samples to examine her use of language in these other contexts. Results should then help determine additional IEP goals and objectives.

Review Questions

1. What are some questions that should be asked in the parent interview as part of the initial speech/language

evaluation that might reveal some early etiological risk factors in Elena's early development? Identify questions related to both prenatal, perinatal and postnatal development.

2. What difficulties might a student like Elena have given that she struggles to formulate syntactically and semantically accurate sentences? How might this weakness impact Elena's academic and social performance?

3. Given the struggles that Elena has both socially and academically, who are the professionals with whom Elena should work? If she receives intervention from a variety of related professionals, why is it important for these professionals to work collaboratively as part of an interdisciplinary team?

Case Study 2: Jake's Case History

Jake is currently attending high school and is in the 10th grade. Jake is the product of a full-term pregnancy with no reported exposure to known gestational risk factors.

The delivery was complicated by the umbilical cord being wrapped around his neck during labor. Apgar scores were remembered to be normal and birth weight was reported at 7.5 pounds. Jake experienced chronic ear infections. Developmental milestones were within normal limits with the exception of speech, which was delayed. Jake said his first word at 1 year of age, but was not using more than one word utterances by 18 months, as which time his pediatrician referred his family to the Infants and Toddlers Program (ITP). Jake's speech and language skills were evaluated through ITP at 22 months of age. Results revealed that his receptive language skills were average, but his expressive language skills were at the 12-month level. As a result, he received early intervention and a re-evaluation at age 4 stated that speech and language skills were "within normal limits." The family history is significant for speech problems in the father and paternal uncle and depression in the maternal aunt.

Prior to entering kindergarten, Jake participated in a universal screening for all students beginning kindergarten. At that time, the school found that he was struggling with phonological awareness skills, including rhyming, segmenting initial and final phonemes, and syllabication. As a result, he worked with the reading specialist in the classroom as part of his school system's participation in the RtI program. He continued this type of work in 1st grade and by the end of that, reports stated that he was reading "slightly below grade level" in reading, adding that he had some difficulties in letter/sound correspondence.

Throughout elementary and middle school, Jake worked with an outside tutor for what his parents say was "homework help," as it often took Jake a long time to complete his homework, especially as the amount increased in middle school. He benefited from having his parents read chapters from his textbooks out loud to him, but also needed them read several times in order to understand the content. On his quarterly report card in 8th grade, Jake's teachers noted that he seemed to have trouble understanding the information presented in textbooks, especially science and social studies, and that his answers to comprehension questions related to curricular material were often vague and lacked the appropriate amount of details. Jake's parents stated that he was never an avid reader and only read books when required to do so.

A full psycho-educational evaluation was completed in 9th grade at which time Jake was diagnosed with a learning disability. While he was not diagnosed with dyslexia specifically, the evaluator noted that Jake struggles significantly with decoding, which clearly impacts his ability to comprehend text that he is required to read. In other words, Jake was exerting so much effort to decode the words that it interfered with his ability to adequately process and comprehend the material. Due to the difficulties with both processing and comprehension, the psychologist recommended a full language evaluation to determine Jake's current language functioning.

Jake was cooperative during all three evaluation sessions. Overall language skills were in the below average to the average range. Receptive language skills ranged from slightly below average to average range, whereas expressive language skills were significantly below average. Weakness was indicated in auditory memory for sentences, following oral directions containing linguistic concepts, expression of word definitions, sentence formulation, sentence assembly, and word retrieval. Additional informal assessment examined Jake's academic performance through a portfolio assessment of his work in 9th grade, as well as a curriculum-based language assessment (CBLA) of his current work in 10th grade. Results of both informal measures revealed significant difficulty in Jake's understanding and production of expository text discourse, particularly with his textbooks. Even when presented in context, Jake had difficulty understanding the new and unfamiliar vocabulary words often bolded in chapters, and was not using any strategy successfully to help him comprehend the information.

Jake's struggles with both decoding and comprehending text are having a significant impact on his academic performance as well as his self-esteem, as he is putting forth as much effort as he can but still not succeeding. Although having information read to him or listening to information audibly helps, he needs direct and explicit intervention on developing and using strategies to improve his comprehension of the material presented, as well as his written production of expository discourse. It is essential that the school-based SLP work collaboratively with Jake's classroom teachers and parents to help facilitate Jake's use of these strategies across all subject areas.

Review Questions

1. List all the different types of reading tasks that a high school student must complete as part of his or her academic work. How are these tasks similar and how are they different? As a school-based SLP, why would it be important to understand these similarities and differences and how might this understanding impact intervention?

2. It is stated that Jake's self-esteem is low. Why do you think this is? What, if anything, should be done to address this area?

3. Jake benefits from having text read to him or listening to text. Research forms of technology that Jake could use other than having a person read information aloud to him.

Case Study 3: Maria's Case History

Maria is currently in 5th grade at a private school and transitioning to middle school. In 3rd grade, a full psychoeducational evaluation was completed by an independent evaluator, at which time Maria was diagnosed with ADD and a learning disability in the area reading. For the past two years Maria has been working with a tutor to strengthen both her decoding and comprehension skills. During her transition meeting to middle school, Maria's 5th grade teacher reported that while Maria has done well with some of the comprehension skills targeted, she continues to struggle with more abstract comprehension tasks. Her teacher noted that whenever Maria is asked to answer more inferential questions, she struggles significantly, often answering with facts from the text but not answering the questions. In classroom discussions, Maria's participation is limited and when she does participate, her teacher reported that her comments are often off-topic or only partial answers to the prompt. In addition, her teacher noted that when Maria answers either orally or in writing, her sentences are usually short and lack the details necessary to make them adequate. Based on this feedback, a full language evaluation was recommended to obtain a more comprehensive understanding of Maria's language skills.

A review of Maria's early speech and language developmental milestones was unremarkable; she reportedly met all of these milestones within the expected age range and was described as a "very chatty little girl." There is also no reported family history of learning or speech/language difficulties. Maria is the oldest of three siblings. She reportedly takes medication daily for management of her ADD.

Maria was cooperative over the two language evaluation sessions, but became visibly frustrated as the items moved from concrete to more abstract language tasks. Selected subtests from the *Comprehensive Assessment of Spoken Language* (CASL) were administered to examine Maria's ability to comprehend and use abstract and figurative language as compared to her ability to comprehend and use more concrete language. As evident from her scores, Maria did significantly better with the more concrete linguistic subtests, performing solidly in the average to high average range. Her performance on receptive measures was not as strong as the syntactic complexity of the stimulus items increased; similarly, performance on the use of abstract linguistic forms such as idioms, sarcasm and figurative language was also in the low average range. Maria often asked for repetition of the items presented and became visibly frustrated, (e.g., shaking her head, laying her head on the desk saying "That doesn't make sense"). As the level of linguistic complexity increased, Maria frequently asked how much longer she had, adding that her "head was starting to hurt."

Based on the results of this language evaluation, Maria was diagnosed with a language disorder specifically in her understanding and use of complex and abstract language. This diagnosis was in addition to her learning disability, resulting in an overall diagnosis of a language learning disability. Since Maria attends a private school where there is not a school-based speech-language pathologist, it was recommended that she work with a private SLP who will be able to use curriculum-based materials to address Maria's struggles. Even though this intervention will not take place at Maria's school, it will be necessary for the SLP to communicate and collaborate with Maria's classroom teacher(s) to ensure that strategies targeted in individual therapy are encouraged and used in classroom tasks. Maria's individual therapy objectives should include her ability to recognize the use of abstract language so that she can begin to use strategies targeted. In addition, her use of more complex syntactical structures in both oral and written expression should be a focus of individual therapy.

Review Questions

1. Why is it important for Maria's SLP to use curriculum-based materials in therapy? What types of materials should these include?

2. What, if any, effect does Maria's diagnosis of ADD have on her language performance?

3. What types of informal evaluation tasks could have been done as part of the language assessment to supple-

ment the standardized testing results from the CASL? What information would these informal measures yield?

References

Allen, M. M., Ukrainetz, T. A., & Carswell, A. L. (2012). The narrative language performance of three types of at-risk first-grade readers. *Language, Speech, and Hearing Services in Schools, 43,* 205–221. doi:10.1044/0161-1461/2011/11-0024

American Speech-Language-Hearing Association. (1990). A model for collaboration service delivery for students with language learning disorders in public schools. *ASHA, 33,* 44–50.

American Speech-Language-Hearing Association. (1993). Definitions of communication disorders and variations. *Asha Practice Policy.* doi:10.1044/policy.RPI1993-00208

American Speech-Language-Hearing Association. (1998). *Operationalizing the NJLCD definition of learning disabilities for ongoing assessment in schools* [Relevant paper]. Retrieved from http:// www.asha.org/policy. doi:10.1044/policy.RP1998-00130

American Speech-Language-Hearing Association. (2000). *Guidelines for the roles and responsibilities of speech-language pathologists with respect to reading and writing in children and adolescents.* Rockville, MD: Author. doi:10.1044/policy.GL2001-00062

Anastasiow, M. (1986). *Development of disability: A psychobiological analysis to special education.* Baltimore, MD: Paul H. Brookes.

Apel, K., Diehm, E., & Apel, L. (2013). Using multiple measures of morphological awareness to assess its relation to reading. *Topics in Language Disorders, 33*(1), 42–56. doi:10.1097/TLD.0b013e318280f57b

Aram, D., Morris, R., & Hall, N. (1992). The validity of discrepancy criteria for identifying children with developmental language disorders. *Journal of Learning Disabilities, 25,* 53–65.

Badian, N. A., McAnulty, G. B., Duffy, F. H., & Als, H. (1990). Prediction of dyslexia in kindergarten boys. *Annals of Dyslexia, 40,* 152–169.

Bashir, A., & Scavuzzo, A. (1992). Children with language disorders: Natural history and academic success. *Journal of Learning Disabilities, 25,* 53–65.

Bateman, B. (1965). *The Illinois Test of Psycholinguistic Abilities in Current Research: Summaries of studies* (ERIC Document Reproduction Service No. ED011417).

Berninger, V. W., Hart, T., Abbott, R., & Karovsky, P. (1992). Defining reading and writing disabilities with and without IQ: A flexible, developmental perspective. *Learning Disabilities Quarterly, 15*(2), 103–118.

Bissex, G. (1980). Patterns of development in writing: A case study. *Theory Into Practice, 19*(3), 197–201.

Brinton, B., & Fujiki, M. (1989). *Conversational management with language-impaired children.* Rockville, MD: Aspen.

Büttner, G., & Hasselhorn, M. (2011). Learning disabilities: Debates on definitions, causes, subtypes, and responses. *International Journal of Disability, Development and Education, 58*(1), 75–87. doi:10.1080/1034912X.2011.548476

Büttner, G., & Shamir, A. (2011). Learning disabilities: Causes, consequences, and responses. *International Journal of Disability, 58*(1), 1–4. doi:10.1020/1034912X.2011.548450

Cahan, S., Fono, D., & Nirel, R. (2010). The regression-based discrepancy definition of learning disability: A critical appraisal. *Journal of Learning Disabilities, 45*(2), 170–178. doi:20.1177/0022219409355-480

Cantwell, D., & Baker, L. (1992). Association between attention-deficit hyperactivity disorder and learning disorder. *Journal of Learning Disabilities, 24,* 88–95.

Casey, J. E. (2012). A model to guide the conceptualization, assessment, and diagnosis of nonverbal learning disorder. *Canadian Journal of School Psychology, 27*(1), 35–57. doi:10.1177/0829573512436966

Centers for Disease Control and Prevention. (2014). *Lead.* Retrieved from http://www.cdc.govnceh/lead/

Chappel, G. (1985). Description and assessment of language disabilities of junior high school students. In C. Simon (Ed.), *Communication skills and classroom success* (pp. 207–242). Eau Claire, WI: Thinking Publications.

Colmar, S. (2011). A book reading intervention with mothers of children with language difficulties. *Australasian Journal of Early Childhood, 36*(2), 104–112.

Conderman, G. (1995). Social status of sixth- and seventh-grade students with learning disabilities. *Learning Disability Quarterly, 18*(1), 13–24.

Coufal, K. (1993). Collaborative consultation: An alternative to traditional treatment for children with communicative disorders. *Dissertation Abstracts International, 51*(2), 694.

Danforth, S. (2011). Learning from Samuel Kirk's 16 versions of learning disability: A rejoinder to Mather and Morris. *Intellectual and Developmental Disabilities, 49*(2), 120–126. doi:10.1352/1934-9556-49.2.120

Denckla, M. (1981). Minimal brain dysfunction and dyslexia: Beyond diagnosis by exclusion. In M. Blau, I. Rapin, & M. Kinsbourne (Eds.), *Child neurology* (pp. 471–479). New York, NY: Spectrum.

Denton, C. A. (2012). Response to intervention for reading difficulties in the primary grades: Some answers and lingering questions. *Journal of Learning Disabilities, 45*(3), 232–243. doi:10.1177/0022219412332155

Donahue, M., & Bryan, T. (1984). Communicative skills and peer relations of learning disabled adolescents. *Topics in Language Disorders, 4*(2), 10–21.

Duchan, J. F., Hewitt, L. E., & Sonenmeier, R. M. (1994). Three themes: Stage two pragmatics, combating marginalization, and the relation of theory and practice. In J. F. Duchan, L. E. Hewitt, & R. M. Sonnemeier (Eds.), *Pragmatics: From theory to practice* (pp. 1–9). Englewood Cliffs, NJ: Prentice-Hall.

Dudley-Marling, C., & Searle, D. (1988). Enriching language learning environment for students with learning disabilities. *Journal of Learning Disabilities, 21*(3), 140–143.

Ehren, B. J., Montgomery, J., Rudebusch, J., & Whitmire, K. (2005). Responsiveness to intervention: New roles for speech-language pathologists. *Journal of Educational Psychology, 78,* 358–364. Retrieved from http://www.asha.org/SLP/schools/prof-consult/NewRolesSLP/children.

Foster, W. A., & Miller, M. (2007). Development of the literacy achievement gap: A longitudinal study of kindergarten through third grade. *Language, Speech, and Hearing Services in Schools, 38,* 173–181. doi:10.1044/0161-1461(2007/018)

Frith, U. (1985). The usefulness of the concept of unexpected reading failure: Comments on "reading retardation revisited." *British Journal of Developmental Psychology, 3*(1), 15–17.

Fuchs, D., & Fuchs, L. S. (2006). Introduction to response to intervention: What, why, and how valid is it? *Reading Research Quarterly, 41*(1), 93–99. doi:10.1598/RRQ.41.1.4

Fuchs, L. S., & Vaughn, S. (2012). Responsiveness-to-intervention: A decade later. *Journal of Learning Disabilities, 45*(3), 195–203. doi:10.1177/0022219412442150

Gentry, J. R. (1978). Early spelling strategies. *Elementary Schools Journal, 79*(2), 88–92.

Gentry, J. R. (1982). Developmental spelling assessment. *Diagostique, 8*(1), 52–61.

Gerber, A. (1993). *Language-related learning disability.* Baltimore, MD: Paul H. Brookes.

Gerber, A., & Bryan, D. (1981). *Language and learning disability.* Baltimore, MD: University Park Press.

Goldstein, S., & Reynolds, C. R. (1999). *Handbook of neurodevelopmental and genetic disorders in children.* New York, NY: Guilford Press.

Graves, A. W., Brandon, R., Duesbery, L., McIntosh, A., & Pyle, N. B. (2011). The effects of tier 2 literacy instruction in sixth grade: Toward the development of a response-to-intervention model in middle school. *Learning Disability Quarterly, 34*(1), 73–86. doi:10.1086/659036

Gregg, N., & Scott, S. S. (2000). Definition and documentation: Theory, measurement, and the courts. *Journal of Learning Disabilities, 33*(1), 5–13.

Gresham, F. M., & Vellutino, F. R. (2010). What is the role of intelligence in the identification of specific learning disabilities? Issues and clarifications. *Learning Disabilities Research & Practice, 25*(4), 194–206. doi:10.1111/j.1540-5826.2010.00317

Hall, P., & Tomblin, J. (1978). A follow-up study of children with articulation and language disorders. *Journal of Speech and Hearing Disorders, 43,* 227–241.

Hamersky, J. (1993). *Vocabulary maps: Strategies for developing word meanings.* Eau Claire, WI: Thinking Publications.

Hamersky, J. (2000). *Vocabulary maps: Strategies for developing word meanings.* Eau Claire, WI: Thinking Publications.

Hammill, D. (1993). A brief look at the learning disabilities movement in the United States. *Journal of Learning Disabilities, 26,* 295–310.

Haynes, W. O., & Pindzola, R. H. (2012). *Diagnosis and evaluation in speech pathology* (8th ed.). Boston, MA: Pearson Education.

Hutson-Nechkash, P. (1990). *Storybuilding: A guide to structuring oral narratives*. Eau Claire, WI: Thinking Publications.

Ikeda, M. J. (2012). Policy and practice considerations for response to intervention: Reflections and commentary. *Journal of Learning Disabilities, 45*(3), 274–277. doi:10.1177/002221 9412442170

Interagency Committee on Learning Disabilities. (1987). *Learning disabilities: A report to the U.S. Congress* (p. 222). Bethesda, MD: National Institutes of Health.

Kaderavek, J., & Sulzby, E. (2000). Narrative production by children with and without specific language impairment: Oral narratives and emergent readings. *Journal of Speech, Language, and Hearing Research, 43*, 34–48.

Kamhi, A. G., & Catts, H. W. (1989). *Reading disabilities: A developmental language perspective*. Boston, MA: College-Hill Press.

Katims, D. S. (1999). Emergence of literacy in preschool children with disabilities. *Language Disorders Quarterly, 17*(1), 58–69.

Kavale, K. A., & Forness, S. R. (2000). What definitions of language disorders say and don't say: A critical analysis. *Journal of Learning Disabilities, 33*(3), 239–256.

Kirby, J. R., Deacon, S. H., Bowers, P. N., Izenberg, L., Wade-Woolley, L., & Parrila, R. (2012). Children's morphological awareness and reading ability. *Reading and Writing: An Interdisciplinary Journal, 25*(2), 389–410. doi:10 .1007/s11145-010-9276-5

Kirk, C., & Gillon, G. T. (2009). Integrated morphological awareness intervention as a tool for improving literacy. *Language, Speech, and Hearing Services in Schools, 40*, 341–351. doi:10 .1044/0161-1461(2008/08-0009)

Koutsoftas, A. D., & Gray, S. (2012). Comparison of narrative and expository writing in students with and without language-learning disabilities. *Language, Speech, and Hearing Services in Schools, 43*, 395–409. doi:10.1044/ 0161-1461(2012/11-0018)

Lahey, M., & Bloom, L. (1994). Variability and language learning disability. In G. Wallach & K. Butler (Eds.), *Language learning disability in school-aged children and adolescents*. New York, NY: Macmillan.

Larson, V., & McKinley, N. (1987). *Communication assessment and intervention strategies for adolescents*. Eau Claire, WI: Thinking Publications.

Launer, P. (1994). Keeping on track to the twenty-first century. In G. Wallach & K. Butler (Eds.), *Language learning disability in school-aged children and adolescents*. New York, NY: Macmillan.

Leonard, L. (1986). Conversational replies of children with specific language impairment. *Journal of Speech and Hearing Research, 29*, 114–119.

Maehler, C., & Schuchardt, K. (2011). Working memory in children with learning disabilities: Rethinking the criterion of discrepancy. *International Journal of Disability, Development and Education, 58*(1), 5–17. doi:10.1080/10349 12X.2011.547335

Mathinos, D. A. (1988). Communicative competence of children with learning disabilities. *Journal of Learning Disabilities, 21*, 437–443.

McTear, M. F. (1985). *Children's conversations*. Oxford, UK: Blackwood.

Mercer, C. D., King-Sears, P., & Mercer, A. R. (1990). Learning disability definitions and criteria used by state education departments. *Learning Disability Quarterly, 20*, 43–60.

Moyle, J., Stokes, S. F., & Klee, T. (2011). Early language delay and specific language impairment. *Developmental Disabilities Research Reviews, 17*, 160–169. doi:10.1002/ddrr.1110

National Joint Committee on Learning Disabilities. (1991). Learning disabilities: Issues on definition. *ASHA, 33*(Suppl. 5), 18–20.

National Joint Committee on Learning Disabilities. (1998). Operationalizing the NJLCD definition of learning disabilities for ongoing assessment in schools. *ASHA, 40*(Suppl. 18), III-258a-258g. doi:10.1044/policy.RP1998-00130

National Joint Committee on Learning Disabilities. (2005). *Responsiveness to intervention and learning disabilities*. Retrieved from http:// www.ldonline.org/article/Responsiveness_ to_Intervention_and_Learning_Disabilities

National Joint Committee on Learning Disabilities. (2007). *Learning disabilities and young children: Identification and intervention* [Technical report]. Retrieved from http://www.asha .org/policy/TR2007-00307.htm

National Joint Committee on Learning Disabilities. (2011a). Learning disabilities: Implications for policy regarding research and practice. *Learning Disability Quarterly, 34*(4), 237–241. doi:10.1177/0731948711421756

National Joint Committee on Learning Disabilities. (2011b). Comprehensive assessment and evaluation of students with learning disabilities: A paper prepared by the National Joint Committee on Learning Disabilities. *Learning Disability Quarterly, 34*(1), 3–21. Retrieved from http://www.cldinternational.org/Publications/LDQ.asp

Nelson, N. W. (1994). Curriculum based language assessment and intervention across the grades. In G. Wallach & K. Butler (Eds.), *Language learning disabilities in school-aged children* (pp. 104–131). New York, NY: Macmillan.

Nelson, N. W. (2010). *Language and literacy disorders: Infancy through adolescence.* Boston, MA: Allyn & Bacon.

Nippold, M. A., Mansfield, T. C., Billow, J. L., & Tomblin, J. B. (2008). Expository discourse in adolescents with language impairments: Examining syntactic development. *American Journal of Speech-Language Pathology, 17,* 356–366. doi:1058-0360/08/1704-0356

Ofiesh, N. (2006). Response to intervention and the identification of specific learning disabilities: Why we need comprehensive evaluations as part of the process. *Psychology in the Schools, 43*(8), 883–888. doi:10.1002/pits

Owens, R. E., Jr. (2010). *Language disorders: A functional approach to assessment and intervention* (5th ed.). Boston, MA: Pearson Education.

Owens, R. E., Jr. (2012). *Language development: An introduction* (8th ed.). Boston, MA: Pearson Education.

Paul, R., & Norbury, C. F. (2012). *Language disorders from infancy through adolescence: Listening, speaking, reading, writing and communicating* (4th ed.). St. Louis, MO: Mosby Elsevier.

Paul, R., & Roth, F. P. (2011). Characterizing and predicting outcomes of communication delays in infants and toddlers: Implications for clinical practice. *Language, Speech, and Hearing Services in Schools, 42,* 331–340. doi:10.1044/0161-1461(2010/09-0067)

Rice, M., Sell, M. A., & Hadley, P. A. (1990). The social interactive coding system: An on-line clinically relevant descriptive tool. *Language, Speech, and Hearing Services in Schools, 21,* 2–14.

Richardson, S. D. (1992). Historical perspectives on dyslexia. *Journal of Learning Disabilities, 25,* 40–47.

Rissnam, B. (2010). Nonverbal learning disability explained: The link to shunted hydrocephalus. *Research Journal of Learning Disabilities, 39,* 209–215. doi:10.1111/j.1468.3156.2010.00652.x

Roth, F., & Speckman, M. (1985). *Story grammar analysis of narratives produced by learning disabled and normally achieving students.* Paper presented at the Symposium on Research in Child Language Disorders, Madison, WI.

Roth, F. P., & Speckman, N. J. (1989). The oral syntactic proficiency of learning disabled students: A spontaneous story sampling analysis. *Journal of Speech and Hearing Research, 32,* 67–77.

Roth, F. P., Speckman, N. J., & Fye, E. C. (1995). Reference cohesion in the oral narratives of students with learning disabilities and normally achieving students. *Language Disabilities Quarterly, 18*(1), 25–40.

Rourke, B. P. (1989). *Nonverbal learning disability: The syndrome and the model.* New York, NY: Guilford Press.

Satz, P., & Morris, R. (1981). Learning disability subtypes: A review. In F. J. Prizollo & M. C. Wittrock (Eds.), *Neuropsychological and cognitive processes in reading.* New York, NY: Academic Press.

Sawyer, D. (1985). Language problems observed in poor readers. In C. Simon (Ed.), *Communication skills and classroom success.* Eau Claire, WI: Thinking Publications.

Schoenbrodt, L., Kumin, L., & Sloan, J. (1997). Learning disability existing concomitantly with communication disorder. *Journal of Learning Disability, 30*(3), 264–281.

Seifert, K., & Espin, C. (2012). Improving reading of science text for secondary students with learning disabilities: Effects of text reading, vocabulary learning, and combined approaches to instruction. *Learning Disability Quarterly, 35*(4), 236–247. doi:10.1177/0731948712444275

Smith, T. E., Dowdy, C. A., Polloway, E. A., & Blalock, G. B. (1999). *Children and adults with learning disabilities.* Boston, MA: Allyn & Bacon.

Snowling, M. J., & Hulme, C. (2012). Interventions for children's language and literacy difficulties. *International Journal of Language & Communication Disorders, 47*(1), 27–34. doi:10.111/j.1460-6984.2011.00081.x

Sohlberg, M., & Mateer, C. (1989). The assessment of cognitive-communication features and head injury. *Topics in Language Disorders, 9*(2), 15–33.

Sowan, N. A., & Stember, M. L. (2000). Effect of maternal prenatal smoking on infant growth and development of obesity. *The Journal of Perinatal Education, 9*(3), 22–29.

Sparks, R. L., & Lovett, B. J. (2009). College students with learning disability diagnoses: Who are they and how do they perform? *Journal of Learning Disabilities, 42*(6), 494–510. doi:10.1177/0022219409338746

Srivastava, P., & Gray, S. (2012). Computer-based and paper-based reading comprehension in adolescents with typical language development and language-learning disabilities. *Language, Speech, and Hearing Services in Schools, 43,* 424–437. doi:10.1044/0161-1461 (2012/10-0108)

Supple, M. D. M., & Söderpalm, E. (2010). Child language disability: A historical perspective. *Topics in Language Disorders, 30*(1), 72–78. doi:10.1097/tld.0b013e3181d0a13e

Torgesen, J. K. (1986). Learning disabilities theory: Its current state and future prospects. *Journal of Learning Disabilities, 19*(7), 399–407.

U.S. Department of Education, Office of Special Education Programs. (2006). *Identification of specific learning disabilities.* Retrieved from http://idea.ed.gov/explore/view/p/%2Cro ot%2Cdynamic%2CTopicalArea%2C13%2C

U.S. Office of Education. (1976). Education of handicapped children: Assistance to states: Proposed rulemaking. *Federal Register, 41*(230), 52404–52407.

Vandewalle, E., Boets, B., Ghesquière, P., & Zink, I. (2012). Development of phonological processing skills in children with specific language impairment with and without literacy delay: A three-year longitudinal study. *Journal of Speech, Language, and Hearing Research, 55*(4), 1053–1067. doi:10.1044/1092-4388(2011/10-0308)

van Kleek, A., & Schuele, C. M. (2010). Historical perspective on literacy in early childhood. *American Journal of Speech-Language Pathology, 19,* 341–355. doi:10.1044/1058-0360(2010/09-0038)

Volden, J. (2004). Nonverbal learning disability: A tutorial for speech-language pathologists. *American Journal of Speech-Language Pathology, 13,* 129–141. doi:10.1044/1058-0360

Wagner, R. K., & Torgesen, J. K. (1987). The nature of phonological processing and its causal role in the acquisition of reading skills. *Psychological Bulletin, 101*(2), 192–212.

Wallach, G. P., & Butler, K. G. (1994). *Language learning disabilities in school-age children and adolescents.* New York, NY: Macmillan.

Wankoff, L. S. (2011). Warning signs in the development of speech, language, and communication: When to refer to a speech-language pathologist. *Journal of Child and Adolescent Psychiatric Nursing, 24,* 175–184. doi:10.111/ j.1744-6171.2011.00292.x

Ward-Lonergan, J. M., & Duthie, J. K. (2013). Expository discourse intervention for adolescents with language disorders. *Perspectives on Language Learning and Education, 20,* 44–56. doi:10.1044/lle20.2.44

Washburn, E. K., Joshi, R. M., & Binks-Cantrell, R. S. (2011). Teacher knowledge of basic language concepts and dyslexia. *Dyslexia, 17,* 165–183. doi:10.1002/dys.426

Watson, S. M. R., Gable, R. A., Gear, S. B., & Hughes, K. C. (2012). Evidence-based strategies for improving the reading comprehension of secondary students: Implications for students with learning disabilities. *Learning Disabilities Research & Practice, 27*(2), 79–89. doi:10.1111/j.1540-5826.2012.00353

West, J. F., & Cannon, G. S. (1988). Essential collaborative consultation competencies for regular and special educators. *Journal of Learning Disabilities, 21,* 56–63.

Westby, C. (1984). Development of narrative language abilities. In G. Wallach & K. Butler (Eds.), *Language learning disabilities in school-age children* (pp. 103–127). Baltimore, MD: Williams & Wilkins.

Wiig, E., & Semel, E. (1984). *Language assessment and intervention for the learning disabled* (2nd ed.). New York, NY: Merrill.

CHAPTER 3

Intellectual Disability

Libby Kumin

Chapter Objectives

Upon completing this chapter, the reader should be able to:

1. Classify intellectual disability according to IQ score and/or according to levels of support needed in daily life. Understand the different systems for classifying intellectual disabilities.
2. Describe specific syndromes resulting from prenatal, birth, or postnatal etiologies that result in intellectual disability
3. Describe the complex conditions that are related to intellectual disabilities
4. List etiologies, characteristics, and associated medical conditions in children with Down syndrome and their impact on speech and language
5. List etiologies, characteristics, and associated conditions for children with fragile X syndrome and other low incidence disorders and their impact on speech and language
6. Discuss assessment of communication disorders in children with Down syndrome, fragile X syndrome, and other intellectual disabilities

7. Develop and understand treatment protocols for children with Down syndrome, fragile X syndrome, and other intellectual disabilities
8. Identify the difficulties encountered in school and daily life related to language disorders in children with intellectual disabilities

Introduction

Many people with disabilities have difficulties with the tasks of daily living. Intellectual Disability (ID) or Intellectual Developmental Disorder is the term used when people demonstrate substantial limitations in intellectual functioning and adaptive behavior in the areas of conceptual (e.g., receptive and expressive language), social (e.g., ability to follow rules, interpersonal skills), and practical adaptive (e.g., using the telephone, using transportation) skills. This disability originates during the developmental period (DSM-V, 2013). Until 2010, the term mental retardation was used to describe this category of disability (Shapiro & Batshaw, 2011). The classic system of defining intellectual disability was based on standardized tests of intelligence. The population with intellectual disability was generally divided into three levels based on the severity of the intellectual impairment (Batshaw, Roizen, & Lotrecchiano, 2013). Mild intellectual disability is most common, affecting over 85% of people diagnosed with the disability. Mild ID is defined as an IQ score 2 to 3 standard deviations below the mean IQ score of 100, that is, an IQ score of 75 or below. The levels that are used to differentiate the groups can be found in Table 3–1.

Sometimes the IQ categories of individuals with severe and profound intellectual disabilities are combined as the severe and profound handicaps (SPH) group. But what do these levels mean? How do they help us understand how a child functions in daily life? These levels are not always meaningful or helpful when planning services for a child and his or her family. Many IQ tests are language based, so children with language and speech difficulties will often score at a lower level than they would score on a nonverbal IQ test. For example, a child with Down syndrome who was enrolled in the speech and language center was tested by the school psychologist using the Wechsler Intelligence Test for Children (WISC). The result was an IQ score of 50. At the suggestion of the speech-language pathologist (SLP), the psychologist retested the child using a nonverbal IQ test, the Leiter International Scale, and the same child had an IQ of 79. A score of 79 would place that child in the low normal intelligence range, not in the range of someone with intellectual disability. Children whose native language is not English may also have scores that are not accurate representations of their overall level of function in daily life because of their limitations in understanding and using the English language. That is an important consideration when assessing whether a child has intellectual disability. Test results are usually reported as mental age scores (MA) or intelligent quotient (IQ) scores. Mental age is a test construct, which means that the individual answered the same number of items correctly on a standardized IQ test as the average for the test norms collected. But, it is not accurate to equate mental age with level of function. A 15-year-old who has 15 years of life experience but has test scores with a mental age of 10 does not function in daily life the same as a typically developing 10-year-old. So, the label of ID, based on IQ test scores, is not always definitive.

For these and other reasons, in 1992, the American Association on Mental Retardation (AAMR) (Schalock, Baker, & Croser, 2002) expanded the definition of MR (the designated term used at that time) so that it would focus on assessing how the person functions in daily living, and the type and level of support that the person needs to function effectively, rather than relying on a test score to define the categories or levels of MR. They also stated four important assumptions that are essential to ensure that the label of MR (now ID) is used appropriately. In 2002,

Table 3–1. Levels of Intellectual Disability (IID)

Level	IQ Score
Mild	50–75
Moderate	35–49
Severe	34 or below
Profound	need full assistance with self-help skills

a fifth assumption was added (Luckasson et al., 2002). The five assumptions are:

1. Limitations in present functioning must be considered within the context of community environments typical of the individual's age peers and culture.
2. Valid assessment considers cultural and linguistic diversity, as well as differences in communication, sensory, motor, and behavioral factors.
3. Within an individual, limitations often coexist with strengths.
4. An important purpose of describing limitations is to develop a profile of needed supports.
5. With appropriate personalized supports over a sustained period, the life functioning of the person with MR generally will improve.

The AAMR expanded diagnostic criteria, in addition to standardized test results of intelligence and adaptive skills, employs a process of evaluating the individual's strengths and needs. The person's strengths and needs are described, in a variety of ways, across four dimensions:

1. Intellectual and adaptive behavior skills
2. Psychological/emotional considerations
3. Physical/health/etiological considerations
4. Environmental considerations

The descriptions may be based on observations, interviews with key people in the person's life, interviews with the person, interacting with the person in his or her daily life, and formal testing. Based on this analysis of strengths and needs, an interdisciplinary team determines the person's needs for support across the four dimensions. Supports are the resources and individual strategies and services that are needed to promote the development, education, interests, and well-being of an individual with ID. In 2002, an expanded system of supports was proposed that includes the need for support in the areas of human developmental, education and school learning, home living, community living, health and safety, behavior, social interaction, and protection and advocacy. Each support is classified as one of four levels of intensity:

- Intermittent: Support on an "as needed basis." The person may need support to find a new job or new housing, but the support would be needed occasionally, not on a regular basis. The support may be needed in times of crisis.
- Limited: Support may be needed for a limited time span. For example, during the transition from school to work, there will be a need for on-the-job training with a job coach. This level of support will be needed for a limited amount of time.
- Extensive: Support is needed on a daily basis for a specific area or for several areas of daily function. The person may have different levels of need for supports in different areas of daily function. For example, she or he may need assistance with transportation, but may not need assistance with bathing, dressing, and grooming.
- Pervasive: Support that is needed on a constant basis across environments and all life areas.

So, there are different routes to the diagnostic label of ID, based on testing and necessary supports for living.

The current widely accepted definition of Intellectual Disability (aka Intellectual; Developmental Disorder) is defined in the DSM-V (American Psychological Association [APA] 2013). This definition is based on a combination of test results and adaptive difficulties, with the need for supports, in the activities of daily living. According to DSM-V, the following three criteria must be met for a diagnosis of Intellectual Disability:

A. Deficits in intellectual functions such as reasoning, problem solving, planning, abstract thinking, judgment, academic learning, and learning from experience, based on both clinical assessment and individualized standardized intelligence testing.
B. Deficits in adaptive functioning; that result in failure to meet developmental and sociocultural standards for personal independence and social responsibility. Without ongoing support, the adaptive deficits limit functioning in one or more activities of daily life such as communication, social participation, and independent living, across multiple environments, such as home, school work, and community.
C. Onset of intellectual and adaptive deficits during the developmental period (DSM-V, 2013, p.33).

The severity levels in the DSM-V definition are based on adaptive functioning and the need for supports in the conceptual, social, and practical domains. Severity levels are classified as mild, moderate, severe, and profound.

The condition described above is currently labeled as Intellectual Disability (ID). In 2010, the American Academy on Mental Retardation (AAMR) changed its title to the American Academy of Intellectual and Developmental Disability (AAIDD) and updated and published definitions and information in Intellectual Disability: Definition, Classification, and Systems of Supports (11th edition). Earlier definitions of ID had been based on IQ scores but the 2002 AAMR definition and the 2010 revisions were based on the level of assistance and support the person needed in daily living. In the same year (2010), President Obama signed a law passed by Congress known as Rosa's law, which eliminated the terms "MR" and "mentally retarded" from federal education, health, and labor laws. The story behind the passage of this law is interesting and illustrates the power of citizen advocacy. Senator Barbara Mikulski introduced the law in the United States Senate in November 2009. The law is named after Rosa Marcellino, a child from Edgewater, Maryland. Senator Mikulski met Rosa's mom at a school meeting, and Nina Marcellino said her youngest child, who has Down syndrome, had been labeled as a child with MR in her Individual Education Plan at school. Nina didn't allow the "R-word" in her house and none of Rosa's three siblings used that word to describe their sister. Children in school sometimes referred to Rosa as "retarded" or a "retard" and that was hurtful and demeaning. Nina teamed up with other parents and their Maryland state delegate, Ted Sophocleus, who agreed to hold a hearing to change the terminology in Maryland State Law. At the hearing, Rosa's 11-year-old brother urged members of the General Assembly to change the terminology because, he said, "What you call people is how you treat them." Senator Mikulski promised Rosa's mom that if the law passed in Maryland, she would fight to change the terminology at a federal level. Rosa's Law passed the Maryland General Assembly and was signed by Governor Martin O'Malley in April 2009. "Just like Rosa's

Law hit a chord in Maryland, it hit a chord in the U.S. Senate," Senator Mikulski said. "This law takes 'mentally retarded' out of the federal law books and replaces it with 'intellectual disability,' a change that will have a positive effect on more than 6 million Americans. This law is about families fighting for the respect and dignity of their loved ones. It was driven by a passion for social justice and compassion for the human condition. And it's a perfect example of citizen advocacy." The bill's passage (PL 111-256) resulted in changes in federal laws including the Individuals with Disabilities Education Act, The law mandated changes in terminology at the federal level affecting federal agencies and federal legislation. Intellectual disability is included as a category within the definition of a child with a disability (section 602) in the Individual with Disabilities Education Act (IDEA 2004). ID is characterized by significantly sub average intellectual functioning, that is, an IQ score of 70 to 75 or below, existing concurrently with limitations in two or more adaptive skill areas, that is, communication, self-care, functional academics (reading, writing, basic math), self-direction, home living, social skills, community use, health and safety, leisure, and work.

But the term mental retardation/MR is still used in many settings and situations, and in many countries outside of the United States.

Etiology

There are many causes of intellectual disability, including genetic syndromes, prenatal trauma, infections and other problems during pregnancy, trauma such as anoxia (lack of oxygen) at birth, and postnatal problems such as illness, injury, and environmental toxins such as lead poisoning (Batshaw, Roizen, & Lotrecchiano, 2013). Biomedical, social, behavioral, and environmental risk factors can increase the chances that an individual will show intellectual disability. Some problems are preventable, such as lead poisoning or alcohol or substance abuse by the mother. These conditions are discussed in other chapters. Some problems, such as hypothyroidism and Rh-incompatibility, can be controlled through medical testing and treatment and prenatal care. Genetic causes account for approximately 45% of cases of intellectual disability (Batshaw, Roizen, & Lottrecchiano, 2013). Two common genetic syndromes that result in intellectual disability are Down syndrome and fragile X syndrome. Because individuals with Down syndrome comprise the largest group of individuals with ID with a genetic etiology, the focus of this chapter will be on children with Down syndrome. The chapter also includes a discussion of fragile X syndrome, which is the largest inherited cause of ID. For both populations, etiologies, medical difficulties, clinical symptoms, and behavioral characteristics, and communication, language, and speech symptoms will be discussed. Assessment and treatment of communication, language and speech problems are presented and discussed. The largest environmental cause of ID, fetal alcohol syndrome and substance abuse, is discussed in another chapter.

Down Syndrome

Down syndrome is a genetically based syndrome that affects an individual's overall development, including speech, language, and communication development and function. Incidence is estimated at one in 700 live births, with 3,000 to 5,000 infants born with Down syndrome every year (Bull & The Committee on Genetics, 2011; NDSC, 2013). Although it was first described by Dr. John Langdon Down in 1866, it was not until 1959 that Dr. Jerome Lejeune identified the underlying chromosomal abnormality, an additional 21st chromosome. There are three different types of chromosomal abnormalities that may be the underlying cause of Down syndrome in an individual: trisomy 21, translocation, and mosaicism.

Approximately 95% of children with Down syndrome have an extra 21st chromosome in each cell, for example, each cell has 47 chromosomes instead of the usual 46 chromosomes. This is known as trisomy 21 or nondisjunction trisomy 21. It results from nondisjunction, or a failure of the 21st chromosome to separate correctly during cell division in the fertilized egg. Approximately 3% to 4% of children with Down syndrome have an extra chromosome 21 in which the long arm attaches or translocates onto another chromosome, usually chromosome 14, 21, or 22. This is known as translocation. Approximately 1% to 2% of children with Down syndrome have an extra chromosome in some cells, but not all cells, for example, some cells have 46 chromosomes, but other cells have 47 chromosomes. This type is known as mosaicism. This means that fewer cells are affected, as compared to trisomy 21 (Bull & The Committee on Genetics, 2011).

Though the etiology of Down syndrome is known, the cause of the extra chromosome is not known. Older mothers have a higher risk of having a child with Down syndrome, but it is estimated that over 80% of babies born with Down syndrome have mothers under age 35 (NDSC, 2013). Paternal factors may play a role as well. Some researchers believe that environmental factors may have an influence. Others have theorized that hormonal problems, immunological problems, viral infections, and/or pollutants may result in the extra chromosome. Exactly how the extra chromosomal material affects development and function is not totally understood. Some researchers feel that there is a dosage effect of the extra material, for example, the extra chromosomal material affects the development of each organ system. Others feel that the extra chromosome results in incomplete development of the embryo. In the year 2000, as part of the human genome initiative, chromosome 21 was mapped. Research is now moving more quickly, but there is still an incomplete understanding of the genetic basis of Down syndrome.

Definition of the Disorder: Medical and Behavioral Definitions

How does the extra chromosome in Down syndrome affect development and function? How does the genotype (genetic changes) affect the phenotype (developmental, communicative, and behavioral)? There are a wide variety of physical and mental characteristics that may occur in individuals with Down syndrome, including physical signs, associated medical conditions, and behavioral and learning characteristics. Approximately 60 clinical signs of Down syndrome have been identified. Before there were tests to determine genetically that a child had Down syndrome, the diagnosis was made on the basis of the presence of seven or more of the clinical signs. An individual with Down syndrome may have few or many signs and medical problems. Some of the more common signs include:

- Underdevelopment of the midface (midface hypoplasia)
- Flattening of the back of the head
- Slanting of the eyelids (palpebral fissures)
- Skin folds at the inner corner of the eyes (epicanthal folds)
- Colored spots in the iris of the eye (Brushfield spots)
- Small upper jaw (maxilla) relevant to the lower jaw (mandible)
- Depressed bridge of the nose
- Small outer ears (tops may fold over)
- Small narrow ear canals
- Single line across the palm of the hand (simian crease)
- Low muscle tone (hypotonia)
- Loose ligaments (ligamentous laxity)
- Decreased muscle strength
- Short arms and legs
- Short stature

Associated Medical Conditions

There are many associated medical conditions seen in individuals with Down syndrome, which must be monitored and treated by the pediatrician and other medical specialists (Bull & The Committee on Genetics, 2011). Hearing problems are very common in individuals with Down syndrome, and they impact speech and language development (Roizen, 1997; Shott, 2000, 2006; Shott, Joseph, & Heithaus, 2001). Other common medical and health concerns include:

- Congenital heart disease, including endocardial cushion defect, ventricular septal defect, and atrial septal defect
- Gastrointestinal abnormalities

- Metabolic difficulties
- Thyroid problems, especially hypothyroidism
- Celiac disease
- Enlarged tonsils and adenoids
- Skeletal difficulties, including atlantoaxial instability (neck alignment problem)
- Higher incidence of seizure disorders
- Higher incidence of leukemia
- Sleep apnea
- Hearing problems, including excess fluid, conductive and sensorineural hearing loss
- Visual problems, including congenital cataracts, strabismus, nystagmus, nearsightedness, and farsightedness
- Periodontal disease
- Skin conditions

The American Academy of Pediatrics published extensive guidelines for medical evaluation and treatment of children with Down syndrome in 2011 (Bull & The Committee on Genetics, 2011). See resources at the end of the chapter.

Communication Strengths and Challenges for Children with Down Syndrome

There is no single pattern of communication impairment in children with Down syndrome; however, there are areas of strength and weakness that commonly occur in many children. But these difficulties may manifest in different symptoms. For example, most children with Down syndrome have difficulties with speech intelligibility, but for one child, this may manifest as articulation and fluency difficulty, whereas for another child, resonance problems will be the major symptom (Berglund, Eriksson,& Johansson, 2011; Kumin, 2012, 2000). Speech and language development is greatly influenced by input from a child's environment. Children learn speech and language by watching and listening to the people in their environment, and then trying to make sense out of what they see and hear. Many children with Down syndrome have difficulty with sensory input and processing systems, and this will impact speech and language development. For example, hearing may be affected by excess fluid buildup in the ears, or the child may be tactilely defensive and seek to avoid oral experiences; these factors will impact speech and language development.

Early development is asynchronous in children with Down syndrome, for example, progress is not the same in all developmental areas. Children with Down syndrome may be more advanced in gross motor development than they are in speech (Winders, 2014). They usually learn better through the visual channel (reading and visual models) than they do through the auditory channel (verbal instructions) (Hopmann & Wilen, 1993; Kumin, 2012). Speech and language development is usually more delayed than would be predicted by cognitive level. Language impairment may be linguistic-specific impairment, as children with Down syndrome are usually more advanced in vocabulary skills than they are in morphosyntactic skills (Fowler, 1990, 1995; Kumin, Councill, & Goodman, 1999; Kumin, Goodman, & Councill, 1998). Receptive language skills are usually far more advanced than expressive language skills, so that children with Down syndrome understand more than they can say (Fidler, Most, & Philosky, 2009; Kumin, 2012; Miller, 1992, 1995, 1999; Miller, Leddy, Miolo, & Sedey, 1995).

Speech is usually the most difficult channel for communication for children with Down syndrome, far more difficult than sign language or picture communication systems (Kouri, 1989), and speech intelligibility is a major problem for children with Down syndrome (Kumin, 1994, 2014a).

The difficulties in expressive language and intelligibility often lead professionals to underestimate the intelligence and capabilities of children with Down syndrome (Chapman, Seung, Schwartz, & Bird, 1998; Chapman, Schwartz, & Bird, 1991; Kumin, 2012). Even when children with Down syndrome increase their expressive language skills, their effectiveness in communicating with others depends, to a large extent, on whether their speech can be understood (Chapman, Seung, Schwartz, & Bird, 1998). When you cannot understand what someone is saying, it is very difficult to assess the person's abilities. Speech and language testing that uses verbal language instructions and expressive language output responses as the measure may not be accurate in assessing the child's receptive language level and/or reading level. If we ask the child to give us a verbal answer and the answer is incorrect, we cannot assume that he or she does not know the answer, only that he or she cannot tell us the answer. This impacts testing as well as educational opportunities. In the classroom, materials often need to be modified to accommodate the visual strengths and auditory and verbal difficulties of children with Down syndrome. Materials that use pictures or written instructions can enable the child to demonstrate knowledge and mastery of skills.

Communication difficulties may also relate to behavior difficulties. When children cannot express their needs, they may use behavior such as screaming or running out of the room as a substitute strategy to express frustration and make needs known. A functional behavioral assessment (FBA) can analyze the situations that come before and after the behavior and draw some conclusions regarding the function that the behaviors are serving for the child. Behavioral evaluations should always consider whether communication difficulties are affecting the behaviors exhibited (Crimmins, 1999; McGuire & Chicoine, 2006). Behavioral treatment plans should provide augmented and assistive communication, when appropriate, to enable the child to communicate her or his needs.

Characteristics of Down Syndrome

The following are characteristics of children with Down syndrome that affect language, speech development and skills, hearing and auditory skills, voice, and fluency.

Language

Children with Down syndrome have more difficulty with expressive language than receptive language. In a classic study, Miller (1988) found that more than 75% of his subjects demonstrated deficits in language production when compared to language comprehension and cognitive skills, and that the expressive language difficulties increased over time (Miller, 1988). Since that study, many other researchers and clinicians have confirmed that receptive language skills are usually more advanced than expressive language skills (Abbeduto et al., 2001; Abbeduto &

Murphy, 2004; Chapman & Hesketh, 2000; Chapman, Schwartz,& Bird, 1991; Chapman, Seung, Schwartz,& Bird, 1998; Fidler, Most, & Philosky, 2009; Fowler, 1999; Jenkins, 1993; Kumin,1996, 2012; Miller, J.F., 1988, 1992, 1995; Petursdottir & Carr, 2011; Rice, Warren,& Betz, 2005; Roberts, Price, & Malkin, 2007; Rondal, 1988). In addition to the receptive and expressive channel (modality) differences, there are also linguistic differences. Studies comparing semantic and syntactic development in children with Down syndrome demonstrate that syntax is a far more difficult area for children with Down syndrome (Chapman & Hesketh, 2000; Fidler, Most, & Philofsky, 2009; Fowler, 1990, 1995; Miller, 1988) than semantics. The abstract nature of grammar and the sequencing skills required appear to be related to this difficulty. Pragmatics and social language skills are reported to be a strength for children with Down syndrome (Cebula, Moore, & Wishart, 2010; Fidler, Most, Booth-LaForce, & Kelly, 2008; Guralnick, 1995; Kumin, 2002, 2010; Kumin, Goodman, & Councill, 2010).

Language level is often more impaired than would be expected by the child's cognitive level. That means that if a language-based test is used to assess cognition, the conclusion may be that the cognitive level of the child is lower than it actually is. Most testing involves language, both in giving instructions and in giving responses. Bray and Woolnough (1988) reported that 11 children from ages 12 to 16 that they studied spoke primarily in single-word utterances. Research has found that adolescents with Down syndrome use shorter phrases and sentences as evidenced by a significantly shorter mean length of utterance (MLU) than typically developing adolescents matched for mental age (MA) or adolescents with ID due to other causes (Rosin, Swift, Bless, & Vetter, 1988). More recent research has found that children and adolescents keep learning and progressing in the area of morphosyntax and that, in studies of narrative output, the stimuli used to elicit the narrative made a difference (Miles, Chapman, & Sindberg, 2006; Robin, Chapman,& Warren, 2008; Thodardotter, Chapman, & Wagner, 2002). The finding of shorter mean length of utterance is probably not only related to difficulties with syntax, but also related to difficulties with speech production, short-term memory, as well as difficulty encoding the language message (Chapman & Hesketh, 2001, 2000; Fidler, Most, & Philofsky, 2009; Jarrold & Baddeley, 2002a, 2002b; Kanno & Ikeda, 2002; Kumin, 2012). School performance is based on language; for learning, for following instructions, and for interacting with other children and teachers and school staff. Thus, having difficulty with language presents many problems for children with Down syndrome during the school years (Kumin, 2001, 2012).

Semantics

Researchers find that vocabulary development and the words included in the early vocabularies of children with Down syndrome are similar to those of typically developing children (Cardoso-Martins, Mervis, & Mervis, 1985; Gillham, 1979; Kumin, Council, & Goodman, 1998, 1999; Mervis, 1997), but that there is a slower rate of development (Cardoso-Martins et al., 1985; Kumin et al., 1998, 1999; Miller, 1995). There is also wide variability in vocabulary development in children with Down syndrome, ranging from rates of vocabulary growth consistent with mental age (Kumin, Council, & Goodman,

1998, 1999; Miller, 1995) to severe delays in vocabulary development.

When young children use their first spoken or signed word, they show that they can connect a symbol with an object, person, or event. There is no definitive research finding related to the age of use of the first sign or first word. The literature documents a wide range of first spoken words in young children with Down syndrome. Gillham cites the first spoken word at an average age of 18 months in children with Down syndrome (Gillham, 1979). Although other researchers have found a range from 1 to 5 years for the first spoken word. However, children with Down syndrome are often able to sign vocabulary words to identify toys or people, and to make requests before 12 months of age (Buckley, 2000; Buckley & Bird, 2001; Kumin, 2012; Kumin, Goodman, & Councill, 1991).

In the area of semantics, there have been a variety of research approaches used. Studies of semantic development in children with Down syndrome match experimental and control groups by chronological age, mental age, linguistic age, or mean length of utterance (MLU). Chronological age (CA) and mental age (MA) matching both generally show delays in vocabulary development for children with Down syndrome, though MA is a better predictor of vocabulary development level. Studies that match by linguistic age or mean length of utterance (length of average output) generally get results that show vocabulary development level in children with Down syndrome closer to the matched group. Miller (1987) studied expressive vocabulary in children with Down syndrome 2 to 12.5 years (CA) and typically developing children matched by mental age or MLU using a 30-minute language sample taken while the children were conversing with a parent. Results showed that when children were matched by MA, children with Down syndrome produced fewer different words than children with typical development, but when children were matched by MLU, children with Down syndrome produced significantly more different words. This may be reflective of findings that suggest that syntactic development and MLU are areas of greater difficulty for children with Down syndrome than their cognitive level would suggest. Matching by MLU would therefore be sampling children who are at a more advanced language level than matching by mental age. A classic study by Rondal (1988), which matched children with Down syndrome and children with typical development by linguistic stage, found that children with Down syndrome had a broader vocabulary and used a greater number of different words than typically developing children who were at that same linguistic stage. Because children with Down syndrome were older at each linguistic stage, Rondal felt that the results reflected the influence of life experience.

Typically developing children combine words into two-word phrases when they have a 50-word vocabulary at an average age of 19 months to 2 years of age. When do children with Down syndrome shift from single-word to multiword utterance usage? In children with Down syndrome, multiword utterances usually occur later and when children have larger single-word vocabularies. Rondal (1988) documented the use of multiword utterances at ages 4 to 5, Buckley at 3 years (Buckley, 2000), and Kumin, Councill, and Goodman (1998) between ages 4 and 5 years. Though typically developing children combine words when they have a 50-word vocabulary, there is a wider range of ages when children with Down syndrome begin to combine words. Buckley reported a range of 21 words to 109 words, with an average of approximately 100 single words before children begin to combine those words into 2 word phrases (Buckley, 1993). Kumin et al. (1998) found significant expressive vocabulary growth in children with Down syndrome from ages 1 to 8 years; however, there was a great deal of variability and a wide range of expressive vocabulary usage. Miller (1988) also noted variability and found that although some children with Down syndrome were delayed in lexical development, others were using the same average number of words as typically developing children.

Syntax

Morphosyntax, including word roots, prefixes, suffixes, word order, and sentence composition, are difficult areas for children with Down syndrome. They have greater difficulty in developing prepositions and connectives and other function words (Fowler, 1990; Kumin, Councill, & Goodman, 1998, 1999; Miller, 1987, 1988). Fowler (1990, 1995) believes that a specific deficit in syntax learning based on underlying sequencing difficulties is a major language learning problem in children with Down syndrome but Chapman and her colleagues have noted that morphosyntax keeps improving and that adults are capable of producing complex sentences in their narratives (Miles, Chapman, & Sindberg, 2006; Robin, Chapman,& Warren, 2008; Thodardotter, Chapman,& Wagner, 2002) It is also possible that syntax presents more difficulty because it is more abstract, or because word endings such as suffixes and verb tense markers tend to be said with decreased volume, making it more difficult for children to hear these word endings (Kumin, 2012). Grammatical markers and word order become a concern when children are using longer, more complex utterances, and more complex utterances are more difficult for children with Down syndrome, so there may be multiple reasons why morphosyntax is a difficult area of language for individuals with Down syndrome. Researchers have not found definitive conclusions that can lead us to appropriate assessment and treatment strategies. There is a need for further research.

What has been identified as a vocabulary delay in children with Down syndrome may be affected by the specific difficulties in learning vocabulary words with grammatical meanings. Kumin et al. (1998) found a significant difference between the expressive vocabulary usage of referential vocabulary words (labels) and grammatical vocabulary words. Children with Down syndrome use significantly more labels than grammatical classification terms. Grammatical and morphosyntactic markers are not used by the majority of children with Down syndrome until at least age 5. Some children with Down syndrome use plurals between ages 4 and 5, but even at age 5 they are not routinely using plurals. Because plural usage is documented through speech, this finding may also be related to phonological and articulatory development. Whether the child uses final consonant deletion and whether the child can produce the /s/ and /z/ sound in the final position in words can impact on whether the child is perceived, during testing, to use plurals in speech. In analyzing expressive speech, we judge whether children are using plurals by whether they include a final /s/ (as in tops), final /z/ (as in cars), or final /ez/ (as in houses). Perhaps they are trying to use plurals, but because they leave out or cannot say certain final consonants, we assume that they are not using the plural marker. Though children can remember and talk about a past event between ages 3 and 4, 77% are still not using past-tense morphosyntactic markers (e.g., *ed*) by age 5 (Kumin et al., 1998). The concept of possession is mastered several years before children begin to use possessive markers (e.g., *'s*). Children with Down syndrome appear to understand concepts related to past, future, and possession, but do not use grammatical markers expressively to mark these concepts until much later. There is a need for further research in the area of syntax in children with Down syndrome.

Pragmatics

Pragmatics and social interactive language are strengths for children with Down syndrome. Though they may have difficulty with specific pragmatics skills, children with Down syndrome seek social interactions and use gestures (e.g., waving, high 5) and facial expressions (e.g., smiling and frowning) to enhance their verbal language. In fact, most research on pragmatics in children with Down syndrome compares social interactive language in children with Down syndrome, autism spectrum disorders, and fragile X syndrome, and finds that individuals with Down syndrome are more advanced than the other populations. But, because the results are based on comparisons of the three groups, rather than separate analyses, they probably overestimate the pragmatic skills of individuals with Down syndrome, that is, they confuse sociability with social skills. Mundy, Sigman,

Kasari, and Yirmiya (1988) found that young children with Down syndrome show strength in nonverbal social inter-actional skills. Thus, though we may need to teach them "how to" use language in certain situations, children with Down syndrome "want to" interact and com-municate with others (sociability). Chil-dren with Down syndrome generally use gestures appropriately. Attwood (1988) found that children with Down syndrome also respond appropriately to instrumen-tal gestures (e.g., come here). But, children with Down syndrome may need help in learning how to make requests (Attwood, 1988; Mundy et al., 1988). Research shows that children with Down syndrome learn and respond well to social scripts (Kumin, 2010; Kumin, Goodman, & Councill, 2010; Loveland & Tunali, 1991). Because many conversational interactions are repeated over and over again in daily life (e.g., greetings, answering a telephone), chil-dren with Down syndrome can learn and practice these skills as social scripts. So, pragmatics is a relatively strong area for most children with Down syndrome when compared to other language areas, but children have more difficulty with advanced pragmatics skills. The areas of difficulty are generally those that involve the use of figurative and abstract language such as conversational skills, narrative discourse, or metalinguistic (language analysis) skills (Kumin, 2010; Kumin, Goodman, & Councill, 2010).

When young children with Down syndrome have great difficulty with social language interactions, further test-ing is indicated. The American Academy of Pediatrics reports that 1% of children with Down syndrome have co-occurring autism, but some researchers have esti-mated the co-occurrence as high as 10% (Bull & The Committee on Genetics, 2011;

Capone, 2002; Capone et al., 2005, 2006, 2007; Carter et al., 2007; Kent, Evans, Paul, & Sharp, 1999). This group may experi-ence difficulty with pragmatic language and social interaction skills. Autism is discussed in detail in a separate chapter of this book.

Speech Development

Research on early sound production dem-onstrates similar patterns of development for vowels and consonants during the first 15 months of age, and similar sounds in babbling and the occurrence of redupli-cated canonical babbling for children with Down syndrome and typically developing children. Emergence of phonemes in chil-dren with Down syndrome in their early language productions follows a definite order, but there is a wide range of age of emergence, from 10 months to 8 years of age (Kumin, Councill, & Goodman, 1994).

There are many factors that influence speech production ability. Young children with Down syndrome often have fluid in the ear (estimates of 50–70% of the popu-lation), with fluctuating hearing loss that will affect speech sound development (Bull & The Committee on Genetics, 2011; Kumin, 2012; Shott, 2006). Difficulty with phonemic processing and sequencing will affect auditory discrimination and production of sounds (Fowler, 1990; Jar-rold & Baddeley, 2002). Hypotonia (i.e., low muscle tone) will affect the precision and accuracy of speech sound produc-tion, as well as voice, resonance, and flu-ency (Kumin, 2012, 2014a; Leddy, 1999; Rosenfeld-Johnson, 1999). Children with Down syndrome often have difficulty with planning and sequencing motor movements (i.e., developmental apraxia of speech), which affects consistency and accuracy of speech production, especially as words and phrases increase in length (Kumin, 2005, 2006b, 2014a; Kumin & Adams, 2000). In almost all children with Down syndrome, speech is affected, and in many children, difficulty with speech intelligibility is a problem (Kumin, 1994, 2000, 2006a, 2012). The physical findings (both anatomical and physiological) and the difficulty with neuromotor and neurosensory function result in combinations of symptoms that directly affect speech. For example, low muscle tone and mouth breathing related to swollen tonsils and adenoids result in open mouth posture, which will affect articulation (e.g., the child's ability to produce the /s/ and /z/ sounds correctly).

Articulation and Phonology

Producing correct sounds and sound combinations in speech is often difficult for children with Down syndrome, and they often continue to use phonological processes, the simplification rules that children use as they learn speech sounds, longer than other children. Dodd (1976) reported that children with Down syndrome show twice as many articulation errors and almost twice as many inconsistent substitutions as children with ID due to other causes, matched for mental age. Rosin, Swift, Bless, and Vetter (1988) found that consonant articulation at the word level shows significantly more errors for adolescents with Down syndrome than other adolescents with ID. Stoel-Gammon (1980, 1997, 2001) has described the phonological patterns observed and has noted more articulation errors in conversation than in isolated sound production.

The most frequent phonological process (i.e., simplification rule) used by individuals with Down syndrome from ages 13 to 22 is final consonant deletion,

followed by consonant cluster reduction (Sommers, Patterson, & Wildgen, 1988). Initial cluster reduction and stopping are also used by younger children with Down syndrome, ages 3 to 4.6 (Bleile & Schwartz, 1984). More phonological processes are used as the length and complexity of the speech output increase, that is, more phonological processes are used in connected language samples than in picture naming or imitative naming (Sommers et al., 1988). Phonological processes are used beyond the expected age by children with Down syndrome (Bleile, 1982; Stoel-Gammon, 2001, 1997). At ages 1.5 to 2, children with Down syndrome and typically developing children showed no significant qualitative or quantitative differences in phonological processes used, but by age 4, the children with Down syndrome showed quantitative differences, that is, they continued to use phonological processes at about the level of the typically developing child ages 2 to 2.5 (Smith & Stoel-Gammon, 1983). The most frequent phonological processes used by children with Down syndrome are:

- Final consonant deletion (saying "boo" for "boot")
- Consonant cluster reduction (saying "gas" for "glass")
- Stopping (saying "toup" for "soup")
- Fronting (saying "doe" for "go")
- Backing (saying "ko" for "toe")
- Weak syllable deletion (saying "nanas" for "bananas")

Speech Intelligibility

Intelligibility of speech is a major problem for children with Down syndrome. Rosin et al. (1988) found that adolescents with Down syndrome had more difficulty with intelligibility of speech than a matched group of adolescents with ID due to other etiologies.

Speech intelligibility is defined as how clearly a person speaks so that his or her speech is comprehensible to a listener (Kumin, 2000, 2006b, 2012, 2014a; Leddy, 1999). The presence of difficulties with speech intelligibility in children with Down syndrome is cited in the research literature in clinical reports (Chapman et al., 1995, 1998; Horstmeier, 1988; Miller, Leddy, & Leavitt, 1999; Swift & Rosin, 1990; Rosin et al., 1988; Swift & Rosin, 1990) and in surveys of families (Kumin, 1994). In the classic survey study of 937 families (Kumin, 1994), over 95% of the respondents reported that their children had difficulty being understood by people outside of their immediate circle sometimes or frequently. When the age groups were examined individually, in every age group, over 50% of the parents indicated that the children had difficulty with intelligibility of speech frequently. Only approximately 5% of parents reported that their children rarely or never had difficulty in being understood. Speech intelligibility is a widespread problem in children with Down syndrome. Anatomical and physiological factors, neurofunctional patterns, and perceptual symptoms contribute to difficulty in speech intelligibility for individuals with Down syndrome (Kumin, 2001b, 2006a).

Anatomical and Physiological Factors

Clinicians and researchers note anatomical and physiological differences in individuals with Down syndrome that make speech difficult (Miller & Leddy, 1999; Miller, Leddy, & Leavitt, 1999). Structural differences such as a high narrow palatal arch, irregular dentition and an open bite, or a relatively large tongue (in relation to the size of the upper and lower jaw) contribute to difficulties with speech. Physiological differences such as low tone in the oral facial muscles and lax ligaments in the temporomandibular joint play a role. Hypotonia (low muscle tone) contributes to difficulty in articulation. Most children with Down syndrome also have a history of otitis media with effusion, which affects phonetic processing as the child is learning language.

Hearing and Auditory Skills

The incidence of both conductive and sensorineural hearing loss is increased in individuals with Down syndrome (Bull & The Committee on Genetics, 2011; Roizen et al., 1992; Shott, 2000, 2006; Shott, Joseph, & Heithaus, 2001). Children with Down syndrome have a history of persistent otitis media with effusion and fluctuating hearing loss (Shott, 2000). Hearing aids, assistive listening devices, and classroom amplification systems can help. Children with Down syndrome also have greater difficulties with auditory-motor and auditory-vocal processing than with visual-motor and visual-vocal processing (Hopmann & Wilen, 1993; Pueschel, Gallagher, Zastler, & Pezzulo, 1987). Their visual-motor skills are relatively strong and they learn best through the visual channel. These differences between auditory and visual skills should be considered when planning educational and treatment programs (Buckley, 1986, 2000; Kumin, 2012).

Neurofunctional Patterns

Neurofunctional patterns will have an effect on production of the sounds of speech, as well as on respiration, voice, resonance, and fluency. Problems with any of these areas can impact on speech intelligibility. Oral motor problems, such as dysarthria, affect the strength and precision of muscle movement, resulting in speech that sounds thickened or imprecise. When muscle function is affected, the problem is consistent for all of the activities that would involve that muscle, so if lip muscles are affected, eating and keeping the lips closed would be affected as well as speech sound production (Kumin, 2014a).

Developmental apraxia of speech (DAS), or any other synonymous label, describes an inability of a child to voluntarily program, combine, organize, and sequence movements necessary for speech tasks (Kumin, 2001b, 2002, 2006b). Historically, children with Down syndrome have been excluded from such studies. This is because the original researchers who defined developmental apraxia of speech included in their studies only subjects who met the following criteria: normal intelligence, absence of hearing loss, and absence of muscle weakness or paralysis. Their results and definitions of DAS were not generalized beyond the original subject groups. Children with Down syndrome frequently have hearing loss (Bull & The Committee on Genetics, 2011; Roizen et al., 1992; Shott, 2000; Shott, 2006), mild to moderate intellectual disability (Bull & The Committee on Genetics, 2011; Cohen, 1999), and low muscle tone (Bull & The Committee on Genetics, 2011; Pueschel et al., 1987; Winders, 2014). Without the diagnosis being made, assessment and treatment programs have generally failed to address the motor-planning difficulties that are experienced by many children with Down syndrome (Kumin, 2001a, 2006b, 2012). Rosin and Swift (1999), writing about planning treatment for Jay, a young man with Down syndrome, state:

There are aspects of Jay's speech that are consistent with characteristics reported for children with developmental apraxia of speech. . . . Regardless of whether the diagnosis of developmental apraxia of speech is appropriate for Jay, associated therapy techniques can be applied to his intervention. (p. 144)

Some current definitions of motor-planning difficulties are beginning to include children with Down syndrome within the populations that experience motor-planning disorders. A study by Kumin and Adams (2000) documented that seven children with difficulties with speech intelligibility who were tested with the Apraxia Profile demonstrated test results indicative of DAS. There is a rich body of treatment literature for children with DAS that can and should be used to help children with Down syndrome who have difficulty with motor planning.

Voice

Voice production may be affected in several ways. Researchers report hoarse and breathy voice quality in some children with Down syndrome. The volume of the voice may be too loud, too soft, inconsistent, and uncontrolled, or inappropriate to the occasion (e.g., screaming in school). Often this is not due to respiratory or voice production difficulties, but is related to the child's lack of awareness of volume. Some children shout and misuse their voice (vocal abuse). Resonance patterns vary. Some children are hyponasal. They sound as if they have a cold all of the time. This is often due to swollen tonsils and adenoids. Other children are hypernasal. This is often due to a high palatal vault, short palate, or weak muscles in the palate and pharyngeal wall (velopharyngeal insufficiency). A comprehensive medical ENT (ear, nose, and throat) evaluation to examine causes for some of these conditions is always needed before a speech assessment and before a treatment plan is developed.

Fluency

Stuttering or dysfluency is more prevalent in people with Down syndrome (Bray, 2007; Fawcett & Virij-Babul, 2006; Fidler, Most, & Philosky, 2009; Kumin, 2012). Incidence of stuttering is estimated at 45% to 53% in individuals with Down syndrome (Devenny & Silverman, 1990; Fawcett & Virji-Babul, 2006). Results of parent surveys indicate that parents report that their children have difficulty with stuttering (Kumin, 1994). Sometimes there is fluency difficulty as the child is developing language. But, more frequently, the fluency difficulty does not become evident until the child is using longer phrases and sentences and more complex language output. Devenny and Silverman (1990) suggest that there is a breakdown of the neural organization of speech at the consonant level, which results in verbal fluency difficulties. Elliott and colleagues hypothesize that there is a dissociation between right hemisphere speech perception and left hemisphere speech production in individuals with Down syndrome, which makes it difficult for them to complete any task that involves both speech perception and production (Elliott, Weeks, & Elliot, 1987; Heath & Elliott, 1999; Weeks, Chua, & Elliott, 2000), and affects the ability to produce fluent speech (Heath & Elliot, 1999).Van Borsel suggests that the dysfluency is more representative of a pattern of

cluttering (Van Borsel, 2008). There is no general agreement among researchers and clinicians as to whether the fluency difficulty is based on motor performance difficulty or on language load and complexity. Clinically, we are able to document that the fluency patterns that we are seeing in children with Down syndrome (ages 7–15) present the same characteristics as stuttering seen in younger typically developing children. Stuttering is one condition that affects the smooth flow of speech. Prosody is the general term for the rhythm of speech output. Prosody includes pitch and inflection. It includes whether the voice goes up at the end of the sentence for a question or down for a statement. Children with Down syndrome may have a rapid rate, a slow rate, or an uneven and changing rate of speech. Prosody and rate patterns are not well documented in the literature.

Overview of Team Approaches to Assessment and Intervention

Difficulties with speech and language are affected by difficulties with sensory processing, low muscle tone, hearing loss, short-term memory, and other. Because of the complex interaction of these difficulties and their effect on language and speech development and skills, there is a need for a multidisciplinary team approach. Because the therapy needs will be ongoing and will affect function in daily life, the family should always be included in the team. As previously discussed, speech is an output system, but, in order for speech to develop, there must be well-functioning sensory input systems, such as vision and hearing, and adequate sensory processing skills. Vision and hearing must be tested and monitored frequently.

In infancy, difficulty with feeding is often noted (Bull & The Committee on Genetics, 2011; Medlen, 2006). Because feeding uses the same structures and many of the same muscles as speech, early intervention for feeding can help develop the mechanism that will be used later in development for speech (Kumin & Bahr, 1999). The family provides speech and language stimulation at home, and can provide practice as well as feedback. There needs to be a close working relationship between families and SLPs (Kumin, 1994, 2012). In infancy and toddlerhood, members of the team might include:

- Speech-language pathologist
- Occupational therapist
- Feeding specialist
- Sensory processing disorder specialist
- Audiologist
- Family
- Pediatrician
- ENT (otorhinolaryngologist)

Most young children with Down syndrome will be ready to use language before they are able to speak. The SLP and family may want to consult with an augmentative communication (AAC) or assistive technology specialist, in order to design an effective sign language, picture board, communication app, or high-technology communication system to help the child continue to communicate during the period when he or she is learning speech. During the school years, the regular education teacher, special education teacher, and school administrators would be part of the planning team. An individualized education plan (IEP) would be developed for the child, which would include school-based speech-language pathology treatment. According to IDEA,

speech-language pathology services in the schools are designed to help children make progress in the regular educational curriculum. Criteria for eligibility for school services focus on providing access to the curriculum. Children with Down syndrome may need to continue to receive services outside the school environment through medical and rehabilitation centers, universities, and private practices, in addition to school services, in order to address all of their communication needs.

Psychosocial Issues— Functioning in the Home and Community Environments

There has been a revolution in the field of ID in the past 25 years. Federal legislation in the United States now mandates that a free, appropriate public education be provided for every child, including children with special needs. More and more children with Down syndrome are being included in regular education classrooms during all or part of the school day. Children in special education are being integrated with other children for lunch, recess, music, art, and other school activities. Children are being included in the community in scouting, religious activities, and other community events. These activities present many opportunities for speech and language practice and growth. But there are major differences in the opportunities for inclusion from state to state county to county, and country to country. Research in the United States and the United Kingdom has documented that inclusion (aka mainstream education) positively affects language and social skills (Buckley, Bird, & Sacks, 2006; Buckley, Bird, Sacks, & Archer, 2006; Guralnick, 1995). In adulthood, individuals with

Down syndrome are living with support or independently in community settings, and working within the community in supported or competitive employment settings. In adulthood, communication abilities, especially speech intelligibility, impact on employment opportunities and on the quality of life (Kumin, 2012).

Speech and Language Skills: Evaluation and Treatment for Children with Down Syndrome

Children with Down syndrome have individual and complicated patterns of strengths and challenges related to communication, language, and speech. There are no evaluation methods or test instruments that are designed specifically for children with Down syndrome. The following discussion, while focusing on children with Down syndrome, could apply to children with ID due to other causes. Evaluation and treatment are part of the same process leading to more effective functional speech and language skills and evaluation needs to be an ongoing process in order to ensure that treatment meets the child's current communication needs. The speech and language evaluation should be the first step in the treatment planning process. The evaluation should clearly describe the child's communication and explore the best channels and approaches for that child, so that treatment can be planned to address any difficulties that a given child is experiencing. The purpose of a speech and language evaluation is to get an accurate picture of the child's present communication function in daily living activities, including those in the home, school, and community. The instruments that are chosen will vary depending on the cognitive level of the child, as well as

whether the child is using speech, sign language, picture communication systems, or other forms of assistive technology. The evaluation should document the speech and language skills that the child has mastered and those that are difficult for her or him. This is difficult to accomplish when testing individuals with Down syndrome because:

- They may have difficulty following test instructions because of auditory or visual processing problems.
- They may have difficulty responding to questions if speech is the response mode on the test.
- They may have difficulty generalizing their skills from a real-life situation to a testing situation.
- They may not perform well with an unfamiliar examiner in an unfamiliar situation
- There is a wide range of communication abilities in children with Down syndrome. Some children may be speaking in sentences and participating in complex conversations, whereas other children will be nonverbal or at a one- or two-word level.

These factors make it very important to collaborate with families to get a more accurate picture of the child's functional communication abilities (Kumin & Mason, 2011; Miller, Sedey, & Miolo, 1995). The SLP can request that the family bring video or audiotapes to the evaluation to assist in assessing the child's communication patterns at home. Informal assessment techniques that involve the family can provide valuable information. Checklists such as the MacArthur-Bates Communicative Development Inventories (2007) can be used to help the parents document the child's communication abilities in the home and community setting. Observations of parents and their child communicating (preferably observation through a one-way mirror) may be part of the assessment. If possible, speech and language evaluation should be conducted over several sessions in a familiar environment with familiar people. Research has shown that the testing performance of a child with a language disorder is affected by whether the child knows the person doing the evaluation. Studies have shown that children with communication difficulties perform more poorly with unfamiliar examiners than with familiar examiners (Fuchs, Fuchs, Power, & Dailey, 1985). Expressive language is especially affected when the setting or examiners are unfamiliar.

In children with Down syndrome, there are usually difficulties in multiple systems that impact on speech and language (Cleland, Wood, Hardcastle, Wishart, & Timmins, 2010; Timmins et al., 2009). Children with Down syndrome may have difficulty with sensory reception, processing, and memory (visual, auditory, tactile), as well as oral motor, oral motor sequencing, language encoding, and word retrieval (Cleland et al., 2009; Kumin, 1996, 2012, 2014a, 2014b, 2014c; Nash & Snowling, 2008). They may also have difficulty with respiration, phonation, resonance, and articulation, which will affect speech and speech intelligibility (Barnes et al., 2009; Cleland et al., 2009; Dodd & Thompson, 2001; Kumin, 2000; Nash & Snowling, 2008; Roberts et al., 2005; Timmins et al., 2010). A comprehensive speech and language evaluation should include assessment of oral motor, speech, receptive and expressive language, and pragmatics skills (Kumin, 1999, 2012).

For infants and toddlers, feeding evaluation and sensory processing evaluation may be done by speech-language pathologists with advanced specialty training, or by occupational therapists, feeding therapists, neurodevelopmental specialists, or sensory processing disorder specialists with advanced specialty training in these areas. This information is essential to plan appropriate and effective treatment programs. For school-age children, evaluation should also include assessment of language and literacy skills (Buckley, 2001; Buckley, Bird & Byrne, 1996), as well as curriculum-based language skills (Kumin, 2001, 2008). Referrals should be made for audiological evaluation and otolaryngological evaluation (ENT). Referrals for neurological evaluation and evaluation of sensory processing skills should be made as needed.

An evaluation should include:

1. Case history
2. Observation of family and child interacting and communicating
3. Family interview
4. Play or conversation (as appropriate for age and developmental level)
5. Formal testing
6. Informal testing
7. Consultation with family
8. Written diagnostic report

The following speech and language skills should be evaluated through case history, observation, and/or testing, for all children with Down syndrome at that stage of development. Information on associated areas, such as audiological status and sensory processing skills, should be evaluated by specialists through referral, and considered when designing the speech and language treatment plan.

During the period from birth to when the child is able to use single words to communicate, evaluation should include assessment of:

- Prespeech skills
  1. Respiration
  2. Feeding
  3. Oral motor skills
- Pragmatics skills
- Prelanguage skills
- Receptive language skills
- Expressive language skills

The above areas can be assessed by the SLP using case history information, observation, and formal and informal testing. For example, it can be observed whether the infant makes requests, and how those requests are made. Does the infant point or look at the object, make grunting noises, say an approximation of the word, or actually say the word? Family reports can help to corroborate the observation. A battery such as the MacArthur Communicative Development Inventory (a parent survey) can be used to document the communication requesting behavior. A test such as the Communication and Symbolic Behavior Scale, which has items designed to elicit requesting behaviors, can be used to assess the infant-toddler. The Rossetti Infant-Toddler Scale can be used to assess communicative behaviors, and parent-infant interaction. This assessment instrument provides for scoring to be based on observed, elicited, or reported behaviors resulting in scores that reflect the child's daily functional level in multiple settings and at multiple times, in addition to performance during the testing session. The Receptive-Expressive Emergent Language Scale (REEL) may be used to structure a comprehensive parent inter-view to assess communication function in the home environment. Consultations with occupational therapists, audiologists, otolaryngologists, and pediatricians may be indicated to determine sensory skills and hearing status. This information will be essential for appropriate treatment planning.

During the period when the child is using single words through the period when he or she is using multiword utterances, the child's skills in vocabulary, pragmatics, oral motor, and articulation/phonology should be determined. Mean length of utterance should be determined using a language sample. There is no formal test designed for children with Down syndrome so language tests developed for typically developing children will be used. There are currently no test norms developed for children with Down syndrome, so scoring is based on norms representing development in typical children. Tests used during this period may include the current versions of the Preschool Language Scale (PLS), Communication and Symbolic Behavior Scale, Clinical Evaluation of Language Function-Preschool (CELF-Preschool), Hawaii Early Learning Profile, Mac Arthur Communicative Development Inventory, Sequenced Inventory of Communication Development (Revised), Test of Early Language Development, Goldman-Fristoe Test of Articulation, Khan-Lewis Phonological Analysis, Peabody Picture Vocabulary Test, Receptive One-Word Picture Vocabulary Test, and the Expressive One-Word Picture Vocabulary Test. Hearing status and sensory processing skills should be monitored through consultation with specialists as during the earlier period.

During the preschool through kindergarten years, the child with Down syndrome is often speaking in multiword utterances, phrases, and short sentences. Morphosyntax and narrative discourse skills are usually not yet mastered and would be difficult to test at this stage because of difficulties with expressive language, as well as speech intelligibility. Areas assessed should include receptive language skills, expressive language skills, vocabulary, concept development (colors, shapes, and other early learning skills), pragmatics skills, and speech skills, including articulation, oral motor skills, and speech intelligibility. The tests cited above can also be used during the preschool and kindergarten years.

During the elementary and middle school years, children will have a wide range of functional communication abilities, as well as a variety of school experiences. Some children will be included in the regular education classroom, receiving any special education services within the classroom. Other children will be split between a regular classroom and a resource room for special help during the day. Others will be in a special education classroom with children who have a variety of disabilities. Still others will be in a special education classroom designed exclusively for children with ID. Other children will be in a separate special education school. Testing during the school years should include assessment of:

- Receptive language skills
  1. Comprehension
  2. Semantics
  3. Morphology/Syntax
- Expressive language skills
  1. Semantics
  2. Morphology
  3. Syntax
  4. Mean length of utterance

- Pragmatics skills
  1. Social interactive skills
  2. Communication activities of daily living
  3. Requests
  4. Narrative discourse skills
  5. Clarification strategies/repairs
- Educational Language Skills
  1. Language of the Curriculum
  2. Language of Instruction in the Classroom
  3. Language of the Hidden Curriculum
  4. Language of Testing
  5. Language of Classroom Routines
  6. Social Interactive Communication
- Speech skills
  1. Articulation
  2. Phonological processes
  3. Speech Intelligibility
  4. Oral motor skills
  5. Motor planning skills
  6. Voice
  7. Resonance
  8. Fluency

Communication needs and communication skills are different in infancy, toddlerhood, childhood, adolescence, and adulthood. This is true for everyone, including people with ID. For people with Down syndrome who often experience difficulties with speech and language skills, it is essential to consider how to help them develop effective communication skills that will meet their needs at all ages and stages of life. Treatment planning for children with Down syndrome and children with ID due to other causes should focus on the child's short-term communication needs for school and daily living as well as long-term considerations for functional communication in school and later in the workplace and the community.

From what we know now, there is going to be a wide range of communication abilities in people with Down syndrome. We do not want to limit any child. For most toddlers and young children, assistive communication systems (e.g., sign language) will be needed to support communication until and while the young children are learning to speak, but the need will fade as speech develops and improves. There is no hard and fast rule as to how far any individual child will progress. We need to learn more about the population, but focus on the individual so that we can maximize communication abilities and help each child reach her or his potential.

For some children and adults with Down syndrome, speech that can be easily understood is a reality by later childhood and adolescence. For some children and adults, complex language that is able to convey and support the rich experiences of daily living is a reality. They are able to have long conversations and are able to clearly tell about an event they attended or a book they read. Some children and adolescents have short MLUs and short conversations with only two or three conversational turns. For other children, their speech is difficult to understand and they need assistance in communication. For a small number of individuals, assistive communication systems and devices (AAC) will be needed to serve as their primary communication system to enable them to communicate effectively. Treatment programs must therefore be based on ongoing evaluation of the communication needs and communication skills of the individual child (Kumin, 2008, 2012).

In the 1950s and 1960s when many individuals with Down syndrome lived in institutions, there was little or no for- mal speech-language pathology services. With the passage of Public Law 94-142 in 1975, speech-language pathology services could be written into the IEP plan for school-aged children. During that period, treatment for children with Down syndrome involved general language stimulation. Behavior modification methods were often used. Early intervention services did not begin until the passage of PL 99-457 in 1986 when states were provided with the opportunity to apply for grants to develop programs for children from birth to 3 years of age. Treatment targeting speech, early language intervention, feeding therapy, prespeech activities, and oral motor treatment began to be used. But, even now, some school systems do not include speech-language pathology services in early intervention; some include evaluation, but not treatment. Some systems provide testing at age 3 years but delay direct SLP services until beyond 3. All services, according to the law, need to be planned individually for the child based on his or her needs, but that is not always the case.

The Individuals with Disabilities Education Act (IDEA 2004) provides mandates for special education and related services (SLP is considered a related service) and is the current federal legislation that guides the IEP process.

Inclusion in education and in community life is fairly recent, beginning with supports available through PL 94-142 and continuing through IDEA 2004. We have barely had one full generation of individuals with Down syndrome who have had the benefits of a comprehensive approach to speech and language development from early intervention through inclusion and special education and related services in elementary, middle, and high school. Some adolescents and adults are now attending specially designed post-secondary programs at community colleges and universities. We cannot predict how far people can go, with the benefits of early stimulation, treatment to support oral motor skills and speech development, transitional communication systems, improved educational opportunities, improved employment opportunities, and a wide range of social and recreational opportunities in the community.

Treatment

There are many different approaches to speech and language treatment that can be used, sometimes simultaneously, as part of a comprehensive individually designed program. In early intervention, feeding therapy, stimulation of communicative intent and other language precursors, and oral motor treatment is begun. Sign language, picture communication, or a low-tech or high-tech transitional communication system is introduced at about 8 months to 12 months of age once the child has mastered the prelanguage skills. Providing a transitional communication system is very important until the child is neurophysiologically able to speak (Kumin, 2012). Though speech is the most difficult communication system for children with Down syndrome, over 95% of children with Down syndrome will use speech as their primary communication system. Total communication (use of sign language plus speech) (Thompson, Cotnoir-Bichelman, McKerchar, & Dancho, 2007; Toth, 2009), communication boards, the Picture Exchange Communication System (PECS) (Bondy & Frost, 2001), communication apps for the iPad, Smartphones, or high tech communication devices may be used as communication systems until the child is ready and able to transition to speech (Green, 2011). A transitional communication system enables the child to continue to progress in language while not yet able to speak, and provides a means of communicating with others to prevent frustration (Kumin, 2012; Kumin et al., 1991; Toth, 2009). Combinations of systems can be used. For example, a child might learn to sign "juice" but when you and he are at the refrigerator door, you might have three picture magnets on the refrigerator with orange, apple, and grape juice, and the child might use the magnet pictures as a communication board. Parents often fear that using sign- or a picture-based communication system will slow their child's progress toward speech. This has not been found to be true. Actually, the opposite is true. Research has shown that children with Down syndrome will discontinue using the sign when they can say the word so that it is understandable to those around them (Beukelman & Mirenda, 1998; Light & Binger, 1998).

The young child with Down syndrome is usually far more advanced in receptive language skills than in expressive language skills, but both areas are usually targeted in therapy. Receptive language therapy may focus on auditory memory and on following directions, which are important skills for the early school years. It will also focus on concept development such as colors, shapes, directions (top and bottom), and prepositions through practice and play experiences. Expressive language therapy may include semantics and expanding the mean length of utterance, and will begin to include grammatical structures (word order) and word endings (such as plural or possessive). Once the young child begins to use single words (in sign or speech), treatment will proceed to stimulate both horizontal and vertical growth in language. Treatment may address single-word vocabulary (semantic skills) in many thematic and whole language activities, such as cooking, crafts, play, and trips. Thus there may be a great deal of horizontal vocabulary growth. Treatment will also target increasing the length of phrases and the combinations of words that the child can use (vertical development); this is known as increasing the mean length of utterance. There are many meaningful relations that the child learns in two-word phrases (e.g., agent-action, posses-sion, negation), and then further expands into three-word phrases. We have found that a pacing board provides a visual and motoric cueing system that capitalizes on the strengths of children with Down syndrome, and helps children to expand the length of their utterances (Kumin, Councill, & Goodman, 1995). A pacing board is usually a rectangular piece of tag board with separate circles that represent the number of words in the desired utterance (e.g., "throw ball" would have two dots). The pacing system concept can also be implemented by putting a dot under each word in a book as shown in Figure 3–1.

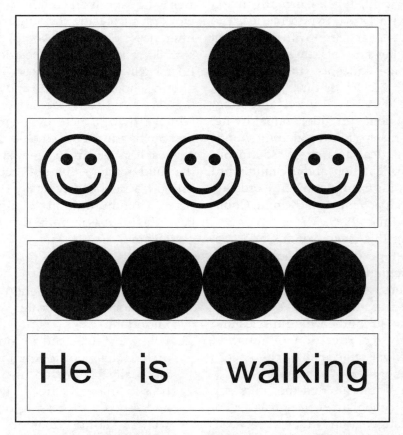

Figure 3–1. Example of 2-word pacing board, 3-word pacing board, and pattern practice pacing board.

Pragmatics skills such as asking for help, appropriate use of greetings, requests for information or answering requests as well as role playing different activities of daily living may be addressed. Again, play activities such as dressing and undressing a doll, crafts activities such as making a card, or cooking activities such as making cupcakes may be used. The same activity may target semantic, syntactic, and pragmatics skills (e.g., how many cupcakes should we make, what color frosting should we use, following the directions to make the cupcakes). Prior to the 1980s, it was considered unlikely or even impossible for children with Down syndrome to read (Buckley,1984; Buckley & Bird, 1993; Elkins & Farrell, 1994). Currently, many children with Down syndrome learn to read effectively at a 3rd to 5th grade level or even higher, and this can help in learning language concepts (Buckley, 1984, 1995, 2012; Buckley & Bird, 1993; Buckley & Buckley, 2011). It also is important for employment and independent living. Reading can help children identify sounds for phonological awareness, sound out words for articulation, and use multiword utterances, for example, when words are used with a pacing board (Kumin, Councill, & Goodman, 1995).

During this stage, sounds and specific sound production would be targeted; articulation therapy could begin. But the therapy would also include oral motor exercises and activities on an ongoing basis to strengthen the muscles and improve the coordination of muscles. Intelligibility is the goal of the speech component of therapy.

During the years that the child is in elementary school, there is a great deal of growth in language and in speech. Speech-language treatment may involve collaboration with the teacher and may be based in the classroom. Often, the curriculum becomes the material used for therapy. This makes sense, because school is the child's workplace, and success in school greatly affects self-esteem. Receptive language therapy becomes more detailed and advanced (Kumin, 2001, 2008; Miller, 1988), including following directions with multiple parts, similar to the instructions given in school. Receptive language therapy might include comprehension exercises, reading and experiential activities, and specific comprehension of vocabulary, morphology, and syntax. Ex-pressive language therapy focuses on more advanced topics in vocabulary, similarities and differences, morphology, and syntax. Expressive language work might also include work on increasing the length of speech utterances. The pacing board, re-hearsal, scaffolds, and scripts have been found helpful in facilitating longer speech utterances.

In school, both inside and outside of the classroom (bus, recess, lunch, after-school activities, there are language skills that can be addressed to help a child progress, especially in inclusive settings where the child is interacting with regular education teachers and typically developing peers. Communication skills that have been identified as important to school success in are:

1. Appropriate behavior (This is often related to communication skills. All behavior communicates something important.)
2. Following rules and routines (When a child does not follow the rules, it is usually blamed on his unwillingness to follow the rules. Hearing loss and sensory processing disorder, as well as auditory memory problems are underlying factors that need to be considered.)

3. Flexibility (Is the child able to adapt when rules and situations change, such as during assemblies or fire drills or when he needs to transition from one activity to another—from reading to math or from lunch to physical education.)
    - Able to deviate from routines when necessary, and
    - Able to make transitions.
4. Receptive language skills
    - Has good listening skills,
    - Able to follow teacher instructions,
    - Able to follow long, complex directions, and
    - Able to recognize when there is a communication breakdown and what needs repair.
5. Expressive language skills
    - Able to answer questions
    - Able to ask for help
    - Able to ask questions
    - Able to share information verbally
    - Knows how to introduce and sustain topics
    - Able to request clarification when direction is unclear
    - Able to repair conversational breakdowns
    - Able to change registers to communicate with peers & school personnel (uses language appropriate for the situation).
6. Interpersonal skills
    - Participates in peer routines at lunch, recess, and in class
    - Able to interact verbally and socially with peers
    - Able to interact verbally with adults
    - Able to decode and understand the teacher's nonverbal cues
    - Understands turn-taking rules
    - Takes turns appropriately in conversation

- Knows how to request a turn
- Uses appropriate greetings for different situations
- Focuses attention on speaker/eye contact
- Understands the background that someone brings to communication (knows the level and amount of information the listener needs or the speaker needs to provide)

7. Academic skills
    - Understands the teacher's expectations for performance in an activity
    - Understands the teacher's expectations for the form and complexity of a response
    - Completes assignments well and in a timely manner
    - Uses appropriate learning strategies
    - Uses effective organizational skills
    - Knows test-taking strategies
    - Uses textbooks and reference books effectively

In addition, students need to understand and use the language of the curriculum in classroom, homework, and testing situations. Textbooks and testing procedures rely heavily on language abilities in speaking and writing, listening, and following instructions that are often presented verbally.

Curriculum-based language skills are a focus in therapy. During the school years, there are a variety of approaches that can be used in treatment. Therapy may be programmed based on linguistic skills, that is, there may be individual goals for semantics (vocabulary), morphosyntax (language structure), pragmatics (social language interaction and conversation), and phonology (sounds of the language). This is a bottom-up approach in which the parts are learned and then combined into the whole. So, a therapy objective may be: "Joan will use the correct ending for plurals 80% of the time in sentences," or "Josh will correctly use vocabulary words pertaining to transportation 80% of the time in sentences." Therapy may also focus on different channels. The goals for therapy may target auditory skills or speech and oral motor skills, or encoding a language message, or producing a language message. In general, children with Down syndrome have stronger visual learning skills and more difficulty with auditory learning skills so visual organizers can help them to learn. One channel, such as reading, may be used to assist another channel such as expressive language or written language. Therapy may also be approached through the needs of the curriculum. In this approach, vocabulary would be taught based on the vocabulary that the child needs for success in science or social studies. The therapy may be proactive, teaching in advance the language skills that the child will need for the curriculum, or reactive, targeting areas of difficulty as they occur and providing assistance with study skills and strategies to meet classroom expectations or to overcome difficulties when they occur. The SLP can also suggest adaptive and compensatory strategies such as seating in front of the room, or using a peer tutor, visual cue sheets, and the like (Kumin, 2001a, 2008, 2012).

Language and literacy are often addressed in a combined approach in which reading, understanding, writing, and expressive language are taught as a whole (Buckley, 1995, 2001, 2006, 2012; Buckley & Bird, 1993; Buckley, Bird, & Byrne, 1996). This often is based on children's literature and thematic activities accompanying the books (e.g., a book about weather might also involve weather reporting, building a weather station, drawing pictures or taking photographs of different weather conditions). Meaningful multisensory experiences are used to teach concepts, and the subject matter may be based on the curriculum or on following the child's interests.

Pragmatics becomes very important during this stage; using communication skills in real life in school, at home, and in the community is the goal. Therapy might address social interactive skills with teachers and peers, conversational and narrative discourse skills, how to make requests, how to ask for help to understand material in school, how to clarify what was said when the teacher or other students do not understand what was meant, and so on. As the child matures, the communicative activities of daily living will change. Treatment and/or home practice must keep pace with the child's communication needs at every stage.

Speech skills with emphasis on articulation and intelligibility would be targeted in therapy during this period. An individual analysis of oral motor strengths and challenges is important to determine what specific skills need to be addressed. For example, does the child have low muscle tone or muscle weakness in the oral facial area? Does the child have difficulty with motor coordination? Does the child have difficulty with motor planning? Are other speech areas such as voice and fluency affecting intelligibility? Each of these areas can be worked on if they are impacting on communication ability for an individual child.

The major difference between inclusion in elementary school and middle school is that, in middle school the child must adjust to different teachers, their expectations, and their teaching styles. The IEP can include assistance with these tasks. Reading skills and writing skills need be sufficient to help the student learn the curriculum material. Various organizational supports can be provided through the IEP. One of the areas in which speech-language pathologists can be helpful is in consulting, or collaborating with the classroom teachers. Together they can determine what kinds of adaptations, scaffolds, and learning assistance will enable the adolescent to learn most effectively.

In middle school and high school, the major change is that the student must be able to decode and respond to language from multiple teachers and peers, and use expressive language in a variety of school and community-based situations (Kumin, 2001, 2008, 2012). This can be difficult. The student must be able to follow teacher instructions, which may vary from subject to subject. They must be able to adapt to different expectations of teachers in different subject areas. They must be able to understand language of the classroom and curriculum, and be able to shift language tasks. They must be able to decode teacher's cues and other students' cues. They must be able to succeed with class assignments. The students must be able to ask questions and seek clarification and to answer questions and make repairs. In inclusion, higher-level language skills may be needed to meet the educational demands of the curriculum. If this is not possible, alternative goals or alternative skill development must be included in the IEP. The teenage years are a time of social growth. The adolescent must be able to talk about teen topics, to understand idiomatic and abstract language and jokes. One focus in therapy may be to practice conversational skills and to role-play various social situations. Clarity and understandability of speech become more critical. So, the focus is on

the areas of pragmatics and speech intelligibility. In the work on conversational and social skills, the SLP may use materials that are designed for children and adolescents with autism, but work effectively for adolescents with Down syndrome. The most active clinicians/researchers in pragmatics and social skills are Carol Gray (http://www.thegraycenter.org) and Michelle Garcia-Winner (http://www.socialthinking.com). When a transition plan is written at age 14, communication needs for postsecondary education and employment should be considered in the planning process and treatment should address speech and language as needed.

Speech and language treatment is complex and can include different approaches, a variety of goals, and many different activities. The goal is to find treatment approaches and methods that will enable each child to reach his or her communication potential.

Fragile X Syndrome

Fragile X syndrome is the most common inherited cause of intellectual disability. Incidence has been estimated at 1 in 3,600 to 4,000 in males and 1 in 4,000 to 6,000 in females (National Fragile X Foundation, 2013). In addition, about 1 in 260 women and 1 in 800 men are carriers, and could pass the condition on to their children. It is a condition that is greatly underdiagnosed. Symptoms are subtle, and may vary widely from person to person; symptoms may accompany other conditions, making it difficult to identify by symptoms (Bailey & Nelson, 1995). Though genetic testing is available and can give a definitive diagnosis, it is not done routinely. Estimates are that 80% to 90% of people with fragile X syndrome are not correctly identified and diagnosed. It is not unusual for families to have 8 to 10 consultations with different physicians and other specialists before the correct diagnosis is made (Hagerman & Hagerman, 2002).

Causes of Fragile X Syndrome

Fragile X syndrome is caused by a defect in the FMR1 gene (Fragile X Mental Retardation-1), which is located on the long arm of the X chromosome. In 1991, Drs. Ben Oostra, David Nelson, and Stephen Warren identified this gene, which is involved in manufacturing a protein that helps messages travel through the nervous system (Hagerman & Hagerman, 2002; Hagerman & Silverman, 1991). The FMR1 protein helps to shape the connections between neurons that underlie learning and memory, so when the protein manufacture is shut down through fragile X syndrome, there is a negative effect on learning, memory, and communication. People who have a permutation (i.e., the FMR1 gene is damaged but functioning) are known as carriers. Carrier men pass this permutation to all of their daughters. A child of a woman who is a carrier has a 50% chance of inheriting the gene. The FMR-1 gene includes a DNA sequence of cytosine, guanine, and guanine (CGG). In the general population, the number of COG sequence repeats ranges from 6 to 50. In permutations (in carriers), there are 50 to 200 repeats. In full mutations, there are over 200 COG sequence repeats. A full mutation shuts the FMR1 gene down, and results in fragile X syndrome. Males have XY sex chromosomes, whereas females have XX sex chromosomes. Males inherit the X chromosome from their mothers and the Y chromosome from their fathers, whereas females inherit an X chromosome from each parent. Because males have only one X chromosome, when they inherit the defective FMR1 gene, they have a full mutation and demonstrate symptoms of fragile X syndrome. Females have two X chromosomes, and that seems to dilute the effects; each body cell needs to use only one of the X chromosomes, so some symptoms appear to be reduced.

Since 1992, there is a genetic test to diagnose fragile X syndrome. It is a blood test that can diagnose both permutations (carriers) and the full mutation present in fragile X. Because it is difficult to diagnose fragile X syndrome from symptoms, physicians recommend that any young child with unexplained developmental delay or ID be tested for fragile X syndrome (Hagerman & Hagerman, 2002).

Symptoms of Fragile X Syndrome

Fragile X syndrome is difficult to diagnose by symptoms. The physical and behavioral symptoms that occur in individuals with fragile X syndrome may also be found in individuals in the general population. Physical symptoms of fragile X syndrome may include:

- Long, thin face
- Large ears
- Flat feet
- Hyperextensible joints
- Machrochidism (large testicles in boys)
- Simian crease or Sydney line (single crease on the upper part of the palm)
- Hallucal crease (single crease across the ball of the foot)

Medical and behavioral symptoms may include:

- Otitis media
- Attention deficit and hyperactivity disorder
- Anxiety
- Impulsivity
- Sensory defensiveness
- Hyperarousal
- Autism
- Intellectual disability (moderate to severe)
- Low muscle tone
- Language difficulties
- Speech difficulties including dysfluency, articulation, and voice disorders
- Learning disabilities
- Seizures
- Sleep disturbances
- Anxiety
- Unstable mood
- Aggression
- Emotional problems

There is currently no direct medical treatment or cure for fragile X syndrome. Research is currently directed toward finding a way to prevent the FMR-1 gene from turning off. Current treatment is to improve and/or control the symptoms and to address the co-occurring conditions such as autism. Symptoms are managed by an interdisciplinary team including physicians, educators, speech-language pathologists, occupational therapists, specialists in sensory processing disorders, psychologists, and psychiatrists. Behavioral management tools may include drug and/or other medical management in addition to therapeutic interventions. Challenging behavior may be related to difficulties in communication experienced by children with fragile X syndrome (Reichle & Wacker, 1993). Aggression is a problem and there is a compounding effect that leads to the acting out behavior. Sleep disorders, sensitivity to sensory stimuli, and a tendency toward hyperarousal can result in rapid loss of capacity for self-regulation, manifesting in aggressive outbursts directed to the self or others. Sensory processing difficulties impact on many of the behavioral symptoms observed (Kranowitz, 2005; Miller, 2007).

Difficulty handling transitions, new environments, and changes in routine can exacerbate the behavioral outbursts. Although all children with disabilities are guaranteed a free appropriate public education by the Individuals with Disabilities Education Act (IDEA 2004), there is no specific category within the definition of Child with a Disability for children with fragile X syndrome. Usually, the symptoms that affect academic learning and behavior in school are used as the identifying category. So, children with fragile X syndrome may be classified under the category of intellectual disability, autism, speech and language impaired, or emotional disability.

The goal of assessment in children with fragile X syndrome is to identify the cognitive, communication and behavioral symptoms, and manifestations so they can be addressed in treatment. Treatment is based on a detailed interdisciplinary assessment of behavioral triggers, communication skills, sensory issues, and co-occurring conditions such as autism, ADHD, and anxiety. There is a high incidence of co-occurring autism, generally reported as co-occurring in 25% to 30% of the fragile X population (Bailey et al., 1998; Hagerman & Hagerman, 2002). But if the co-occurrence of fragile X syndrome with pervasive developmental disorder (PDD) is used instead, the estimate has been as high as 50% (Demark, Feldman, & Holden, 2003; Harris et al., 2008; Philofsky, Hepburn, Hayes, Hagerman, & Rogers, 2004).

The most recent guidelines for assessment were developed by Dowling and Barbouth for the National Fragile X Foundation (2012). The most recent guidelines for treatment were developed by Picker and Sudhalter for the National Fragile X Foundation (2012).

Treatment should include:

- A sensory diet developed by the OT
- A Functional Behavioral Analysis of the antecedents and triggers that result in behavioral difficulties and a treatment plan to minimize or avoid the triggers
- An effective communication system, which may be speech or an augmentative/alternative communication system (AAC)
- Self-awareness training and self-calming routines
- Feeding therapy to focus on sensory and oral motor issues
- Adaptations and modifications in the IEP to facilitate learning

There are usually different severity patterns in boys and girls, with the presenting symptoms in boys tending to be more severe. Most boys with fragile X syndrome have ID. Though about one-third of girls do have ID, it tends to be milder. The other 66% of girls with fragile X syndrome have average IQ or learning disabilities. They may also have difficulty in attention, executive function, visual-spatial skills, math, and exhibit signs of shyness and social anxiety (Roberts, Hennon, & Anderson, 2003). Behavioral prob-

lems and emotional problems are common in both groups (Picker & Sudhalter, 2012; Weber, 2000).

Speech and Language Difficulties

There is a wide variety of symptoms and difficulties related to speech and language development, as well as functional communication in daily living (Schopmeyer & Lowe, 1992). Often, speech and language difficulties are among the first symptoms noted, and children are referred to speech-language pathology services before the diagnosis of fragile X syndrome has been made. Differences between males and females have been noted, with the communication problems being more widespread and more severe in males. Males with fragile X syndrome typically have communication problems (Abbeduto & Hagerman, 1997). The incidence of co-occurrence of fragile X syndrome and autism is higher in males (Bailey, Mesibov, Hatton, Clark, Roberts, & Mayhew, 1998; National Fragile X Foundation, 2013). Males from ages 2 to 7 with fragile X syndrome show significant language delays in semantics and morphosyntax, and difficulties with gestures, reciprocity, and symbolic play skills (Roberts, Chapman, & Warren, 2008; Roberts, Mirrett, & Burchinal, 2001). On the Communication and Symbolic Behavior Scale, they show relative strengths in verbal and vocal communication (Roberts, Mirrett, Anderson, Burchinal, & Neebe, 2002). Speech intelligibility is a major issue (Barnes et al., 2009; Hagerman & Hagerman, 2002; Paul, Cohen, Breg, Watson, & Herman, 1984; Scharfenaker, 2012). Conversational speech is often unintelligible (Roberts, Hennon, & Anderson, 2003). Speech is often dysfluent including sound, word, and phrase repetitions and a pattern of cluttering. Difficulties with articulation and phonology, oral motor skills, and motor planning skills have been documented (Roberts, Hennon, & Anderson, 2003). Adolescent and adult males with fragile X syndrome demonstrate speech patterns characterized by fluctuating rate, and frequent perseveration of words, sentences, and topics. Perseveration may be severe and interferes with communication (Finestack, Richmond, & Abbeduto, 2009; Martin et al., 2012). Though they may have fairly good intelligibility in single words, they generally have poor intelligibility in connected speech (Paul, Cohen, Breg, Watson, & Herman, 1984; Roberts et al., 2007; Roberts, Chapman, & Warren, 2008). Oral motor difficulties are common with difficulty in repetition of multisyllabic word sequences, and motor planning problems.

There have been conflicting findings related to semantics with some research documenting delays in vocabulary (Abbeduto & Hagerman, 1997) and others documenting high receptive vocabulary scores (Scharfenaker, 2012). Morphosyntax has been found by some researchers to be appropriate for the nonverbal mental age level (Finestack, Richmond, & Abbeduto, 2009; Roberts, Hennon, & Anderson, 2003; Sharfenaker, 2012), but other researchers have reported lower scores and greater difficulty (Roberts, Price, et al., 2007; Rice, Warren, & Betz, 2005). Researchers agree that there are difficulties in pragmatics including difficulty with staying on topic and the frequent occurrence of tangential comments (Abbeduto & Sterling, 2011; Scharfanaker, 2012; Sudhalter & Belser, 2001). Some of the more common speech and language symptoms in males are listed in Table 3–2. In females, the speech and language symptoms tend to be milder.

Some of the more common speech and language symptoms in females are presented in Table 3–2.

Treatment for Children with Fragile X Syndrome

There is no established protocol for assessment in children with fragile X syndrome. Often communication difficulties are the first sign that there is a problem. There is a need for a comprehensive evaluation of speech, oral motor, articulation, and language skills including phonology, morphology, syntax, semantics and pragmatics, and both receptive and expressive language skills. Treatment for individuals with fragile X syndrome focuses on targeting each symptom that is manifested in that individual. If ID is evident, special education would help the child learn. If learning disabilities are evident, treatment would target the learning disability. Medications and specialized treatment methods are used to help control the emotional and behavioral symptoms. Researchers are trying to find new genetic and pharmacological treatments that can address the underlying genetic problem. Currently, there are research treatment initiatives in three areas: gene therapy, gene repair, and psychopharmacology. Gene therapy seeks to insert a functional FMR1 gene into the brain of individuals with fragile X syndrome. Gene repair strategies seek to turn the FMR1 gene back on, so that it can produce the protein for the cell. Psychopharmacological approaches seek to treat the symptoms and improve daily function for individuals with fragile X syndrome.

Finestack, Sterling, and Abbeduto (2013) found that there are specific language profiles that can distinguish children

Table 3–2. Speech and Language Characteristics of Children With Fragile X Syndrome

Males	Females
Delayed onset of expressive language	Expressive language difficulties
Syntax difficulty	Auditory memory difficulties
Delays in expressive vocabulary	Difficulty staying on-topic
Receptive/expressive language gap	Use of tangential language
Pediatric verbal apraxia	
Cluttering	
Poor language organization skills	
Reduced speech intelligibility	
Fast, uneven rate of speech	
Echolalia	
Perseveration	
Disturbed speech rhythm	
Hoarse and breathy voice	
Pragmatic difficulties	
Gaze aversion	
Difficulty staying on-topic	
Turn-taking difficulties	

with fragile X syndrome from those with Down syndrome.

Therapeutic approaches target the behavioral, emotional, and communication difficulties experienced by individuals with fragile X syndrome (Abbeduto & Sterling, 2011), that is, they focus on the symptoms. Co-occurring conditions including autism and sensory processing difficulties affect communication function and need to be addressed by the multidisciplinary team. Many children with fragile X syndrome have sensory processing difficulties, that is, they have difficulty in organizing sensory input from the environment. This may affect the sensory information received through hearing, vision, touch, movement, and balance. Many children feel overwhelmed by sights, sounds and movement in their environment. For example, if a child does not process auditory stimuli accurately, raindrops can sound like bullets and would be very frightening. The occupational therapist works on sensory processing problems with the child and family. Often a cotreatment model where the SLP and OT treat the child together is used. If that is not possible, then close collaboration and consultation is needed because the sensory processing issues need to be considered when designing and implementing speech and language treatment. Some children with fragile X syndrome have strong visual skills and verbal imitations skills, and these strengths can be used in therapy. See Table 3–2 for speech and language characteristics in males and females with fragile X syndrome.

Behavioral characteristics observed in children with fragile X syndrome may include hand flapping, hand biting, perseveration, poor eye contact, and tantrums (Bailey et al., 1998). Overall behavioral patterns may include short attention span, hyperactivity, difficulty in relating to other people, anxiety, hypervigilance, depression, and autism spectrum disorder. These symptoms make it more difficult to learn in school and to interact socially in the community. Psychologists and special educators will directly target these symptoms in treatment.

Some children with fragile X syndrome will use sign language or an augmentative communication system to communicate, but most will communicate by using speech. Speech and language development is often severely delayed, especially in males. Perseveration and echolalia may be present. Speech is often difficult to understand because of the presence of rapid rate of speaking, cluttered speech, poor eye contact, and difficulty with staying ontopic (Roberts et al., 2003). Thus, speech intelligibility is a major problem. Speech-language pathology treatment will target the specific areas of communication difficulty for the individual. If the child has hypotonia (low muscle tone) in the oral facial muscles, the child would need exercises to help strengthen the muscles to improve speech. If speech is unintelligible, the SLP would need to investigate the reasons for the lack of intelligibility. Is cluttering the problem? Is the child talking too rapidly?

The treatment program is always individually designed for the child's strengths and challenges. The treatment program may include:

- Oral motor planning (childhood apraxia of speech) therapy
- Receptive language skills
- Expressive language skills
- Assistive technology for communication
- Conversational skills
- Nonverbal communication skills, including eye contact
- Treatment to decrease rate of speaking
- Treatment for cluttering
- Treatment to reduce perseveration
- Treatment to reduce echolalia

Treatment goals must be individualized, but there are some general strategies that can address the learning and communication challenges of children with fragile X syndrome. Visual cues can be very helpful. For young children, this might include pictures of relevant vocabulary, pictures of requests (help me, juice please), visual schedules to help with transitions, and pictures to help children follow directions. For older children, visual cues for classroom routines and behaviors (quiet, line up), as well as cues to help them learn the curriculum in science and social studies, may be needed. Girls often have difficulty with social situations, and as a result develop anxiety about participating in those situations, avoiding conversations when possible. Lunch and recess are good times to practice social skills. Children with fragile X syndrome seem to learn best in real-life activities and situations. Role-playing using props and social scripts can be used if it is not possible to use the real situation.

One of the difficulties in designing treatment programs is that children with fragile X syndrome are often not identified at an early age. It is important to begin treatment early because speech is a motor output system that is based on sensory input and learning from the language environment. Because most infants and toddlers with fragile X syndrome have sensory processing difficulties, they find it difficult to learn from their environment without sensory processing treatment. A comprehensive early intervention language treatment program would involve collaboration between the SLP, occupational therapist (or sensory processing disorders specialist), special educator or developmental specialist, assistive technology specialist, pediatrician, and family. Boys with fragile X syndrome often have complicated communication problems that are affected by physical, oral motor, and speech intelligibility concerns, as well as attentional and behavioral concerns. Girls may have mild speech problems or have good verbal skills, but both girls and boys often have difficulty in pragmatic (social interactive) speech. Speech-language pathology services cannot address all of the complex factors that may be affecting communication in the classroom or the community. A comprehensive language intervention program during the school years would involve collaboration between the SLP, occupational therapist, special educator, regular educator, pediatrician, and family.

With early diagnosis and comprehensive medical and therapeutic treatment, there is hope that the individual with fragile X syndrome can live a full and productive life. The outcome is generally better for children and adults with fragile X syndrome who do not have co-occurring autism (Kauffman et al., 2004; Lewis et al., 2006; Philofsky, Hepburn, Hayes, Rogers, & Hagerman, 2004). Through early intervention and continued communication, psychological, and educational assistance through the school years, children with fragile X syndrome can reach their potential.

Case Study 1

This case study is designed as a Think Aloud to facilitate understanding of how a clinician might think through a case. The clinician's thoughts are shown in italics.

Sara is a 2-year 9-month old bright active girl with Down syndrome. She is currently enrolled in the special education early intervention program through the local school system for 3 mornings a week. She also works with a speech-language pathologist in private practice once a week. Her mother is involved in the private practice sessions, which are based on a coaching model, and mom follows through with home activities.

The Rossetti Infant-Toddler Language Scale was used to assess Sara's current level of language. *(SLP notes: This is a criterion referenced instrument that assesses Interaction-Attachment, Pragmatics, Gesture, Play, Language Comprehension, and Language Expression. It is designed to provide a comprehensive analysis of a child's language development by using a scoring system that gives credit for behaviors that are observed during the session by the examiner, and behaviors reported by the parents/caregivers, in addition to the behaviors that can be elicited during the testing session. Results document the child's mastery of skills in each of the areas assessed at three-month intervals. It is a good scale to use for young children beginning to use verbal language, so it is a good choice to assess Sara).*

Results indicate levels of performance in the following areas:

Interaction Attachment—Sara's responses reflect a well-functioning reciprocal relationship between she and her mom. Mother responds to signs and to speech attempts. Mom also provides models for verbalizations.

Pragmatics—This subtest assesses the way the child uses language to communicate with others in a social manner. Sara approaches peers and plays alongside them. Some hugs were observed, but no verbal interactions.

Gesture—This subtest assesses the child's use of gesture to express thought and intent prior to the consistent use of spoken language. Sara uses a combination of signs, pantomime and words to communicate.

Play—This subtest assesses the changes in a child's play that reflect the development of representational thought with this subtest. Sara uses adaptive play with objects. She will pretend to drink from a cup. She does not use representational or dramatic play. She will carry a doll or stuffed animal by the hand, but will not pretend to feed them or put them to sleep. When a play situation has cues, for example, baskets are set up on the floor, and she is shown a model of the SLP throwing the ball into the baskets, Sara will follow the model and engage in the task.

Language Comprehension—This subtest assesses the child's understanding of verbal language with and without linguistic cues. Sara appears to understand single words when the referent is present in the environment. She can point to pictures of familiar objects and familiar people in photos.

Language Expression—This subtest assesses the child's use of preverbal and verbal behaviors to communicate with others. Sara uses about 60 signs and 10 words to communicate at present.

Informal observation of play and a case history completed by the parents were used to further analyze Sara's performance and to assist in IFSP planning. Sara appears to have mastered the language precursors. She understands communicative intent, and can initiate a communication interaction. Her receptive language skills are good, and she was observed to follow directions well. It is reported that she has no difficulty following directions at preschool when models are provided. On informal testing, Sara was able to follow one-stage commands, but could not follow two-stage commands. She is able to use turn-taking in play and in sound-making. She was observed to use joint attention, visual tracking, and reciprocal gaze. She was attentive to her mom's requests, and followed verbal commands to come over for a snack, and to pick up her sweater. She appeared to hear instructions, and turned to localize a sound source. She appears to have mastered the cognitive precursors for language including object permanence, cause and effect, means-end, and referential knowledge. She will search for a hidden object. Sara can develop a plan to get what she cannot reach, for example, she will climb on to the counter with a stool to reach the cookie jar. Sara understands the relationship between a symbol and its referent. She uses signs meaningfully. In the last year, she has progressed from using 5 signs to using 60 signs appropriately. Sara is actively using sign language and saying some single words. She is able to imitate motor actions.

(SLP notes: Because Sara understands the symbol-referent relationship and currently has 60 signs, goals for therapy should address both horizontal language development (more words and concepts) and vertical development (increase MLU by teaching and stimulating two-word combinations.)

IFSP goals for receptive and expressive language are:

1. Sara will use a combination of signs and word approximations to request and comment 5 or more times a day for 3 days.
2. Sara will produce 10 verbal word approximations for common objects/ actions in her environment 5 or more times a day for 3 days.
3. Sara will produce 5 different descriptive words 3 or more times a day for 3 days.
4. Sara will model 3 or more different descriptive words in combination with object words 3 times a day for 3 days. These may be sign or verbal approximations such as big car.

(SLP notes: Judging by Sara's present language performance, the prognosis is good that she will be successful in reaching those goals and mastering the skills.)

The IFSP document lists the family's strengths and needs, but there also needs to be specific goals for parent education, sharing of information, and involvement as active members of the treatment team.

There needs to be an IFSP goal for frequent (once weekly or at least 2–4 times monthly) information sharing and a home practice program. The family is willing to work with Sara and they need to have more specific information, not just a general request to stimulate language. Although the mom communicates regularly with the private SLP, the early intervention program is center based and does not work directly with family members. One way to share information would be to keep parents in the loop and send a quick email as the objectives listed in the IFSP are addressed in treatment (e.g., which action words were worked on this week, or which descriptive words, which single words were combined into two-word combinations, and were they combined through sign or speech?).

The objectives for receptive language address yes/no head shaking responses, and following novel directions using gestural and contextual cues.

1. Sara will follow 2-step directions with verbal and gestural, as well as contextual cues, in 3 out of 4 opportunities for 5 days.
2. Sara will respond to yes/no questions by shaking her head appropriately in 3 out of 4 opportunities for 5 days.

(SLP notes: The family needs information and modeling on what kinds of cues will be used, and on what questions are most successful in eliciting yes/no responses for Sara.)

In the area of social interaction/pragmatics, Sara needs help with initiating interactions. She will currently respond to peers when they ask for a turn, and will engage with them in activities such as rolling a ball back and forth, but she will not initiate social interactions.

1. Sara will initiate greetings routines with peers in 2 out of 3 opportunities a week for 2 weeks.
2. Sara will initiate and maintain a turn-taking game with a peer for 3 or more turns 2 or more times a week for 2 weeks.

(SLP notes: School-home communication is important. Parents should be taught to use the same cues and assists that are being used in school. Sara is in a playgroup and this goal can be addressed during daily life, as well as in school.)

Speech appears to be emerging for Sara. She is using a variety of vowels and is consistently using /b/, /p/, /m/, /n/, /d/, and /h/. She is using /w/ as a substitute for the /l/ sound. In the assessment session, she was observed to imitate CV (consonant-vowel), VC, CVC, and CVCV combinations, and some individual words such as pop when popping bubbles that were floating in front of her. There are no signs of childhood apraxia of speech at this time. She appears to be able to get her message across through a combination of signs, vocalizations, gestures, and words. Her motor skills for walking and climbing are very good, so she is often able to get things she wants by herself rather than needing to rely on asking for them.

Recommendations/Goals

It is strongly recommended that Sara receive SLP services through the early intervention program three times weekly. Ongoing family coaching and information sharing can be part of the early intervention program or through private practice, but it is important that it continue. In the state in which Sara's family resides, there is an option, at the age of 3, to move on to the IEP planning/treatment process or stay with the IFSP planning/treatment process until age 4. It is recommended that the family choose to stay with the IFSP planning/treatment process.

(SLP notes: With Sara, and with most young children with Down syndrome, the family is an extremely important member of the intervention team. Because children with DS have difficulty in generalizing skills, practice needs to be part of daily living situations, not limited to treatment sessions only. The IFSP documents the families' strengths and needs, and provides for more family involvement.)

1. There is a need to stimulate and increase Sara's speech and language development horizontally and vertically.
2. Horizontal development will address increasing the number of single words Sara can understand and use. This can be accomplished through play activities (e.g., games, toys) and real life experiences (going to stores, park, playground). Reading can also be used to help develop the concepts. Words and concepts that need to be part of Sara's core vocabulary are words that will help her communicate more effectively, for example, if Sara is enrolled in a swimming class, water and swimming would be important concepts in her world; if she has pets, their names should be on her list.
3. Vertical language development will focus on expanding the mean length of utterance to two- and three-word phrases. Imitation with expansion and the pacing board can be used to help Sara begin to use two-word signed and spoken utterances.
4. Sara is using a variety of consonant and vowel sounds individually and

in combination. Use books and real-life experiences to help reinforce the sound combinations that she can currently say. Here are some children's books that focus on the specific sounds that she can already say:

The /p/ Sound

Bang, Molly. *The Paper Crane.*

Carle, Eric. *Pancakes, Pancakes.*

De Paola, Tomie. *Pancakes for Breakfast.*

McPhail, David. *Pigs Aplenty, Pigs Galore.*

Oxenbury, Helen. *Tom & Pippo* (series).

Prelutsky, Jack. *Ride a Purple Pelican.*

Seuss, Dr. *Hop on Pop.*

The /b/ Sound

Bob the Builder (series).

Barton, Byron. *Boats.*

Berenstain, Stan & Jan. *The Berenstain Bears* (series).

Brown, Margaret. *Big Red Barn.*

Carle, Eric. *The Very Busy Spider.*

Carter, David. *More Bugs in Boxes.*

Isadora, Rachel. *Ben's Trumpet.*

Martin, Bill, Jr. *Brown Bear, Brown Bear, What Do You See?*

Potter, Beatrix. *The Tale of Benjamin Bunny.*

The /d/ Sound

Alborough, Jez. *Cuddly Dudley.*

Aliki. *Digging Up Dinosaurs.*

Bridwell, Norman. *Clifford, the Red Dog* (series).

Hines, Anna. *Daddy Makes the Best Spaghetti.*

Kirk, Daniel. *Breakfast at the Liberty Diner.*

McClosky, Robert. *Make Way for Ducklings.*

Shannon, D. *Duck on a Bike.*

The /m/ Sound

Brett, Jan. *The Mitten: A Ukranian Folktale.*

Brown, Margaret. *Goodnight Moon.*

Day, Alexandra. *Carl's Masquerade.*

Dunrea, Olivier. *Mogwogs on the March.*

Gag, Wanda. *Millions of Cats.*

Guarino, Deborah. *Is Your Mama a Llama?*

McCloskey, Robert. *Make Way for Ducklings.*

Kellogg, S. *The Missing Mitten Mystery.*

McCloskey, Robert. *One Morning in Maine.*

Shulevitz, Uri. *One Monday Morning.*

5. There is a need to expand Sara's sound repertoire. When I analyze the sounds she can currently produce, I find that she is able to make sounds that are produced in the front of the mouth, sounds made with lip rounding (/p/), sounds made with tongue tip elevation (/d/), and the glottal sound /h/. She is not yet making sounds that have placement in the

back of the mouth such as /k/ or /g/. She is able to move the soft palate and close off the velopharyngeal sphincter, that is, she can make both oral and nasal sounds such as /b/ and /m/. She is able to make both voiced /b/ and voiceless /p/ sounds. She is making stop plosive sounds, which means that she can stop the airstream and explode the sound. She is not currently making fricative sounds such as /f/, /v/, /th/, or /s/. These are sounds that develop later for all children. They involve sending the airstream slowly between partially closed articulators.

According to the movements and manner of the sounds Sara is making, the next sounds targeted should be /t/ and /l/. She has the correct place for these sounds and the correct manner for /t/. Because she can elevate the tongue for the /d/ sound, that should carry over to the /l/ sound. The /w/ substitution for the /l/ sound can be worked on through an articulation approach teaching the manner of productions for liquid sounds, or through a phonological processes approach working on the process of gliding the liquid. Here are some children's books to help the teacher and family get started, so that Sara can hear the sounds in many different contexts in the stories:

The /t/ Sound

Baker, Alan. *Two Tiny Mice.*

Brett, Jan. *The Mitten: A Ukranian Folktale.*

Crowe, Robert. *Tyler Toad and the Thunder.*

Isadora, Rachel. *Ben's Trumpet.*

Lester, Helen. *Tacky the Penguin.*

McClosky, Robert. *Time of Wonder.*

Mosel, A. *Tikki Tikki Tembo.*

The /l/ sound

Brown, Marc. *Pickle Things.*

Guarino, Deborah. *Good-Night Owl!*

Kraus, Robert. *Leo the Late Bloomer.*

Lionni, Leo. *Little Blue and Little Yellow.*

Martin, Bill & Archambault, John. *Listen to the Rain.*

Mayer, Mercer. *Liza Lou and the Yeller Belly Swamp.*

Waber, Bernard. *Lyle, Lyle Crocodile* (series).

Sara is making good progress in receptive and expressive language. She is increasing the number of sounds she can make and is beginning to use speech to make her wants and needs known. Re-evaluate in one year.

Review Questions

1. What does a diagnosis of ID mean? What are the severity levels of ID? How did the diagnosis help her qualify for early intervention services?

2. How can we describe the different levels of support that a person with ID may need? How do communication skills affect the need for support for the child? What kinds of support do the parents need to help their child learn to speak?

3. What do we mean when we say that treatment is based on the communication patterns of the child and must be individually designed.

4. What are common co-occurring conditions, for example, OME for Down syndrome and autism for fragile X syndrome? How do these co-occurring conditions affect communication?

5. What is the role of the SLP working as part of the multidisciplinary assessment and treatment team for children with Down syndrome during IFSP planning and early intervention?

6. How was children's literature used in Sara's speech and language treatment program?

Case Study 2: Down Syndrome

Becky is a 9-year-old girl with Down syndrome. Testing soon after birth revealed the etiology to be trisomy 21. Becky was born with cardiac problems (atrial-ventricular septal defect and endocardial cushion defect), which were surgically corrected at 6 months of age. For the first 16 months of life, Becky was breastfed, but experienced some difficulty with sucking early on. Feeding therapy was helpful during this period. Becky did not have difficulty transitioning to a cup or to solid food. It was very difficult to bathe Becky as she did not like to be touched, especially around the mouth, face, and head. So, shampooing her hair became an ordeal for her mother. Early intervention focused on sensory processing and physical therapy, in addition to speech-language pathology services. Becky had chronic fluid in her middle ear, which resulted in a moderate fluctuating conductive hearing loss. Early speech-language pathology services worked on auditory stimulation, turn-taking, oral motor stimulation, and language stimulation through play and musical activities.

Becky was taught the signs "more" and "all done" at about 9 months of age, and a total communication program was instituted. Becky began speaking using single words to communicate at age 2. Speech-language pathology treatment focused on the oral motor foundations for articulation and vocabulary development.

At age 3.6, Becky began to combine words into two-word phrases, increasing her communication skills. She was advancing in pragmatics, and was included in a regular preschool program two days weekly and received special education services in a special preschool setting three days weekly. Speech-language pathology treatment targeted names, objects, colors, shapes, numbers, prepositions, and functional vocabulary skills such as social greetings. Becky began kindergarten at age 6, and remained in kindergarten for two years. During this period, she began to read, which helped facilitate vocabulary development. In kindergarten, she had difficulty with transitioning from one activity to another and in following directions. She was not willing to move from one activity to another. When a functional behavioral assessment was completed, it was determined that communication difficulties were affecting her behavior in the classroom. A positive behavior support plan for Becky included use of a picture activity schedule to help with transitioning, and a visual cueing system to help her with following instructions.

In first grade, Becky was on grade level in reading, but had difficulty with mathematics. She learned to add and subtract, but had difficulty following the instructions on worksheets. She also had difficulty paying attention in class and staying focused on the assignments to complete them. A medical and psychological evaluation determined that she had attention deficit disorder, which was treated with medication. The SLP worked with the special education and regular education teacher to modify worksheets for Becky in class. Fewer items were included on worksheets, and instructions were shortened and simplified and always included a sample question and answer.

Becky is now in third grade. She is included in the regular classroom, and receives special education and speech-language pathology services within the classroom. Becky communicates primarily through speech, but she is often difficult to understand. Articulation, use of phonological processes, and speech intelligibility are being addressed in treatment. She uses an assistive listening device in class, and has preferential seating. She enjoys social studies and reading, but has difficulty with mathematics and science. In therapy, the SLP helps Becky with the vocabulary that she needs to learn for her subjects. The focus of treatment is on what is needed for the classroom: vocabulary, following instructions, and learning the routines of the class. One of the annual goals addresses speech intelligibility and another addresses grammar, which is difficult for Becky. Testing reveals receptive language scores at age 7.6, and expressive language scores at the age 5 level. Becky speaks in five- to six-word utterances. She is beginning to retell stories that she has read. Socially, she does well with greetings and social language, but has difficulty with requests, idioms, and colloquial expressions.

Review Questions

1. How do the labels of ID and Down syndrome affect school placement and inclusion for Becky?

2. Describe the development of Becky's receptive language and expressive language skills. Is there a receptive-expressive gap in Becky's language skills?

3. Did Becky's language development follow the same path as language development in typical children?

4. What was the relationship between communication and behavior? How were the results of the functional behavior analysis applied to develop a plan to help Becky?

Case Study 3: Fragile X Syndrome

Frank is an 8-year-old boy with fragile X syndrome. At age 3, Frank was not yet speaking. When his parents tried to communicate with him, Frank would look away. He would sometimes use gestures, but it was difficult for his parents to figure out what he was trying to tell them. He often moved his hands in front of his eyes, and seemed to block out the world. He was hyperactive, and had frequent tantrums. He was impulsive and was covered with bumps and bruises from his many daredevil episodes. Frank's parents talked with the pediatrician, who sent them home, telling them that Frank would outgrow this phase. When they did not see positive change after six months, they decided to change pediatricians. The new physician sent them for a developmental evaluation, which included speech-language pathology. The conclusion was that Frank had a developmental delay, and had some symptoms of pervasive developmental disability. Frank began receiving occupational therapy, therapy for sensory processing disorders, and speech-language pathology services. Sometimes, the therapies were integrated, and Frank would be working on articulation while he was lying on a big orange ball. He appeared to be more comfortable when he was rolling on the ball or swinging. The movement seemed to help him learn.

By age 5, Frank had made some progress, but was still lagging far behind his peers. He was communicating primarily through pointing. He was using two to three words and some sounds, but was perseverating on those words. He was having great difficulty making sounds and had a limited repertoire of sounds. He had poor lip closure with some drooling. From ages 3 to 5, Frank had six ear infections (serous otitis media) and they seemed to last a long time. Frank's parents were concerned about his development. His mother was worried that he was not getting enough to eat. Frank would only eat macaroni and cheese. If his mom tried to add peas and carrots, he would refuse to eat. Frank was thin, and had a long face and big ears. A more detailed evaluation was suggested by the therapy team. Frank's pediatrician ordered further testing, including DNA analysis. The parents waited anxiously for the results. After two weeks, the genetic testing revealed that Frank had fragile X syndrome.

A referral was made for an assistive technology evaluation. Frank began using a Touch Talker communication device. He began with just two pictures, juice, and his favorite toy truck. For the first time, people could understand what he was trying to tell them. He did not need to drag his mom to the refrigerator. He could tell her when he was thirsty. Frank began using spoken words along with the device, and appeared more motivated to communicate. The SLP noted that the lim-

ited number of sounds that Frank made, his inconsistent sound production, and his effortful attempts at speaking suggested a diagnosis of motor-planning difficulties. She began using specialized methods to teach him to speak that focused on the length and complexity of the words. It is an approach used for children who have been diagnosed with developmental apraxia of speech. This seemed to help Frank. He was more successful in his speech attempts. The combination of using the Touch Talker and speaking enabled him to be understood and communicate his needs. Sensory integration treatment helped Frank, and he began to participate more at school. Frank was enrolled in a special education class within his regular neighborhood school. His favorite activity was center time, because there was a learning center about transportation. Frank loved airplanes, and he always tried to be the first one at the transportation center. There were books about airplanes, and he would put on the earphones and listen to the story. Sometimes, he would just look at the pictures and turn the pages. He was fascinated by the movements of the propellers. When he played with the toy planes, he would spin the propellers and make whirring sounds. His family often took him to a small local airport, so he could watch the planes. It was difficult to get Frank to leave the airport. He loved those planes!

Presently, at age 8, Frank is using a combination of speech and assistive technology to communicate. It is still difficult to understand his speech, but he is successful at communicating using his augmentative communication device. He is making educational progress. Classroom modifications and adaptations are used to help him learn. Transitions are difficult for him, so he uses picture schedules to help him with transitions in class. When the class has reading time, Frank can participate now. Oral reading is difficult for him, but the teacher has input repeated phrases from books into Frank's augmentative communication device. When the class reads *Chicken Soup with Rice*, Frank pushes the button on his AAC device, and "says" the words right along with the other children. His favorite subject is social studies. He is doing a report now on the Wright brothers, and has been making a paper model of their plane with his dad. Math is difficult for Frank, and the teacher is using visual cues and computer-based learning to help him. Frank's parents still have concerns, but they can see that he is making progress. They hope that he will be able to communicate through his speech. They hope that he will be able to continue learning. They hope he will be able to live and work in his neighborhood when he grows up. They hope that he has a bright future ahead.

Review Questions

1. When Frank's parents changed pediatricians he was identified as having ID and other labeled conditions. How did his treatment plan change based on the diagnoses?

2. What kinds of augmentative/alternative communication were provided for Frank?

3. What was the impact of AAC usage with Frank?

4. How did Frank's therapy plan change when the diagnosis of motor planning difficulties was given?

5. What was the role of the SLP working as part of the multidisciplinary assessment and treatment team for children with fragile X syndrome such as Frank during the school years? What information can the SLP provide to help the team in planning the IEP?

6. What is a classification system that can be used to describe the role of language at school?

References

Abbeduto, L., & Hagerman, R. J. (1997). Language and communication in fragile X syndrome. *Mental Retardation and Developmental Disabilities Research Reviews, 3,* 313–322. doi:10.1002/(SICI)1098-2779(1997)3:4<313::AID-MRDD6>3.0.CO;2-O

Abbeduto, L., & Murphy, M. (2004). Language, social cognition, maladaptive behavior, and communication in Down syndrome and fragile X syndrome. In M. L. Rice & S. F. Warren (Eds.), *Developmental language disorders: From phenotypes to etiologies.* Mahwah, NJ: Erlbaum.

Abbeduto, L., & Sterling, A. (2011). Language development and fragile X syndrome. *Perspectives on Language Learning and Education, 15,* 57–97, doi:10.1044/lle18.3.87

American Psychiatric Association. (2013). *Diagnostic and statistical manual of mental disorders* (5th ed.). Washington, DC: Author.

Attwood, A. (1988). The understanding and use of interpersonal gestures by autistic and Down's syndrome children. *Journal of Autism and Developmental Disorders, 18,* 241–257. doi:10.1007/BF02211950

Bailey, D., Mesibov, G., Hatton, D., Clark, R., Roberts, J., & Mayhew, L. (1998). Autistic behavior in young boys with fragile X syndrome. *Journal of Autism and Developmental Disorders, 28,* 499–508. doi:10.1023/A:1026048027397

Barnes, E., Roberts, J., Long, S., Martin, G., Berni, M., & Sideris, J. (2009). Phonological accuracy and intelligibility in connected speech of boys with fragile X syndrome or Down syndrome. *Journal of Speech, Language and Hearing Research, 52,* 1048–1061. doi:10.1044/1092-4388(2009/08-0001)

Batshaw, M., Roizen, N., & Lotrecchiano, G. (2013).*Children with disabilities: A medical primer* (7th ed.). Baltimore, MD: Brookes.

Beukelman, D., & Mirenda, P. (1998). *Augmentative and alternative communication: Management of severe communication disorders in children and adults* (2nd ed.). Baltimore, MD: Paul H. Brookes.

Berglund, E., Eriksson, M.,& Johansson, I. (2001). Parental reports of spoken language skills in children with Down syndrome. *Journal of Speech, Language and Hearing Research, 44,* 179–191. doi:10.1044/1092-4388(2001/016)

Bleile, K. (1982). Consonant ordering in Down's syndrome phonology. *Journal of Communication Disorders, 15,* 275–285. doi:10.1016/0021-9924(82)90010-7

Bleile, K., & Schwarz, I. (1984).Three perspectives on the speech of children with Down's syndrome. *Journal of Communication Disorders, 17,* 87–94. doi:10.1016/0021-9924(84)90014-5

Bochner, S., Outhred, L., & Pieterse, M. (2001). A study of functional literacy skills in young adults with Down syndrome. *International Journal of Disability, Development and Education, 48,* 67–90. doi:10.1080/10349120120036314

Bondy, A., & Frost, L. (2001). *A picture's worth: PECS and other visual communication strategies in autism.* Bethesda, MD: Woodbine House.

Bray, M. (2007). *Speech production in people with Down syndrome. Proceedings from: The Down Syndrome Research Directions Symposium.* Retrieved from http://www.down-syndrome .org

Bray, M., & Woolnough, L. (1988). The language skills of children with Down's syndrome aged 12 to 16 years. *Child Language Teaching and Therapy, 4,* 311. doi:10.1177/026565908800400305

Brownell, R. (2000a). *Expressive One-Word Picture Vocabulary Test-Second Edition.* Novato, CA: Academic Therapy Publications.

Brownell, R. (2000b). *Receptive One-Word Picture Vocabulary Test-Second Edition.* Novato, CA: Academic Therapy Publications.

Buckley, S. (1984). *Reading and language development in children with Down's syndrome: A guide for parents and teachers.* Portsmouth, UK: Down's Syndrome Project.

Buckley, S. (1993a). Developing the speech and language skills of teenagers with Down syndrome. *Down Syndrome Research and Practice, 1*(2), 63–71. doi:10.3104/reports.12

Buckley, S. (1993b). Language development in children with Down's syndrome: Reasons for optimism. *Down's Syndrome: Research and Practice, 1,* 3–9. doi:10.3104/reviews.5

Buckley, S. (1995a). Improving the expressive language skills of teenagers with Down syndrome. *Down Syndrome Research and Practice, 3*(3), 110–115. doi:10.3104/reports.57

Buckley, S. (1995b). Teaching children with Down syndrome to read and write. In L. Nadel & D. Rosenthal (Eds.), *Down syndrome: Living and learning in the community,* 158–169. New York, NY: Wiley-Liss.

Buckley, S. (1996). *Reading before talking: Learning about mental abilities from children with Down's syndrome.* University of Portsmouth Inaugural Lecture, Portsmouth, UK.

Buckley, S. (2000). *Speech and language development for individuals with Down syndrome: An overview.* Portsmouth, UK: The Down Syndrome Educational Trust.

Buckley, S. (2001). *Reading and writing for individuals with Down syndrome: An overview.* Portsmouth, UK: The Down Syndrome Educational Trust.

Buckley, S. (2012). *Programme to teach literacy skills.* Portsmouth, UK: The Down Syndrome Educational Trust.

Buckley, S., & Bird, G. (1993). Teaching children with Down's syndrome to read. *Down's Syndrome: Research and Practice, 1,* 34–41. Retrieved from http://www.down-syndrome.net/library/periodicals/dsrp/01/1/034/

Buckley, S., & Bird, G. (2001). *Speech and language development for infants with Down syndrome.* Portsmouth, UK: The Down Syndrome Educational Trust.

Buckley, S., Bird, G., & Byrne, A. (1996). The practical and theoretical significance of teaching literacy skills to children with Down syndrome. In J. Rondal & J. Perera (Eds.), *Down syndrome: Psychological, psychobiological and socioeducational perspectives* (pp. 119–128). London, UK: Whurr.

Buckley, S., Bird, G., & Sacks, B. (2006). Evidence that we can change the profile from a study of inclusive education. *Down Syndrome Research and Practice, 9,* 51–55. doi:10.3104/essays.294

Buckley, S., Bird, G., Sacks, B., & Archer, T. (2006). A comparison of mainstream and special education for teenagers with Down syndrome: Implications for parents and teachers.

Down Syndrome Research and Practice, 9, 54–67. doi:10.3104/reports.295

Buckley, S., & Buckley, F. (2011). *See and learn.* Portsmouth, UK: The Down Syndrome Educational Trust.

Bull, M., & The Committee on Genetics. (2011). Health supervision for children with Down syndrome [Clinical report]. *Pediatrics,128*(2), 393–406.

Bzoch, K. R., League, R., & Brown, V. L. (2003). *Receptive-Expressive Emergent Language Test, Third Edition.* Austin, TX: Pro-Ed.

Capone, G. (2002). Down syndrome and autistic spectrum disorders. In W. Cohen, L. Nadel, & M. Madnick (Eds.), *Down syndrome: Visions of the 21st century.* New York, NY: J. Wiley & Sons.

Capone, G., Goyal, P., Ares, W., & Lannigan, E. (2006). Neurobehavioral disorders in children, adolescents, and young adults with Down syndrome. *American Journal of Medical Genetics Part C- Seminars in Medical Genetics, 142C*(3), 158–172. doi:0.1002/ajmg.c.30097

Capone, G., Grados, M., Kaufmann, W., Bernad-Ripoll, S., & Jewell, A. (2005). Down syndrome and comorbid autism-spectrum disorder: Characterization using the aberrant behavior checklist. *American Journal of Medical Genetics Part A 134A*(4), 373–380. doi:10.1002/ajmg.a.30622

Cardoso-Martins, C., Mervis, C. B., & Mervis, C. A. (1985). Early vocabulary acquisition by children with Down syndrome. *American Journal of Mental Deficiency, 90,* 177–184.

Carter, J., Capone, G., Gray, R., Cox, C. S., & Kaufmann, W. E. (2007). Autistic-spectrum disorders in Down syndrome: Further delineation and distinction from other behavioral abnormalities. *American Journal of Medical Genetics Part B-Neuropsychiatric Genetics, 144B*(1), 87–94. doi:10.1002/ajmg.b.30407

Cebula, K. R., Moore, D. G., & Wishart, J. G. (2010). Social cognition in children with Down's syndrome: Challenges to research and theory building. *Journal of Intellectual Disability Research, 54*(2), 113–134. doi:10.1111/j.1365-2788.2009.01215.x.

Centers for Disease Control. (2011). *Facts about Down syndrome.* Retrieved from http://www.cdc.gov/ncbddd/birthdefects/DownSyndrome.html

Chapman, R., Schwartz, S., & Bird, E. R. (1991). Language skills of children and adolescents with Down syndrome I: Comprehension. *Journal of Speech and Hearing Research, 34,* 1106–1120. doi:10.1044/jshr.3405.1106

Chapman, R., Seung, J., Schwartz, S., & Bird, E. R. (1998). Language skills of children and adolescents with Down syndrome II: Production deficits. *Journal of Speech, Language and Hearing Research, 41,* 861–873.

Chapman, R. S., & Hesketh, L. J. (2000). Behavioral phenotype of individuals with Down syndrome. *Mental Retardation and Developmental Disabilities Research Reviews, 6,* 84–95. doi:10.1002/1098-2779(2000)6:2<84::AID-MRDD2>3.3.CO;2-G

Chicoine, B., & McGuire, D. (2010). *The guide to good health for teens and adults with Down syndrome.* Bethesda, MD: Woodbine House.

Cleland, J., Wood, S., Hardcastle, W., Wishart, J., & Timmins, C. (2010). The relationship between speech, oromotor, language and cognitive abilities in children with Down's syndrome. *International Journal of Language and Communication Disorders, 45*(1), 83–95. doi:10.3109/13682820902745453http://eresearch.qmu.ac.uk/1656/

Crimmins, D. (1999). Positive behavioral support: Analyzing, preventing, and replacing problem behaviors. In T. Hassold & D. Patterson (Eds.), *Down syndrome: A promising future together* (pp. 127–132). New York, NY: Wiley-Liss.

Denmark, J. L., Feldman, M. A., & Holden, J. J.(2003). Behavioral relationship between autism and fragile X syndrome. *American Journal of Mental Retardation, 108,* 314–326. doi:10.1352/0895-8017(2003)108<314:BRBAAF>2.0.CO;2

Devenny, D. A., & Silverman, W. P. (1990). Speech dysfluency and manual specialization in Down's syndrome. *Journal of Mental Deficiency Research, 34,* 253–260. doi:10.1111/j.1365-2788.1990.tb01536.x

Dodd, B. (1976). A comparison of the phonological systems of mental age matched, normal, severely subnormal and Down's syndrome children. *British Journal of Disorders of Communication, 1,* 27–42. doi:10.3109/13682827609011289

Dodd, B., & Thompson, L. (2001). Speech disorder in children with Down's syndrome. *Journal of Intellectual Disability Research, 45*(4), 308–316. doi:10.1046/j.1365-2788.2001.00327.x

Dowling, M., & Barbouth, D. (2012). *Consensus of the Fragile X Clinical & Research Consortium Practices. Assessment of Fragile X Syndrome*. Walnut Creek, CA: National Fragile X Foundation.

Dunn, M., & Dunn, L. M. (2007). *Peabody Picture Vocabulary Test-4*. Circle Pines, MN: AGS.

Elkins, J., & Farrell, M. (1994). Literacy for all? The case of Down syndrome. *Journal of Reading, 38*, 270–280.

Elliott, D., Weeks, D. J., & Elliott, C. L. (1987). Cerebral specialization in individuals with Down's syndrome. *American Journal on Mental Retardation, 92*, 263–271.

Fawcett, S., & Virji-Babul, N. (2006). Integrated therapy for stuttering and expressive syntax in Down syndrome: A case report. *International Journal on Disability and Human Development, 5*(4), 391–396. doi:10.1515/IJDHD.2006.5.4.391

Fenson, L., Dale, P. S., Reznick, J.S., Thal, D., Bates, E., Hartung, J. P., . . . Reilly, J. S. (1993). *The MacArthur Communicative Development Inventories: User's guide and technical manual*. San Diego, CA: Singular Publishing Group.

Fidler, D., Most, D., & Philosky, A. (2009). The Down syndrome behavioural phenotype: Taking a developmental approach. *Down Syndrome Research and Practice*, 37–44. doi:10.3104/reviews.2069

Fidler, D. J., Most, D. E., Booth-LaForce, C., & Kelly, J. (2008). Emerging social strengths in young children with Down syndrome at 12 and 30 months. *Infants and Young Children,33*, 303–315. doi:10.1097/01.IYC.0000324550.39446.1f

Finestack, L., Richmond, E., & Abbeduto, L. (2009). Language development in individuals with fragile X syndrome. *Topics in Language Disorders, 29*, 133–148. doi:10.1097/TLD.0b013e3181a72016

Finestack, L., Sterling, A., & Abbeduto, L. (2013). Discriminating Down syndrome and fragile X syndrome based on language ability. *Child Language, 40*(1), 244–265. doi:10.1017/S0305000912000207

Fowler, A. E. (1990). Language abilities in children with Down syndrome: Evidence for a specific syntactic delay. In D. Cicchetti & M. Beeghley (Eds.), *Children with Down syndrome: A developmental perspective* (pp. 302–328). Cambridge, UK: Cambridge University Press.

Fowler, A. E. (1995). Linguistic variability in persons with Down syndrome: Research and implications. In L. Nadel & D. Rosenthal (Eds.), *Down syndrome: Living and learning in the community* (pp. 121–131). New York, NY: Wiley-Liss.

Fowler, A. E. (1999).The challenge of linguistic mastery in Down syndrome. In T. J. Hassold (Ed.), *Down syndrome: A promising future, together* (pp. 165–182). New York, NY: Wiley-Liss.

Fuchs, D., Fuchs, L., Powers, M., & Dailey, A. (1985). Bias in the assessment of handicapped children. *American Educational Research Journal, 22*, 185–197. doi:10.3102/00028312022002185

Furuno, S., O'Reilly, K., Hosaka, K., Inatsuka, T., Zeisloft-Fabley, B., & Allman, T. (1988). *Hawaii Early Learning Profile*. Palo Alto, CA: VORT.

Garcia-Winner, M. *Specialist in teaching children how to think socially and handle social situations*. Retrieved from http://www.socialthinking.com

Gillham, B. (1979). *The first words language programme: A basic language programme for mentally handicapped children*. London, UK: George Allen &Unwin.

Goldman, R., & Fristoe, M. (2000). *Goldman –Fristoe Test of Articulation* (2nd ed.). Circle Pines, MN: American Guidance Service.

Gray, C. *Specialist in social stories*. Retrieved from http://www.thegraycenter.org

Green, J. (2011). *The ultimate guide to assistive technology in special education*. Waco, TX: Prufrock Press.

Guralnick, M. J. (1995). Peer-related social competence and inclusion of young children. In L. Nadel & D. Rosenthal (Eds.), *Down syndrome: Living and learning in the community* (pp. 147–153). New York, NY: Wiley-Liss.

Hagerman, R. J., & Hagerman, P. (2002). *Fragile X syndrome: Diagnosis, treatment and research* (3rd ed.). Baltimore, MD: Johns Hopkins University Press.

Hagerman, R. J., & Silverman, A. C. (1991). *Fragile X syndrome: Diagnosis, treatment and research*. Baltimore, MD: Johns Hopkins University Press.

Harris, S., Hessl, D., Goodlin-Jones, B., Ferranti, J., Bacalman, S., Barbato, I., . . . Hagerman, R. J. (2008). Autism profiles of males with fragile X syndrome. *American Journal on Mental Retardation, 113*, 427–438. doi:10.1097/00004703-200512000-00026

Heath, M., & Elliott, D. (1999).Cerebral specialization for speech production in persons with Down syndrome. *Brain and Language, 69*, 193–211. doi:10.1006/brln.1998.2131

Hendrick, D. L., Prather, E. M., & Tobin, A. R. (1990). *Sequenced Inventory of Communication Developmen-Revised edition.* Seattle, WA: University of Washington Press.

Hopmann, M. R., & Wilen, E. (1993, March). *Visual and auditory processing in children with Down syndrome: Individual differences.* Presented at the Society for Research in Child Development, New Orleans, LA.

Horstmeier, D. (1988). But I don't understand you—The communication interaction of youths and adults with Down syndrome. In S. Pueschel (Ed.), *The young person with Down syndrome.* Baltimore, MD: Paul H. Brookes.

Hresko, W. P., Reid, D. K., & Hammill, D. D. (1999).*Test of Early Language Development-3rd Edition.* Austin, TX: Pro-Ed.

Jarrold, C., & Baddely, A. D. (2002a). Short term memory in Down syndrome: Applying the working memory model. *Down Syndrome Research and Practice, 7*(1), 17–23. doi:10.3104/ reviews.110

Jarrold, C., & Baddeley, A. D. (2002b). Verbal short-term memory in Down syndrome. *Journal of Speech, Language and Hearing Research, 45,* 531–544. doi:10.1044/1092-4388(2002/042)

Jenkins, C. (1993). Expressive language delay in children with Down's syndrome: A specific cause for concern. *Down's Syndrome: Research and Practice, 1,* 10–14. doi:10.3104/reports.6

Kanno, K., & Ikeda, Y. (2002). Word length effect in verbal short-term memory in individuals with Down's syndrome. *Journal of Intellectual Disability Research, 46,* 613–618. doi:10.1046/j.1365-2788.2002.00438.x

Kaufmann, W., Cortell, R., Kau, A., Bukelis, I., Tierney, E., Gray, R., . . . Stanard, P. (2004). Autism spectrum disorder in fragile X syndrome: Communication, social interaction and specific behaviors. *American Journal of Medical Genetics, 129A,* 225–234. doi:10.1002/ ajmg.a.30229

Kent, L., Evans, J., Paul, M., & Sharp, M.(1999). Comorbidity of autism spectrum disorder in children with Down syndrome. *Developmental Medicine and Child Neurology, 41,* 153–158. doi:10.1017/S001216229900033X

Khan, L. M. L., & Lewis, N. P. (2002). *Khan-Lewis Phonological Analysis, Second Edition.* Circle Pines, MN: American Guidance Service.

Kouri, T. (1989). How manual sign acquisition related to the development of spoken language: A case study. *Language, Speech and Hear-*

ing Services in Schools, 20, 50–62. doi:10.1044/ 0161-1461.2001.50

Kranowitz, C. S. (2005). *The out of sync child: Recognizing and coping with sensory processing disorder* (Rev. ed.). New York, NY: Perigee.

Kumin, L. (1994). Intelligibility of speech in children with Down syndrome in natural settings: Parents' perspective. *Perceptual and Motor Skills, 78,* 307–313. doi:10.2466/pms.1994.78. 1.307

Kumin, L. (1996). Speech and language skills in children with Down syndrome. *MR and Developmental Disabilities Research Reviews, 2,* 109–116. doi:10.1002/(SICI)1098-2779(1996) 2:2<109::AID-MRDD9>3.0.CO;2-O

Kumin, L. (2001a). Speech intelligibility in individuals with Down syndrome: A framework for targeting specific factors for assessment and treatment. *Down Syndrome Quarterly, 6,* 1–8.

Kumin, L. (2001b). *Classroom language skills for children with Down syndrome: A guide for parents and teachers.* Bethesda, MD: Woodbine House.

Kumin, L. (2002a). Maximizing speech and language in children and adolescents with Down syndrome. In W. Cohen, L. Nadel, & M. Madnick (Eds.), *Down syndrome: Visions for the 21st century* (pp. 403–415). New York, NY: Wiley-Liss.

Kumin, L. (2002b). Why can't you understand what I am saying? Speech intelligibility in daily life. *Disability Solutions, 5*(1),1–15.

Kumin, L. (2002c). You said it just yesterday, why not now? Developmental apraxia of speech in children and adults with Down syndrome. *Disability Solutions, 5*(2),1–16.

Kumin, L. (2006a). Differential diagnosis and treatment of speech sound production problems in individuals with Down syndrome. *Down Syndrome Quarterly, 8,* 7–18.

Kumin, L. (2006b). Speech intelligibility and childhood verbal apraxia in children with Down syndrome. *Down Syndrome Research and Practice, 10,* 10–22. doi:10.3104/reports.301

Kumin, L. (2008a). Language intervention to encourage complex use: A clinical perspective. In J. E. Roberts, R. S. Chapman, & S. F. Warren (Eds.), *Speech and language development & intervention in Down syndrome & fragile X syndrome* (pp. 193–218). Baltimore, MD: Paul H. Brookes.

Kumin, L. (2008b). *Helping children with Down syndrome communicate better: Speech and language skills for ages 6–14.* Bethesda, MD: Woodbine House.

Kumin, L. (2010). Social communication skills. *Down Syndrome News, 33,* 86–89.

Kumin, L. (2012a). *Early communication skills for children with Down Syndrome* (3rd ed.). Bethesda, MD: Woodbine House.

Kumin, L. (2012b). Language skills for school success. *Down Syndrome News, 35,* 24–27.

Kumin, L. (2014a). Childhood apraxia of speech: A co-occurring condition that affects speech intelligibility. *Down Syndrome News, 37*(Summer).

Kumin, L. (2014b). Speech intelligibility: Helping children and adults develop and maintain understandable speech. *Down Syndrome News, 37*(Spring).

Kumin, L. (2014c). Perceptual and pragmatic issues in speech intelligibility: What does the listener see and hear? *Down Syndrome News, 37*(Winter).

Kumin, L., & Adams, J. (2000). Developmental apraxia of speech and intelligibility in children with Down syndrome. *Down Syndrome Quarterly, 5,* 1–6.

Kumin, L., & Bahr, D. C. (1999). Patterns of feeding, eating, and drinking in young children with Down syndrome with oral motor concerns. *Down Syndrome Quarterly, 4,* 1–8.

Kumin, L., Councill, C., & Goodman, M. (1994). A longitudinal study of the emergence of phonemes in children with Down syndrome. *Journal of Communication Disorders, 27,* 265–275. doi:10.1016/0021-9924(94)90019-1

Kumin, L., Councill, C., & Goodman, M. (1995). The pacing board: A technique to assist the transition from single word to multiword utterances. *Infant-Toddler Intervention, 5,* 23–29.

Kumin, L., Councill, C., & Goodman, M. (1998). Expressive vocabulary development in children with Down syndrome. *Down Syndrome Quarterly, 3,* 1–7.

Kumin, L., Councill, C., & Goodman, M. (1999). Expressive vocabulary in young children with Down syndrome: From research to treatment. *Infant-Toddler Intervention, 9*(1), 87–100.

Kumin, L., Goodman, M., & Councill, C. (1991). Comprehensive communication intervention for infants and toddlers with Down syndrome. *Infant-Toddler Intervention, 1,* 275–296.

Kumin, L., Goodman, M., & Councill, C. (2010). *Addressing Social Skills in Adolescents/Young Adults with Down Syndrome.* American Speech-Language-Hearing Association, November 2010.

Kumin, L., & Mason, G. (2011). Collaborative planning to teach strategies for the language of testing. *Perspectives in School-Based Issues, 12,* 139–152. doi:10.1044/sbi12.4.139

Leddy, M. (1999). The biological bases of speech in people with Down syndrome. In J. Miller, M. Leddy, & L. A. Leavitt (Eds.), *Improving the communication of people with Down syndrome* (pp. 61–80). Baltimore, MD: Paul H. Brookes.

Lewis, P., Abbeduto, L., Murphy, M., Richmond, E., Giles, N., Bruno, L., . . . Schroeder, S. (2006). Cognitive, language and social-cognitive skills of individuals with fragile X syndrome with and without autism. *Journal of Intellectual Disability Research, 50*(7), 532–545. doi:10.1111/j.1365-2788.2006.00803.x

Light, J., & Binger, C. (1998). *Building communicative competence with individuals who use augmentative and alternative communication.* Baltimore, MD: Paul H. Brookes.

Loveland, K. A., & Tunali, B. (1991). Social scripts for conversational interactions in autism and Down syndrome. *Journal of Autism and Developmental Disorders, 21,* 177–186. doi:10.1007/BF02284758

Luckasson, R., Borthwick-Duffy, S., Buntinx, W., Coulter, D., Craig, E., Reeve, A., . . . Tasse, M. (2002). *ID: Definition, classification and systems of supports* (10th ed.). Washington, DC: American Association on ID/ID.

MacArthur-Bates Communicative Development Inventories. (2007). Baltimore, MD: Brookes.

Martin, G. E., Roberts, J. E., Helm-Estabrooks, N., Sideris, J., Vanderbilt, J., & Moskowitz, L. (2012). Perseveration in the connected speech of boys with fragile X syndrome with and without autism spectrum disorder. *American Journal on Intellectual and Developmental Disabilities,117*(5), 384–399. doi:10.1352/1944-7558-117.5.384

McGuire, D., & Chicoine, B. (2006). *Mental wellness in adults with Down syndrome.* Bethesda, MD: Woodbine House.

Medlen, J. (2006). *The Down syndrome nutrition handbook: A guide to promoting healthy lifestyles.* Portland, OR: Phronesis.

Mervis, C. (1997). *Early lexical and conceptual development in children with Down syndrome.* Presented at the National Down Syndrome Society International Down Syndrome Research Conference on Cognition and Behavior, Florida.

Miles, S., Chapman, R., & Sindberg, H. (2006). Sampling context affects MLU in the language of adolescents with Down syndrome. *Journal of Speech, Language, and Hearing Research, 49*, 325–337. doi:10.1044/1092-4388(2006/026)

Miller, J. (1987). Language and communication characteristics of children with Down's syndrome. In S. Pueschel, C. Tingey, J. E. Rynders, A. C. Crocker, & D. M. Crutcher (Eds.), *New perspectives in Down syndrome*. Baltimore, MD: Paul Brookes.

Miller, J. (1999). Profiles of language development in children with Down syndrome. In J. Miller, M. Leddy, & L. A. Leavitt (Eds.), *Improving the communication of people with Down syndrome* (pp. 11–40). Baltimore, MD: Brookes.

Miller, J., & Leddy, M. (1999). Verbal fluency, speech intelligibility, and communicative effectiveness. In J. Miller, M. Leddy, & L. A. Leavitt (Eds.), *Improving the communication of people with Down syndrome* (pp. 81–92). Baltimore, MD: Paul H. Brookes.

Miller, J., Leddy, M., & Leavitt, L. A. (1999). (Eds.). *Improving the communication of people with Down syndrome*. Baltimore, MD: Paul H. Brookes.

Miller, J., Leddy, M., Miolo, G., & Sedey, A. (1995). The development of early language skills in children with Down syndrome. In L. Nadel & D. Rosenthal (Eds.), *Down syndrome: Living and learning in the community* (pp. 115–119). New York, NY: Wiley-Liss.

Miller, J., Sedey, A., & Miolo, G. (1995). Validity of parent report measures of vocabulary development for children with Down syndrome. *Journal of Speech and Hearing Research, 38*, 1037–1044. doi:10.1044/jshr.3805.1037

Miller, J. F. (1988). Developmental asynchrony of language development in children with Down syndrome. In L. Nadel (Ed.), *Psychobiology of Down syndrome*. New York, NY: Academic Press.

Miller, J. F. (1992). Lexical development in young children with Down syndrome. In R. Chapman (Ed.), *Processes in language acquisition and disorders*. St. Louis, MO: Mosby Yearbook.

Miller, J. F. (1995). Individual differences in vocabulary acquisition in children with Down syndrome. *Progress in Clinical and Biological Research, 393*, 93–103.

Miller, L. (2007). *Sensational Kids: Hope and help for children with sensory processing disorder (SPD)*. New York, NY: G. P. Putnam's Son.

Mundy, P., Sigman, M., Kasari, C., & Yirmiya, N. (1988). Nonverbal communication skills in Down syndrome children. *Child Development, 59*, 235–249. doi:10.2307/1130406

Myers, B., & Pueschel, S. (1995). Major depression in a small group of adults with Down syndrome. *Research in Developmental Disabilities, 16*(4), 285–299. doi:10.1016/0891-4222(95)00015-F

Nash, H. M., & Snowling, M. J. (2008). Semantic and phonological fluency in children with Down syndrome: Atypical organization of language or less efficient retrieval strategies? *Cognitive Neuropsychology, 25*(5), 690–703. doi:10.1080/02643290802274064

Paul, R., Cohen, D. J., Breg, W. R., Watson, M., & Herman, S. (1984). Fragile X syndrome: Its relation to speech and language disorders. *Journal of Speech and Hearing Disorders, 49*, 326–336. doi:10.1044/jshd.4903.328

Petursdottir, A. I., & Carr, J. E. (2011). A review of recommendations for sequencing receptive and expressive language instruction. *Journal of Applied Behavior Analysis, 44*, 859–876. doi:10.1901/jaba.2011.44-859

Philofsky, A., Hepburn, S., Hayes, A., Rogers, S., & Hagerman, R. (2004). Linguistic and cognitive functioning and autism symptoms in young children with fragile X syndrome. *American Journal on Mental Retardation, 109*(3), 208–218. doi:10.1352/0895-8017(2004)109<208:LACFAA>2.0.CO;2

Picker, J., & Sudhalter, V. (2012b). *Consensus of the Fragile X Clinical & Research Consortium Practices. Behavior problems in fragile X syndrome*. Walnut Creek, CA: National Fragile X Foundation.

Pueschel, S. M., Gallagher, P. L., Zastler, A. S., & Pezzulo, J. C. (1987).Cognitive and learning processes in children with Down's syndrome. *Research and Developmental Disabilities, 8*, 21–37. doi:0.1016/0891-4222(87)90038-2

Reichle, J., & Wacker, D., (1993). *Communicative alternatives to challenging behavior: integrating functional assessment and intervention strategies*. Baltimore, MD: Paul H. Brookes.

Rice, M. L., Warren, S. F., & Betz, S. K. (2005). Language symptoms of developmental language disorders: An overview of autism, Down syndrome, fragile X, specific language impairment, and Williams syndrome. *Applied Psycholinguistics, 26*(1) 7–27. doi:10.1017/S0142716405050034

Roberts, J., Chapman, R., & Warren, S. (2008). *Speech and language development and intervention in Down syndrome and fragile X syndrome.* Baltimore, MD: Brookes.

Roberts, J., Hennon, E., & Anderson, K. (2003). Fragile X syndrome and speech and language. *The ASHA Leader.*

Roberts, J., Long, S., Malkin, C., Barnes, E., Skinner, M., Hennon, E., . . . Anderson, K. (2005). A comparison of phonological skills in boys with fragile X syndrome and Down syndrome. *Journal of Speech, Language and Hearing Research, 48*, 980–995. doi:10.1044/1092-4388(2005/067)

Roberts, J., Price, J., Barnes, E., Nelson, L., Burchinal, M., Hennon, E., . . . Hooper, S. R. (2007). Receptive vocabulary, expressive vocabulary, and speech production of boys with fragile X syndrome in comparison to boys with Down syndrome. *American Journal on Mental Retardation, 112*, 177–193. doi:10.1352/0895-8017(2007)112[177:RVEVAS]2.0.CO;2

Roberts, J., Price, J., & Malkin, C. (2007). Language and communication development in DS. *Mental Retardation and Developmental Disabilities Research Review, 13*, 26–35. doi:10.1002/mrdd.20136

Roberts, J. E., Mirrett, P., Anderson, K., Burchinal, M., & Neebe, E. (2002). Early communication, symbolic behavior, and social profiles of young males with fragile X syndrome. *American Journal of Speech-Language Pathology, 11*, 295–304. doi:10.1044/1058-0360(2002/034)

Roberts, J. E., Mirrett, P., & Burchinal, M. (2001). Receptive and expressive communication development of young males with fragile X syndrome. *American Journal on ID/ID, 106*, 216–230. doi:10.1352/0895-8017(2001)106<0216:RAECDO>2.0.CO;2

Roizen, N. (1997). Hearing loss in children with Down syndrome: A review. *Down Syndrome Quarterly, 2*, 1–4. doi:10.1016/S0022-3476(05)81588-4

Roizen, N. J., Wolters, C., Nicol, T., & Blondis, T. (1992). Hearing loss in children with Down syndrome. *Pediatrics, 123*, S9–12. doi:10.1016/S0022-3476(05)81588-4

Rondal, J. A. (1988). Language development in Down's syndrome: A lifespan perspective. *International Journal of Behavioral Development, 11*, 21–36. doi:10.1177/016502548801100103

Rosenfeld-Johnson, S. (1999). *Oral-motor exercises for speech clarity.* Tucson, AZ: Innovative Therapists International.

Rosin, M., Swift, E., Bless, D., & Vetter, D. K. (1988). Communication profiles of adolescents with Down syndrome. *Journal of Childhood Communication Disorders, 12*, 49–64. doi:10.1177/152574018801200105

Rosin, P., & Swift, E. (1999). Communication interventions: Improving the speech intelligibility of children with Down syndrome. In J. Miller, M. Leddy, & L. A. Leavitt (Eds.), *Improving the communication of people with Down syndrome* (pp. 133–159). Baltimore, MD: Paul H. Brookes.

Rossetti, L. (1990). *The Rossetti Infant-Toddler Language Scale.* East Moline, IL: LinguiSystems.

Schalock, R. L., Baker, P. C., & Croser, M. D. (2002). *Embarking on a new century: MR at the end of the twentieth century.* Washington, DC: AAMR.

Scharfenaker, S. (2012). *The fragile X syndrome: Speech and language characteristics.* Retrieved June 21, 2013, from http://www.chp.edu

Schopmeyer, B., & Lowe, F. (1992). *The fragile X child.* Clifton Park, NY: Delmar Learning.

Semel, E., Wiig, E. H., & Secord, W. (2003). *Clinical evaluation of language fundamentals* (4th ed.). San Antonio, TX: The Psychological Corporation.

Shapiro, B. K., & Batshaw, M. L. (2011). Intellectual disability. In R. M. Kliegman, R. E. Behrman, H. B. Jenson, & B. F. Stanton (Eds.), *Nelson textbook of pediatrics* (19th ed., Chap. 33). Philadelphia, PA: Saunders Elsevier.

Shott, S. (2006). Down syndrome: Common otolaryngological manifestations. *American Journal of Medical Genetics, 142C*(3), 131–140. doi:10.1002/ajmg.c.30095

Shott, S. R. (2000). Down syndrome: Common pediatric ear, nose, and throat problems. *Down Syndrome Quarterly, 5*, 1–6.

Shott, S. R., Joseph, A., & Heithaus, D. (2001). Hearing loss in children with Down syndrome. *International Journal of Pediatric Otolaryngology, 1:61*(3), 199–205. doi:10.1016/S0165-5876(01)00572-9

Smith, B. L., & Stoel-Gammon, C. (1983). A longitudinal study of the development of stop consonant production in normal and Down's syndrome children. *Journal of Speech and Hearing Disorders, 48*, 114–118. doi:10.1044/jshd.4802.114

Sommers, R. K., Patterson, J. P., & Wildgen, P. L. (1988). Phonology of Down syndrome speakers, ages 13–22. *Journal of Childhood Communication Disorders, 12*, 65–91. doi:0.1177/152574018801200106

Stoel-Gammon, C. (1980). Phonological analysis of four Down's syndrome children. *Applied Psycholinguistics, 1*, 31–48. doi:10.1017/S0142716400000710

Stoel-Gammon, C. (1997). Phonological development in Down syndrome. *ID/ID and Developmental Disabilities Research Reviews, 3*, 300–306. doi:10.1002/(SICI)1098-2779(1997)3:4<300::AID-MRDD4>3.0.CO;2-R

Stoel-Gammon, C. (2001). Down syndrome phonology: Developmental patterns and intervention strategies. *Down Syndrome Research and Practice, 7*(3), 93–100. doi:10.3104/reviews.118

Sudhalter, V., & Belser, R.C. (2001). Conversational characteristics of children with fragile X syndrome: Tangential language. *American Journal on Mental Retardation, 106*, 389–400. doi:10.1352/0895-8017(2001)106<0389:CCOCWF>2.0.CO;2

Swift, E., & Rosin, P. (1990). A remediation sequence to improve speech intelligibility for students with Down syndrome. *Language, Speech and Hearing Services in Schools, 21*, 140–146.

Thompson, R. H., Cotnoir-Bichelman, N. M., McKerchar, P. M., Tate, T. L., & Dancho, K. A. (2007). Enhancing early communication through infant sign training. *Journal of Applied Behavior Analysis, 40*, 15–23. doi:10.1901/jaba.2007.23-06

Thordardottir, E., Chapman, R., & Wagner, L. (2002). Complex sentence production by adolescents with Down syndrome. *Applied Psycholinguistics, 23*, 163–183. doi:10.1017/S0142716402002011

Timmins, C., Cleland, J., Rodger, R., Wishart, J., Wood, S., & Hardcastle, W. (2009). Speech production in Down syndrome. *Down Syndrome Quarterly, 11*(2), 16–22.

Toth, A. (2009). Bridge of signs: Can sign language empower non-deaf children to triumph over their communication disabilities? *American Annals of the Deaf, 154*(2), 85–95. Retrieved from http://search.proquest.com.ezp.lndlibrary.org/comdisdome/docview/742785695/13553DFB88849713164/25?accountid=12164

Van Borsel, J., & Vandermeulen, A. (2008). Cluttering in Down syndrome. *Folia Phoniatricaet Logopaedica, 60*(6), 312–317. doi:10.1159/00017008

Weber, J. D. (Ed.). (2000). *Children with fragile X syndrome: A parent's guide.* Bethesda, MD: Woodbine House.

Wechsler, D. (2003). *Wechsler Intelligence Scale for Children-Fourth Edition* (WISC-IV). San Antonio, TX: Pearson.

Weeks, D., Chua, R., & Elliott, D. (Eds.). (2000). *Perceptual-motor behavior in Down syndrome.* Champaign, IL: Human Kinetics.

Wetherby, A. M., & Prizant, B. M. (2002).*Communication and Symbolic Behavior Scales Developmental Profile: First Normed Edition.* Baltimore, MD: Paul H. Brookes.

Wiig, E. (2004). *Wiig Assessment of Basic Concepts.* Greenville, SC: Super Duper.

Winders, P. C. (2014). *Gross motor skills in children with Down syndrome: A guide for parents and professionals* (2nd ed.). Bethesda, MD: Woodbine House.

Ypsilanti, A., & Grouios, G. (2008). Linguistic profile of individuals with Down syndrome: Comparing the linguistic performance of three developmental disorders. *Child Neuropsychology, 14*, 148–170.

Zimmerman, I. L., Steiner, V. G., & Pond, R. E. (2011). *PLS-5: Preschool Language Scale-5.* San Antonio, TX: The Psychological Corporation.

PART II

Organic Disorders

CHAPTER 4

Cerebral Palsy

Angela Strauch Lane

Chapter Objectives

Upon completing this chapter, the reader should be able to:

1. Identify cerebral palsy as a nonprogressive motor disorder that varies in severity and characteristics
2. Understand that cerebral palsy can occur before or during birth, or within the first five years of life
3. Identify dysarthria and apraxia as two expressive language disorders that frequently co-occur with cerebral palsy
4. Identify factors associated with cerebral palsy that affect gross motor and fine motor skills, including walking, speaking, and eating
5. List several impairments that frequently co-occur with cerebral palsy
6. Describe interventions, such as surgery, augmentative communication, pharmacological approaches, and behavior modification
7. Identify psychosocial issues that affect self-esteem
8. Identify complementary or alternative therapies that are used in the treatment of CP

Introduction

Cerebral palsy (CP) is a motor disorder that presents with a variety of characteristics and secondary disorders. Speech-language pathologists (SLPs) and others who work with this population of people should be aware of the organic bases of this disorder in order to provide effective treatment. This chapter discusses the etiologies and types of cerebral palsy, as well as effective assessment and intervention techniques.

Cerebral palsy is caused by damage to the motor systems of the brain. This damage affects the person's ability to perform basic functions such as walking, swallowing, and speaking. In order to understand how cerebral palsy affects speech, it is necessary to review the neurology of the speech process.

Neurology of the Speech Process

Speech production is a complex process involving major mechanisms throughout the nervous system. It is produced through the integration of three primary motor systems: the pyramidal system, the extrapyramidal system, and the cerebellar system.

Pyramidal System

The pyramidal system is responsible for voluntary movement of the speech muscles. It is composed of three important pathways, the corticospinal, corticobulbar, and corticopontine tracts, which aid in the transmission of messages to other parts of the nervous system. Damage to these tracts can cause severe upper and lower motor neuron disorders.

Neurons are the basic nerve cells of the nervous system that are responsible for receiving and transmitting neural behaviors, including speech, language, and hearing. They transmit neural impulses, or electrical signals, to glands, muscles, and other neurons. Neurons contain two processes, the dendrites and the axon. Dendrites are projections from the neurons that receive neural stimuli. In contrast, the axon is a projection that conducts a nerve impulse away from the neuron and synapses, or transmits a nerve impulse to another neuron, a gland, or a muscle (Webb & Adler, 2008). In order to understand the speech motor disorders of children with CP, it is necessary to discuss two neuron groups, the upper and lower motor neurons.

The neurons along the corticobulbar tract, which send axons from the cerebral cortex to the nuclei (a group of nerve cells in the central nervous system that have the same function) in the brainstem, are called upper motor neurons. These neurons are contained within the brain, brainstem, and spinal cord. Neurons that send motor axons to the peripheral nerves (cranial and spinal nerves) are called lower motor neurons.

Damage to the upper and lower motor neurons can greatly affect speech production (Brookshire, 1997; Freed, 2011). When there is damage anywhere along the corticobulbar tract, upper motor neuron damage occurs. As a result, the muscles become spastic, or tight. Spastic muscles are characterized by resistance to movement, called hypertonia. The effects of upper motor neuron damage on speech include slow speech characterized by limited flexibility of the articulators and decreased flexibility of the speech muscles.

When a lesion occurs in the pathway of the lower motor neurons, neural impulses are not transmitted to the muscles (denervation). As a result, a flaccid paralysis causing low muscle tone, or hypotonia, occurs. Fasciculations, or muscle twitches, in the articulators are often seen in cases of lower motor neuron damage (Seikel, King, & Drumright, 2010). In addition, vocal quality, respiration, resonance, coordination, and articulation are affected (Duffy, 2012).

Extrapyramidal System

The extrapyramidal system is responsible for regulating extraneous movements. It is involved with maintaining proper tone and posture and changing facial expressions. One important component of the extrapyramidal system is the basal ganglia, a group of subcortical nuclei that influence the initiation and maintenance of movement. Damage to the basal ganglia can result in dyskinesias (involuntary movement disorders), including reduction in movement (akinesia), excess movement (hyperkinesia), and too little movement (hypokinesia) (Webb & Adler, 2008). The damage also produces uncoordinated speech that results in the production of imprecise consonants and ultimately reduces intelligibility (Workinger, 2005).

Cerebellar System

The cerebellar system works in conjunction with the pyramidal and extrapyramidal systems to provide the coordination for motor speech. It is divided into three lobes: the anterior lobe, which is responsible for regulating posture, tone, and trunk control; the posterior lobe, which regulates coordination of muscle movement; and the flocculondular lobe, which controls equilibrium. The cerebellar system provides smooth, coordinated, and precise movements required for connected speech production. Damage to this system can cause ataxic dysarthria, adiadochokinesia (the inability to perform rapid alternating muscle movements), hypotonia, or intention tremors (Duffy, 2012). All of these impairments negatively affect speech production.

These three systems play an integral part in the motor processes involved in speaking. When a person is asked a question, the message is received and comprehended in Wernicke's area, a speech and language center in the temporal lobe responsible for comprehension. In order for the person to respond, the message travels through the arcuate fasciculus, a long subcortical tract that connects the posterior and anterior speech and language areas in the cerebrum, to Broca's area in the frontal lobe. Broca's area is a speech and language center that is important for the expression of language. It is here that the verbal response is developed.

Once the response is developed, the brain sends the message to the corticobulbar tract. Through the corticobulbar tract,

impulses are sent to the cranial nerves, which originate in the brainstem and provide sensory and motor information to the oral, pharyngeal, and laryngeal musculature. The cranial nerves are identified by their names and by a roman numeral. Those involved in speech production include (a) trigeminal—V, (b) facial—VII, (c) glossopharyngeal—IX, (d) vagus—X, (e) accessory—XI, and (f) hypoglossal—XII. Duffy (2012) discussed the individual functions of each of these nerves that combine to form the process of speech. These functions are shown in Table 4–1.

Consequences of Cerebral Palsy

The National Dissemination Center for Children with Disabilities (2010) describes cerebral palsy as a condition caused by damage to the parts of the brain that control motor function, and may occur before, during, or soon after birth. "Cerebral" refers to the brain and "palsy" to a disorder of movement or posture. These disorders are not caused by problems in the muscles or nerves. Instead, damage to motor areas in the brain disrupts the brain's ability to control movement and posture adequately. In other words, it is not the muscles or the nerves themselves that have something wrong with them. It is the damaged parts of the brain that send the wrong messages to the muscles. CP results in difficulty producing, preventing, or controlling movement. It cannot be cured since damaged cells are unable to regenerate (Stanton, 2012).

When CP occurs before or during birth, it is called congenital CP. Acquired CP is the name given to the disorder when it occurs after birth. However, it can be

Table 4–1. Cranial Nerves Involved in Speech Production

Nerve	Motor Functions	Sensory Functions	Effects of Damage
Trigeminal Nerve V	Innervates muscles of mastication and the mylohyoid, anterior belly of the digastric, the tensor tympani (muscle involved in hearing), and the tensor veli palatini (muscle involved in raising the velum).	Transmits pain, thermal and tactile sensation from the face and forehead, mucous membranes of the nose and mouth, and conveys deep pressure and kinesthetic information from the teeth, gums, hard palate, and temporomandibular joint.	Paresis (weakness) or paralysis of muscles of mastication on the affected side of the body, can cause the mandible to hang open or move slowly with decreased range of motion, ultimately affecting place and manner of articulation.
Facial Nerve VII	Innervates the stapedius muscle (involved in hearing) and the muscles of facial expression.	Involves the provision of taste to the anterior two-thirds of the tongue. Does not have a clear role in speech.	Paralyzes muscles on the entire ipsilateral (same side) side of the face, resulting in facial asymmetry.
Glossopharyngeal Nerve IX	Provides motor supply to the stylopharyngeus muscle (muscle of the pharynx) and upper constrictor muscles of the pharynx.	Transmits sensory information from the pharynx, tongue, and eustachian tubes.	Causes reduced pharyngeal sensation and a decreased gag reflex.
Vagus Nerve X	Innervates the muscles of the soft palate, pharynx, and larynx.	Provides sensation from the palate, pharynx, and larynx.	Affects resonance, phonation, voice quality, and swallowing and causes decreased peristalsis for bolus transport.
Accessory Nerve XI	Innervates sternocleidomastoid and trapezius muscles.	None	Reduces head rotation and the ability to elevate shoulder on the affected side.
Hypoglossal Nerve XII	Innervates all intrinsic muscles and all but one extrinsic muscle of the tongue.	None	Causes atrophy, weakness, and fasciculations (uncontrollable twitching) of the tongue.

acquired only until a person reaches age 5. It is believed that injuries to the brain that occur after age 5 result in neurological impairments similar to those observed in adults. Therefore, the damage to the brain would be considered a stroke or traumatic brain injury (Pellegrino & Dormans, 1998a; Stanton, 2012).

United Cerebral Palsy (2012) estimates that between 1.5 to 2.0 million children and adults in the United States currently have CP. In addition, 10,000 infants and babies are diagnosed with CP annually. One would assume that these statistics would decrease as medical improvements are made. However, medical advances have saved the lives of children who previously would have died at birth (Miller & Bachrach, 2006; Stanton, 2012); thus, the incidence of CP has remained constant.

Causes of Cerebral Palsy

Congenital Etiologies

It is estimated that up to 50% of cases of CP have no known cause (Stanton, 2012). Through their research, Rosenbaum and Rosenbloom (2012) have found that establishing the cause of CP is typically challenging. However, preconceptual (before conception), prenatal (before birth), and perinatal (during birth) risk factors have been identified, which can present as single, isolated factors or as a combination of multiple potential risk factors (Moreno-De-Luca, Ledbetter, & Martin, 2012).

Preconceptual Risk Factors

There are several factors that can increase the risk of a child developing CP. These include poor socioeconomic status, mater-

nal smoking or alcohol use, high blood pressure, and diabetes (Rosenbaum & Rosenbloom, 2012). In addition, a gene on chromosome 2q24–25 has been linked with symmetrical spastic CP (McHale, Mitchell, & Bundey, 1999). The role of genomic anomalies has not been widely researched in CP. However, it is estimated that many CP diagnoses that are attributed to prenatal causes may actually be due to genomic abnormalities (Moreno-De-Luca, Ledbetter, & Martin, 2012). Clearly more research needs to be conducted to obtain a full understanding of the roles genes play in the diagnosis. However, prevention prior to conception is within the control of the mother, and can be addressed to minimize the risks.

Prenatal Risk Factors

A variety of prenatal issues can present an increased risk for CP. These include:

- Brain malformations
- Maternal infections such as toxoplasmosis and rubella
- Metabolic conditions
- Fetomaternal hemorrhage
- Cytomegalovirus (CMV)

Rh incompatibility has long been a risk factor; however, testing for this condition has become part of regular prenatal care in the United States. As a result, Rh incompatibility can be diagnosed via a blood test and treated if identified early in the pregnancy (Miller & Bachrach, 2006).

Perinatal Risk Factors

Perinatal causes account for 10% to 15% of all cases of CP, and typically are the result of issues during labor and delivery (Reddihough, 2011). When an infant is born prematurely, the blood vessels in the brain are very fragile and may bleed into the ventricles (inner fluid spaces) of the brain. As a result, an intraventricular hemorrhage (IVH) may occur. An IVH is defined as bleeding into the normal fluid spaces (ventricles) within the brain and occurs when blood vessels in the brain burst. When the IVH is severe, it frequently causes neurological damage and often results in the occurrence of CP (Pellegrino & Dormans, 1998a; Pishva, Parsa, Saki, & Saki, 2012).

The cause of CP in a full-term baby is frequently related to hypoxic-ischemic encephalopathy (HIE), which is a brain dysfunction caused by insufficient oxygen and blood flow during the birth process. For example, meconium aspiration syndrome is a condition where aspiration of the first bowel movement occurs during labor and delivery. This condition causes respiratory compromise and frequently results in HIE. HIE commonly occurs when the umbilical cord is wrapped around the child's neck during labor and delivery. The developmental stage of the full-term baby's brain makes the child vulnerable to damage in the basal ganglia. Therefore, CP in full-term babies is typically characterized by uncoordinated and uncontrolled muscle movements (Pellegrino & Dormans, 1998a; Stanton, 2012). Perinatal stroke is often a cause of CP in a full-term baby (Raju, Nelson, Ferriero, & Lynch, 2007; Rosenbaum & Rosenbloom, 2012). The stroke results from occlusion of a major blood vessel as the result of an embolism or thrombosis (Rosenbaum & Rosenbloom, 2012). Although risk factors for a perinatal stroke have been identified, there are no reliable predictors on which to base prevention and treatment. As a result, the incidence of perinatal stroke remains very high (Raju et al., 2007).

Acquired Etiologies

According to United Cerebral Palsy (2012), approximately 1,200 to 1,500 young children are diagnosed with CP each year. Acquired CP can result from severe brain infections (meningitis, encephalitis), a lack of oxygen to the brain (asphyxia), or traumatic brain injury, either accidental or non-accidental (Rosenbaum & Rosenbloom, 2012). Levin (2006) reported that many third world countries continue to experience outbreaks of cerebral malaria and other infectious diseases, which are common causes of postnatally acquired CP.

Classification of Cerebral Palsy

Because motor ability and coordination vary greatly in children with CP, it is difficult to classify the various types (Miller & Bachrach, 2006; Rosenbuam & Rosenbloom, 2012). Classification involves the site of lesion and effects on movement and the identification of affected extremities. When classifying CP by the site of the lesion, professionals use the terms *spastic, athetoid, ataxic,* and *mixed.* Figure 4–1 depicts the percentage of the population that exhibits each type of CP.

Spastic Cerebral Palsy

Spastic CP occurs when there is damage to the pyramidal system of the brain. It is the term used to describe muscle tone that is hypertonic. It is the most common form of CP, as it occurs in 70% to 80% of all cases (United Cerebral Palsy, 2012). A person with spastic CP presents with impaired control of voluntary movements due to rigid muscles that are permanently

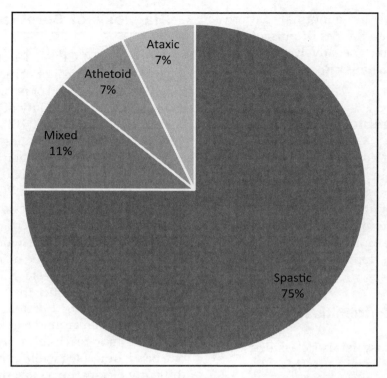

Figure 4–1. Prevalence of the types of cerebral palsy. This figure demonstrates the percentage of the population that exhibits each type of cerebral palsy.

contracted. Attempts to complete a motor activity result in increased tensing of the muscles. For example, when people with spastic CP attempt to drop an object from their hand, the muscles become tighter and prohibit the release of the object.

Athetoid Cerebral Palsy

Athetoid CP is the result of damage to the extrapyramidal system. It results in mixed (sometimes hypertonic and sometimes hypotonic) muscle tone and impairs the person's ability to control involuntary movements. It affects 5% to 10% of persons with CP. Athetoid CP is characterized by slow, writhing, involuntary movements.

These uncontrolled movements make it difficult for the person to grasp objects, such as eating utensils, and to coordinate muscles for ambulation (walking). The muscles of the face and tongue can also be affected, resulting in grimaces, odd facial expressions, or drooling (Pincus, 2000; Yong-Tae, & Brennan, 2008).

Ataxic Cerebral Palsy

Ataxic CP is caused by damage to the cerebellum and affects coordination. It is characterized by hypotonia and affects 5% to 10% of the CP population. Persons with ataxia present with unsteady, shaky movements, or tremors. They typically demonstrate an abnormal pattern of movement and a loss of muscular coordination, which negatively affect ambulation (Rosenbaum & Rosenbloom, 2012).

Mixed Cerebral Palsy

People who exhibit a combination of two or more of the types of CP (spastic, athetoid, ataxic) are said to have mixed CP. This form of impairment results in a mixture of hypertonicity (high tone or tightness of the muscles) and hypotonicity (low tone or floppiness of the muscles).

Affected Extremities

Cerebral palsy is also classified by the extremities that are affected:

- Hemiplegia—one arm and one leg on the same side of the body are affected
- Diplegia—both legs are involved, but the arms are not affected
- Triplegia—three limbs are affected
- Quadriplegia—all four extremities are affected

Following this dual-descriptive model, a doctor would be able to classify the disorder based on both site of lesion and affected extremities. For example, a person with tight muscles and involvement of only the legs is classified as having "spastic diplegia." Similarly, a person with rigidity and involvement of all four limbs has "spastic quadriplegia." CP can affect a person's motor skills mildly or severely. The location and extent of the brain injury determine the severity of the CP.

Diagnosis of Cerebral Palsy

The diagnosis of CP is a lengthy process requiring a great deal of observation over time. Adverse prenatal or perinatal events can increase the possibility of CP (Rosenbaum & Rosenbloom, 2012). However, three main factors contributing to the diagnosis of CP are the acquisition of developmental milestones, muscle tone, and muscle function (Miller & Bachrach, 2006; Stanton, 2012). Developmental milestones include reaching for toys, sitting, crawling, walking, and speaking a first word. Because these milestones are based on motor function, delays may suggest CP. Parents will typically begin to notice that their child's motor skills may be different from those of other children around 6 months of age. The child may reach for a toy with only one hand, drag a leg while crawling, have difficulty picking up a crayon, or demonstrate excessive drooling (Mayo Clinic, 2010). As the infant matures, the concern of CP may arise as development of milestones becomes increasingly delayed.

Observation of muscle tone and function are two other important factors in the diagnosis of CP. Abnormal muscle tone, atypical movements, and lasting infantile reflexes are red flags for the diagnosis. Some of these abnormalities include:

- Variable muscle tone—tone may change from floppy to stiff
- Asymmetry of movement—one side of the body moves more easily than the other
- Weak oral motor skills—poor tongue and lip control, especially during feeding
- Persistent primitive reflexes—reflexes like the asymmetric tonic neck reflex (ATNR) and Babinski

reflex persist longer than 6 months and 1 year of age, respectively

Some symptoms of CP can occur during the first six months of life. The infant may demonstrate difficulty with head control, overextension of the back and neck, crossed or scissored legs, and floppy or stiff muscle tone (Centers for Disease Control and Prevention, 2012). These symptoms alone are not sufficient for the diagnosis of CP, as they must accompany muscular issues and delayed developmental milestones. The use of magnetic resonance imaging (MRI) and computerized topography (CT) scans assists physicians in ruling out other motor impairments when the diagnosis of CP is questionable.

Characteristics of Children with Cerebral Palsy

The characteristics of children with CP vary based on the site and severity of the brain damage. Typically, deficits can be found in four areas of functioning: motor, sensory, cognitive/linguistic, and other co-occurring impairments.

Motor Impairments

Cerebral palsy is solely a motor disorder that affects people's abilities to control their muscles. It is not the direct cause of cognitive, visual, hearing, or attention impairments. Therefore, understanding how CP affects gross and fine motor functions is critical. In the following sections the affected motor area is described followed by some suggested adaptations or treatments to improve functionality.

Gross Motor: Lower Extremities

The gross motor impairments of the lower extremities (legs) vary greatly. Some children with CP require the use of a wheelchair, walker, or cane. Others walk with a distorted gait or without any noticeable impairment. The rigidity of the muscles frequently causes the feet to turn inward or the legs to "scissor," or cross, when the child attempts to walk. In contrast, CP may also cause the child to take uncontrolled and uncoordinated large steps when walking. A prosthetic device called an ankle foot orthosis (AFO) or brace is used to maintain the proper positioning of the ankle and calf.

Commonly, children with CP develop hip and pelvic deformities, as well as tight hamstring, calf, and ankle muscles. Hip deformities are the second most common orthopedic issue in children with CP (Stanton, 2012). Very often, the child's hip may become dislocated due to increased muscle tone. A regular course of muscle stretching or splinting can reduce the possibility of dislocation. However, surgical intervention is often required to decrease the tone. Botox, or botulism, is used to paralyze a muscle group and allow for increased range of motion. Because Botox intervention is temporary, it is not considered a long-term solution. However, it can aid in delaying surgery. Surgical interventions include clipping a muscle, such as the hamstring, to facilitate stretching and improve mobility. Selective dorsal rhizotomy (SDR) is a surgical intervention that involves cutting the nerve rootlets along the spinal cord that are damaged and causing spasticity. Although studies have shown that SDR improves gross motor function in the short term, there is not significant evidence that demonstrates positive long-term effects (Grunt, Becher, & Vermeulen, 2011). Another surgical procedure is placement of a Baclofen pump. Baclofen is a muscle relaxant that reduces spasticity throughout the body. During this procedure, the surgeon places a pump that is about 3 inches wide in the child's stomach. The pump then continuously delivers Baclofen into the fluid surrounding the child's spine. A benefit to the pump is that is allows for a low dose of Baclofen to be delivered continuously, as opposed to a higher monthly dose that is offered orally and can cause side effects. The Baclofen needs to be refilled every one to six months, depending on the dose. Research has indicated that the placement of a Baclofen pump does not increase the mortality rate of individuals with CP, and may even suggest an increase in life expectancy (Krach, Kriel, Day, & Strauss, 2010).

For children with more severe motor deficits, spinal deformities are common (Stanton, 2012). These include:

- *Scoliosis:* where the spine to distorted in an S-curve.
- *Thoracic kyphosis:* where the upper spine is distorted, causing a rounded back.
- *Lumbar lordosis:* where the lower spine is distorted, causing convexity in front.

Each of these conditions negatively affects gross motor function, and may require surgical management.

Gross Motor: Trunk Control

Impaired trunk control in children with CP is determined by the location and severity of the motor impairment (Heyrman et al., 2013). Poor trunk control affects sitting, walking, proprioception

(awareness of body in space), and balance (Figure 4–2). Hippotherapy, or therapeutic horseback riding, has been found to be an effective means for improving balance and postural control in children with CP (Zadnikar & Kastrin, 2011). According to the American Equestrian Alliance (n.d.), hippotherapy uses the multidimensional movement of the horse to provide sensory input to the child with CP. As a result, the child must development new movement strategies in order to stay on the horse, thereby improving trunk control. In addition, hippotherapy has been found to affect perceived self-competence and social acceptance for children with mild CP (Frank, McCloskey, & Dole, 2011).

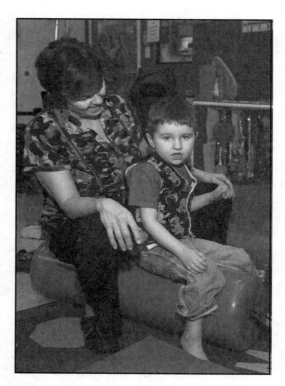

Figure 4–2. An occupational therapist assists a boy with cerebral palsy in improving balance and trunk control. Printed with permission from Kate Higgins.

Fine Motor: Upper Extremities

In most cases, CP affects both the lower and upper (arms) extremities. Weakness or tightness of the muscles makes even the simplest tasks difficult. Fine motor deficits of the upper extremities affect the children's abilities to dress themselves, toilet themselves, write, feed themselves, and use simple tools such as scissors. It is not uncommon for the wrists to be "stuck" in a pronated, or downward, position. This prohibits the rotation of the wrist and makes daily tasks, such as self-feeding, difficult. Hand and wrist splints are often utilized to ensure the proper positioning of the fingers and wrist. In addition, adaptive equipment, such as adapted scissors, built-up handle spoons, crayon holders, slant boards, and pencil grips can be used to assist children with CP in independently completing common fine motor tasks.

Fine Motor: Speech

The speech characteristics of people with CP are as varied as those of CP itself. For many people with the disorder, speech is affected mildly or not at all. Mild articulation errors caused by hypertonicity or hypotonicity may be present. For others, their speech is severely impaired by one of two speech motor disorders called dysarthria and apraxia.

Dysarthria is considered to be the most frequently occurring speech disorder in children with CP (McNeil, 2009). It is defined as a group of motor disorders characterized by disturbed muscle control resulting from damage to the central or peripheral nervous system or to the speech musculature. This disorder affects the strength, tone, range, steadiness, and accuracy of movements required for res-piration, phonation, articulation, resonance, and prosody (Duffy, 2012). It can result in paralysis, decreased range, force, intelligibility, timing, and regulation of speech muscles (Carter, Yorkston, Strand, & Hammen, 1996; Yorkston, Beukelman, Strand, & Hakel, 2010). The types of dysarthria vary depending on the site of the brain damage. Seikel, King, and Drumright (2010) discussed the varieties of dysarthria that are most common in children with CP. These include spastic, flaccid, and ataxic dysarthrias.

- Spastic dysarthria—caused by bilateral damage to the upper motor neurons of the pyramidal and extrapyramidal tracts. Characteristics include decreased muscle tone and range, dysphagia, articulation errors, hypernasality, decreased rate of speech, a perceptually harsh and strained vocal quality, and decreased variation in loudness. Spastic dysarthria is most commonly seen in children with spastic CP.
- Flaccid dysarthria—caused by damage to the extrapyramidal system (lower motor neuron lesion). As a result, flaccid dysarthria often causes damage to the cranial nerves that innervate the muscles of speech. Characteristics include hypotonic muscle tone, dysphagia, articulation disorders, involuntary movements, hypernasality, breathiness, stridor, prevocalizations, and monotone pitch and loudness. Flaccid dysarthria is most commonly seen in children with athetoid CP.
- Ataxic dysarthria—caused by damage to the cerebellar system. Characteristics include articulation

and prosody errors, tremors, increased rate of speech, impaired production of repetitive sounds, unequal stress, and loudness and pitch variability. Speech appears to be explosive. Ataxic dysarthria is most commonly seen in children with ataxic CP.

If more than one system of the brain is damaged, mixed dysarthria can occur. As a result, a child with CP might demonstrate some characteristic of spastic, flaccid, and/or ataxic dysarthrias. Given the similarities among all three types of dysarthria, differential diagnosis cannot be determined by articulatory errors alone. Site of lesion, etiology, and speech characteristics, such as vocal and prosodic features, play a vital part in the perceptual judgment of the dysarthrias (Duffy, 2012).

Apraxia is defined as an impaired ability to execute complex coordinated movements of speech in the absence of muscular or sensory impairment (Freed, 2011). In other words, it is a disorder of motor planning rather than that of muscle weakness. It is caused by a lesion in the motor areas of the brain. Though there are several different types of apraxia, the most common type seen in children with CP is childhood apraxia of speech. Childhood apraxia of speech (CAS) is defined as "a neurological childhood (pediatric) speech sound disorder in which the precision and consistency of movements underlying speech are impaired in the absence of neuromuscular deficits (e.g., abnormal reflexes, abnormal tone)" (American Speech-Language-Hearing Association, 2007, pp. 3–4). It is characterized by vowel and consonant production errors, atypical errors in repeated attempts at pronouncing syllables, irregular prosody (intonation of speech), and poor transi-

tion between sounds and syllables when coarticulation is involved (Teverosky, Bickel, & Feldman, 2009). CAS is identified only by irregular prosody and atypical sound errors that cannot be attributed to dysarthria.

It is often difficult to differentiate apraxia of speech from dysarthria. Observations of subtle differences must be made to determine the correct diagnosis. Apraxia is characterized by inconsistent speech errors and articulatory movements, whereas the speech errors of dysarthria are more consistent and involve distorted sounds. In addition, people with dysarthria demonstrate some impairment of the nonspeech musculature (weakness, paralysis, or involuntary movement). The completion of a motor speech assessment is essential to observe speech production at various levels of complexity (Patel et al., 2013). The information gathered from this assessment will assist the SLP in differentiating between apraxia and dysarthria.

Fine Motor: Respiration

The respiratory system is made up of the upper airway (nose, mouth, pharynx, and larynx) and the lower airway (tracheal tree and lungs). Normal respiration involves three phases of breathing: quiet, forced, and speech breathing. During quiet breathing, there is active inspiration and passive expiration. Forced breathing consists of active inspiration and exhalation. Finally, speech breathing uses active inspiration and expiration against the resistance of the vocal folds (Dikeman & Kazandjian, 2003). For children with CP, the processes of respiration are not as clearly defined. Respiration is often compromised by immature lungs and respiratory distress, asthma, aspiration pneumonia, sleep apnea (intermittent interruptions of breathing during sleep), and chronic obstructive pulmonary disease (COPD), an irreversible lung disorder. Some respiratory issues are outgrown, whereas others persist and compromise respiration severely enough to require intervention. Two types of respiratory management are tracheostomy and ventilation.

A tracheotomy is the surgical placement of a plastic or metal tube through the outer surface of the neck and into the trachea to create an airway (Dikeman & Kazandjian, 2003). The stoma (hole), which remains after the procedure, is called a tracheostomy. Placement of a tracheostomy tube provides a secure airway, long-term access to the airway, and an interface if ventilation becomes necessary (Bove & Sherif Afifi, 2010; Driver, 2000). Following the surgery, airflow is diverted through the tracheostomy tube and out of the neck, rather than through the upper airway. Medical complications due to tracheostomy placement are common, and often result in hospital emergency admissions, increased length of stay, and readmissions (Graf, Montagnino, Hueckel, & McPherson, 2008). If a tracheostomy tube is placed and the child is unable to maintain adequate respiratory functioning, mechanical ventilation may be required.

Mechanical ventilation is the process by which negative or positive pressure is provided to assist or substitute for the inspiratory muscle function needed for breathing (Bach & Ishikawa, 2000; Cairo, 2012). This support is necessary when the normal exchange of air in and out of the lungs is compromised and hypoventilation (inadequate ventilation) occurs. The process of mechanical ventilation begins when a ventilator machine is attached to the tracheostomy by a plastic coil tube. A preset volume of oxygen is delivered into the lungs to inflate them. The lungs then begin to deflate passively and air leaves the lungs. The ventilator then repeats the cycle (Dikeman & Kazandjian, 2003). Mechanical ventilation assists in maintaining the respiratory process when the child is unable to control it himself or herself. Both the tracheostomy tube and mechanical ventilation alter the process by which air enters and leaves the body. Therefore, use of these interventions affects speech and feeding and swallowing.

Effects on Speech. Tracheostomy placement negatively affects expressive language development, including phonation, vocal quality, and articulation (Van Roeyen, 2010). The presence of a tracheostomy tube with a cuff, an internal balloon that surrounds the outer portion of the tracheostomy tube, and ventilator prohibits or reduces airflow to the upper airway. Therefore, the vocal folds do not vibrate and sound production does not occur. To allow for the production of speech, one-way speaking valves can be attached to the tracheostomy tube (when mechanical ventilation is not required). One example of a speaking valve is the Passy-Muir Tracheostomy Speaking Valve. This valve consists of a thin silicone membrane that opens on inhalation and allows air to enter the lungs through the tube. The membrane closes on exhalation, resulting in the diversion of air upward through the larynx and out the nose and mouth. This process provides the airflow necessary for speech production. Although children with CP may need to build up strength to use the valve for speech, most are able to use it after a period of adjustment (Johns Hopkins Medicine, n.d.). Before a speaking valve can be placed, an assessment of oral motor function and upper airway status must occur. Contraindications for valve placement include severe laryngeal obstruction, excessive secretions, significant aspiration, absence of a swallow reflex, and bilateral adductor vocal cord paralysis (Van Roeyen, 2010). A trial of finger occlusion should occur when the cuff is deflated to determine if the person can independently produce sound. This process involves the manual occlusion of the tracheostomy so the air in the person's lungs is forced into the upper airway. If this trial is successful, a speaking valve is not required.

Speech production in conjunction with mechanical ventilation requires the deflation of the cuff. The purpose of the cuff is to prevent air from escaping around the tube when the air is moving from the lower to upper airway and to reduce the risk of aspiration. The deflation of the cuff allows air to rise to the upper airway and vibrate the vocal folds (Dikeman & Kazandjian, 2003). Given the cuff's protective purpose, its deflation could cause respiratory compromise. For some children, the respiratory situation is too compromised to allow for the placement of speaking valve or cuff deflation. In those cases, alternate forms of communication must be explored.

Effects on Feeding and Swallowing. The coordination of respiration and swallowing are essential in the oral feeding process. For children who have depended on a tracheostomy tube or mechanical ventilation since birth, feeding and swallowing can be severely impaired. When food is introduced, lack of experience may cause oral defensiveness. In addition, limited experience with handling secretions may cause desensitization or decreased glottic closure and affect the swallowing process.

The placement of a tracheostomy tube can negatively impact swallowing. It is possible for the tracheostomy tube to "anchor" the larynx and cause reduced laryngeal elevation and epiglottic closure during a swallow. In addition, a lack of airflow through the pharynx and larynx can cause desensitization of those areas and increased risk of aspiration. The use of a speaking valve equalizes air pressure, increases sensation in the upper airway, and has been shown to improve the child's swallow ability for some bolus types (Suiter & Leder, 2007).

The process of swallowing involves several fine motor functions, including: (a) forming of the bolus (a chewed piece of food ready to be swallowed) intra-orally, (b) propelling the bolus posteriorly, (c) raising the larynx, (d) closing the velopharyngeal port, (e) inverting the larynx, and (f) closing the true vocal folds. When muscle function is affected, swallowing becomes more difficult and less effective. For children with CP, weakness of the muscles of the lips, tongue, and pharynx inhibits the production of a strong swallow, leaving residue in the mouth and throat. Swallow function and airway protection can also be compromised by delayed reflex and decreased glottic closure, which may allow food or liquid to enter the airway. One must review the process of a normal swallow, in order to determine how the swallow function is impaired. Sherif Afifi (2010) discussed the three phases of the swallow: oral preparatory phase, pharyngeal phase, and esophageal phase.

Oral Phase. The oral phase of the swallow begins when the bolus of food is placed in the mouth, is moistened, masticated, and formed into a bolus. The tongue presses the bolus of food against the hard palate and thrusts it posteriorly to the hypopharynx, or portion of the throat below the base of the tongue. At the same time, the velum or soft palate rests against the base of the tongue to prevent food from entering the nasal cavity. As the bolus passes through the faucial arches, the pharyngeal phase begins.

Pharyngeal Phase. The pharyngeal phase begins as the bolus moves from the pharynx to the esophagus via contraction of the constrictor muscles. The larynx begins to move anteriorly and superiorly and the epiglottis inverts to protect the trachea. The arytenoids rock forward toward the epiglottis and the true vocal folds and epiglottis close. Intraoral pressure forces the bolus down while the pharyngeal constriction assists in the clearance of the bolus. The respiratory area of the medulla is inhibited during a swallow, so that breathing does not occur. This action, which takes one second to complete, is referred to as deglutition apnea. At this time, the esophageal phase begins.

Esophageal Phase. During the esophageal phase, the bolus of food passes through the opening at the top of the esophagus called the cricopharyngeal sphincter, or upper esophageal sphincter (UES). This sphincter is typically closed and seals off the entrance to the esophagus. It is the elevation of the larynx in conjunction with the relaxation of the UES that allows food to enter the esophagus. The food is then propelled through the lower esophageal sphincter (LES) into the stomach via esophageal peristalsis.

Fine Motor: Feeding

It is estimated that 30% to 40% of children with CP present with feeding difficulties due to oral motor and swallowing dysfunction (Sullivan, 2009a). Many of these children require assistance with feeding

and a prolonged feeding time. Variable muscle tone can affect chewing pattern, amount of food intake, swallowing ability, and the likelihood of aspiration. Decreased tongue strength can cause a forward thrusting of the tongue that pushes the food anteriorly toward the lips and limits the lateralization of the bolus to the teeth for mastication. Consequently, a sucking pattern is observed where the tongue mashes the bolus against the hard palate, and the food is swallowed without having been chewed. An open mouth posture is common in children with CP as low tone in the mandible and lips inhibits closure and results in drooling and anterior bolus leakage. If the muscles of the larynx and epiglottis are weak, insufficient protection of the airway occurs. Similarly, high muscle tone can restrict jaw movement for chewing, constrict the pharynx, and make swallowing laborious. If a child presents with an unsafe swallow, is unable to receive sufficient nutrition orally, and requires an excessively long period for feeding, then an alternate method of nutrition may be indicated (Sullivan, 2009b). These methods include the placement of tubes through the nose (nasogastric tube) or directly into the stomach (gastrostomy tube). Liquid nourishment is then sent through the tube into the person's body to ensure proper nutrition. The decision to place a gastrostomy tube is often a difficult one. Very often, caregivers feel as if they are giving up or failing if they choose an alternate means of feeding for their child. Conversely, other caregivers see the placement of a feeding tube as the end of a long struggle with feeding issues. In general, the impact of a feeding tube is a positive one (Sullivan, 2009b).

Feeding issues not related to swallowing are prevalent in the child with CP. High muscle tone or extraneous movements cause the child to burn excessive calories and develop weight issues. A strong gag reflex or hypersensitivity to temperature, texture, and taste can result in a lack of food intake (Strudwick, 2009). Feeding programs are often developed to ensure proper nutrition. They may consist of foods high in calories to supplement weight loss or varying textures of foods (i.e., pureed foods, thickened liquids) to assist in decreasing sensitivity.

If feeding becomes compromised by weakness of the muscles involved in swallowing, alternate feeding techniques must be considered. When the coordination of swallowing is lacking, food, liquid, or saliva may penetrate be aspirated into the lungs. Penetration occurs when the food or liquid enters the laryngeal vestibule but does not reach the vocal folds. Aspiration takes place when the food or liquid enters the laryngeal vestibule and passes below the vocal cords into the trachea and lungs (Strudwick, 2009). The symptoms of aspiration include coughing, gagging, choking while eating, runny nose, throat clearing, wet/gurgly voice quality, and difficulty breathing when eating. For children without a strong cough or gag reflex, aspiration can be "silent" or unnoticeable because no symptoms are observed. When dietary changes are unsuccessful at eliminating the aspiration, a feeding tube is considered.

Fine Motor: Acuity and Visual-Motor Impairments

Visual impairments are frequently reported in children with CP (Workinger, 2005). A variety of factors predispose a person to visual difficulties, including prematurity and a lack of oxygen to the brain, which result in damage to the retina, optic nerve, or occipital lobe. In the educational system, a child is considered to have a visual impairment when it interferes with the ability to learn (Miller & Bachrach, 2006). Marasini, Paudel, Adhikari, Shrestha, and Bowan (2011) identified ocular issues that significantly affect the vision of children with CP. These include:

- Strabismus—an eye muscle imbalance resulting in inward or outward turning of one eye. It is frequently referred to as "cross-eye" and can cause double vision.
- Nystagmus—an eye disorder that causes jerking movements of the eye in either a vertical or a horizontal direction.

Most visual impairments can be corrected with surgery, corrective lenses, or eye patching. Visual deficits experienced by children with CP affect not only motor function, but also perceptual skills.

Sensory Impairments

Visual-Perceptual Impairments

Visual impairments often affect the sensory organization of the child with CP. For example, nystagmus may alter balance and cause a delay in motor milestones such as crawling and walking. Diplopia, or double vision, distorts vision and makes it difficult to discriminate between foreground and background. Consequently, the child may frequently trip over objects (Blacklin, 1998). Children with hemiplegia frequently experience hemianopia, which is decreased vision or blindness in half the visual field of one or both eyes. They may experience visual neglect or frequently trip and fall (National Institute of Neurological Disorders and Stroke, 2012). Pellegrino and Dormans (1998a) described these other sensory visual impairments that frequently affect children with CP:

- Refractive errors—which include nearsightedness, farsightedness, and astigmatism or distorted vision.
- Retinopathy of prematurity—which is a condition that commonly occurs in children born prematurely and results from oxygen-related damage to the blood vessels of the retina. It frequently causes severe visual impairments, including blindness.
- Optic atrophy—which is damage to the optic nerve that prohibits the brain from receiving visual stimuli and transferring it into a visual image.
- Cortical blindness—which is caused by damage to the brain that prohibits the conversion of visual stimuli into a visual image. In other words, the eye and optic nerve are functioning properly, but are not receiving the visual messages from the brain.

Visual-perceptual impairments play a role in the child's ability to operate a power wheelchair, walk, complete spatial activities (i.e., puzzles), and reach for objects.

Hearing Impairments

Hearing impairment is not common in children with CP, but it does occur (Rosenbaum & Rosenbloom, 2012). There are two types of hearing impairments, sensorineural and conductive. A sensorineural hearing loss occurs when the inner ear or auditory nerve is damaged. A conductive hearing loss is caused by a problem in the outer or middle ear that prohibits the conduction of sound into the inner ear or auditory nerve. A mixed hearing loss can occur when a person with a sensorineural hearing loss develops a conductive hearing loss. The severity of hearing impairments ranges from slight to profound and can negatively affect the speech and language of the child with CP.

Auditory Processing

Auditory processing disorder (APD) is the inability of the brain to process incoming auditory signals (Cohen, 2012). For children with CP, APD is often observed. In these cases, hearing is found to be within normal limits, but the children have difficulty understanding speech. As a result, children with ASD demonstrate increased distractibility and fatigue, poor volume control, decreased short-term memory, difficulty completing multistep tasks, and organizational deficits (Holland, 2011). Compensatory strategies, such as use of an assisted listening device or preferential classroom seating, are utilized to decrease the severity of these deficits (Bellis, 2003)

For a more in-depth discussion on APD, you may refer to the APD chapter, Chapter 9, in this book.

Sensory Integration

Children with CP frequently demonstrate sensory integration dysfunction, which is the inability of the brain to process information sent by the senses (Associated Conditions of Cerebral Palsy, n.d.). As a result, proprioception is often affected. It's very common for children with CP to lean to one side when sitting, and to be completely unaware of their postures. Tactile defensiveness is another common sensory impairment. The feeling of wet paint on their hands or feet often results in a sensory integration "overload" that causes crying, refusing to participate in the activity, or attempting to remove the paint from the body part. Continued experiences with varied textures assist the children in decreasing the defensiveness.

Cognitive/Linguistic Impairments

Cognition

Intelligence can be defined as the ability to reason, conceptualize, solve problems, think, and adapt in the environment (Blacklin, 1998). It is determined based on a standard test of intelligence that measures the intelligence quotient (IQ). People who achieve a score between 70 and 130 on an IQ test are said to have normal intelligence. When the score falls below 70, the person is considered to have an intellectual disability. Intellectual disability is a term used to describe deficits in the areas of cognitive skills and adaptive behavior (American Association on Intellectual and Developmental Disabilities, 2011). For a more complete discussion of intellectual disability please refer to Chapter 3 on Intellectual Disabilities. The causes of intellectual disability are similar to those of CP; however, it is the location of lesion in the brain that differentiates the disorders. Due to damage to the brain, some form of intellectual disability (mild, moderate, or severe) is found in two-thirds of people with CP (Miller & Bachrach, 2006; National Institute of Neurological Disorders and Stroke, 2012). Physical limitations make it difficult to test the cognition of a person with CP. The inability to speak or complete a motor task may impede testing and produce a score that is not commensurate with true cognitive ability.

Assumptions regarding cognition can have negative effects on a child with CP's development. If a caregiver believes that a child has an intellectual disability, he or she may not provide adequate cognitive stimulation. Children who are unable to speak are often classified as having poor receptive language skills as well. However, this is frequently not the case. It is imperative that children with CP are offered the same opportunities as children who speak, especially when cognitive levels are unknown (Stanton, 2012).

When cognitive deficits are present, children with CP often demonstrate difficulty with executive function and working memory. These deficits become more apparent once the children begin school. They might have difficulty initiating tasks, using problem solving skills, monitoring behavior, and making decisions. Jenks, de Moor, and van Lieshout (2009) found that children with CP who present with these deficits tend to demonstrate problems completing arithmetic tasks. It is also suggested that the presence of executive dysfunction may result in learning and socialization issues for children with CP (Bottcher, Flachs, & Uldall, 2010). Compensatory strategies, such as verbal prompting, the use of checklists, behavior redirection, and tasks broken down into steps, are utilized to minimize the effects of executive function and working memory deficits.

Because CP is a motor disorder, it does not necessarily manifest itself as a cognitive disorder. Many children with CP do not demonstrate any cognitive deficits. They are impaired only by their motor function and are able to succeed in the cognitive tasks of daily life. For example, athetoid CP results from damage to the basal ganglia and/or cerebellum, which regulate voluntary movement but do not play a role in cognition. As a result, cognitive skills are not typically affected in children with athetoid CP. However, Turner, Paradiso, Marvel, and Pierson (2007) did identify that damage to the cerebellum may result in emotional lability.

Language and Communication Impairments

Language is the symbol system that allows an individual to talk, read, write, comprehend, and learn (Beukelman & Mirenda, 2013). It can be receptive (comprehension) or expressive (output), verbal or nonverbal. Language can include gestures, words, head shakes, and reaching. The five general systems of language are:

- Phonology—the sound system
- Morphology—form
- Syntax—grammar
- Semantics—meaning
- Pragmatics—social aspects/language use

According to Brookes and Kempe (2012), the development of language is influenced by several factors. First, reciprocal interaction between a child and parent is an essential element. Parents assist in stimulating the child's language by reacting to verbal and nonverbal communication. When communicating with an unresponsive child, parents often become frustrated by the lack of communication and limit their own interaction. Without reciprocity from the parent, it is difficult for normal language and communication skills to develop. A second factor in the development of language is interaction within society. In order to communicate successfully with others, children must learn the rules of the shared language. If one communication partner does not follow the rules, then there is a communication breakdown. To avoid this, children develop intersubjectivity, which is a mutual awareness between conversation partners that they have a shared understanding of the situation (Brookes & Kempe). A final factor affecting language development is language experience. Children learn language by modeling their peers. For children with CP, motor and cognitive deficits limit their interactions with peers and the opportunities for language development (Brooks & Kempe).

Language deficits associated with CP have several possible etiologies, which include damage to the language-processing areas of the brain, intellectual disability, hearing and vision loss, and attention disorders. The specific language impairments developed by the child with CP depend on the site of the lesion in the brain.

Learning Disabilities

When a child demonstrates difficulty storing, processing, and producing information, he may have a learning disability (Lerner & Johns, 2011). The result is an impaired ability to read, write, organize, spell, reason, and listen. The two main areas of dysfunction associated with learning disabilities are processing and discrepancies in achievement. A person with an LD processes information differently than people not affected by the disorder. Processing involves the reception, use, storage, retrieval, and expression of information. When processing is impaired, the result is compromised understanding and use of written and spoken language. The discrepancy occurs between the person's ability and achievement. Despite normal cognitive functioning, the LD impairs performance and the child appears to be lower functioning. The characteristics of LD often become apparent when the child begins elementary school and demonstrates difficulty attaining academic skills (Lerner & Johns, 2011).

Consequences of a learning disability can include dyslexia (severely impaired reading skills), dysgraphia (severely impaired writing skills), and difficulty with reading comprehension, written and oral expression, and auditory processing. For a more complete understanding of LD please refer to Chapter 2.

Other impairments can occur in conjunction with CP that are neither motor- nor sensory-based. However, like the motor and sensory disorders, these impairments affect the child's social skills, academic achievement, and daily functioning. These additional impairments include growth issues, seizures, behavioral issues, and attention deficits.

Additional Impairments

Growth Issues

Delayed growth can be caused by poor nutrition or neurological factors. Hormone imbalances caused by damage to the brain may also stunt growth (Miller & Bachrach, 2006). Hamza, Ismail, and Hamed (2011) found that Growth Hormone Deficiency (GHD) is prevalent in children with CP and could be a contributing factor to short stature. Because swallowing difficulties are common, the child may not take in enough nutrition to increase height or weight. Muscles that are too weak or too tight also affect the growth of the child. Meals commonly take an hour to complete, with little food having been ingested. Poor lip closure and a tongue thrust also contribute to the loss of food. Therefore, the child does not receive adequate calories and nutrition to grow at a normal rate. For children with CP, low weight is frequently associated with an increased number of concurrent chronic medical conditions (Brooks, Day, Shavelle, & Strauss, 2011). As a result, medical management for children with growth issues is essential to determine possible etiologies.

Seizures

Seizures occur when there is an episode of disorganized activity in the brain that results in abnormal involuntary movements or alterations of consciousness (Pellegrino & Dormans, 1998b). They may involve one or both hemispheres of the brain and range in severity from mild to severe. Grand mal seizures typically occur in children with CP. This type of seizure involves the entire body and includes a loss of consciousness, alternating rigidity and relaxation, and periods of lethargy or disorientation (Miller & Bachrach, 2006). Myoclonic seizures are less severe and include brief periods of involuntary jerking of the arms and legs. Most seizures can be controlled with medication. Children with hemiplegia who experienced a perinatal stroke are at a high risk for developing epilepsy. However, prognosis for seizure remission is good via pharmacological intervention (Wanigasinghe et al., 2010).

Behavioral Issues

Behavioral issues are not any more common in children with CP than in children with normal development; however, they do occur. One type of behavior problem is self-injurious behaviors (SIB), which are chronic and repetitive behaviors that a person inflicts on self to cause physical harm. They include head banging; pinching, biting, cutting, burning, and scratching oneself; and repeated vomiting (Miller & Bachrach, 2006; Whitlock, 2010). Behavior modification programs are required to decrease the behaviors.

Children with CP have limited control over their environment. Their physical impairments limit their ability to react when upset (e.g., run out of the room) or to break a rule (e.g., purposefully run the wrong way in a race). To compensate, they often develop behavioral control issues. For example, the child may not open his mouth during feeding as a way to manipulate the environment. He may drive in the wrong direction during a power wheelchair race or ignore verbal directions. The opposite behaviors may be seen in more passive children. Some children are content to sit in a room without causing disruption. Their low affect and docile nature sometimes compromise their success in school. If a child does not require a great deal of attention, he or she may be ignored by a caregiver or teacher and receive limited interaction.

For nonverbal children with severe motor impairment, communicating pain can be a difficult task. Parkes et al. (2008) found that these children demonstrate increased behavioral difficulties when in severe pain. Acute and chronic pain is often expressed via challenging behavior (Dubois, Capdevila, Bringuier, & Pry, 2010). The development of a high or low technology communication system could provide a means for expressing pain, and ultimately decreasing negative behaviors.

Attention Deficits

Attention Deficit Hyperactivity Disorder (ADHD) or Attention Deficit Disorder (ADD) affects approximately 20% of children with CP (Gillette Center for Cerebral Palsy, 2009). These disorders are characterized by increased impulsivity and distraction, difficulty following directions and taking turns, and difficulty completing tasks that require sustained attention. In addition, if the child is verbal he may be overly talkative. These difficulties affect academic progress, social interactions, and self-control. For children with CP, attention deficits further segregate them from their nondisabled peers. These deficits impact their ability to make friends, play with others, and follow the rules of a game. Impulsivity can impact test scores when the child chooses an answer before fully processing the information. Group participation in class is difficult for children with CP as they daydream or call out an answer instead of raising their hand. These impairments in attention may help to explain why children with CP demonstrate increased social and learning issues (Bottcher et al., 2010). Medication and compensatory strategies can be used to assist the child in decreasing attention deficits and improving academic and social skills. The varying impairments associated with CP make the input of numerous professionals essential. These professionals interact to provide comprehensive assessment and therapeutic services for the child.

Microcephaly

Microcephaly is a disorder that develops as a result of brain damage, which restricts the brain's ability to grow. Characteristics of microcephaly include a small head and a backward sloping forehead. In addition, it often results in an intellectual disability, seizures, and hyperactivity (Stanton, 2012). There is currently no treatment for microcephaly.

Hydrocephaly

Hydrocephaly is an increased build-up of cerebrospinal fluid in the skull. It is first identified when the upper part of the child's head grows in size and is no longer proportionate with the face. Hydrocephaly can cause an intellectual disability, although treatments have been identified. The most common treatment is placement of a shunt (or valve) in the brain that releases the excess fluid. However, careful consideration regarding shunt placement must be made because they often cause infections and require additional surgeries (Stanton, 2012).

Interdisciplinary Management

An interdisciplinary evaluation of the child with CP is essential to determine strengths and weaknesses and identify the need for intervention. Although CP itself is not progressive, there are many co-occurring impairments that affect cognition and communication. For example, most learning disabilities are not identified until the child is close to age 5. The course of CP is difficult to predict due to the variability of the co-occurring impairments. Therefore, consistent monitoring provides for early identification of changes in functioning. The input of professionals representing various areas of expertise assists in determining and maintaining the most appropriate services for the child. These professionals include:

- Orthopedic Specialist: a doctor who specializes in medical and surgical treatment of the bones, joints, and ligaments
- Developmental pediatrician: a doctor who works with children with developmental disabilities
- Physical therapist: a therapist who provides assessment and intervention for gross motor impairments
- Occupational therapist: a therapist who provides assessment and

intervention for fine motor impairments
- Speech-language pathologist: a therapist who provides assessment and intervention for speech, language, oral motor, and communication skills
- Social worker: a person who assists families in coping with their social, emotional, physical, or financial needs
- Special educator: a person who provides specialized education services for people with emotional, physical, or social disabilities
- Behavioral therapist: a therapist who develops plans and provides services for the remediation of negative behaviors.
- Psychologist: a person who provides counseling and makes recommendations for issues relating to behavior

Team Approaches

Given the complex needs of children with CP, a team approach to care is essential. Historically, a multidisciplinary team approach was the standard, and was made up of team members who provided services independently of each other. This model was often criticized due to the fact that collaboration among professionals was limited and the needs of the "whole child" were not taken into account (Stanton, 2012). More recently, the interdisciplinary team approach has gained popularity. This type of intervention involves team members working together to solve issues and problems. For example, an occupational therapist and a speech-language pathologist collaborate on a child's feeding assessment to ensure that fine motor and swallowing issues are both addressed appropriately. The interdisciplinary teams work closely together and are considered to be more forward thinking (Stanton, 2012).

Some of the most important people involved in the interdisciplinary management are the child's family members.

Family Involvement

Family members play an important role in the management of the child's intervention. Although the interdisciplinary team of professionals can make suggestions for the child, it is family who ultimately makes the decisions regarding the child's care. In addition, the family is responsible for following through on the therapy recommendations. For example, the child may need to wear braces every night to lengthen the hamstrings or drink thickened liquids to prevent aspiration. Active family participation and support assist in creating the most complete and appropriate program for the child. As a result, the Family-Centered Service (FCS) approach has gained popularity in service delivery. In this model, the family is seen as the expert regarding the child's needs, and the family and professionals collaborate closely (Jeglinsky, Autti-Ramo, & Brogren Carlberg, 2011). FCS offers an opportunity for family members to play an integral role in therapeutic and educational decisions regarding the child.

Assessment

Assessment entails collecting reliable and valid information and interpreting it so as to make an informed decision about something (Shipley & McAfee, 2008). The con-tinued assessment of children with CP is essential due to the variable nature of the co-occurring impairments. For children with CP, the speech and language assessment process can be a long one. Impulsivity, attention difficulties, behavioral issues, cognitive impairment, and physical limitations may play a part in complicating the assessment. The assessment process, completed by a speech-language pathologist (SLP), involves two types of testing: formal (standardized) and informal (naturalistic). Both components are necessary to ensure that the SLP gains the whole picture of the child's skills.

Formal Testing

Formal or standardized testing is important in identifying the child's strengths and weaknesses. These test results provide a comparison of the child's abilities with those of same-aged peers (Beukelman & Mirenda, 2013). However, language tests for children with severe CP are rare (Geytenbeek et al., 2010) and, therefore, the children's true skills may not be represented. For example, a child's dysarthric speech may negatively affect the outcome of expressive language testing or physical limitations may limit the manual manipulation of objects required for some testing items. However, formal tests such as the Preschool Language Scales (PLS-5, Zimmerman, Steiner, & Pond, 2011) and the Clinical Evaluation of Language Fundamentals (CELF-5, Semel, Wiig, & Secord, 2013) should be used whenever possible to obtain standardized scores. A complete formal assessment by the SLP should test several areas, including:

- Receptive language
- Expressive language

- Speech/Communication skills
- Vocabulary
- Pragmatics
- Oral motor skills
- Memory
- Auditory comprehension
- Literacy

It is important for the evaluator to note any characteristics that may be indicative of a learning disability, as the child would benefit from early intervention. In addition, any behavioral issues, distractibility, or impulsivity should be documented during testing, as they could negatively affect school performance.

For children with CP who demonstrate physical limitations, distractibility, or increased response time, modifications within the formal assessment process may be necessary to assist them in completing the test items. These modifications may include:

- A quiet room without distractions
- Testing broken down into several sessions to avoid fatigue
- Repetition of directions for children with auditory processing difficulties
- Frequent redirection to task
- Enlargement of testing pictures for children who are visually impaired
- Use of eye gaze when physical impairments limit pointing abilities
- Untimed testing for those children with physical impairments or delayed processing

In addition, assistive technology can be beneficial for children with CP when they are completing standardized tests (Warschausky et al., 2012). The use of a word processor for completing tasks, an augmentative and alternative communication device, or an alternate access method (i.e., eye gaze, switch access, head mouse) can provide the child with a means for demonstrating true language skills.

The results of standardized testing do not always coincide with the child's functional potential. A child who achieves a high score in a quiet testing area may not be able to perform in a classroom full of distractions. In addition, a child who does not test well might be stronger in the functional use of the skills. It is important to note that while standardized measures may be used, modifications need to be listed, and the results must be interpreted cautiously as the "standardization" was not adhered to. Therefore, the use of informal testing is essential to gain information about the child in her or his naturalistic setting.

Informal Testing

The use of informal or naturalistic testing provides the SLP with information regarding the child's performance when no testing demands are placed on him or her. Although this type of testing does not provide the examiner with age equivalents or standard scores, it gives a more accurate picture of the child's functional use of speech and language skills in the naturalistic setting (Shipley & McAfee, 2008). Two types of informal testing are interview and behavioral observation.

Interviews

The interview can offer valuable insights into speech and language that cannot be obtained through standardized tests. For children who do not perform well in a testing situation, the parent interview is essential for providing information regarding the child's true skills. It is important, however, that the clinician record that this information was by parent report and not directly observed. Though parent report of children's language skills is often a valid proxy, parents may have the tendency to exaggerate their child's skills. Therefore, the use of "by report" will qualify the information.

Interviews with teachers are also important. Like the parent, the teacher interacts with the child on a daily basis and becomes aware of her or his strengths and weaknesses. The information provided by the teacher will be helpful in determining classroom modifications and functional speech and language goals that will enhance classroom learning.

Behavioral Observations

The SLP should also observe the child in a variety of settings to determine how effectively he or she communicates and understands in each one. Behavioral and pragmatic observations provide essential information that standardized tests may not (American Speech-Language-Hearing Association, n.d.). Playtime provides a good opportunity to observe the child's behavior in a naturalistic setting or for the older student a classroom or lunchroom observation may be helpful.

Given the large number of variables included in observation interpretation, it is necessary to complete several observations in a variety of settings. Once the assessment process is complete, specific goals for speech and language intervention are created and implemented.

Intervention

Though CP is not progressive, it requires intervention that will assist in maintaining or improving the child's current level of functioning. The SLP, in conjunction with other professionals, is responsible for several aspects of the child's intervention. These areas include speech, language, oral motor/feeding, and communication.

Speech Disorders

Speech disorders may include developmental articulation errors and motor speech disorders (dysarthria and apraxia). Traditional articulation therapy can be utilized when the articulation errors are developmental in nature and not associated with motor involvement. Intervention for motor speech disorders is more complicated. The therapist must focus on improving oral motor skills, respiration, vocal quality, and resonance. One therapy intervention used to treat dysarthria in children with CP is the Lee Silverman Voice Treatment (LSVT) LOUD (http://www.lsvtglobal.com/). The rationale of the program is that if the child speaks in a loud voice, he improves respiratory, laryngeal, and articulatory function, which improves speech intelligibility. The outcomes of LSVT LOUD have yielded positive results, as participants have shown improvement on certain aspects of vocal functioning (Fox & Boliek, 2012). For children with apraxia, the Prompts for Restructuring Oral Muscular Phonetic Targets (PROMPT) program is frequently used. PROMPT utilizes touch to cue the child's articulators to produce the sounds of a word. According to The Prompt Institute (n.d.), the technique develops motor control and encourages accurate oral muscular movements while discouraging unnecessary muscle movements. Speech-language pathologists must complete an intense training program before providing PROMPT services. If the motor speech disorder is too severe and not improving with intervention, then alternate forms of communication should be considered.

Communication

Communicative impairments can occur as a result of a motor speech disorder, placement of a tracheostomy tube, cognitive delay, or other impairment. When traditional speech and language therapy techniques are unsuccessful, alternative forms of communication can be explored. Augmentative and alternative communication (AAC) "involves attempts to study and when necessary compensate for temporary or permanent impairments, activity limitations, and participation restrictions of individuals with severe disorders of speech-language production and/or comprehension, including spoken and written modes of communication (American Speech-Language-Hearing Association Special Interest Division 12, 2005, p. 1). It can be broken down into the follow categories (Binger, Kent-Walsh, Ewing, & Taylor, 2010):

- No tech: AAC that is nonelectronic
- Low-tech: simple electronic devices
- High-tech: more expensive and sophisticated devices

The purpose of AAC is to augment (supplement) or act as an alternative to speech. For example, a child with CP can use an AAC device to interact with friends, participate in the morning opening exercises, and make choices throughout the day. Communication intervention is an essential part of intervention due to the number of children with CP who have impaired speech skills. Alternative forms of communication not only provide the child with a means of expression, they also assist in improving self-concept when they are used to answer questions in class.

There are a variety of AAC devices available to individuals with communi-cation impairments. These devices vary in size and shape, and offer language systems that utilize letters, words, and/or preprogrammed phrases. They are also referred to as Speech Generating Devices (SGD). Manufacturers such as DynaVox Technologies, Prentke Romich Company, and Tobii Assistive Technology, Inc., have created high-tech AAC devices that are dedicated, or used solely for the purpose of speech generation (Figure 4–3). Health care organizations typically cover most or all of the cost of a dedicated AAC device. AAC manufacturers have recently introduced integrated devices, which offer access to computer and Internet functions, in addition to communication. However, health care organizations typically refuse to cover the cost of integrated devices. Medicare guidelines for AAC funding state that any devices that are capable of running software for purposes other than speech generation do not meet the criterion for funding (Centers for Medicare and Medicaid Services, 2001). As a result, manufacturers have produced dedicated AAC devices, which can become integrated for a fee after the device has been delivered to the individual. This way, the health care organization will cover the cost of the device, and the individual will have access to the computer functions offered by the device.

Since the release of the Apple iPad in April 2010, it has become a very popular communication tool. In a survey of SLPs working in the school system, it was noted that 40% of participants who use the iPad in therapy are using it for AAC purposes (Fernandes, 2011). The iPad is a cost-effective device that can meet many communication needs and is socially acceptable (Alliano, Herriger, Koutsoftas, & Bartolotta, 2012). For children with CP, it is often difficult to feel accepted by

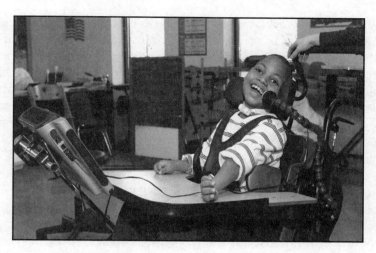

Figure 4–3. A young boy with cerebral palsy uses a high-technology AAC device to communicate his wants and needs. Printed with permission from Kate Higgins.

a peer group. The use of an iPad, which is becoming popular in classrooms and society in general, can assist the child with CP in feeling more similar to and accepted by peers. There are a variety of AAC apps (or programs) that have been designed for the iPad. The vocabulary on these apps ranges from simple preprogrammed messages (Tap to Talk), to word-based configurations (Verbally and TouchChat HD with WordPower), to letter-based programs (Speak It!), and finally to complex language that allows for preprogrammed and novel phrases (Proloquo2Go).

The benefit of using the iPad as an AAC device as compared to using dedicated AAC devices or low-technology strategies has yielded variable results. In a study of five elementary school children with autism and other developmental disabilities, Flores et al. (2012) found that the children's communication behaviors either improved or stayed the same when using the iPad as opposed to low technology picture cards. Many professionals in the field of AAC have reported a prefer-

ence for the iPad due to their familiarity with the device and the cost. However, other professionals prefer recommending dedicated AAC devices due to their many capabilities (i.e., environmental controls) and insurance company funding. The final recommendations for an AAC device should be made based on each child's individual strengths and needs (Chaffee et al., 2011).

Unfortunately, the iPad is not produced by an AAC manufacturer who might be more aware of health care funding guidelines. As a result, the iPad is considered to be an integrated device and is not routinely funded through health care. The burden then falls on the family and/or support staff to locate funding for the iPad. Another concern regarding use of the iPad is limited access methods. The iPad is accessed through direct access using a finger or specialized stylus. Many children with CP present with motor deficits that would make finger isolation, stylus use, and target accuracy difficult. Access via scanning is available using

Bluetooth switches, but very few communication apps are switch accessible. In order for the iPad to meet the needs of children with speech and motor deficits, app developers must begin to incorporate alternate access methods (Chapple, 2011). Although the iPad may offer advantages over dedicated devices, such as decreased cost, global acceptance, and ease of use, it may not always be the best choice for a child with complex communication needs. Because an iPad is an appealing, low-cost, readily available tool, many SLPs are recommending its use for their students without a formal assessment. An assessment provides essential feature matching information, which can identify an appropriate AAC device and reduce abandonment of the communication system (McBride, 2011). An individualized assessment is essential to determine the most appropriate AAC device for the child with CP (Bradshaw, 2013).

Therapeutic intervention for AAC should focus on mastering four areas of communicative competence: linguistic, operational, social, and strategic (Beukelman & Mirenda 2013; Light, 1989; Light, Arnold, & Clark, 2003; Light, Roberts, Dimarco, & Grenier, 1998). These four essential components are described below:

- Linguistic competence: mastering the sound, syntax, and semantics of the native language
- Operational competence: mastering the technical skills needed to accurately access and AAC system
- Social competence: mastering skills of social interaction, including initiating and terminating communication.
- Strategic competence: mastering the compensatory strategies needed to repair communication breakdowns.

AAC devices can provide increased socialization and improved self-esteem for children with communication disabilities (Uliano et al., 2010). For children with CP, they can be an invaluable resource, whether augmenting the speech of a dysarthric child, acting as an alternate to speech, or providing access to computer functions.

Language Disorders

The language impairments of children with CP vary depending on the severity of involvement. Language intervention focuses on improving skills in the areas of pragmatics, receptive and expressive language disorders, and oral motor and feeding disorders.

Pragmatics

According to McTear and Conti-Ramsden (2007), children with pragmatic deficits often have difficulty making friends in school, coping with daily social interaction, and satisfying the social rules of language. For children with CP, speech impairments and a lack of social interaction may further limit the use of pragmatics. The role of the SLP is to present the child with social situations to allow for increased conversational opportunities and experience. These should occur in small group or classroom settings to ensure that all of the child's pragmatic needs are being addressed. This type of intervention supports a functional approach to pragmatic improvement.

Receptive and Expressive Language

Deficits in the areas of receptive and expressive language are common in children with CP due to developmental disabilities, learning disabilities, or lack of experience. The characteristics of the language disorder are typically determined by the severity of the CP. For example, verbal abilities tend to be stronger than nonverbal abilities in high functioning children with CP. In more severe cases of CP, impaired verbal and language skills are negatively affected by articulation deficits (Straub & Obrzut, 2009). Because language is a crucial part of academics (i.e., spatial and temporal concepts in math, descriptive concepts and writing stories in English, and following complex directions in science), the SLP frequently works in conjunction with the child's teacher. The SLP can introduce strategies that the child can generalize to the classroom. In addition, the SLP can provide support in the classroom to ensure that the child keeps pace with peers.

Children with CP often demonstrate deficits in vocabulary skills. Vocabulary is developed through experiences such as social interaction and exploring new situations. For children with CP, some of these experiences may be limited due to physical impairments. The SLP works to improve the child's vocabulary by providing these experiences through thematic units (i.e., all vocabulary is associated with one topic), reading books, and first-hand experiences. When poor vocabulary skills are related more to neurological deficits than to a lack of experience, the SLP must provide the child with compensatory strategies in conjunction with the experiential intervention.

Oral Motor/Feeding

Poor oral motor skills affect the child's ability to speak, eat, swallow, and manage drooling. The creation and execution of a personalized oral motor stimulation treatment program can result in decreased drooling and improved biting, spoon feeding, chewing, and drinking skills in children with CP (Sigan et al., 2013). The SLP customizes an oral motor stimulation program consisting of deep pressure and stroking of the lips, tongue, cheeks, and gums. The deep pressure assists in improving muscle tone, while the stroking works to provide sensory input and alleviate oral defensiveness. The use of Chewy Tubes™ and food wrapped in cheesecloth can encourage a rotary chewing pattern. Programs such as the Beckman Oral Motor Protocol (http://www.beckmanoralmotor.com/) train clinicians on assessment and intervention for oral motor deficits. Through this program, clinicians develop competency in oral motor stimulation techniques for feeding intervention.

The benefits of oral motor stimulation programs for feeding have been debated. A review of the literature reveals that oral motor stimulation programs have played a major role in speech-language pathology treatment for many years, and that many prominent SLPs have advocated their use for feeding and swallowing treatments (Marshalla, 2008). However, Arvedson, Clark, Lazarus, Schooling, and Frymark (2010) found that there is insufficient data to determine the effects of oral motor exercises on children with sensorimotor deficits. With a lack of evidence based practice, additional research is needed to determine the benefits of an oral motor stimulation treatment program for children with CP.

The SLP works in conjunction with the occupational therapist to determine a feeding protocol, or program, for the child. For some children with impaired chewing and swallowing patterns, modifications to their diet are necessary. A complete feeding assessment will reveal the most appropriate food and liquid textures. In addition, the result of a videofluoroscopy can provide the clinician with valuable information regarding function of the anatomical structures used for feeding (Strudwick, 2009). Based on the information obtained, an appropriate feeding protocol can be generated.

When creating a feeding protocol, the SLP should be sure to include information about the texture of the food and liquid, as well as feeding techniques. Recommended food textures could be regular, bite size, chopped, ground, or pureed, based on the child's needs. In addition, if the child has difficulty handling thin liquids, a thickener such a Thick-It™ or Thicken Up™ can be utilized. Using the thickener, liquid textures can become nectar consistency honey consistency, or pudding consistency. Use of a liquid thickener decreases the incidence of anterior liquid loss and provides the child with increased time to control the liquid before swallowing. Verbal cueing techniques, which encourage the child to take small bites and sips, eat slowly, chew thoroughly, and sit upright can assist in decreasing the possibility of choking and aspiration. Intervention may also include the introduction of adaptive equipment to assist the child in feeding herself or himself. Scoop dishes provide a "lip" for easier, scooping, built-up handle spoons offer an improved grip, and cut-out cups made of flexible plastic with space for the nose discourage the child from tilting his head backward when drinking (Strudwick, 2009).

Poor saliva management or drooling is common in children with CP and should be addressed as part of the oral motor intervention. Reid, McCutcheon, Reddihough, and Johnson (2012) found that drooling is prevalent in 40% of children with CP and is associated with poor oral motor function. Open mouth posture, reduced swallowing, and poor head control are also factors in excessive drooling, since the child

in unable to control manage the saliva. Strudwick (2009) identified three treatment options for saliva management:

- Oral motor therapy: this intervention includes strengthening the articulators and has demonstrated short-term success.
- Pharmacological intervention: the use of prescription drugs, such as hyoscine, can decrease reduce the production of saliva.
- Botulinum toxin injections: this procedure injects botox into the select salivary glands and reduces the production of saliva. Side effects could include dysphagia and weak chewing.

The SLP plays many roles in the intervention of the child with CP. However, each role is an important one. These children adapt to new situations more successfully when they receive early intervention. Through the early intervention process, the child receives the modifications needed to be mobile, to communicate, to feed self, and to gain independence. This intervention assists in creating a more positive self-image for the child, which is necessary as he or she enters school. However, children with CP often develop psychosocial issues and require professional intervention due to the physical differences caused by their impairment.

Complementary and Alternative Therapies

Many parents of children with CP choose to explore alternatives to traditional therapies in an attempt to improve their child's gross motor, fine motor, and speech skills. These alternatives, called Complementary and Alternative Medicines (CAM), are utilized in conjunction with conventional medical treatment or as an alternative to them (Workinger, 2005). CAM have produced varied results and are not always supported by the medical community.

Hyperbaric Oxygen Therapy

Hyperbaric Oxygen Therapy (HBOT) is the process whereby the amount of oxygen in the blood is increased, thereby delivering supplementary oxygen to the body's cell and tissue (Workinger, 2005). The rationale for use of HBOT in children with CP is that the damage to the brain occurs due to lack of oxygen to the developing brain, and that there are areas around the brain that can be restimulated. Therefore, if additional oxygen is forced into the circulatory system under pressure, then the body's overall concentration of oxygen is increased, and improved brain function occurs (Rosenbaum & Rosenbloom, 2012). However, this theory has flaws. Nelson (2003) found that, despite common belief, CP is rarely caused by a perinatal lack of oxygen to the brain, and that most CP is predetermined prior to birth. Research on HBOT does not support any evidence-based benefits (Bell, Wallace, Chouinard, Shevell, & Racine, 2011), nor does it show improved gross motor function in children with spastic CP (Lacey, Stolfi, & Pilati, 2012). Serious consideration of the possible benefits and risks should be taken before parents enroll their child in HBOT.

Conductive Education

Developed by Dr. Andras Peto in the 1950s, Conductive Education (CE) seeks to overcome motor disorders rather than to treat or to compensate for them (Stanton, 2012). The program, which is in session 12 hours a day, is implemented by "conductors" who work to improve the children's motor skills through goal-oriented activities. Learning takes place in groups, as opposed to individual therapy. Motor tasks are broken down into basic steps, and music and rhythm are utilized to augment the learning process. Children are encouraged to use their own self-determination and problem solving skills to overcome motor deficits. Conductors provide limited assistance in completing tasks, and independence is promoted (Stanton). For example, children sit on benches during activities. They are required to use problem solving and motor skills to keep themselves upright. This task can be very difficult for a child with a severe motor impairment.

The benefits of CE are disputable. Its use of group education has been shown to promote improved social interaction and increased mobility in familiar environments (Hamid, Leila, Awat, Susan, & Hussein, 2009). In addition, results of CE show improved hand function and completion of Activities of Daily Living (ADLs) (Blank, von Kries, Hesse, & von Hoss, 2008). However, there is no evidence that suggests that CE results in better outcomes than traditional therapy (Darrah, Wiart, Magill-Evans, Ray, & Andersen, 2004; Oldman & Oberg, 2005; Tuersley-Dixon & Frederickson, 2010). One criticism of the program is that it accepts only those children who demonstrate a certain level of intellectual and physical disabilities, thus resulting in a higher success rate. In addition, CE has been viewed as a means for attempting to force the child with CP to adapt to society norms, as opposed to society adapting (Stanton, 2012). Although the benefit can be debated, the CE program provides children with CP an alternate method for improving overall motor and intellectual functioning.

Constraint-Induced Movement and Language Therapies

Based on animal studies, Constraint-Induced Movement Therapy (CILT) has been utilized for many years with individuals who have suffered a stroke, developed hemiplegia, and maintain at least minimal use of the affected hand. In CIMT, the less affected hand/arm is restrained for up to 6 hours a day for 2 weeks so that the individual is required to use the affected hand. The rationale behind this program is that increased use of the affected hand will improve hand function and increase bilateral use of the hands (Rosenbaum & Rosenbloom, 2012). Although studies of CIMT have shown significantly improved use of hand function through behavior change (i.e., use of the affected hand), it is unclear if the changes are caused by the constraint or by increased intensity of services (Taub, 2012).

Modeled after CIMT, Constraint-Induced Language Therapy (CILT) is a group therapy where individuals are permitted to provide only verbal responses. Use of nonverbal communication, such as gestures and writing, is prohibited. Sessions last for up to 3 hours per day and occur 5 days a week. CILT has been studied extensively and has shown to be an effective tool for improved language output, especially for individuals with nonfluent chronic aphasia (Raymer, 2009). Again, the intensity and frequency of services could be the impetus for improved language output. Mozeiko, Coelho, and Myers (2011) determined that individuals with aphasia who received intensive CILT services (30 hours over two weeks) showed more improvement in discourse than those who received distributed CILT (30 hours over 10 weeks). Intensity of services appears to be an essential factor in CILT, and the same gains could possibly be reached with traditional speech-language services of the same intensity. Currently, use CILT for children with CP is limited, and could be considered only for those children who demonstrate the necessary speech skills.

Pyschosocial Issues

Young children with cerebral palsy are frequently unaware that they are different from other children their age. Their determination and ability to modify tasks lead them to the belief that they can do whatever their friends do. As they enter school, they become increasingly aware of their disability. It is not uncommon for children with CP to ask when they can stop using a walker or start writing with a pencil. Since many children with CP do not have cognitive impairments, they begin to realize that this disorder is permanent and that it makes them different from others. Therefore, building self-esteem is essential for children with CP so they feel a sense of belonging and develop relationships with their peer group.

School Age

When children with CP enter elementary school, they begin to develop an awareness of their differences. They may be unable to attend their community school with their siblings and friends because it is not accessible. Participation in gym, music, or art classes may be difficult due to motor impairments. At this age, these children should be given information about their disability so they can develop personal motivation and investment in dealing with their personal issues (Trachtenberg & Rouse, 1998).

People outside of the home environment, like classmates, may not be as accepting as family members. Children may tease or exclude the child with CP from activities. Teachers can play a vital role in assisting the child in development of a sense of belonging by creating situations where she or he can succeed. However, teachers who are unfamiliar with CP may not have the knowledge of adaptations that can assist the inclusion of the child.

Although school-age children with CP begin to recognize their differences, their self-concept is not always negatively affected. Shields, Loy, Murdoch, Taylor, and Dodd (2012) found that global self-worth, image of physical appearance, and behavioral conduct of children with CP did not vary greatly from children without impairment. However, these children reported that they tend to feel less secure in their athletic skills, schoolwork, and peer relationships.

Adolescence

The impairments of CP make adolescence an even more difficult time for the teenager with CP, who must cope with physical differences as well as typical adolescent issues such as identity crises, varied emotions, increased independence, and peer pressure.

During adolescence, teenagers begin to develop a sense of independence by obtaining a driver's license and attending activities without their parents. Motor impairments often prohibit adolescents with CP from gaining this independence. They may be forced to rely on their par-

ents for transportation, assistance with hygiene, or even feeding. All of these factors work to isolate these teenagers from their peer group.

Most adolescents with CP have the same sexual feelings as those of their peers. However, a history of ridicule or rejection may make them unwilling to chance dating (Miller & Bachrach, 2006). Poor self-image caused by delayed growth may also inhibit these teenagers from seeking a relationship.

Peer interaction and acceptance is an important aspect of adolescence. Adolescents with CP consider sense of belonging and being believed in by others as determining factors in success in life (Kang et al., 2012; King, Cathers, Polgar, MacKinnon, & Havens, 2000). Self-concept can play a significant role in this feeling of acceptance. Youths with CP who judge themselves to be competent as a friend tend to be more willing to participate in activities and, ultimately, to develop more peer relationships (Kang et al., 2012). Support from family, teachers, and counselor can promote a positive self-image and encourage the development of these very important friendships.

It is during the adolescent years that most parents seek counseling for their children with CP. The social and emotional issues that they face may become too overwhelming for the teenagers and their families. Therefore, professional advice is invaluable in assisting the teenagers in pursuing activities in which they can be successful.

Young Adulthood

The transition to adulthood continues to be a social and emotional trial for young adults with CP. It is during this time that they may desire to move out of their parents' house and into an independent setting. However, it is often difficult for these young adults to take control of their lives or for their parents to relinquish the decision-making role (Rosenbaum & Rosenbloom, 2012). It is, though, an essential shift in social dynamic so that the young adult with CP can begin to develop his own identify. During this time, people determine their career path in life. Career choices may be limited more by motor impairments than by cognitive issues. Assistive devices are available to increase employment opportunities for people with CP and to integrate them into a workplace. For example, voice recognition software allows a person to use the voice as a replacement for hands when creating a word processing document. In addition, joysticks, similar to those on power wheelchairs, serve as an alternate access method for persons who have difficulty controlling a computer mouse.

For adults with CP, quality of life is primarily influenced by the attitudes they have toward themselves and the attitudes of other people. The participation of all parties involved and the acceptance of professional guidance can assist the person with CP and loved ones in overcoming the physical limitations associated with CP (Miller & Bachrach, 2006).

The impairments of CP can deeply affect the social and emotional well-being of anyone diagnosed with the disorder. Familial acceptance, professional advice, and participation in activities for people with disabilities (i.e., Special Olympics) can assist in building a strong self-image. A positive self-concept will lead the person with CP to personal and professional success.

Conclusion

The effects of CP vary from one child to another. The severity and location of the brain damage play a major role in the manifestation of the CP. The effects of the disorder can range from complete physical and cognitive involvement to a barely noticeable limp. Each child is unique and his or her needs should be assessed and met based on specific strengths and needs.

Cerebral palsy can severely affect language and speech production, communication, and swallowing. These impairments can impact the child's socialization, academics, and vocation goals. Therefore, timely assessment and intervention play an integral part in preparing the child for the future. Due to the multiple impairments that can co-occur, assessment and intervention must be ongoing processes.

Family members play an important role in supporting the child with CP. Once family members accept and understand the child's disability, they can work to assist the child in understanding the disorder and creating a positive self-concept. Parent advocacy helps the child receive beneficial services. The most successful interdisciplinary team is one that includes the parents. The team of people who work with children with CP is an interdisciplinary group of professionals who work together to meet the child's needs. Frequent cotreatment and consultations occur to ensure that comprehensive treatment is provided.

The occurrence of CP has remained constant over the past several years due to medical advances that have decreased the morbidity rate of newborns. Because CP is not curable, continued development of assistive devices, medical and surgical interventions, alternative therapies, knowledgeable professionals, and acceptance are essential in helping the person with CP meet personal and professional goals.

Case Study 1

The following case study shows the thinking of the speech-language pathologist throughout the assessment process. The commentary is noted in the italicized text.

Sabrina, a 2-year, 6-month-old female presented with athetoid CP when she was enrolled in a nonpublic special education preschool. She was born at 39 weeks gestation. However, her umbilical cord was wrapped around her neck during birth and, as a result, she experienced a hypoxic-ischemic encephalopathy. Sabrina demonstrated hypotonia, and motor skills were characterized by writhing in the extremities and fine motor deficits. Sabrina was nonambulatory and was positioned in a Kid Cart (a pediatric wheelchair). She could not sit independently. Speech skills were judged to be poor. At that time, intelligibility of speech was judged to be 50% for familiar listeners and 10% for unfamiliar listeners. At the time of her admission, Sabrina demonstrated an expressive language disorder, dysarthria, and oral motor deficits.

This child had received in-home early intervention services prior to her admission. However, speech and feeding skills remained poor. She was able to produce vowel sounds with varying intonations, but did not make any consonant sounds. The SLP observed that receptive language skills appeared to be good, as Sabrina was able to follow single-step commands and attempted to respond to questions using vocalizations. Her good receptive language skills will assist Sabrina in grasping the articulation and feeding techniques she learns in speech therapy. Oral motor and swallowing deficits were also observed. There were concerns over Sabrina's low weight, poor head and trunk control, and inability to feed herself. In addition, behavioral issues were noted, as Sabrina frequently refused to follow directions. Given her feeding issues, Sabrina was placed in a one-on-one feeding environment so that her specific needs could be addressed by an SLP. To encourage Sabrina to eat, she was read a book during lunch. When distracted by the book, she would willingly accept food. Use of the book as a reinforcer was faded as behavioral issues decreased.

Sabrina lives with her parents in a two-story townhouse. She does not have any siblings. Her parents were not pleased with the intensity of services she was receiving through the Infants and Toddlers program, so they decided to investigate a nonpublic school placement. They were anxious for her to receive intensive occupational therapy, physical therapy, and speech-language therapy services. It was reported that Sabrina demonstrated above average cognitive and receptive language skills, and was beginning to identify letters.

Both of Sabrina's parents are active in her care. Her mother works days shift hours and her father works on the weekends so that one of them is home with her at all times. Prior to her admission to the nonpublic school, Sabrina was receiving in-home therapy services and her parents participated actively in them. Sabrina's parents are very open to alternative therapies, and immediately inquired about conductive education and AAC. Given her parents' support of AAC, Sabrina was immediately introduced to PECS so that she could communicate basic wants and needs. Reportedly, Sabrina's parents have been reading books to her since she was in infant and she has begun to demonstrate emerging basic literacy skills. Because Sabrina's parents are active and involved in her care, the SLP can exploit this to help generalize skills in the home environment.

Initial Evaluation Results

The first formal assessment was completed one week after school admission. The Preschool Language Scales–5th Edition (PLS-5) Core Subscales were administered over one session. Arm support was provided for some auditory comprehension subtest items when Sabrina was unable to independently point to the desired choice. Results of the Auditory Comprehension subtest revealed that Sabrina demonstrated receptive language skills on a 2-year, 8-month level, with a standard score of 98 and a percentile rank of 45. Expressive language skills were found to be on a 1-year, 7-month level with a standard score of 70 and a percentile rank of 2. Severe dysarthria negatively affected expressive output.

The Auditory Comprehension subtest measures the child's ability to understand language. Tasks evaluate precursors for language development, comprehension of vocabulary, various concepts, grammatical structure, and complex information. Sabrina was able to understand quantity concepts, pronouns, and negatives in sentences, which are skills at the 36- to 41-month level. She demonstrated difficulty following two-step related commands without cues.

The Expressive Communication subtest determines the child's ability to communicate with others. Tasks measure social communication, the ability to use concepts, to describe objects, to express quantity, and to use sentence structure. Sabrina's skills

on this subtest were negatively affected by her severe dysarthria. She demonstrated an ability to protest by vocalizing, to vocalize two different vowel sounds, to seek attention from others, to approximate a vocabulary of at least on word, to use vocalizations to request food or toys, and to approximate the names of objects in photos. A scatter of skills was observed due to Sabrina's difficulty producing consonant sounds. Sabrina had difficulty babbling two syllables together, extending a toy to show others, producing a variety of consonant sounds, producing consonant-vowel combinations, and using plurals.

Speech/Voice/Fluency

Articulation skills were not formally assessed due to Sabrina's lack of consonant sound production. She presented with severe dysarthria and decreased respiration. Vocal quality was perceived to be breathy with decreased intensity. Dysfluent speech was not observed.

Oral-Motor/Swallowing

An informal oral-motor evaluation was completed. Weakness and decreased coordination of the articulators was observed. Sabrina demonstrated difficulty with lip pursing and retraction, tongue lateralization and elevation, and smoothly opening/closing her jaw. A high palate was observed. Pureed food was presented on a mothercare spoon. Sabrina did not demonstrate lip closure around the spoon. She was unable to lateralize the food, and a mashing pattern was noted. Anterior liquid loss and coughing was noted when thin liquids were presented. Her swallow appeared to be weak but occurred without delay. Sabrina refused to eat unless she was distracted by a book during the meal.

Hearing

A formal hearing evaluation was not completed. However, Sabrina did not appear to demonstrate hearing deficits as we she was able to localize to sound and to respond to auditory directions.

Summary

Impairments: Expressive language disorder, Oral-motor dysfunction, Dysarthria, Pragmatic deficits

The PLS-5 Core Subscales were administered so the SLP could obtain information regarding Sabrina's language skills. Sabrina's parents had reported that their daughter was very intelligent, but unable to demonstrate true skills due to her motor and speech deficits. During testing, Sabrina appeared very eager to participate. She was seated in a modified chair that offered trunk and head support. Given her motor deficits, the use of arm support was utilized to assist Sabrina in choosing the desired choice. This technique is an approved accommodation for PLS-5 administration. Sabrina required occasional breaks due to variable attention to task. She benefited from having a few pages of a story read aloud, and was motivated to complete additional tasks so that she could hear more of the story. Following each test item in the Auditory Comprehension subscales, Sabrina responded quickly. She benefited from verbal cues to look at each picture before making a choice. However, her answers were typically correct, even when she appeared to be impulsive. Receptive language skills were found to be age appropriate. She was able to successfully complete subtest items on a 3 to 3½-year level. Sabrina's parents had reported that she was beginning to identify letters of the alphabet, and this was observed during test administration. The results of the Expressive Communication portion of the PLS-5 revealed that Sabrina's dysarthria and oral motor dysfunction negatively affected expressive language skills. She attempted to approximate words, but a lack of consonant production resulted in decreased intelligibility. Poor respiration and decreased volume negatively affected intelligibility as well. As a result, Sabrina was unable to respond to many test items, including "use of plurals" and "answering questions." Given her poor expressive language and speech skills, the SLP recommended a formal AAC assessment. This SLP acknowledged that accessing the AAC device would be a challenge for Sabrina, and recommended that an OT participate in the evaluation. Results of the oral motor assessment revealed that Sabrina did not demonstrate chewing skills, and food and liquid loss was significant. Because she was enrolled in a full-day school program, it was essential that a feeding protocol be created immediately so that staff members could safely feed her. Her protocol included adaptive feeding equipment, including a left curved spoon with a built-up handle, a scoop dish, and a cut-out cup. To decrease the possibility of choking, she was offered a pureed diet and nectar thick liquids. A goal was created to increase Sabrina's food to a ground texture. Given the fact that Sabrina demonstrated age appropriate cognitive skills but significant motor deficits, she tended to "act out" via negative behavior. She frequently refused to eat, roll off her cot at nap time, and put her head on her desk. A meeting has been scheduled to plan for Sabrina's transition from an IFSP to an IEP. Specific recommendations for speech-language therapy, occupational therapy, physical therapy, and special education services will be developed at that time. Immediate goals for speech-language therapy include the following.

Recommendations/Goals

It is highly recommended that Sabrina receive speech and language services two to three times per week. The following goals should be addressed during therapy.

Maximize Expressive Language Abilities

1. To produce 5 consonant sounds.
2. To produce 5 consonant vowel combinations.
3. To approximate 20 words.
4. To approximate 2 word phrases.
5. To answer WH questions.
6. To initiate a turn-taking game or social routine.
7. To use words for a variety of pragmatic functions.
8. To participate in an Augmentative and Alternative Communication (AAC) assessment.

Maximize Oral-Motor/ Feeding Abilities

1. To improve tongue strength via tongue elevation, protrusion, and lateralization exercises.
2. To improve lip strength via lip pursing and retraction exercises.
3. To tolerate 3 ounces of ground texture food.
4. To tolerate 3 ounces of nectar thick liquid.
5. To self-feed ¼ of each meal.

Maximize Pragmatic Skills

1. To establish and maintain eye contact for 5 seconds.
2. To respond to questions.
3. To maintain attention to a task for 2 minutes.

Review Questions

1. What information would you give parents of a child with CP and dysarthria to convince them that use of an AAC device would encourage rather than discourage natural speech production?

2. How can new advances in technology assist doctors in predicting, and possibility preventing, the prenatal risk of CP?

3. Discuss why a high incidence (75%) of Intellectual Disability co-occurs with CP.

4. When assessing a child with CP, do you think it is most beneficial to compare the child's skills with those of same age nondisabled peers (through standardized testing) or to use informal testing to gain knowledge of functional skills? Why?

5. Why after age 5 does a child receive a diagnosis of TBI rather than CP after an injury?

6. Discuss the pros and cons of letting a child with spastic quadriplegia who has severe motor involvement and normal cognitive skills attend an included or regular school classroom rather than a special needs school or classroom.

7. How would poor trunk control, weak oral motor skills, and poor hand skills negatively affect a child with CP's ability to feed himself or herself?

8. How could participation in complementary/alternative therapies negatively and positively affect a child's progress in standard therapies?

9. Name 5 impairments that co-occur with CP and discuss how they could

negatively affect speech and language skills.

10. At what point in speech and language intervention should AAC devices be considered for a child with CP and dysarthria? Why?

Case Study 2: The Effects of CP on a School-Age Child

Tameka is a 7-year-old female who presents with spastic quadriplegia. Therefore, her motor impairment is characterized by muscle rigidity in all four extremities and limited range of motion. Her co-occurring impairments include strabismus, developmental delay, reactive airway disease, and status postorthopedic surgery.

Tameka was born prematurely at 26 weeks' gestation and developed respiratory distress syndrome (RDS), a pulmonary disease caused by pneumonia, aspiration, or a traumatic injury that often results in respiratory failure or pulmonary edema. She was diagnosed with retinopathy of prematurity that did not severely impair her vision. However, strabismus and refractive errors are noted and have been corrected with surgery and glasses, respectively.

Due to her motor impairments, Tameka is unable to sit independently or walk. She uses a power wheelchair for mobility, which she operates with a joystick. When she began using her power chair, Tameka demonstrated visual-perceptual difficulties that caused her to veer to the left and bump into walls. A large orange line was painted in the middle of the hallway as a guide for Tameka when she drove her wheelchair. This cue assisted her in paying attention and improving her "driving"

skills. Ankle foot orthoses (AFOs) are worn to maintain proper positioning of Tameka's ankles and feet. Due to increased tightness in her hamstrings and calves, she underwent muscle lengthening surgery in September 2000. This is a process where the muscles are clipped to allow for stretching and lengthening. Periodically, Tameka receives botox injections that paralyze her rigid muscles and cause them to relax slightly. The effect of each injection lasts approximately 6 months.

Tameka's hand skills are poor due to low tone. She is unable to dress herself independently or write. She uses a portable word processor to complete any written work. Hand splints are utilized to maintain proper finger and wrist positioning. Tameka cannot straighten her arms completely to give a hug, but is able to hug with her arms bent. The grasp she maintains is tight and often difficult for her to release voluntarily. Tameka's favorite activity in occupational therapy is painting her therapist's fingernails. While Tameka is having fun, her therapist is improving Tameka's grasp on objects and her fine motor skills.

Tameka demonstrates poor oral motor skills that result in feeding issues. Due to a history of aspiration, her food is chopped and her liquids are slightly thickened. She uses a scoop dish, curved spoon, feeding platform (to raise her bowl), and two-handled cup to improve her self-feeding skills.

Tameka receives individual speech and language therapy two times per week and therapy within her classroom setting one time per week. Speech skills are affected by dysarthria. Her speech is characterized by imprecise sound production and final consonant deletion. Vocal quality is normal except for occasional breathiness. Intelligibility of speech is judged to be fair to good and has improved over the past few years.

Receptive language skills are on a 4- to 4.5-year level. Tameka demonstrates difficulty following complex directions and understanding quantity concepts, passive voice sentences, and part/whole relationships. She requires the repetition of oral directions. Tameka is distracted by noises outside of her classroom and requires frequent redirection to task. Expressive language skills are on a 2.5- to 3-year level and are negatively affected by dysarthria, which influences the length and syntax of her sentences. Tameka demonstrates difficulty using prepositions and answering "wh" questions. Her conversational speech is characterized by sentences of four to five words in length, which frequently begin with "I" (i.e., "I want that toy," "I go my house"). She is able to ask answer simple questions and maintain eye contact. Topic maintenance skills are poor. Vocabulary skills coincide with Tameka's language skills.

Tameka receives services in a special education classroom with one teacher, one teacher's aide, and seven children with disabilities. She learns math, reading, writing, and English, but at a much slower pace than her nondisabled peers. Tameka learns most successfully through functional activities in the classroom and appears to have difficulty grasping abstract concepts. She is learning to spell and completes all of her written homework and class work on her word processor.

Tameka requires the assistance of a teacher's aide for toileting and for food setup in the cafeteria. She suffers from chronic asthma and receives nebulization treatments (the process by which medication is administered in a mist form through the nose and mouth) three times per day.

Family support is limited. Tameka's mother frequently misses her daughter's meetings and often fails to give Tameka her glasses. Communication between home and school is poor.

Tameka is an outgoing and determined child. She has become very independent and often says, "I can do it myself." She appears unaware of her differences and has developed a positive self-concept. Tameka attends music and art classes with her nondisabled peers. They accept her because she is so friendly and willing to participate. Her peers are anxious to carry Tameka's books or hand her project supplies. The children enjoy sitting next to Tameka and gladly oblige when she asks them to hold her hand. When Tameka becomes excited, the muscles in her extremities tighten, resulting in arm and leg extension.

Tameka demonstrates typical characteristics of a child with CP. Her gross and fine motor skills, vision, speech, language, attention, pragmatics, and feeding skills are all affected by the disorder. She is part of a special education classroom due to her co-occurring developmental delay. Tameka receives physical, occupational, and speech and language therapies and is followed by an orthopod. Her impairments will not progress, but Tameka will require intervention for the remainder of her life to maintain her skills.

Review Questions

1. As Tameka's SLP, what aspect of language do your believe is most important to focus on this time?

2. Develop one measureable long-term goal and three measureable short-term goals for each of the following

areas: phonology, syntax, semantic, and pragmatics. Provide a rationale for each goal.

3. What oral motor exercises can be implemented to assist Tameka in strengthening oral musculature, specifically the articulators?

4. To decrease Tameka's risk of aspiration, are there any additional measures that you can take to ensure safe swallowing? Consider Tameka's language skills and muscle tone.

5. How might you approach Tameka's uninvolved family in an effort to include them in decisions? Is it appropriate to encourage them to become more involved in Tameka's therapy routines?

Case Study 3: The Effects of CP on an Adolescent

Donny is a 16-year-old male who presents with spastic quadriplegia and severe to profound intellectual disability. He has received special education services in a self-contained classroom since age 3. In addition, speech-language therapy, physical therapy, and occupational therapy are provided on a consultative basis.

Donny's motor skills are severely impaired. He has limited use of his upper and lower extremities bilaterally due to high muscle tone. Donny uses a manual wheelchair and is dependent for mobility. His physical therapist attempted training with a power chair, but she was unable to identify a body part that would consistently operate the controls. To allow Donny the opportunity to bear weight and stretch his hamstring and calf mus-

cles, he is often placed in a prone stander. This device allows him to stand up while straps support his back and legs. However, he can stay in this device for only 20 minutes before fatigue sets in.

Donny's hand skills are poor. Due to high muscle tone, he is unable to grasp an object for more than 10 seconds. Therefore, he is unable to feed or dress himself, or complete simple craft activities. Donny's teacher uses adapted equipment to allow him to participate in classroom activities. When Donny is required to cut paper, his teacher attaches battery-powered scissors to a communication switch. Donny's activation of the switch powers the scissors as his teacher guides them over the paper. This technique provides Donny with control over the situation and allows him to participate in the activity.

Donny's oral motor skills are weak. He demonstrates an open mouth posture and high tone in his cheeks and tongue. He uses his tongue to mash the food against his hard palate. He does not lateralize the food or chew. His occupational therapist began placing small pieces of toast on Donny's molars to encourage chewing. Donny has eaten regular chopped foods for most of his life. His SLP began to observe coughing and a wet vocal quality after Donny ate. Donny was referred for a modified barium swallow (MBS), a test that utilizes barium-coated food and X-ray machines to observe the patient's swallow. The results of the MBS showed that Donny was aspirating regular textured foods and thin liquids. Therefore, he was put on a pureed diet with thickened liquids. Because his diet modifications, Donny's coughing has decreased and vocal quality has improved.

Donny is dependent on others for toileting and bathing. He is unable to indicate that he has to go to the bathroom, so he wears adult diapers throughout the day. A bath chair, a chair with supports that sits in the bathtub, is used to assist Donny's mother in bathing him. However, since Donny entered his teenage years, it has become more difficult for his mother to lift him in and out of his bath chair. Eventually, she will require human or mechanical assistance in transporting her son in and out of his chair.

Speech skills are limited. Due to weak oral musculature and high tone, Donny is able to produce only one word ("yeah") and vocalizations. He has used a communication device since age 8. At the time, the device was programmed with four pictures that allowed Donny to communicate basic wants and needs. With daily practice and encouragement, he now has 20 pictures per page. Donny is able to navigate independently throughout the various pages on his device using visual scanning and a switch that he accesses with his head. His doctors initially gave Donny the diagnosis of severe to profound intellectual disability. However, use of the communication device has allowed Donny to display his cognitive skills accurately. He has begun sight reading words, telling the weather, making choices, and reporting sports scores. Use of the communication device has increased Donny's participation in social and academic classroom activities.

Standardized testing reveals that Donny's receptive language skills are on a 3- to 3.5-year level. However, informal observations suggest that these skills are higher. As previously stated, Donny is able to use his communication device to identify letters and colors and to make decisions. Due to physical limitations, he is not able to complete many of the items on standardized tests accurately. Therefore, observing Donny's functional comprehension of language appears to be the most effective way to obtain information regarding his strengths and needs. Expressive language skills are on a 6-month to 1-year level and are negatively affected by Donny's poor speech skills.

Donny receives special education services in a self-contained classroom that consists of 10 students, one special educator, and three teacher's assistants. Although positioning, toileting, and eating occupy a large portion of his day, Donny also receives instruction on current events, sequencing, colors, numbers, and spelling. He appears to enjoy learning and likes to use his communication device to be the first student to answer a question. When Donny is age 21, he will graduate from his school. However, the transition process has already begun so that Donny will have a smooth transition to his next placement. He will either attend an adult day program or be employed at a sheltered workshop where he can complete simple computer activities.

Donny has a great deal of family support. His mother is a single parent who gave birth to Donny when she was 16 years old. She receives assistance from family members, but prefers to be her son's main care provider. Donny's mother is a strong advocate for her son, as she attends all of his meetings and verbalizes concerns. Though her literacy skills are limited, she learned how to program Donny's communication device so that he could share his home experiences with classmates. Financially, Donny's mother relies on her son's social workers to assist in securing funds for a wheelchair ramp, bath chair, and accessible van. Donny has a strong relationship with his mother and squeals with joy when her name is mentioned.

Donny is an outgoing and friendly teenager. He likes to listen to rock music, report the baseball scores, and use his friendly smile to flirt with girls. Like any teenager, Donny is emotional and becomes upset when his routine is interrupted. He enjoys private time in his room as much as socializing with friends. As his verbal abilities have increased through the use of his communication device, so has his interaction with others. His mother hopes that one day Donny will be able to be a greeter at a department store. She feels that he can use his communication device and welcoming brown eyes to greet the customers as they enter the store. Donny's strong personality and determination will assist him as he prepares to transition to adulthood.

Though Donny's CP affects his mobility, speech, feeding skills, and independence, he is just like any other teenager. Adapted equipment, supportive family, intensive therapy, and caring teachers have given Donny a strong foundation for the future. His determination and easygoing personality will assist him in living a happy and satisfying life.

Review Questions

1. In addition to coughing and a wet vocal quality after eating, what other signs and symptoms might you look for to identify penetration and/or aspiration?

2. What would you say to Donny's mother to explain why his diet texture was changed from regular to pureed?

3. Based on Donny's current interests, design a functional 30-minute lesson plan that is engaging and motivating. Provide a rationale for each activity.

4. As mentioned, Donny's standardized test scores do not accurately reflect his functional comprehension of lan-guage. Why is informal observation so important, and what information can it provide you that a standardized test cannot?

5. What strategies can you use to assist Donny in transitioning in and out of his speech and language therapy sessions?

References

Alliano, A., Herriger, K., Koutsoftas, A. D., & Bartolotta, T. E. (2012). A review of 21 iPad applications for augmentative and alternative communication purposes. *Perspectives on Augmentative and Alternative Communication, 21*(2), 60.

American Association of Intellectual and Developmental Disabilities. (2011). *FAQ on AAIDD Definition on Intellectual Disability*. Retrieved from http://www.aaidd.org/IntellectualDisabilityBook/content_7473.cfm?navID=36

American Equestrian Alliance. (n.d.). *Therapeutic Riding Program*. Retrieved from http://www.americanequestrian.com/hippotherapy.htm

American Speech-Language-Hearing Association. (n.d.). *Directory of speech-language pathology assessment instruments introduction*. Retrieved from http://www.asha.org/SLP/assessment/Assessment-Introduction/

American Speech-Language-Hearing Association. (2005). *Roles and responsibilities of speech-language pathologists with respect to augmentative and alternative communication* [Position statement]. Retrieved from http://www.asha.org/policy/PS2005-00113.htm

American Speech-Language-Hearing Association. (2007). *Childhood apraxia of speech* [Technical report]. Retrieved from http://www.asha.org/policy/PS2007-00277. htm

Arvedson, J., Clark, H., Lazarus, C., Schooling, T., & Frymark, T. (2010). The effects of oral-motor exercises on swallowing in children: An evidence-based systematic review. *Developmental Medicine & Child Neurology, 52*(11), 1000–1013. doi:10.1111/j.1469-8749.2010.03707.x

Associated Conditions of Cerebral Palsy. (n.d). *Sensory of perception impairments*. Retrieved from http://www.associatedconditionsofcere bralpalsy.com/sensory.html

Bach, J. R., & Ishikawa, Y. (2000). Respiratory insufficiency: Pathophysiology, indications, and other considerations for intervention. In D. C. Tippett (Ed.), *Tracheostomy and ventilator dependency* (pp. 47–64). New York, NY: Thieme.

Bell, E., Wallace, T., Chouinard, I., Shevell, M., & Racine, E. (2011). Responding to requests of families for unproven interventions in neurodevelopmental disorders: Hyperbaric oxygen 'treatment' and stem cell 'therapy' in cerebral palsy. *Developmental Disabilities Research Reviews, 17*(1), 19–26. doi:10. 1002/ddrr.134

Bellis, T. J. (2003). *Assessment and management of central auditory processing disorders in the educational setting: From science to practice.* San Diego, CA: Delmar Cengage Learning.

Beukelman, D., & Mirenda, P. (2013). *Augmentative & alternative communication: Supporting children & adults with complex communication needs* (4th ed.). Baltimore, MD: Paul H. Brookes.

Binger, C., Kent-Walsh, J., Ewing, C., & Taylor, S. (2010). Teaching educational assistants to facilitate the multisymbol message productions of young students who require augmentative and alternative communication. *American Journal of Speech-Language Pathology, 19,* 108–120.

Blacklin, J. S. (1998). Your child's development. In E. Geralis (Ed.), *Children with cerebral palsy: A parents' guide* (2nd ed., pp. 193–230). Bethesda, MD: Woodbine House.

Blank, R., von Kries, R., Hesse, S., & von Voss, H. (2008). Conductive education for children with cerebral palsy: Effects on hand motor functions relevant to activities of daily living. *Archives Physical and Medical Rehabilitation, 89,* 251–259.

Bottcher, L., Flachs, E., & Uldall, P. (2010). Attentional and executive impairments in children with spastic cerebral palsy. *Developmental Medicine & Child Neurology, 52*(2), e42–e47.

Bove, M., & Sherif Afifi, M. (2010). Tracheotomy procedure. In L. L. Morris & M. Sherif Afifi (Eds.), *Tracheostomies: The complete guide* (pp. 17–40). New York, NY: Springer.

Bradshaw, J. (2013). The use of augmentative and alternative communication apps for the iPad, iPod and iPhone: An overview of recent developments. *Tizard Learning Disability Review, 18*(1), 31–37. doi:10.1108/13595471311295996

Brooks, J., Day, S., Shavelle, R., & Strauss, D. (2011). Low weight, morbidity, and mortality in children cerebral palsy: New clinical growth charts. *Pediatrics, 128*(2), e299–e307. doi:10.1542/peds.2010-2801

Brooks, P., & Kempe, V. (2012). *Language development.* West Sussex, UK: John Wiley & Sons.

Brookshire, R. H. (1997). *Introduction to neurogenic communication disorders.* St. Louis, MO: Elsevier Mosby.

Cairo, J. M. (2012). *Pilbeam's mechanical ventilation: Physiological and clinical applications* (5th ed.). St. Louis, MO: Elsevier Mosby.

Carter, C. R., Yorkston, K. M., Strand, E. A., & Hammen, V. L. (1996). Effects of semantic and syntactic context on actual and estimated sentence intelligibility of dysarthric speakers. In D. A. Robin, K. M. Yorkston, & D. R. Beukelman (Eds.), *Disorders of motor speech* (pp. 67–87). Baltimore, MD: Paul H. Brookes.

Centers for Disease Control and Prevention. (2012). *Facts about cerebral palsy.* Retrieved from http://www.cdc.gov/NCBDDD/cp/facts.html

Centers for Medicare and Medicaid Services. (2001). *National coverage determination for speech generating devices.* Retrieved from http://www.cms.gov/medicare-coverage-database/details/ncd-details.aspx?NCDId=274&ncd ver=1&bc=AgAAgAAAAAAA&

Chaffee, S., Guistwite, C., Pfister, M., Horan, K., Azeles, L., Dalmas, N., . . . Smith, P. (2011). *Cost/Benefit analysis of using the iPad versus the Dynavox as an AAC device.* Poster session presented at the American Speech-Language Hearing Association Annual Convention, San Diego, CA.

Chapple, D. (2011). The evolution of augmentative communication and the importance of alternate access. *Perspectives on Augmentative and Alternative Communication, 20,* 34–37. doi:10.1044/aac20.1.34

Cohen, L. (2012). *Exploring auditory processing disorder* [Kindle iPad version]. Retrieved from http://www.amazon.com

Darrah, J. J., Wiart, L. L., Magill-Evans, J. J., Ray, L. L., & Andersen, J. J. (2012). Are family-centered principles, functional goal setting and transition planning evident in therapy services for children with cerebral palsy? *Child:*

Care, Health and Development, 38(1), 41–47. doi:10.1111/j.1365-2214.2010.01160.x

Dikeman, K. J., & Kazandjian, M. S. (2003). *Communication and swallowing management of tracheostomized and ventilator-dependent adults* (2nd ed.). Clifton Park, NY: Delmar Learning.

Driver, L. E. (2000). Pediatric considerations. In D. C. Tippett (Ed.), *Tracheostomy and ventilator dependency* (pp. 193–235). New York, NY: Thieme.

Dubois, A., Capdevila, X., Bringuier, S., & Pry, R. (2010). Pain expression in children with intellectual disability. *European Journal of Pain, 14,* 654–660.

Duffy, J. R. (2012). *Motor speech disorders: Substrates, differential diagnosis, and management* (3rd ed.). St. Louis, MO: Elsevier Mosby.

Fernandes, B. (2011). iTherapy: The revolution of mobile devices within the field of speech therapy. *Perspectives on School-Based Issues, 12*(2), 35–40. doi:10.1044/sbi12. 2. 35

Flores, M., Musgrove, K., Renner, S., Hinton, V., Strozier, S., Franklin, S., . . . Hil, D. (2012). A comparison of communication using the Apple iPad and a picture-based system. *AAC: Augmentative and Alternative Communication, 28*(2), 74–84. doi:10.3109/07434618.2011.644 579

Fox, C., & Boliek, C. (2012). Intensive voice treatment (LSVT LOUD) for children with spastic cerebral palsy and dysarthria. *Journal of Speech, Language, and Hearing Research: JSLHR, 55*(3), 930–945. doi:10.1044/1092-4388 (2011/10-0235)

Frank, A., McCloskey, S., & Dole, R. (2011). Effect of hippotherapy on perceived self-competence and participation in a child with cerebral palsy. *Pediatric Physical Therapy, 23*(3), 301–308.

Freed, D. B. (2011). *Motor speech disorders: Diagnosis and treatment* (2nd ed.). Clifton Park, NY: Delmar Cengage.

Geytenbeek, J., Harlaar, L., Stam, M., Ket, H., Becher, J.G., Oostrom, K., . . . Vermeulen, J. (2010). Utility of language comprehension tests for unintelligible or non-speaking children with cerebral palsy: A systematic review. *Developmental Medicine & Child Neurology, 52*(12), 1098.

Gillette Center for Cerebral Palsy. (2009). *A guide to understanding cerebral palsy.* Retrieved from http://www.gillettechildrens.org/fileup load/understand_cerebral_palsy.pdf

Graf, J. M., Montagnino, M. S., Hueckel, R., & McPherson, M. L. (2008). Pediatric tracheostomies: A recent experience from one academic center. *Pediatric Critical Care Medicine, 9,* 96–100.

Grunt. S., Becher, J., & Vermeulen, R. (2011). Long-term outcome and adverse effects of selective dorsal rhizotomy in children with cerebral palsy: A systematic review. *Developmental Medicine and Child Neurology, 53*(6), 490–498.

Hamid, D., Leila, D., Awat, F., Susan, A., & Hussein, B. (2009). Effect of the Bobath technique, conductive education and education to parents in activities of daily living in children with cerebral palsy in Iran. *Hong Kong Journal of Occupational Therapy, 19,* 14–19. doi:10.1016/S1569-1861(09)70039-7

Hamza, R., Ismail, M., & Hamed, A. (2011). Growth hormone deficiency in children and adolescents with cerebral palsy: Relation to gross motor function and degree of spasticity. *Pakistan Journal of Biological Sciences, 14*(7), 433–440.

Heyrman, L., Desloovere, K., Molenaers, G., Verheyden, G., Klingels, K., Monbaliu, E., . . . Feys, H. (2013). Clinical characteristics of impaired trunk control in children with spastic cerebral palsy. *Research in Developmental Disabilities, 34*(1), 327–334.

Holland, J. (2011). *Train the brain to hear: Brain training techniques to treat auditory processing disorders in kids with ADD/ADHD, low spectrum autism, and auditory processing disorders.* Boca Raton, FL: Universal.

Jeglinsky, I. I., Autti-Rämö, I. I., & Brogren Carlberg, E. E. (2012). Two sides of the mirror: Parents' and service providers' view on the family-centeredness of care for children with cerebral palsy. *Child: Care, Health and Development, 38*(1), 79–86. doi:10.1111/j.1365-2214.2011.01305.x

Jenks, K. M., de Moor, J., & van Lieshout, E. M. (2009). Arithmetic difficulties in children with cerebral palsy are related to executive function and working memory. *Journal of Child Psychology and Psychiatry, 50*(7), 824–833. doi:10.1111/j.1469-7610.2008.02031.x

Johns Hopkins Medicine. (n.d.). *Tracheostomy and a passy-muir valve.* Retrieved from http://www.hopkinsmedicine.org/tracheostomy/living/passey-muir_valve.html

Kang, L. J., Palisano, R. J., King, G. A., Chiarello, L. A., Orlin, M. N., & Polansky, M. M.

(2012). Social participation of youths with cerebral palsy differed based on their self-perceived competence as a friend. *Child: Care, Health and Development, 38*(1), 117–127. doi:10.1111/j.1365-2214.2011.01222.x

King, G., Cathers, T., Polgar, J. M., MacKinnon, E., & Havens, L. (2000). Success in life for older adolescents with cerebral palsy. *Qualitative Health Research, 10,* 734–749.

Krach, L., Kriel, R., Day, S., & Strauss, D. (2010). Survival of individuals with cerebral palsy receiving continuous intrathecal baclofen treatment: A matched-cohort study. *Developmental Medicine & Child Neurology, 52*(7), 672–676. doi:10.1111/j.1469-8749.2009.03473.x

Lacey, D., Stolfi, A., & Pilati, L. (2012). Effects of hyperbaric oxygen on motor function in children with cerebral palsy. *Annals of Neurology, 72*(5), 695–703. doi:10.1002/ana.23681

Lerner, J., & Johns, B. (2011). *Learning disabilities and related mild disabilities: What's new in education* (12th ed.). Belmont, CA: Wadsworth.

Levin, K. (2006). I am what I am because of who we all are: International perspectives on rehabilitation: South Africa. *Pediatric Rehabilitation, 9,* 285–292.

Light, J. (1989). Toward a definition of communicative competence for individuals using augmentative and alternative communication systems. *Augmentative and Alternative Communication, 5,* 137–144.

Light, J., Arnold, K., & Clark, E. (2003). Finding a place in the "social circle of life." In J. C. Light, D. R. Beukelman, & J. Reichle (Eds.), *Communicative competence for individuals who use AAC: From research to effective practice* (pp. 361–397). Baltimore, MD: Paul H. Brookes.

Light, J., Roberts, B., Dimarco, R., & Greiner, N. (1998). Augmentative and alternative communication to support receptive and expressive communication for people with autism. *Journal of Communication Disorders, 31,* 153–180.

Marasini, S., Paudel, N., Adhikari, P., Shrestha, J., & Bowan, M. D. (2011). Ocular manifestations in children with cerebral palsy. *Optometry & Vision Development, 42*(3), 178–182.

Marshalla, P. (2008). Oral motor treatment vs. non-speech oral motor exercises. *Oral Motor Institute, 2*(2). Retrieved from http://www.oralmotorinstitute.org

Mayo Clinic. (2010). *Cerebral palsy.* Retrieved from http://www.mayoclinic.com/health/cerebral-palsy/DS00302/DSECTION=symptoms

McBride, D. (2011). AAC evaluations and new mobile technologies: Asking and answering the right questions. *Perspectives on Augmentative and Alternative Communication, 20,* 9–16. doi:10.1044/aac20.1.9

McHale, D., Mitchell, S., & Bundey, S. (1999). A gene for autosomal recessive symmetrical spastic cerebral palsy maps to chromosome Zq 24–25. *American Journal of Human Genetics, 64,* 526–532.

McNeil, M. R. (2009). *Clinical management of sensorimotor speech disorders* (2nd ed.). New York, NY: Thieme.

McTear, M., & Conti-Ramsden, G. (2007). *Pragmatic disability in children: Assessment and intervention.* Hoboken, NJ: Wiley.

Miller, F., & Bachrach, S. J. (2006). *Cerebral palsy: A complete guide for caregiving* (2nd ed.). Baltimore, MD: Johns Hopkins University Press.

Moreno-De-Luca, A., Ledbetter, D., & Martin, C. (2012). Genetic insights into the causes and classification of cerebral palsies. *Lancet Neurology, 11*(3), 283–292. doi:10.1016/S1474-4422(11)70287-3

Mozeiko, J., Coelho, C., & Myers, E. (2011). *A comparison of intensity for constraint induced language therapy in aphasia.* Retrieved from http://aphasiology.pitt.edu/archive/00002293/

National Dissemination Center for Children with Disabilities. (2010). *Cerebral palsy disability fact sheet #2.* Retrieved from http://nichcy.org/wp-content/uploads/docs/fs2.pdf

National Institute of Neurological Disorders and Stroke. (2012). *Cerebral palsy: Hope through research.* Retrieved from http://www.ninds.nih.gov/disorders/cerebral_palsy/detail_cerebral_palsy.htm#211403104

Nelson, K. (2003). Sounding board. Can we prevent cerebral palsy? *New England Journal of Medicine, 349*(18), 1765–1769.

Oldman, P., & Oberg, B. (2005). Effectiveness of intensive training for children with cerebral palsy—a comparison between child and youth rehabilitation and conductive education. *Journal of Rehabilitation Medicine, 37,* 263–270.

Parkes, J., White-Koning, M., Dickinson, H. O., Thyen, U., Arnaud, C., & Beckung, E. (2008). Psychological problems in children with cerebral palsy: A cross-sectional European study. *Journal of Child Psychology and Psychiatry, 49,* 405–413.

Patel, R., Connaghan, K., Franco, D., Edsall, E., Forgit, D., Olson, L., . . . Russell, S. (2013). "The caterpillar": A novel reading passage for assessment of motor speech disorders. *American Journal of Speech-Language Pathology, 22*(1), 1–9. doi:10.1044/1058-0360(2012/11-0134)

Pellegrino, L., & Dormans, J. P. (1998a). Definitions, etiology, and epidemiology of cerebral palsy. In J. P. Dormans & L. Pellegrino (Eds.), *Caring for the children with cerebral palsy* (pp. 3–30). Baltimore, MD: Paul H. Brookes.

Pellegrino, L., & Dormans, J. P. (1998b). Making the diagnosis of cerebral palsy. In J. P. Dormans & L. Pellegrino (Eds.), *Caring for the children with cerebral palsy* (pp. 31–54). Baltimore, MD: Paul H. Brookes.

Pincus, D. (2000). *Everything you need to know about cerebral palsy.* New York, NY: Rosen.

Pishva, N., Parsa, G., Saki, F., Saki, M., & Saki, M. (2012). Intraventricular hemorrhage in premature infants and its association with pneumothorax. *Acta Medica Iranica, 50*(7), 473–476.

Prompt Institute. (n.d.). *What is prompt?* Retrieved from http://promptinstitute.com/index. php ?page=what-is-prompt3

Raju, T., Nelson, K., Ferriero, D., & Lynch, J. (2007). Ischemic perinatal stroke: Summary of a workshop sponsored by the National Institute of Child Health and Human Development and the National Institute of Neurological Disorders and Stroke. *Pediatrics, 120*(3), 609–616.

Raymer, A. (2009, February 10). Constraint-induced language therapy: A systematic review. *The ASHA Leader.*

Reddihough, D. (2011). Cerebral palsy in childhood. *Australian Family Physician, 40*(4), 192–196.

Reid, S. M., McCutcheon, J., Reddihough, D. S., & Johnson, H. (2012). Prevalence and predictors of drooling in 7- to 14-year-old children with cerebral palsy: A population study. *Developmental Medicine & Child Neurology, 54*(11), 1032–1036.

Rosenbaum, P., & Rosenbloom, L. (2012). *Cerebral palsy: From diagnosis to adult life.* London, UK: Mac Keith.

Seikel, J. A., King, D. W., & Drumright, D. G. (2010). *Anatomy and physiology for speech, language, and hearing* (4th ed.). Clifton Park, NY: Delmar Cengage.

Semel, E., Wiig, E. H., & Secord, W. A. (2013). *Clinical evaluation of language fundamentals* (5th ed.). San Antonio, TX: Psychological Corporation.

Sherif Afifi, M. (2010). Functional anatomy of the airway. In L. L. Morris & M. Sherif Afifi (Eds.), *Tracheostomies: The complete guide* (pp. 1–16). New York, NY: Springer.

Shields, N., Loy, Y., Murdoch, A., Taylor, N. F., & Dodd, K. (2007). Self-concept of children with cerebral palsy compared with that of children without impairment. *Developmental Medicine & Child Neurology, 49*(5), 350–354.

Shipley, K., & McAfee, J. (2008). *Assessment in speech-language pathology: A resource manual* (4th ed.). Clifton Park, NY: Delmar Cengage.

Sigan, S. N., Uzunhan, T. A., Aydinli, N., Eraslan, E., & Caliskan, M. (2013). Effects of oral motor therapy in children with cerebral palsy. *Annals of Indian Academy of Neurology, 16*(3), 342–346.

Stanton, M. (2012). *Understanding cerebral palsy: A guide for parents and professionals.* London, UK: Jessica Kingsley.

Straub, K., & Obrzut, J. E. (2009). Effects of cerebral palsy on neuropsychological function. *Journal of Developmental and Physical Disabilities, 21*(2), 153–167. doi:10.1007/s10882-009-9130-3

Strudwick, S. (2009). Oral motor impairment and swallowing dysfunction: Assessment and management. In P. B. Sullivan (Ed.), *Feeding and nutrition in children with neurodevelopmental disability* (pp. 35–56). London, UK: Mac Keith.

Suiter, D., & Leder, S. (2007). Contribution of tracheotomy tubes and one-way speaking valves to swallowing success. *Topics in Geriatric Rehabilitation, 23*(4), 341–351.

Sullivan, P. (2009a). Feeding and nutrition in neurodevelopmental disability: An overview. In P. B. Sullivan (Ed.), *Feeding and nutrition in children with neurodevelopmental disability.* (pp. 8–20). London, UK: Mac Keith.

Sullivan, P. (2009b). Gastrointestinal disorders: Assessment and management. In P. B. Sullivan (Ed.), *Feeding and nutrition in children with neurodevelopmental disability.* (pp. 106–117). London, UK: Mac Keith.

Taub, E. (2012). The behavior-analytic origins of constraint-induced movement therapy: An example of behavioral neurorehabilitation. *Behavior Analyst, 35*(2), 155–178.

Teverosky, E., Bickel, J., & Feldman, H. (2009). Functional characteristics of children diagnosed with childhood apraxia of speech. *Disability and Rehabilitation, 31*(2), 94–102.

Trachtenberg, S. W., & Rouse, C.F. (1998). The family. In J. P. Dormans & L. Pellegrino (Eds.), *Caring for the children with cerebral palsy* (pp. 429–445). Baltimore, MD: Paul H. Brookes.

Tuersley-Dixon, L., & Frederickson, N. (2010). Conductive education: Appraising the evidence. *Educational Psychology in Practice, 26,* 353–373.

Turner, B. M., Paradiso, S., Marvel, C. L., & Pierson, R. (2007). The cerebellum and emotional experience. *Neuropsychologia, 45*(6), 1331–1341.

Uliano, D., Falciglia, G., Del Viscio, C., Picelli, A., Gandolfi, M., & Passarella, A. (2010). Augmentative and alternative communication in adolescents with severe intellectual disability: A clinical experience. *European Journal of Physical and Rehabilitation Medicine, 46*(2), 147–152.

United Cerebral Palsy. (2012). *Cerebral palsy fact sheet.* Retrieved from http://www.ucp-cm.org/uploads/media_items/cp-fact-sheet.original.pdf

Van Roeyen, L. S. (2010). Special considerations for the child with a tracheostomy. In L. L. Morris & M. Sherif Afifi (Eds.), *Tracheostomies: The complete guide* (pp. 243–264). New York, NY: Springer.

Wanigasinghe, J., Reid, S., Mackay, M., Reddihough, D., & Harvey, S. (2010). Epilepsy in hemiplegic cerebral palsy due to perinatal arterial ischaemic stroke. *Developmental Medicine and Child Neurology, 52*(11), 1021–1027.

Warschausky, S., Van Tubbergen, M., Asbell, S., Kaufman, J., Ayyangar, R., & Donders, J. (2012). Modified test administration using assistive technology: Preliminary psychometric findings. *Assessment, 19*(4), 472–479.

Webb, W. G., & Adler, R. K. (2008). *Neurology for the speech-language pathologist* (5th ed.). St. Louis, MO: Elsevier Mosby.

Whitlock, J. (2010). Self-injurious behavior in adolescents. *PLoS Medicine, 7*(5), e1000240. doi:10.1371/journal.pmed.1000240

Workinger, M. (2005). *Cerebral palsy resource guide for speech-language pathologists.* Clifton Park, NY: Delmar Learning.

Yong-Tae, L., & Brennan, P. (2008). Cerebral palsy. In W. R. Frontera, J. K. Silver, & T. D. Rizzo (Eds.), *Essentials of physical medicine and rehabilitation* (2nd ed., pp. 627–634). Philadelphia, PA: Saunders.

Yorkston, K., Beukelman, D., Strand, E., & Hakel, M. (2010). *Management of motor speech disorders in children and adults* (3rd ed.). Austin, TX: Pro-Ed.

Zadnikar, M., & Kastrin, A. (2011). Effects of hippotherapy and therapeutic horseback riding on postural control or balance in children with cerebral palsy: A meta-analysis. *Developmental Medicine & Child Neurology, 53*(8), 684–691. doi:10. 1111/j.1469-8749.2011.03951.x

Zimmerman, I. L., Steiner, V. G., & Pond, R. E. (2011). *Preschool Language Scales* (5th ed.). San Antonio, TX: Psychological Corporation.

CHAPTER 5

Cleft Lip and Palate

Kathleen Siren

Chapter Objectives

Upon completion of this chapter, the student should be able to:

1. Describe the general embryological development of the lip and palate
2. Explain patterns of cleft lip and cleft palate and the classification terms used to describe clefts
3. Discuss both genetic and environmental factors involved in lip and palate clefts
4. List and briefly describe five common syndromes and one sequence that likely involve clefts of the lip and/or palate
5. Describe resonance, articulation, and voice disorders associated with cleft palate or a history of cleft palate
6. Discuss feeding, hearing, and dental difficulties likely for individuals with cleft palate or a history of cleft palate
7. Describe the team approach to management of an individual with a cleft palate, with particular emphasis on the roles of the speech-language pathologist and audiologist
8. Describe both direct and indirect instrumental procedures that may be

used to assess velopharyngeal function during speech
9. Discuss timing of primary and secondary surgeries for cleft lip and cleft palate
10. Provide examples of common surgical techniques for primary cleft palate surgery and for secondary surgical management of velopharyngeal dysfunction
11. Discuss prosthetic management options prior to, or in place of, secondary surgical management for individuals with velopharyngeal dysfunction
12. Discuss possible psychosocial issues affecting individuals born with clefts of the lip and/or palate as well as parents and family members of these individuals

Introduction

Individuals born with a cleft palate face numerous challenges to normal speech and hearing development. As such, speech-language pathologists (SLPs) and audiologists are important members of cleft palate teams. These teams of professionals provide ongoing interdisciplinary assessment and intervention for individuals with a cleft palate or a history of cleft palate. Additionally, SLPs and audiologists who are not members of a cleft palate team will undoubtedly see clients with a history of cleft palate. These professionals must be able to provide information to the client and family and to make appropriate referrals. This chapter provides an overview of cleft lip and palate, including how and why clefts occur, the effects on speech and hearing, and the team approach to assessment and intervention.

Embryology and Physiological Anomalies

Cleft lip and cleft palate occur when there is a disruption in development of the oral cavity during gestation of the embryo. To understand how and why clefts occur, it is necessary to have a basic understanding of embryological development of the lip and palate. The following sections discuss general embryology of the lip and palate; development of the lip and primary palate specifically, development of the secondary palate; and the embryological basis of clefts of the lip and palate. Though students are familiar with the terms *hard palate* and *soft palate,* the distinctions used here will be *primary palate* and *secondary palate.* These terms do not refer to the same structures. The terms *primary palate* and *secondary palate* are based upon embryological development. The embryonic structure called the primary palate consists of the middle portion of the lip and a wedge-shaped portion in the anterior of the palate extending posteriorly to the incisive foramen (a small hole in the bone underlying the alveolar ridge area). The secondary palate is the portion of the palate posterior to the incisive foramen.

Embryology of the Lip and Palate

The formation of the facial structures depends on neural crest cells that develop in the embryo and migrate at different rates during embryological development. Specifically, the first neural crest cells to reach the facial area migrate over the top of the cranial end of the embryo. These cells form the frontonasal process, or frontonasal prominence. This frontonasal process eventually forms the outer nose as well as the middle two-thirds of the upper lip and anterior portion of the palate (primary palate). Other neural crest cells reach the facial area by migrating via a longer route around the primitive facial area. These cells eventually form a series of paired arches. These pairs include one pair, the mandibular arches, each consisting of a lower mandibular process and an upper maxillary process. The paired maxillary processes eventually form the sides of the upper lip. On either side of the embryonic tongue, two palatine processes, or palatal shelves, project medially from the maxillary processes. These palatal shelves eventually form the posterior portion of the palate (secondary palate). These facial processes and palatal shelves merge, or fuse, from the sixth through the 12th weeks of embryological development.

Formation of the Primary Palate (Including the Lip)

During the sixth week of gestation, the frontonasal process and the paired maxillary processes begin to fuse. The formation of the primary palate begins at the incisive foramen with fusion proceeding anteriorly on both sides to form the premaxilla, consisting of the anterior portion of the hard palate and maxilla, and the alveolar ridge. Fusion then proceeds to form the base of the nose. Finally, the frontonasal process and the maxillary processes fuse to form the philtral lines on both sides of the upper lip. This completes the formation of the upper lip.

Formation of the Secondary Palate

Initially, the palatal shelves hang down vertically on either side of the embryonic tongue. During the seventh or the eighth week of gestation, the palatal shelves rise to a horizontal position. This occurs at nearly the same time that the embryonic tongue begins to drop down. During the eighth to the ninth week, the palatal shelves begin to fuse. This fusion takes place in an anterior to posterior direction. That is, initially the palatal shelves fuse with the primary palate, and then continue to join and fuse with each other from the incisive foramen posteriorly with formation of the uvula occurring last. Additionally, the nasal septum and vomer bone move down and fuse on the superior surface of the palatal shelves. The secondary palate is completely formed somewhere between the 10th and the 12th weeks of gestation.

The Embryology of Clefts

During embryological development, disruptions may occur that impair the fusion of the processes and associated structures. If neural cell migration or palatal shelf movement is disrupted or delayed, clefts can occur where processes and structures do not fuse. Thus, clefts generally follow fusion lines from the incisive foramen out to the periphery (Figure 5–1). Clefts of the lip or primary palate occur when the frontonasal process fails to meet or fuse entirely with the maxillary processes on either or both sides. Clefts of the secondary palate occur when the palatal shelves fail to elevate, join medially, or completely fuse.

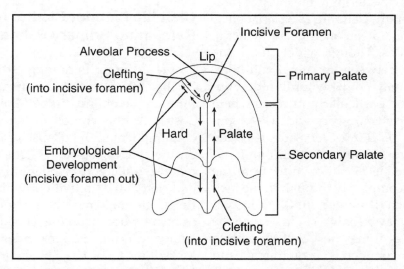

Figure 5–1. Embryological development proceeds from the incisive foramen outward to the periphery. Clefts begin at the periphery and extend inward toward the incisive foramen. Reprinted with permission from Kummer, A. W. *Cleft Palate and Craniofacial Anomalies: The Effects on Speech and Resonance* (3rd ed.). Clifton Park, NY: Cengage Learning, 2014.

Classification of Clefts

Though clefts generally follow a predictable pattern, describing clefts in different individuals is not an easy task. Clefts can vary along several dimensions. This section discusses general issues related to the classification of clefts.

Clinicians and researchers have proposed numerous classification systems over the years to describe clefts. Most systems were elaborations of the basic dichotomy of cleft lip (with or without cleft palate) versus cleft palate only (Peterson-Falzone, Hardin-Jones, & Karnell, 2009). The most universally accepted system is one proposed by Kernahan and Stark (1958), which classifies clefts based upon embryological development (Kummer, 2014). In Kernahan and Stark's system, clefts of the primary palate are those anterior to the incisive foramen, including clefts of the lip. Clefts of the secondary palate are those posterior to the incisive foramen. Generally, clefts are also classified as either unilateral, on one side, or bilateral, on both sides. Though widely used, the distinction between unilateral and bilateral clefts may not be helpful in describing severity, particularly in cases where unilateral clefts are very wide (Peterson-Falzone et al., 2009). Clefts are also often described as "complete" or "incomplete." A complete cleft is an opening from the periphery completely through to the incisive foramen (Kummer, 2014). An incomplete cleft may be only a slight cleft on the periphery, or it may be a cleft through to the incisive foramen with a minimal band or bridge of tissue at some point along the cleft. Thus, these terms may also not always be useful in describing severity.

In an attempt to describe severity of a cleft, clinicians and researchers have developed several classification systems that are elaborations of these basic dichotomous descriptions. However, unless all future readers of a description are familiar with the classification system used, the descriptors may be meaningless. Additionally, clefts may vary in several dimensions: anterior to posterior, width, and depth (Peterson-Falzone et al., 2009). Therefore, it is best to describe a cleft in as much detail as possible.

The following sections will use general classification terms based on Kernahan and Stark's (1958) system. However, clefts of the lip will be discussed separately from other clefts of the primary palate. The rationale for this is that individuals with clefts of the lip without a cleft in the alveolus (or dental arch) rarely have speech problems, whereas individuals with clefts of the alveolus (primary palate) and/or secondary palate often have speech difficulties.

Cleft Lip Without Cleft of the Remaining Primary Palate

Clefts of the lip may range from only a small notch in the lip to a cleft that extends through the philtral lines of the lip to the nostril. A more complete cleft will likely cause flattening or collapse of the nostril on the side of the cleft. Clefts of the lip may be unilateral or bilateral. A unilateral cleft of the lip (with or without additional clefting into the alveolus) more frequently occurs on the left side (Jensen, Kreigorg, Dahl, & Fogh-Anderson, 1988; McWilliams, Morris, & Shelton, 1990). In a bilateral cleft of the lip, the philtral tissue that hangs free is called the prolabium. Occasionally, a small bridge of soft tissue extends across an otherwise open cleft. This is called a Simonart's band.

Clefts of the lip only present cosmetic concerns, but do not generally present serious speech concerns. However, a cleft lip is often accompanied by a cleft through the alveolus.

Cleft of the Primary Palate

Clefts that extend into the alveolus may also range from a small notch to a cleft extending completely through the dental arch. A cleft that extends through the alveolus to the incisive foramen is often called a "complete cleft" or even a "complete cleft lip." Such clefts may also be unilateral or bilateral. When there is a bilateral complete cleft of the lip and alveolus, both the prolabium and premaxilla (the triangular-shaped bone that normally contains the central and lateral maxillary incisors) are unattached and may project anteriorly or appear to be attached to the end of the nose. Figures 5–2 and 5–3 depict infants with unilateral complete clefts of the lip and primary palate. Figure 5–4 shows an infant with a bilateral incomplete cleft of the lip and primary palate. Figure 5–5 illustrates an infant with a bilateral complete cleft of the lip and primary palate.

Due to the course of embryological development, clefts of the alveolus are almost always accompanied by clefts of the lip. However, cleft palate teams have

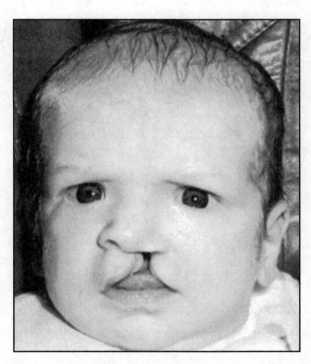

Figure 5–2. Infant with a unilateral complete cleft of the lip and primary palate. Reprinted with permission from Kummer, A. W. *Cleft Palate and Craniofacial Anomalies: The Effects on Speech and Resonance* (3rd ed.). Clifton Park, NY: Cengage Learning, 2014.

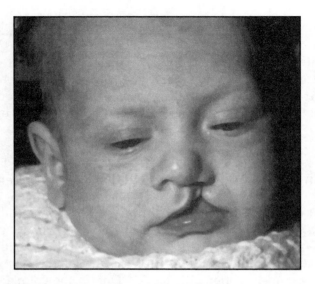

Figure 5–3. Infant with a unilateral complete cleft of the lip and primary palate. Reprinted with permission from Kummer, A. W. *Cleft Palate and Craniofacial Anomalies: The Effects on Speech and Resonance* (3rd ed.). Clifton Park, NY: Cengage Learning, 2014.

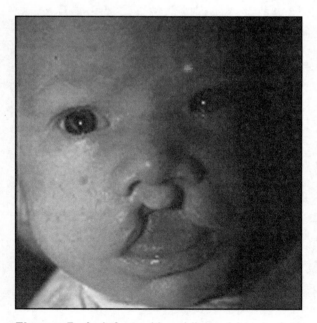

Figure 5–4. Infant with a bilateral incomplete cleft of the lip and primary palate. Reprinted with permission from Kummer, A. W. *Cleft Palate and Craniofacial Anomalies: The Effects on Speech and Resonance* (3rd ed.). Clifton Park, NY: Cengage Learning, 2014.

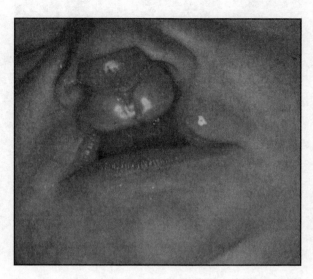

Figure 5–5. Infant with a bilateral complete cleft of the lip. Note the slight forward projections of the prolabium and premaxilla. Reprinted with permission from Kummer, A. W. *Cleft Palate and Craniofacial Anomalies: The Effects on Speech and Resonance* (3rd ed.). Clifton Park, NY: Cengage Learning, 2014.

reported cases of alveolar clefting in the absence of lip clefting (Ranta & Rintala, 1989). Moreover, the majority of individuals with clefts of the primary palate also have clefts of the secondary palate.

Cleft of the Secondary Palate

As with clefts of the primary palate, clefts of the secondary palate may also range from minimal to extensive. A defect in the secondary palate may involve only a small notch in the uvula (bifid uvula). A bifid uvula is not of concern unless it occurs in conjunction with a submucous cleft palate (discussed below). On the other hand, a complete cleft of the secondary palate extends anteriorly all the way to the incisive foramen. Clefts of the secondary palate may also be unilateral or

bilateral. In a unilateral cleft, the vomer bone, or bottom part of the nasal septum, generally fuses to the intact palatal shelf. In a bilateral cleft, the vomer bone fails to fuse to either palatal shelf. Figure 5–6 illustrates a child with a bilateral complete cleft of the secondary palate. Figure 5–7 depicts a child with a bilateral complete cleft of the secondary palate in combination with a bilateral complete cleft of the lip and primary palate.

Submucous Cleft of the Secondary Palate

A submucous cleft palate is a defect in the underlying structures of the secondary palate without a complete opening between the oral and nasal cavities. Thus, though the surface of the palate in the

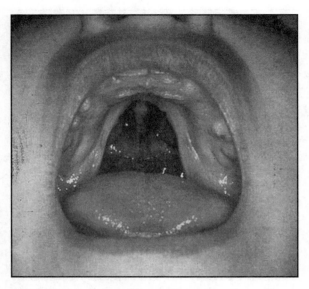

Figure 5–6. Child with a complete bilateral cleft of the secondary palate. Reprinted with permission from Kummer, A. W. *Cleft Palate and Craniofacial Anomalies: The Effects on Speech and Resonance* (3rd ed.). Clifton Park, NY: Cengage Learning, 2014.

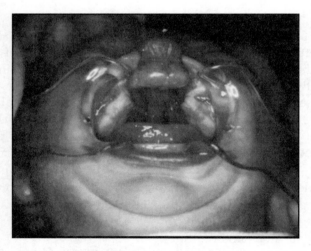

Figure 5–7. Child with a complete bilateral cleft of the secondary palate in combination with a bilateral complete cleft of the lip and primary palate. Reprinted with permission from Kummer, A. W. *Cleft Palate and Craniofacial Anomalies: The Effects on Speech and Resonance* (3rd ed.). Clifton Park, NY: Cengage Learning, 2014.

oral cavity appears to be intact, underlying muscle and bony structures have not entirely fused. Three classic stigmata of a submucous cleft may be identified through oral examination: a bifid uvula, a midline division of the musculature of the soft palate (which may cause the middle of the velum to have a bluish tint), and a notch in the posterior border of the hard palate. SLPs must be aware of submucous clefts, as they can cause the same speech problems as overt clefts.

Describing and classifying clefts is not easy. Likewise, determining the cause of clefting is not straightforward. Clefts may have many different causes, or etiologies, and even with similar causes, resulting clefts may be vastly different across individuals. The following section discusses what is currently known about the etiology of clefts.

Etiology

As with many physiological traits, no single cause can explain clefting in all or even most individuals. Congenital malformations including clefts may be due to genetic, chromosomal, environmental, multifactorial, or unknown causes. However, both genetics and environmental factors may predispose an individual to clefts of the lip or palate. This section covers three areas: genetic and chromosomal bases of cleft lip and palate; environmental factors involved in clefting; and multifactorial inheritance, the most widely accepted theory regarding the etiology of clefts.

Genetic and Chromosomal Bases of Clefts

In some individuals, disorders that include clefting may be caused by a single, abnormal gene. In many cases, these single-gene disorders appear to be autosomal dominant. Autosomal is a term referring to any chromosome that is not a sex chromosome. Thus, such disorders do not vary by gender. In an autosomal dominant disorder, individuals will likely present with the disorder if they receive the abnormal gene from either parent. Additionally, such individuals have a 50% chance of passing the abnormal gene on to each of their offspring. Several single-gene, autosomal dominant disorders that include clefts will be discussed in a later section.

In other individuals, clefts may be part of a chromosomal disorder. In a chromosomal disorder, an individual may be missing part of a chromosome or may have an extra chromosome. Cleft palate has been traced to deletions on chromosomes 2 and 4 and to duplications on chromosomes 3, 7, 8, 10, 14, 16, and 22 (Gangopadhyay, Mendonca, & Woo, 2012). In both single-gene and chromosomal disorders, a cleft of the lip and/or palate is often one potential trait in a series of traits that generally characterize a disorder or syndrome.

Environmental Factors Involved in Clefting

An environmental teratogen is a chemical or physical substance that may disrupt normal embryological development and, therefore, cause a congenital malformation. Studying the effects of suspected environmental teratogens is difficult because experimenters cannot purposefully expose humans to potentially hazardous substances. However, researchers are able to study individuals who have a history of contact with specific substances. Such studies have highlighted several teratogens that appear to be associated with cleft lip and/or palate. Maternal use of alcohol (Grewal, Carmichael, Ma, Lammer, & Shaw, 2008; Munger et al., 1996; Shaw & Lammer, 1999) and maternal use of cigarettes (or exposure to cigarette smoke) (Dixon, Marazita, Beaty, & Murray, 2011; Kohli & Kohli, 2012; Reiter et al., 2012; Shi, Wehby, & Murray, 2008) both appear to be linked to an increased risk for clefts in offspring. Additionally, maternal use of corticosteroids (Carmichael et al., 2007; Edwards et al., 2003; Pradat et al., 2003) and maternal intake of anticonvulsant drugs used to treat epilepsy (Kohli & Kohli, 2012) also appear to increase the risk of clefts.

Researchers have also investigated maternal diet and vitamin intake as potentially related to clefts in offspring. Particularly, folic acid (vitamin B-6) deficiency during pregnancy appears to be linked to a decrease in embryonic cell propagation, with resulting congenital malformations such as clefts (Munger et al., 2004). Studies are equivocal in terms of the effect of folic acid supplementation. Some studies demonstrate a decreased risk of recurrence in subsequent offspring of women who take a folic acid supplement (Jia et al., 2011; Tolarova & Harris, 1995; Wehby et al., 2013). However, other studies do not demonstrate a lower prevalence of clefting in large populations with folic acid supplementation (Bille, Knudsen, & Christensen, 2005; Castilla, Orioli, Lopez-Camelo, Dutra Mda, & Nazer-Herrera, 2003; Hashmi, Waller, Langlois, Canfield, & Hecht, 2005; Ray, Meier, Vermeulen, Wyatt, & Cole, 2003).

Regardless of specific teratogen, the developing embryo is most susceptible to clefts of the lip and/or palate between the fourth and 12th weeks of gestation, the period of time from early neural crest cell migration through the formation of the upper lip and the palate. There do appear to be slight differences between males and females in the timing of embryological fusion. The palatal shelves rise and fuse approximately one week earlier in males (Burdi & Silvey, 1969). The increased time frame for fusion in females may allow for a longer period of time for potential teratogenic agents to affect palatal development. In fact, clefts of the secondary palate occur twice as frequently in females, even though clefts of the lip with or without clefts of the palate occur more frequently in males (Calzolari et al., 1988; Jensen et al., 1988; Maresova, Veleminska, & Mullerova, 2004; Shaw, Croen, & Curry, 1991).

Current Theories Regarding the Etiology of Clefts

Currently, the most popular theory to explain clefts is the multifactorial model of inheritance. This theory holds that clefts are the result of an interaction of several factors, both genetic and environmental. In other words, certain gene combinations may provide a genetic predisposition for a cleft, though a cleft is more likely to result only if certain environmental factors are also present. In this model, if enough predisposing genetic and environmental factors are present, the embryo is pushed over a theoretical threshold and a cleft results. Multifactorial disorders may recur in families both because close relatives have more genes in common and because families are more likely to share similar environmental influences.

The multifactorial model is used to explain clefts that do not occur as part of a syndrome. Clefts that are present as part of a syndrome generally occur based upon a known pattern of inheritance. The following section discusses some syndromes that have clefts of the lip and/or palate as typical characteristics.

Syndromes Associated with Cleft Lip and Palate

A syndrome is a cluster of anomalies that occur together and have a single known, or suspected, cause. It is estimated that there are over 400 syndromes that involve orofacial clefting (Kummer, 2014). A sequence, on the other hand, is a series of secondary anomalies resulting from one initial event or anomaly. Finally, an association is a cluster of anomalies present in two or more individuals, without a known pathogenesis and not identified as either a syndrome or a sequence. With repeated identification and a discovered or suspected etiology, associations may later be identified as

syndromes or sequences. This section discusses five syndromes and one sequence that involve clefts of the lip and/or palate.

Van der Woude Syndrome

Van der Woude syndrome is an autosomal dominant disorder with the affected gene mapped to chromosome 1. This syndrome is one of the most common syndromes involving clefts of the lip and/or palate. Individuals with this syndrome are likely to have pits in the lower lip either externally or internally, cleft lip, and/or cleft palate (including submucous cleft palate) (Figure 5–8). Individuals may also have neonatal teeth or missing teeth. Speech

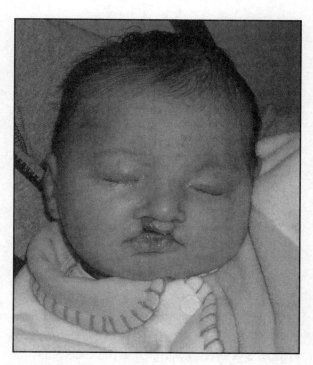

Figure 5–8. Infant with Van der Woude syndrome. Note the bilateral cleft lip and palate and the lower lip pits. Reprinted with permission from Kummer, A. W. *Cleft Palate and Craniofacial Anomalies: The Effects on Speech and Resonance* (3rd ed.). Clifton Park, NY: Cengage Learning, 2014.

problems related to the cleft palate are likely. However, the individual's development is likely to be otherwise normal.

Opitz Syndrome

Opitz syndrome may be caused by an autosomal dominant disorder with the affected gene mapped to chromosome 22 (Robin, Opitz, & Muenke, 1996). The syndrome may also be an X-linked recessive disorder. X-linked recessive disorders generally affect only males. A carrier female will transmit the disorder to 50% of her sons, and 50% of her daughters will be carriers. An affected male will pass the gene to 100% of his daughters. Opitz syndrome is a common cause of cleft lip with

cleft palate (Kummer, 2014). Individuals with this syndrome are likely to have hypertelorism (widely spaced eyes) and hypospadias (malpositioning in the opening of the urethra of the penis in males). Individuals may also have an imperforate anus, undescended testes, and hernias in the area of the groin. In addition to cleft lip with or without cleft palate, these individuals may also have a laryngeal cleft. Those with Opitz syndrome are at risk for learning disabilities, and possibly intellectual disability. Voice and feeding problems may result from the laryngeal cleft, and speech problems are likely if cleft palate is present. Figure 5–9 depicts a boy with Opitz syndrome characterized by a bilateral cleft of the lip and palate (repaired) and hypertelorism.

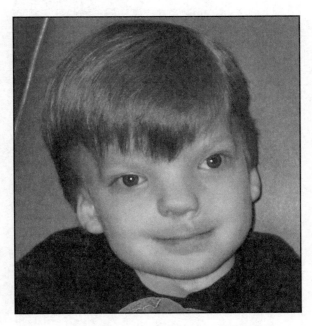

Figure 5–9. A boy with Opitz syndrome. Note the hypertelorism and evidence of cleft lip (repaired at the time of the picture). Reprinted with permission from Kummer, A. W. *Cleft Palate and Craniofacial Anomalies: The Effects on Speech and Resonance* (3rd ed.). Clifton Park, NY: Cengage Learning, 2014.

Pierre Robin Sequence

The initiating event for Pierre Robin sequence is interference with mandible (jaw) development during the ninth week of gestation. However, this interference may result from different causes, including chromosomal abnormalities (Jakobsen et al., 2006) and restriction of growth due to crowding in utero (Kummer, 2014). Once mandibular growth is restrained, the tongue is likely to remain high in the oral cavity, thus interfering with closure of the secondary palate. Therefore, clefts of the secondary palate are common in individuals with Pierre Robin sequence. These are often described as wide, U-shaped or bell-shaped clefts (Kummer, 2014). When infants with Pierre Robin sequence are born, their tongues are often in a posterior position, thus blocking the pharynx and airway. Infants generally require individualized treatment to address breathing and feeding difficulties. Although individuals with isolated Pierre Robin sequence will likely have speech problems related to the cleft palate, attention to early breathing and feeding issues may delay surgical repair of the palate.

Pierre Robin sequence may occur in isolation or may be part of a syndrome, most commonly Stickler syndrome and velocardiofacial syndrome (Izumi, Konczal, Mitchell, & Jones, 2012). (For a review of Pierre Robin sequence, including associated syndromes and management options, see Gangopadhyay, Mendonca, & Woo, 2012.)

Stickler Syndrome

Stickler syndrome is an autosomal dominant disorder with variable expression. That is, individuals with this syndrome vary in terms of which structures and functions are affected, and to what extent they are affected. The syndrome may be caused by mutations on chromosome 6 (Kummer, 2014). Individuals with this syndrome are likely to have cleft palate, possibly as part of Pierre Robin sequence; early and progressive osteoarthritis; sensorineural hearing loss; and progressive myopia with risk of retinal detachments (Snead et al., 2011). Many individuals also have characteristic craniofacial features including a flat midface (resulting from underdevelopment of the maxillary and mandibular regions), prominent eyes, epicanthal folds (folds of tissue in the inner corners of the eyes), and a long philtrum. Individuals with Stickler syndrome do not appear to be at a greater risk for developmental disabilities. However, speech and language problems are likely due to cleft palate and/or hearing loss.

Velocardiofacial Syndrome

Velocardiofacial syndrome is an autosomal dominant disorder with most cases involving a deletion of part of chromosome 22. The features associated with this syndrome are highly variable. Though more than 180 different anomalies and characteristics have been reported, only the most common are discussed here.

Individuals with velocardiofacial syndrome are likely to have velopharyngeal insufficiency either with or without cleft palate. When present, clefts of the secondary palate may occur as part of Pierre Robin sequence. Individuals with velocardiofacial syndrome are also likely to have congenital heart defects. Additionally, certain facial features are often associated with the syndrome. These include, but are not limited to, the following: long face, narrow and downward-slanted eye slits, long maxillary region, wide nasal root, thin upper lip, and small mandible.

Individuals with velocardiofacial syndrome are also likely to have numerous medical problems and developmental disabilities, including language and learning disabilities, intellectual disability, and oral-motor dysfunction. Researchers and clinicians have also reported psychiatric problems, in particular schizophrenia (Chow, Bassett, & Weksberg, 1994; Eliez et al., 2001; Heineman-de Boer, Van Haelst, Cordia-de Haan, & Beemer, 1999; Karayiorgou et al., 1995; Pulver et al., 1994).

Most children with velocardiofacial syndrome will exhibit difficulty sucking, and later difficulty chewing and swallowing, due to poor oral motor skills including poor palatal function. Speech disorders are common due to the same factors.

Fetal Alcohol Syndrome

Fetal alcohol syndrome, or fetal alcohol spectrum disorder, is caused by maternal use of alcohol during pregnancy, especially during the first trimester (Jones & Smith, 1973). Individuals with fetal alcohol syndrome may have cleft lip with or without cleft palate. Most notably, children are small at birth, have microcephaly (small head circumference), short eye slits, a short nose, a flat philtrum, and a thin upper lip, and may have congenital heart defects (Kummer, 2014). Fetal alcohol syndrome may also cause intellectual disability (Jones, 1986) as well as significant behavior problems in older children (Nash, Sheard, Rovet, & Koren, 2008; Streissguth et al., 1991). Speech and language problems may result from developmental disabilities as well as from cleft palate.

For a more complete discussion on fetal alcohol syndrome (FAS), refer to the FAS chapter (Chapter 7) in this text.

Characteristics of Cleft Lip and Palate

In many syndromes other medical conditions require more immediate attention than clefts of the lip or palate. However, whether clefts occur as part of a syndrome or as an isolated occurrence, there are resulting implications for speech, language, hearing, feeding, and often dental, development. This section addresses common characteristics associated with clefts.

Individuals with clefts of the lip and/or palate are a heterogeneous group. Not all individuals will have the same characteristics, and individuals with the same characteristics will not have the same degree of difficulty. Even individuals with similar clefts may have different resulting problems. This section covers the characteristics related to clefts that may adversely impact communication development.

Speech

Because a cleft lip is usually repaired early in infancy, no speech effects generally result. On rare occasion, a repaired lip (particularly if the cleft was bilateral) may be too short for the appropriate production of bilabial sounds (/b, p, m/). However, affected individuals usually can substitute labiodental productions with little perceptual effect on speech production. Rather, most speech problems associated with clefts are related to clefts of the palate.

Individuals with cleft palate are at obvious risk for speech disorders. Most speech disorders resulting from palatal clefts are related to velopharyngeal dysfunction, or the inability to utilize the velum and pharynx to close off the oral cavity from the nasal cavity during speech. As with lip clefts, palatal clefts are usually repaired in infancy. However, individuals who have undergone palatal surgery to close a cleft are sometimes left with a velum that is too short to reach the back pharyngeal wall or with velar musculature too weak to achieve velopharyngeal closure. Additionally, a fistula (a hole between the oral and nasal cavities) may result if an individual fails to heal properly following surgery, or if future growth of the individual weakens prior suture lines. Any open connection between the oral and nasal cavities will result in difficulties with speech. Speech production problems, particularly those associated with velopharyngeal dysfunction, can be classified into three general categories: resonance, articulation, and voice.

Resonance

Resonance is a difficult term to understand. Though the strict definition of resonance refers to an acoustical phenomenon, it is also often used to refer to a perceived quality of the voice that results from vibration of sound in the pharyngeal, oral, and sometimes nasal cavities during speech. Thus, resonance is a term only applied to speech sounds that are voiced. For most voiced speech sounds in English, the sound source generated by vibration of the vocal folds is directed through the pharynx and into the oral cavity. This is accomplished by contact of the velum with the back pharyngeal wall to effec-

tively close off the nasal cavity. Therefore, if an individual cannot effectively close off the nasal cavity during speech, the resonance of the majority of voiced speech sounds will be affected. By contrast, there are only three speech sounds in English that require nasal resonance: (/m, n, ŋ/). To produce these sounds, an individual relaxes the velum and back pharyngeal wall and allows the sound source generated by vocal fold vibration to be directed into the nasal cavity as well.

The most common resonance disorder associated with cleft palate is hypernasality. In hypernasal speech, the sound source generated by vocal fold vibration also flows into the nasal cavity during the production of normally orally resonated sounds. Hypernasality is most obvious perceptually during the production of vowels. This occurs because vowels are voiced, relatively long in duration, and produced with a relatively open vocal tract. Degree of perceived hypernasality will depend to some extent upon size of the opening into the nasal cavity. The American Cleft Palate-Craniofacial Association website (2006) contains samples of men, women, and children with varying degrees of hypernasal speech.

Strangely enough, another resonance disorder that can be associated with cleft palate is hyponasality. In hyponasal speech, normal nasal resonance is not heard due to a partially occluded or blocked nasal passage. Thus, hyponasality will mainly affect production of nasal consonants (/m, n, ŋ/) and surrounding vowels, reducing the nasality normally heard during production. As an example of this, when an individual has a cold, speech is hyponasal due to inflamed tissue and mucus in the nasal passageways. In an individual with a history of a palatal cleft, hyponasality generally results from an obstruction in the nasal cavity or pharynx, such as a deviated septum or hypertrophic adenoids. A type of hyponasality called cul-de-sac resonance is also sometimes heard in individuals with a history of cleft palate. Cul-de-sac resonance occurs when acoustic energy is trapped in a pouch with an entrance but no outlet (Kummer, 2014). In individuals with a history of cleft palate, cul-de-sac resonance may occur due to a number of factors, such as more anterior blockage of the nasal cavity due to a deviated septum. The muffled characteristic of cul-de-sac resonance can be simulated if you produce nasal sounds ("me, me, me, me . . . ") while pinching your nose. Some individuals with a history of cleft will present with mixed hypernasality and hyponasality. Such an individual may have velopharyngeal dysfunction and some form of nasal resistance.

Hypernasality is a direct result of coupling of the oral and nasal cavities or velopharyngeal dysfunction during speech. However, an individual with either problem may still produce speech that is hyponasal due to structural issues such as those discussed above. Thus, though hyponasality and hypernasality are on opposite ends of the resonance continuum, they are not mutually exclusive. SLPs must remember that the presence of hyponasality in any form in an individual's speech does not rule out velopharyngeal dysfunction.

Though resonance disorders affect perceptual qualities of an individual's speech, such changes in the quality of speech are not likely to have a significant effect on intelligibility. That is, though speech may sound "too nasal" or "not nasal enough" to the listener, the speaker is still generally understood. However, when the oral and nasal cavities are coupled, articulation disorders are also likely, and these may have a significant effect on intelligibility.

Articulation

Articulation disorders are common in individuals with palatal clefts or a history of palatal clefts. As with hypernasality, some articulation disorders are a direct result of poor velopharyngeal structure and function, or an existing palatal cleft or fistula. These articulation disorders include nasal emission and weak-pressure consonants. Other articulation disorders result from an attempt by the individual to overcome the faulty velopharyngeal mechanism. These various articulatory substitutions are called compensatory articulation. Still other articulation problems may result from dental anomalies, such as lateralized /s/ production.

Many consonants in English require the buildup of intraoral air pressure for accurate production. These high-pressure consonants include stops, fricatives, and affricatives. In order to build up the required intraoral air pressure, the velopharyngeal mechanism must function appropriately to close off the nasal cavity. Two possible effects on articulation occur when air escapes into the nasal cavity during production of these high-pressure consonants: (1) there is associated nasal emission of air, or (2) the consonants may be produced with weak pressure.

Nasal Emission. Nasal emission is the inappropriate escape of air into the nasal cavity during attempted production of high-pressure consonants. Nasal emission may be inaudible or audible. Inaudible nasal emission occurs with no audible evidence of the air leakage. This type of nasal emission is often called "visible nasal emission" because it can be detected when a cold mirror held under the nose fogs up during production of high-pressure consonants. Audible nasal emission can be detected as a soft sound that is heard as air passes through the nose. Sometimes nasal emission meets some resistance either by a narrow velopharyngeal opening or an obstruction in the nose. This more turbulent flow of air is sometimes referred to as nasal turbulence or a nasal rustle. When air is expelled forcibly through the nose during production of these high-pressure sounds, a noisy, sneeze-like sound results. This is called a nasal, or nasopharyngeal, snort.

Weak-Pressure Consonants. Weak-pressure consonants are another articulation disturbance that may result when individuals with a faulty velopharyngeal mechanism attempt to produce high-pressure consonants. The reduction in available intraoral air pressure for production of these sounds results in consonants that are weak in pressure and intensity and may appear to be completely omitted. Though some investigators and clinicians view weak-pressure consonants as a passive production that is a direct result of velopharyngeal dysfunction (Harding & Grunwell, 1998), others view weak articulation as an active attempt to camouflage the perceptual consequences of velopharyngeal dysfunction (Peterson-Falzone et al., 2009).

The weak production or omission of stops, fricatives, and affricates in an individual's speech is likely to have a significant impact on intelligibility. However, intelligibility is likely to be more severely affected when an individual changes place of production to produce atypical sounds. Such compensatory articulations are discussed next.

Compensatory Articulation. Some articulatory substitutions are clearly compensatory. Compensatory articulation productions are many and varied, though they all have one commonality. They are atypical speech sounds produced by the speaker in an attempt to overcome structural or functional inadequacies. When an individual is unable to achieve intraoral air pressure by closing off the nasal cavity from the oral cavity at the velopharyngeal level, that individual may attempt closure at another point along the vocal tract. Generally, place of articulation for high-pressure consonants is changed from an oral location to a pharyngeal or laryngeal location. The individual is then able to take advantage of air pressure in the pharynx before it is lost at the level of the velopharyngeal valve.

Compensatory productions may include glottal or pharyngeal productions as substitutes for the normally produced sounds. Glottal stops are produced by a forceful release of air trapped beneath the vocal folds. In individuals with clefts or velopharyngeal dysfunction, glottal stops are often substituted for all stops, though they may also be substituted for fricatives and affricates. Pharyngeal productions involve the back of the tongue articulating with the pharyngeal wall. Pharyngeal stops are typically substituted for velar stops (/k, g/). Pharyngeal fricatives and pharyngeal affricates are typically substituted for sibilant sounds (/s/, /z/, /ʃ/ "sh," /ʒ/ "zh," /tʃ/ "ch," /dʒ/ "j") (Kummer, 2014).

Recent evidence from ultrasound imaging suggests that individuals demonstrating compensatory articulation strategies may utilize additional movements that may not be detectable through perception alone. Thus, instrumental analysis may be helpful in determining exact articulator placement (Bressmann, Radovanovic, Kulkarni, Klaiman, & Fisher, 2011).

Articulation Problems Related to Dental Anomalies

Some articulation problems result from the dental anomalies typical of individuals with clefts. Crowding of maxillary teeth and/or a narrow palatal arch may result in dentalized or lateralized distortion of sibilants, particularly /s/, or substitution of a middorsum palatal stop for lingua-alveolar and sometimes velar sounds. A middorsum palatal stop is produced with the back (dorsum) of the tongue up against the middle of the hard palate.

Articulation disorders are likely in individuals with palatal clefts or a history of palatal clefts. It is important that these individuals be seen regularly by an SLP as part of a cleft palate team. Based upon a review of the literature, Peterson-Falzone et al. (2009) report that many individuals with a history of cleft palate will have articulation problems that continue into adolescence. However, they also point out that individuals seen on a regular basis by a cleft palate team are less likely to develop articulation disorders.

Though articulation disorders are many and varied in the cleft population, the relationship between articulation disorders and velopharyngeal dysfunction is relatively clear. However, the relationship between voice disorders and velopharyngeal dysfunction is less clear. The next section addresses voice disorders in individuals with a history of cleft palate.

Voice

It has generally been accepted that voice disorders are more common in individuals with a history of cleft palate or velopharyngeal dysfunction than they are in the general population. However, recent studies do not demonstrate a higher prevalence of voice disorders in the cleft population (Hamming, Finkelstein, & Sidman, 2009; Robison, Todd, & Otteson, 2011). Regardless, individuals with a mildly impaired velopharyngeal mechanism are at increased risk for hyperfunctional use of the voice (Kummer, 2014). This is likely related to increased strain that may potentially be put on the vocal mechanism. That is, individuals with a small velopharyngeal opening may attempt to achieve closure by increasing muscular and respiratory effort. If these individuals persist with hyperfunctional use of the voice, they may develop vocal nodules. Hyperfunctional use of the voice may also occur as a result of aggressive speech therapy for individuals with velopharyngeal dysfunction. For this reason, individuals with a faulty velopharyngeal mechanism must be referred for, and receive, the appropriate treatment.

Some individuals with velopharyngeal dysfunction may present with a soft, breathy voice. This reduced vocal intensity may be a compensatory strategy to reduce the listener's ability to perceive hypernasality and nasal emission (Peterson-Falzone, Trost-Cardamone, Karnell, & Hardin-Jones, 2006). In any case, speech therapy should not be undertaken for voice, or other speech, issues related to velopharyngeal inadequacy when other treatment options are available to address the structural or functional problem.

Language

Though studies throughout the years have resulted in mixed conclusions, children with isolated cleft lip and palate do not appear to be at a higher risk for long-term language delays or disorders. However, when the cleft is associated with a syndrome, developmental and language problems are common and may be associated with intellectual disability or neurological involvement. Still, many factors interact to affect language acquisition and development. Physiological factors such as hearing loss associated with otitis media may impact language acquisition. Additionally, more subtle psychosocial factors, such as multiple hospitalizations, lack of adequate stimulation, and even social isolation, may also influence language development (Kummer, 2014). Therefore, the SLP should carefully monitor language development from infancy through the early school years.

Hearing

Individuals with palatal clefts, or a history of clefts, are at high risk for otitis media and conductive hearing loss. This occurs because of the physiological relationship between the velopharyngeal system and the eustachian tube (Sheer, Swarts, & Ghadiali, 2010). To explain this, a brief review of anatomy and physiology is necessary. The eustachian tube functions to aerate the middle ear cavity, equalize pressure between the middle ear cavity and external atmospheric pressure, and drain middle ear fluid into the nasopharynx. The eustachian tube opens to perform these functions. The muscle responsible for opening the eustachian tube is the tensor veli palatini. In its course, the tensor veli palatini attaches to the lateral wall of the eustachian tube, and upon contraction, opens the eustachian tube. In individuals born without compromise to the velopharyngeal system, the tensor veli palatini muscle courses downward to the palate and fans out along the length of the palate. However, in individuals with a palatal cleft, the tensor veli palatini muscle does not have a stable base (the palate),

and therefore cannot contract effectively to open the eustachian tube. When the eustachian tube cannot function properly, the middle ear is not ventilated. This may lead to bacterial infection and inflammation of the middle ear, a condition referred to as otitis media. The buildup of fluids associated with otitis media results in a temporary conductive hearing loss. In chronic otitis media, permanent damage to the middle ear can result in a permanent conductive hearing loss. In individuals with clefts, the conductive hearing loss is generally bilateral and mild to moderate in degree.

Individuals with clefts are at risk for otitis media from birth, and the risk continues for some individuals through later childhood or early adolescence. Therefore, it is imperative that an otolaryngologist and audiologist follow individuals with clefts, or a history of clefts. Patients should be monitored as early as possible and continuously. When deemed necessary, treatment may involve myringotomies (surgical punctures of the eardrum to drain fluid). Some patients may also require placement of ventilation tubes inserted into the eardrum as an alternate route for aeration of the middle ear. As a preventative measure, breast milk has been shown to decrease the occurrence of middle ear disease in infants with clefts (Aniansson, Svensson, Becker, & Ingvarsson, 2002; Paradise, Elster, & Tan, 1994). Feeding, however, is often a difficult issue in and of itself for children with clefts and their families. The next section briefly covers feeding difficulties for infants with clefts.

Feeding

Infants with lip and/or palatal clefts are likely to have difficulty with the feeding process. For most infants this occurs because they cannot completely close off the oral cavity to create the necessary negative intraoral pressure required for sucking. Specific problems will vary depending upon type and severity of cleft. Because no single feeding method will work with all infants, modifications must be made on a case-by-case basis. This section presents only general information regarding feeding issues for infants with clefts of the lip only, clefts of the secondary palate only, and clefts of the primary and secondary palate combined.

Infants with cleft lip may only have difficulty achieving adequate closure around the nipple of the bottle or breast. Infants with bilateral lip clefts may have more difficulty than infants with a unilateral lip cleft. However, for most infants with cleft lip, normal feeding is still likely. If the infant is breast fed, the breast will likely conform to fill the lip cleft. The mother may also assist the lip closure with her hand (Kummer, 2014). If the infant is bottle fed, use of a soft, wide-based nipple will likely promote success.

Infants with clefting of the secondary palate only will have difficulty achieving intraoral air pressure for sucking due to air leaking through the open cleft into the nasal cavity. Level of difficulty will depend upon extent of the cleft. However, infants with a cleft of the posterior secondary palate only, particularly if the cleft is narrow, may still be able to achieve adequate pressure for sucking. If the cleft does not extend too far forward, infants will be able to compress the nipple against the hard palate. In breast-fed infants, feeding success is more likely due to the infant's ability to position and compress the breast nipple. In bottle-fed infants, nipple modifications and/or feeder systems that assist milk delivery may be necessary. If the cleft is more extensive, more

difficulty is likely for both breast-fed and bottle-fed babies.

Infants with clefting of the primary and secondary palate are likely to have significant difficulty with feeding, particularly if there is also clefting of the lip. These infants are unable to generate negative intraoral air pressure, compress the nipple, or achieve an adequate lip seal. For these infants, a supplemental nursing system and/or a modified feeding device will probably be necessary. In severe cases, orogastric or nasogastric tube feeding may be required. In rare cases, a gastrostomy tube may be needed on a temporary basis.

Because there is no single feeding method that will work for all individuals, infants must be evaluated immediately at birth and followed closely by a pediatrician, nurse, SLP, and/or other professionals as needed. Feeding problems must be addressed early because they are likely to have a negative impact on nutrition, sensory and motor stimulation, parent-infant bonding, and oral motor development (Kummer, 2014).

Dental Anomalies

Individuals with cleft lip and palate, or a history of cleft lip and palate, are at-risk for abnormalities of the teeth and jaws. Problems such as missing, crowded, or rotated teeth are particularly likely when clefts pass through the alveolus. In addition, underdevelopment of the midface region may also cause jaw and teeth occlusion problems. A description of these potential problems and possible treatments is too extensive to provide here. For more in-depth information on dental anomalies and dental management of individuals with clefts, the student should consult the appropriate chapters in Kummer (2014) or Peterson-Falzone et al. (2009) or the numerous journal articles written on this subject.

Coordination of management may involve the orthodontist, a pediatric or family dentist, the oral surgeon, and a prosthodontist if necessary. Furthermore, because dental abnormalities may affect production of speech sounds, an SLP should be consulted, and may provide treatment once the structural problems have been addressed.

Team Assessment and Intervention

The many and varied needs of individuals with clefts of the lip and palate require a team approach to assessment and intervention. This section provides general guidelines for an interdisciplinary approach to evaluation and treatment of individuals with clefts. The role of the SLP is emphasized.

Rationale for a Team Approach

In 1987, the Surgeon General of the United States recognized that patients with special health care needs required comprehensive, coordinated care by a team of professionals (Surgeon General's Report, 1987). Following this report, the American Cleft Palate-Craniofacial Association (ACPA) received funding from the Maternal and Child Health Bureau to address this need. In response, various professionals participated in a consensus conference in 1991 and published a document outlining evaluation and treatment parameters for individuals with clefts or craniofacial anomalies. This document has since been revised (American Cleft Palate-Craniofacial Association, 2009). As outlined in this document, a cleft palate team must consist of a surgeon, an orthodontist, an SLP, and at least one other specialist. A craniofacial team must consist of a craniofacial surgeon, an orthodontist, an SLP, and a mental health professional. Additionally, a team must have a coordinator who schedules visits, documents team recommendations, facilitates communication with the patient and family, and ensures implementation of recommendations. In practice, many other professionals may serve on a team in a permanent or consultative role. Table 5–1 lists professionals likely to be included on a cleft palate or craniofacial team. The patient and his or her family are also key members on any team of care. The wishes of the patient and family must be a part of any treatment decisions (Johansson & Ringsbert, 2004; Knapke, Bender, Prows, Schultz, & Saal, 2010).

A cleft or craniofacial team is generally required for patient management from birth until an individual is physically grown, typically around age 18 to 20 (Kummer, 2014). Individuals will generally be seen by a team one to two times per year when undergoing treatment. If a team is not located near a patient's community, professional(s) near that individual's home may see the patient for routine care. In this case, local professionals must communicate and consult with the team.

An interdisciplinary team approach to assessment and intervention provides many advantages to the patient and family (American Cleft Palate-Craniofacial Association, 2009; Austin et al., 2010; Capone & Sykes, 2007; Vargervik, Oberoi, & Hoffman, 2009). The team performs a comprehensive, coordinated evaluation of

Table 5–1. Professionals on a Cleft Palate or Craniofacial Team

Professional	Role on a Cleft Palate or Craniofacial Team
Team coordinator (nurse or other professional)	• Schedules patients and plans team meetings • Compiles team recommendations and writes reports • Ensures follow-up of recommendations • Represents the team to parents, other professionals, and the community
Plastic surgeon	• Surgically repairs clefts of the lip and palate • Addresses velopharyngeal dysfunction (if surgery indicated) • May perform bone grafts, cranial surgery, or jaw surgery
Oral surgeon	• Performs bone grafts in alveolar cleft area • Performs jaw surgeries
Orthodontist	• Aligns misplaced teeth • Treats dental and jaw malocclusions
Speech-language pathologist (SLP)	• Educates parents regarding speech expectations • Provides information on speech and language stimulation • Evaluates feeding and swallowing • Evaluates speech, language, and resonance • Recommends treatment for disorders identified • Provides therapy as indicated and as appropriate
Psychologist	• Evaluates, and addresses as necessary, the psychosocial needs of the patient and family • Assists in determining readiness for surgical procedures
Social worker	• Helps families deal with issues and stressors related to child's cleft or craniofacial anomaly • May assist with insurance and possible funding sources • May act as team coordinator
Nurse	• Assesses overall physical development • May assist family with feeding in consultation with SLP • Counsels family and answers questions regarding surgical procedures
Pediatrician	• Assesses patient's health, growth, and development • Determines if presurgical medical care is needed
Audiologist	• Tests hearing and middle ear function • Works with otolaryngologist to monitor auditory functioning

Table 5–1. *continued*

Professional	Role on a Cleft Palate or Craniofacial Team
Otolaryngologist	• Monitors hearing and middle ear function • Treats middle ear disease if present • Assesses structural aspects of oral and nasal cavities and upper airway • Treats pharyngeal and laryngeal anomalies and upper airway disorders as needed • May perform surgery for velopharyngeal dysfunction
Pediatric dentist (pedodontist)	• Provides general care of teeth • Ensures development of good oral hygiene habits • May manage misaligned alveolar segments prior to cleft lip surgery • Manages palatal expansion if necessary to treat malocclusion
Prosthodontist	• Restores or replaces teeth • Develops prosthetic devices for teeth and oral structures • Develops devices to assist with velopharyngeal closure • Develops feeding devices if needed
Geneticist	• Assesses patient's genetic background • Counsels patient and family on recurrence risk for future offspring
Neurosurgeon	• Evaluates and assists surgeon in treating patients with craniofacial syndromes involving cranial and brain anomalies
Ophthalmologist	• Evaluates and treats patients with congenital eye anomalies and vision problems

Note. Reprinted with Permission from Kummer, A. W. *Cleft Palate and Craniofacial Anomalies: Effects on Speech and Resonance, Third Edition.* Clifton Park, Cengage Learning, 2014.

the whole child in order to make better decisions with respect to the child and the family. Team assessment is generally accomplished with fewer visits and decreased cost as compared to individual evaluations. The single team coordinator is able to facilitate follow-up and monitor care for the patient and family better than different individuals scheduling numerous visits. Teams are also generally composed of experts in various fields who can provide care based on current, up-to-date information in their field. Finally, teams are generally located in facilities with state-of-the-art equipment and access to educational and psychosocial resources for the patient and the family.

The team approach is also advantageous to the professionals involved. It saves evaluation time, increases interprofessional communication, increases transdisciplinary knowledge, aids collaborative research, and saves time recordkeeping (Kummer, 2014). As a required team member, the SLP can both benefit from, and lend much to, a successful, coordinated team effort. The following section highlights the role of the SLP in team assessment and intervention.

The Role of the Speech-Language Pathologist

For an individual with a cleft palate, one of the main goals of any treatment procedure is accurate speech development. Therefore, an SLP is involved in the team assessment and treatment of an individual with a cleft palate from birth, and will often follow an individual through adolescence or adulthood. Surgeons and prosthodontists will ask the team SLP to assess the individual's speech prior to and following surgical and/or prosthetic procedures. Prosthodontists may have the team SLP present to assess speech production during development and testing of prosthetic devices.

Additionally, another SLP in the child's community may see the child for assessment and/or treatment as needed. In this case, the local SLP must consult with the child's cleft palate management team. If no team is currently managing the child, the SLP should refer the child and family to a cleft palate team. The Cleft Palate Foundation (associated with the American Cleft Palate-Craniofacial Association) is a group dedicated to assisting families and professionals who need information regarding assessment or treatment of individuals with clefts or other craniofacial anomalies. The Cleft Palate Foundation can provide a list of qualified cleft and craniofacial teams in various areas throughout the country. The toll-free number is (800) 24-CLEFT (800-242-5338). The web site is http://www.cleftline.org

This section outlines the procedures involved in the assessment and treatment of speech-language problems associated with cleft palate.

Assessment

The basic protocol for speech-language assessment of an individual with a cleft or history of cleft is not significantly different from a speech-language evaluation of a child without a cleft. However, the challenge is in sorting out the contribution of various etiological factors (structural, functional, behavioral). Etiological differentiation is important because speech therapy should never be initiated until the appropriate professionals have addressed all structural and/or functional concerns. The speech-language assessment should include a clinical history, an orofacial examination, an assessment of resonance, an assessment of articulation, an assessment of voice, and a language screening. A language screening will not be discussed here, as students should be familiar with assessment of language skills in children. This section addresses each of the other areas of assessment with attention given only to those aspects specific to individuals with clefts or suspected velopharyngeal dysfunction.

Clinical History. Because an individual with a history of cleft palate is likely to have had extensive prior medical intervention, it is necessary to obtain all possible information in order to assess the individual's current functioning. A thorough clinical history should include information about the following (Peterson-Falzone et al., 2009):

- Surgical history and surgeries planned for the future
- Medical history, including health problems, frequency of middle ear infections, and feeding history
- History of speech-language therapy, including duration, frequency, and type
- Parental perspective, including experiences, expectations, and knowledge

Orofacial Examination. An orofacial examination (oral-peripheral examination) should always be performed on an individual with a cleft palate or history of cleft palate. Students should be familiar with such an examination. Therefore, the following list is limited to features that may be associated with cleft palate or other craniofacial anomalies (Kummer, 2014; Peterson-Falzone et al., 2009):

- Face: Observe overall structure, symmetry, and muscle tone; observe spacing, size, and structure of eyes; observe shape of nose and note if open-mouth breathing
- Lips: Note lip structure and symmetry; test lip approximation; note presence of internal or external lip pits (Van der Woude's syndrome)
- Teeth: Note bite (occlusion) problems and extra or misplaced teeth; note presence of dental appliances
- Tongue: Judge tongue size relative to oral cavity; note any tongue growths or deviations
- Hard palate: Note contour and width; examine carefully for fistulae; palpate for notch in border (may suggest submucous cleft)

- Tonsils: Note size if present
- Soft palate: Note symmetry, examine for bifid uvula or bluish tone midline (may suggest submucous cleft); examine for fistulae, observe velar movement during sustained phonation ("ah")
- Pharyngeal walls: Note any movement during sustained phonation

Assessment of Resonance. Assessment of resonance involves three steps. First, the SLP must determine if resonance is normal or not. Second, if resonance is judged to be abnormal, the SLP should note the type of abnormal resonance. Third, once type of abnormal resonance is determined, the SLP should estimate degree of severity.

Determining normal versus abnormal resonance is not always an easy task. Nasality in speech occurs along a continuum and is affected by factors such as dialect. Additionally, resonance disorders in an individual may be subtle, may be difficult to distinguish from abnormal voice characteristics, and may be complicated by the presence of unusual articulation errors. Appropriate stimulus materials will help the clinician determine both presence and type of abnormal resonance. The following list provides examples of stimulus items and procedures most helpful in identifying different resonance disorders:

- Hypernasality: The individual should produce words or sentences with vowels and low-pressure consonants (e.g., "Why are you where we were?"). The SLP should listen for increased nasality, particularly during vowel production.

■ Hyponasality: The individual should produce words or sentences with nasal consonants and vowels (e.g., "My mama knew many men."). The SLP should listen for decreased nasality, particularly during nasal consonants and adjacent vowels.

During assessment, an SLP may note both hypernasality and hyponasality in the same individual. This likely indicates velopharyngeal dysfunction with other structural complications. As mentioned previously, the SLP should not interpret the presence of hyponasality as a sign that the individual is able to achieve appropriate velopharyngeal closure. Additionally, if hyponasal speech has a "muffled" quality, cul-de-sac resonance should be noted.

Assessment of resonance should also include a conversational speech sample. Some individuals with small velopharyngeal gaps are able to achieve fairly normal resonance during short productions. However, during conversational speech, resonance disorders may become more obvious.

Once the SLP identifies the presence of hypernasality or hyponasality, degree of severity should be estimated. Some clinicians use a numbered rating scale whereas others use terms such as "mild," "moderate," "severe." If hyponasality is evident, presence or absence of mixed nasality or cul-de-sac resonance may also be noted.

Assessment of Articulation. An articulation assessment should include word or sentence productions as well as a sample of conversational speech. Because individuals with cleft palate may have developmental or phonological errors, an articulation assessment should include all speech sounds. However, in order to identify atypical articulation disorders prevalent in this population (nasal emission, weak-pressure consonants, and compensatory articulation substitutions), the SLP may need to focus on production of high-pressure consonants. High-pressure consonants include stops (/p, b, t, d, k, g/), fricatives (/f, v, θ, ð, s, z, ʃ, ʒ, h/), and affricates (/tʃ, dʒ/). Two formal articulation tests are available that specifically focus on these consonants. These are the Iowa Pressure Articulation Test, a part of the Templin-Darley Tests of Articulation (Templin & Darley, 1960), and the Bzoch Error Pattern Diagnostic Articulation Tests (Bzoch, 1979). However, these tests are limited to single-word productions. Clinicians should also have the individual produce sentences when possible. It is best if stimulus sentences focus on one articulatory placement at a time. Additionally, it may be easier to sort out articulation disorders utilizing voiceless sounds. For example, the sentence, "Try to tell Teddy" assesses the voiceless lingua-alveolar stop.

To test for inaudible nasal emission, the SLP can hold a dental mirror under the client's nose during production of high-pressure consonants. Because no air should be directed out the nose during high-pressure consonant production, if the mirror fogs the SLP can tentatively diagnose inaudible nasal emission. To be done correctly, the mirror must be placed under the nose only during production of the target sound to ensure the condensation is not caused by normal breathing before or after an utterance (Kummer, 2014).

Assessment of Voice. Procedures for a voice screening or voice evaluation are not discussed here. However, some individuals may use a soft voice to mask resonance and articulation disorders.

Additionally, some individuals may develop hyperfunctional use of the voice as a response to an inadequate velopharyngeal mechanism. Thus, differential diagnosis of voice disorders is important for this population.

Intervention

An SLP on a cleft palate team will have an immediate role in early intervention for a child born with a cleft lip and/or palate. This will initially involve parent education. This education should include (Peterson-Falzone et al., 2009):

- Information about the impact of a cleft on the speech structure, and therefore communication development of the child
- Information and guidance in speech and language stimulation techniques
- Information about possible compensatory articulation productions and guidance to avoid reinforcement of these sounds
- Information about expected speech performance after surgical procedures
- Referral for early speech-language intervention if needed

Once information is provided to the parents, the SLP on a cleft palate team continues in an active role in the ongoing surgical, dental, and prosthetic management of the individual. In addition to this involvement in ongoing team treatment of an individual, an SLP may see an individual with a history of cleft for individual speech therapy. However, it is more likely that an SLP in the child's community will provide this therapy. The local SLP must consult with, and report to, the cleft palate team managing the individual in order for treatment to be most effective.

A caveat is in order, particularly for beginning SLPs who may one day find themselves face to face with a client with hypernasality and nasal emission. If an individual produces speech with any of the resonance or articulation characteristics associated with velopharyngeal dysfunction, the SLP should assume that the individual has an underlying structural or functional inadequacy. In this case, the individual should be referred to a cleft-palate team or an otolaryngologist with experience evaluating velopharyngeal function. Speech therapy should never be initiated with an individual who does not have an intact velopharyngeal system. Such therapy will be frustrating at best, futile more likely, and may cause a secondary voice disorder. Individuals with velopharyngeal dysfunction are best treated with surgical or prosthetic management. However, an SLP may be called upon to provide therapy to an individual who produces compensatory articulation errors.

Compensatory articulation productions generally develop because the individual cannot achieve adequate intraoral air pressure to produce the sounds normally. Therefore, the speaker moves place of production posterior to the velopharyngeal area. Though such productions are atypical and may sound odd to a listener, they may result in better use of airflow and therefore improve intelligibility (Kummer, 2014). Therefore, therapy to eliminate compensatory articulation in individuals with an inadequate velopharyngeal mechanism is not advised, particularly if surgery to correct the velopharyngeal dysfunction is planned.

However, there are two instances when therapy for compensatory articulations is warranted. First, in the rare case where velopharyngeal function is unclear, and compensatory articulations are the only speech characteristic, therapy is mandatory. If correction of the compensatory articulation results in normal speech, no additional treatment is necessary. On the other hand, if correction of the compensatory articulation results in articulation that is appropriate in place, but produced with nasal emission, further surgical or prosthetic management of the individual may be needed. Second, if velopharyngeal function is judged to be normal, and compensatory articulations continue, therapy is also necessary. Such productions may now be a learned part of speech production, even in the absence of velopharyngeal dysfunction. The following are suggestions to modify place of production for specific compensatory articulations (Kummer, 2014):

Glottal stops as substitutes for oral stops:

- Have child whisper syllable to prevent glottal closure
- Have child produce stops slowly followed by /h/ before the vowel (i.e., t-ha for ta)

Pharyngeal stops as substitutes for oral stops:

- Have child begin with /ŋ/ ("ng"); then hold nose and drop tongue quickly for /k/ sound

Pharyngeal fricatives as a substitute for sibilant sounds:

- Have child produce fricative sounds first with the nostrils occluded and then with the nostrils open to get a feel for oral versus pharyngeal airflow

- For /s/ production, have child close the teeth and produce a hard /t/; gradually increase duration of sound (/tsssssss/); then eliminate initial /t/
- For /ʃ/ ("sh") production, have child close the teeth, round the lips, and produce a big sigh; work on increasing air pressure
- For /tʃ/ ("ch") production, have child close the teeth and produce a hard /t/ or a loud sneeze

Middorsum palatal stops:

- Have child bite on a tongue blade; then have child produce lingua-alveolar sounds by touching the tongue tip to the tongue blade

Though an SLP may provide therapy on an individual basis, most SLPs who work with individuals with a history of cleft palate do so as members of a cleft palate team. As a required member of a cleft palate or craniofacial team, the SLP has an important and ongoing role in the assessment and intervention for individuals with clefts.

Instrumental Procedures

Although an SLP's trained ear remains the best tool for evaluating velopharyngeal dysfunction, instrumental procedures may provide additional information during assessment and intervention. This section will provide a brief overview of instrumental procedures to assess velopharyngeal function. These procedures can be grouped into two categories. Indirect instrumental procedures provide information about the acoustic and aerodynamic results of velopharyngeal function during speech. Indirect procedures include nasometry and aerodynamic measurement. Direct instrumental procedures allow the examiner to view the velopharyngeal mechanism directly as it functions during speech. Direct procedures include videofluoroscopy and nasopharyngoscopy.

Indirect instrumental procedures provide objective data about the speech output resulting from velopharyngeal function. During nasometry, the individual wears a headset that measures the relative nasal and oral acoustic energy during speech. During aerodynamic assessment, tubes in the nose and mouth connect to pressure transducers to detect airflow and air pressure during speech. Although both nasometry and aerodynamic procedures provide objective data, they do not allow direct visualization of the velopharyngeal mechanism (Kummer, 2014).

Direct instrumental procedures allow the examiner to visualize the velopharyngeal structures during speech. Videofluoroscopy is a specialized x-ray technique providing moving images of the velopharyngeal mechanism during speech production. Multiple views are usually necessary to provide complete information about velopharyngeal function. Nasopharyngoscopy, also an imaging technique, involves insertion of a flexible fiberoptic endoscope through the nose to view velopharyngeal movement from the nasal surface. Though both procedures allow direct visualization of the velopharyngeal function during speech, interpretation of the information provided is based on expertise of the examiner and is therefore somewhat subjective (Kummer, 2014).

Instrumental assessment may be used to confirm or explain an SLP's perceptions of speech production (Peterson-Falzone et al., 2006). Instrumental procedures may also be used to identify the appropriate surgical or prosthetic intervention and to assess results postintervention (Karnell, 2011). The following section discusses surgical and prosthetic management for velopharyngeal dysfunction.

Surgical and Prosthetic Management

In addition to the SLP, the surgeon is another required member of cleft palate and craniofacial teams. Plastic or oral surgeons often work in conjunction with SLPs, orthodontists, and other team members to decide appropriate care of the individual with a cleft. This section discusses general surgical procedures related to clefts of the lip and palate.

There are many different theories regarding timing of surgery and many different surgical procedures. Therefore, this section presents broad guidelines and general standards used in the United States for lip and palate repair. The terms *primary surgery* and *secondary surgery* will be used. These do not correspond to primary palate and secondary palate, but refer to initial surgery (primary surgery) and follow-up surgery (secondary surgery), whether related to clefts of the lip, primary palate, or secondary palate. This section discusses primary and secondary surgery for cleft lip, primary surgery for cleft palate, secondary surgery for velopharyngeal dysfunction, nonsurgical prosthetic management for velopharyngeal dysfunction, and orthognathic surgery.

Primary and Secondary Surgery for Clefts of the Lip

The initial, or primary, surgery to repair cleft lip is referred to as cheiloplasty.

Although cheiloplasty used to be performed during the first few months after birth, most surgeons now perform the surgery when the infant is 10 to 12 months of age (Kummer, 2014). Surgeons often follow the "rule of tens," which states that an infant should weigh at least 10 pounds, be at least 10 weeks of age, and have a hemoglobin of 10 gm before surgery is performed. Prior to the formal lip surgery, particularly for wide clefts, some surgeons attempt to bring the lip into better alignment. This presurgical management may involve taping the lip, utilizing an extraoral or intraoral dental appliance, or pulling the segments of the lip together in a modified surgical procedure.

Two major surgical techniques are widely used to repair a unilateral cleft lip. These are the Millard rotation-advancement technique (Bardach, 1994; Knezevic, Grgurevic, Uglesic, & Grgurevic, 2012; Millard, 1958, 1976; Stal et al., 2009; Trier, 1985) and the Tennison-Randall triangular-flap procedure (Bardach & Salyer, 1987; Brauer & Cronin, 1983; Lazarus, Hudson, Van Zyl, Fleming, & Fernandes, 1998; Randall, 1959, 1990; Tennison, 1952). The Millard technique is used in approximately 80% of unilateral cleft lip surgeries and the Tennison-Randall technique is used in approximately 20% (Kummer, 2014). For bilateral cleft lip repair, the two major surgical techniques are a modification of the Millard technique (Millard, 1977; Noordhoff, 1994) and the Broadbent-Manchester repair (Kummer, 2014).

Children with a cleft lip may also undergo additional, or secondary, surgery. This surgery is largely cosmetic in that it is undertaken to improve lip symmetry, improve nose appearance and symmetry, and reduce scar tissue. Secondary surgery is generally delayed until early school age so that it does not interfere with mid-facial growth.

Primary Surgery for Clefts of the Palate

The initial, or primary, surgery to repair cleft palate is usually performed when the infant is between 9 months and 1 year of age, though surgery may be performed earlier or later. Over the past several decades, cleft palate team members have debated timing of primary palatal surgery. Earlier surgery appears to favor better speech results (Murthy, Sendhilnathan, & Hussain, 2010). However, earlier surgery has also been identified as a potential cause of the restricted growth of the maxilla and mid-facial region often seen in children with a history of cleft palate. Recent research has attempted to determine the contribution of early surgery to restricted mid-facial growth, with mixed findings (Meazzini, Tortora, Morabito, Garattini, & Brusati, 2011; Priya, Reddy, Ramakrishna, & Reddy, 2011; Saperstein, Kennedy, Muliken, & Padwa, 2012; Xu et al., 2012) As more longitudinal data are collected, more precise guidelines may be developed.

Surgery to repair a palatal cleft is called palatoplasty. The oldest and still most widely used technique for palatoplasty is the Von Langenbeck repair (Trier & Dreyer, 1984). Another widely used technique is the Wardill-Kilner V-Y pushback procedure. These repairs attempt to close the palate, but do not address reconstructing the levator sling. In individuals with normal palatal development, the levator veli palatini muscle fuses in the middle of the velum on both sides to form the levator sling, which contracts to assist velopharyngeal closure. In individuals with cleft palate, the levator veli palatini instead inserts into the back of the hard palate. More recently developed techniques attempt to reconstruct the levator sling. Two such techniques are the Furlow

Z-plasty (Furlow, 1986, 1990, 2009) and two-flap palatoplasty (Kummer, 2014).

Approximately 20% to 30% of individuals who undergo primary palatoplasty will still have velopharyngeal dysfunction or velopharyngeal inadequacy following surgery. The resulting velopharyngeal dysfunction may be caused by anatomical factors such as a velum that is too short due to scarring or may be caused by neuromuscular factors such as poor muscle insertion. Regardless of cause, these individuals must undergo some form of secondary management, often in the form of surgery.

Secondary Surgery for Velopharyngeal Dysfunction

In order to diagnose velopharyngeal dysfunction, the child must be able to produce connected speech. For most children, this occurs around age 3. Therefore, although secondary surgery should be performed as soon as possible so that the child does not develop a habit of compensatory articulation, secondary surgery does not usually take place until the child is around ages 3.5 to 4.

Because the goal of secondary surgical procedures is to allow the individual to achieve velopharyngeal closure, these procedures must reduce the size of the current velopharyngeal opening by introducing something into the velopharyngeal space and changing the physiology of the velopharyngeal mechanism. Secondary surgical procedures include a pharyngeal flap, pharyngeal wall augmentation, or sphincter pharyngoplasty.

Pharyngeal Flap

During a pharyngeal flap procedure, a flap of tissue is dissected from the pharyngeal wall, brought forward, and sutured into the velum. This provides a bridge of tissue in the middle of the velopharyngeal port. Pharyngeal flaps can be either inferiorly or superiorly based. Openings are left on both sides of the flap so that normal nasal breathing, as well as production of nasal speech sounds, can occur. During speech, the lateral pharyngeal walls must move medially toward the flap, effectively closing off the velopharyngeal port for nonnasal sounds. Thus, patients are candidates for this procedure only if they have good lateral pharyngeal wall movement (Argamaso et al., 1980).

Pharyngeal Wall Augmentation

Pharyngeal wall augmentation is another procedure surgeons utilize to address velopharyngeal dysfunction following primary palatal surgery. During this procedure, the surgeon injects a substance or material into the posterior pharyngeal wall in an attempt to bring the wall forward. This "bulge" then fills part of the velopharyngeal gap. With adequate velar movement and enough lateral pharyngeal wall movement, the individual can achieve velopharyngeal closure. Various substances have been used for augmentation including collagen, fat, cartilage, silicone, Teflon, Proplast, and calcium hydroxylapatite (Brigger, Ashland, & Hartnick, 2010; Cantarella, Mazzola, Mantovani, Baracca, & Pignataro, 2011; Denny, Marks, & Oliff-Carneol, 1993; Furlow, Williams, Eisenbach, & Bzock, 1982; Lypka et al., 2010; Remacle, Bertrand, Eloy, & Marbaix, 1990; Rossleigh, Purcell, McGlynn, Parkin, & Shield, 2013; Ulkur et al., 2008; Wolford, Oelschlaeger, & Deal, 1989).

Sphincter Pharyngoplasty

A third surgical procedure to achieve velopharyngeal closure is sphincter pharyngoplasty (Jackson, 1985; Orticochea,

1968, 1997; Marsh, 2009). In this procedure, bilateral flaps from the posterior faucial pillars are dissected, rotated, and sutured to a small pharyngeal flap. Once healing occurs, a small round opening remains in the center of the pharynx. This small sphincter closes during speech with contraction of the levator palatini and palatopharyngeus muscles. This procedure may be most useful with individuals with poor lateral pharyngeal wall movement.

Prosthetic Management for Cleft Palate and Velopharyngeal Dysfunction

In some individuals with cleft palate or velopharyngeal dysfunction, surgical management is not an option. In this case, prosthetic management is a good alternative. This section discusses prosthetic management for cleft palate and velopharyngeal dysfunction.

When an individual with cleft palate or velopharyngeal dysfunction cannot undergo surgery, or must wait to undergo surgery, the prosthodontist may develop prosthetic devices to aid an individual in achieving velopharyngeal closure for speech. There are three basic types of speech appliances: a palatal obturator, a speech bulb obturator, and a palatal lift. The prosthodontist may develop combinations of these devices as necessary for patients.

Palatal Obturator

A palatal obturator is a device used to cover a palatal cleft or, more likely, a palatal fistula. A fistula is a hole between the oral and nasal cavities that may result from a surgical suture that did not heal properly, or a suture that opened when growth took place. A palatal obturator looks and fits much like a dental retainer,

though it has additional acrylic on top to cover the palatal opening.

Speech Bulb Obturator

A speech bulb obturator is used to address velopharyngeal dysfunction when the velum is too short to reach the back pharyngeal wall. A speech bulb is a removable device that fits on the teeth. However, the important part of a speech bulb is the posterior extension, on the end of which is an acrylic mass or bulb. The bulb functions to partially occlude the velopharyngeal space. Individuals then utilize lateral pharyngeal wall movement to completely close the space during nonnasal speech production.

Palatal Lift Device

A palatal lift device may be used to address velopharyngeal dysfunction. It also attaches to the teeth and extends in a posterior fashion. However, a palatal lift device involves a rigid posterior extension that serves to lift the velum up and back against the posterior pharyngeal wall. With a palatal lift, the velum is constantly held in a position to achieve velopharyngeal closure. Therefore, a palatal lift is generally only used with individuals who have neurological impairment of velar movement.

In determining treatment options for patients, the prosthodontist works closely with the surgeon. Choice of appropriate initial and follow-up surgical procedures, as well as possible prosthetic device development, is dependent on a careful and complete evaluation of the patient. This involves accurate assessment of velopharyngeal function by physiological evaluation and measurement. Additionally, the SLP will be consulted to assess speech prior to, and following, any treatment procedure. Often the SLP, plastic surgeon, and/or prosthodontist will also work with an oral surgeon for surgeries that involve bony structures. Examples of such orthognathic surgery are described in the next section.

Orthognathic Surgery

Because clefts may affect underlying bony tissues as well as soft tissues, orthognathic surgery, surgery that involves the bones of the upper and lower jaw, is often necessary. Two common types of orthognathic surgery for individuals with palatal clefts are alveolar bone grafting and maxillary advancement.

Alveolar Bone Grafting

Alveolar bone grafting may be necessary due to absence of bone, particularly in alveolar clefts. This surgery attempts to restore the continuity of the alveolus so that the child is less likely to develop crossbite or have missing teeth. Additionally, gaps in the alveolus may result in an oronasal fistula. Timing of surgery to address alveolar gaps is a source of controversy (Trindade-Suedam et al., 2012). Alveolar bone grafting may be done early, often at the same time as primary palatal surgery, and prior to the eruption of the teeth. This is called primary bone grafting. In some individuals, this surgery is postponed until permanent teeth begin to erupt. This is called delayed bone grafting.

Maxillary Advancement

Maxillary advancement surgery may be necessary due to underdevelopment of the midface region. Various midface advancement surgeries attempt to establish an appropriate upper and lower jaw rela-

tionship and improve facial appearance. Maxillary advancement surgery is usually postponed until early adolescence when mandibular growth has occurred.

Though surgical management is but one part of the treatment for individuals with clefts, it is an important one. Appropriate surgery combined with other necessary treatment will have a positive impact on a child's self-image and on how that child functions in the family, and eventually in school and society. The following section discusses psychosocial issues related to individuals with clefts and their families.

Psychosocial Issues

One of the main concerns of parents-to-be is, "Will my child be okay?" The birth of a baby who is "different" is therefore a shock to new parents. Because of the nature of cleft lip and cleft palate, early medical intervention is necessary, which further complicates life with a newborn. As the child grows, the child and the family must deal with both personal issues and societal pressures related to having a craniofacial anomaly. The child must deal with such issues through the school years and beyond. This section examines psychosocial issues related to clefts of the lip and palate and addresses the following topics: initial concerns of the parents, the effect of continued medical management, self-image and socialization, and school adjustment and performance. Discussion of these issues is limited to children with isolated clefts of the lip and/or palate. Children who have other craniofacial anomalies or associated syndromes will likely have additional and more complex psychosocial issues.

Current technology allows some parents to know more about their child before birth. Prenatal imaging techniques such as ultrasound may detect clefts of the lip and some multiple anomaly disorders. Prenatal chromosomal or genetic analysis such as amniocentesis can identify many syndromes. It is likely that studies will begin to look at the psychosocial impact of such knowledge on parents and families (Peterson-Falzone et al., 2009). Currently, however, most literature still focuses on parents' reaction to the birth of a child with a cleft.

Initial Concerns of the Parents

Several reports have documented the various reactions of parents to learning that their infant has a cleft. These reactions may include shock, grief, anger, guilt, depression, and/or fear (Barden, Ford, Jensen, Rogers-Salyer, & Salyer, 1989; Coy, Speltz, & Jones, 2002; Groll-emund, et al., 2010; Johansson & Rings-berg, 2004; Pope, Tillman, & Snyder, 2005; Rosenberg, Kapp-Simon, Starr, Cradock, & Speltz, 2011). For some parents, a period of mourning follows as they adjust to the unexpected situation (van Staden & Ger-hardt, 1995). Adverse effects on the marriage and other family and social relationships might seem likely, though research findings are inconclusive.

Almost immediately, parents of a child with a cleft must begin to deal with management issues. Feeding the infant, usually a pleasant interaction, may be difficult and stressful. The need for explanation and support to relatives and other family members may also take a toll on parents. Additionally, parents must begin to face the extensive medical interventions necessary for their child during the first year of life and beyond. It is important that parents receive immediate sup-port from professionals who can provide accurate information, answer questions, and provide referrals as necessary (Kum-mer, 2014).

The Effect of Continued Medical Management

Infants with clefts of the lip and/or palate face at least one surgery within the first year of life. The first surgery and subsequent hospitalization is a period of high stress for the parents. Though hospital stays are generally more family-friendly today, with less isolation of the child from family, the potential negative effects on parent-infant bonding and family life should still be considered (Peterson-Falzone et al., 2009). The child will most likely require additional surgeries and treatments throughout childhood and adolescence. This is particularly true of a child with a cleft palate. Continued contact with health professionals, and continued emotional and financial demands on the family, may result in the perception of cleft palate as a "chronic medical condition." Therefore, it is important that professionals continue to support the family, and relate to the patient not as a compilation of their physical issues, but as a whole person (Kummer, 2014).

Self-Image and Socialization

Stressors to the child and family continue through the toddler and preschool years. However, during this period of time, the child's self-image is largely developing based upon the parents' behaviors and attitudes. Once a child enters school, self-image and socialization issues take on a more significant role and become more complex (Peterson-Falzone et al., 2009).

As children with a history of clefts enter school, they may still look and/or sound different than their peers. Children who have had clefts of the lip and/or palate tend to have a more negative self-concept and lowered self-esteem compared to peers with no history of physical anomalies (Broder & Strauss, 1989; Kapp-Simon, 1986; Slifer et al., 2003). These children may also be more likely to be teased by their peers (Broder, Smith, & Strauss, 2001). Children with a history of clefts do not typically have as many friends as other age-matched children and, as they get older, tend to be more concerned about interpersonal relationships (Kummer, 2014) and more apprehensive about social interactions (Berger & Dalton, 2011; Dzioba, Husein, Dworschak-Stokan, & Doyle, 2012; Slifer et al., 2004). All of these findings vary by disorder, gender, and age, and are largely influenced by the support the child receives, particularly from family. Self-esteem and socialization issues also have an influence on the child's academic success.

School Adjustment and Performance

Academic achievement is a major focus for children and their families from the time the child enters school throughout the school years. The effects of clefts on academic achievement are difficult to sort out, and are influenced by self-esteem and socialization issues, as well as by societal and cultural views of clefts.

Children with clefts, as a group, achieve below expectations academically when achievement is compared to intellectual skill level (Broder, Richman, & Matheson, 1998; Millard & Richman,

2001). Teachers may underestimate the intellectual skills and abilities of individuals with craniofacial anomalies. Furthermore, both parents and teachers may expect less academically of these individuals. This may result in lower academic aspirations for the child and less favorable evaluations by the teachers (Richman & Eliason, 1982).

Individuals with cleft palate are also more likely to have serious reading disabilities (Richman & Millard, 1997). However, children with a history of cleft may lack self-confidence reading aloud in class, which may adversely affect teacher evaluations and thus stigmatize students as reading disabled (Kummer, 2014). Overall, peers and teachers perceive children with clefts as more inhibited in the classroom (Richman & Eliason, 1982).

There are several variables that interact to affect achievement in school. These include intelligence, language abilities, speech and hearing abilities, the presence or absence of learning disabilities, self-concept, social adjustment to school, and the expectations of peers, parents, and teachers (Peterson-Falzone et al., 2009). It is therefore imperative that cleft palate teams have a psychologist or similar professional address these issues with children and their families. Providing assistance to the child and family will maximize the possibility of the child functioning optimally in the family, school, and community.

Case Study 1: Jared

The following case study includes the SLP's thoughts throughout the assessment process. The SLP's thoughts are in italicized text.

Margaret was an SLP on a cleft palate team in a large metropolitan area. Once each month, patients from around the state came to consult with the team. One such patient was Jared, who lived in a rural area of the state. Jared was 11 years old. He had been born with a cleft of the secondary palate. It was repaired at the age of 8 months, and Jared's speech had progressed well. When Jared was 10 years old, his parents noticed that Jared's speech began to sound different, slightly more nasal. Because of Jared's history, his parents were concerned, so they took him to see an ENT. The ENT noted no problems upon visual examination of Jared's oral structures. The ENT also performed nasoendoscopy and concluded that Jared's velopharyngeal mechanism appeared to be working properly. The ENT referred Jared's parents to an SLP. Jared was evaluated by the local SLP who noted mild hypernasality and began therapy with Jared to work on resonance issues. When Jared came to see the cleft palate team, he had been seen by his local SLP for 1 year. The local SLP's written report to the cleft palate team noted that Jared had been working on "blowing techniques" to help direct airflow out the mouth rather than the nose. The SLP noted limited success and also noted that Jared had begun to have a slightly hoarse quality to his voice. She had referred Jared back to the ENT, who discovered slight edema on Jared's vocal folds. The ENT told the parents to continue to work with the SLP. Jared's parents decided to contact the surgeon who had performed Jared's initial cleft palate surgery. That surgeon referred them to the cleft palate team.

(*Upon review of this client's information, I have several thoughts and some hypotheses. Jared's increased nasality in his speech is a cause for concern. Resonance issues are rarely behavioral, meaning that Jared is not likely making his speech more nasal. Therefore, there is likely something structural going on that is impacting his ability to achieve complete velopharyngeal closure. Given that his surgery was over 10 years ago, it is not likely that there are any current complications of the surgery, or a fistula, or any such occurrence. I am guessing the change has something to do with Jared's growth. It could be that his velopharyngeal closure was always tenuous, and that additional growth, and perhaps a deepening of the back pharyngeal wall, has made velopharyngeal closure less stable. Another possibility at his age is that his adenoids have begun to shrink. This is a normal process during adolescence. In many children, the adenoids assist velopharyngeal closure by creating a "pad" at the location where the velum contacts the back pharyngeal wall. If Jared's adenoids have begun to shrink, and his velopharyngeal mechanism is not able to adapt, this could affect velopharyngeal closure and therefore resonance, resulting in mild hypernasality.*

Regardless of cause of the potential resonance issue, I have concerns about the speech therapy that Jared has been receiving. Although I am sure the local SLP has good intentions, there is no evidence in the literature that techniques such as blowing [often referred to as NSOME, or "nonspeech oral motor exercises"] have any effect on speech. More importantly, if Jared is unable to achieve complete velopharyngeal closure because of anatomy or physiology of the velopharyngeal mechanism, any speech therapy targeting resonance is futile. In fact, such therapy can be detrimental. If Jared has been trying to overcome velopharyngeal insufficiency with extra effort, this could have resulted in hyperfunctional use of the voice. This may be why Jared has swelling on his vocal folds and is sounding hoarse. My strong recommendation is that

Jared undergo a full assessment of function of his velopharyngeal mechanism.)

Through evaluation with nasopharyngoscopy and mulitview videoflouroscopy, the cleft palate team diagnosed Jared with borderline velopharyngeal insufficiency. His velum had good mobility but appeared to be slightly short to make adequate contact with the back pharyngeal wall. Based on the direction of velar movement, the team surmised that Jared's adenoids had been assisting with velopharyngeal closure and had begun to shrink as part of normal adolescence. Jared's speech therapy had been in vain, as his mechanism was not structurally able to achieve velopharyngeal closure. The speech therapy had likely introduced a new voice problem due to Jared's attempts to produce nonnasal speech and the hyperfunctional use of his voice. Because Jared's adenoids had not completely shrunk, the cleft palate team recommended that Jared be fitted with an obturator to temporarily assist with velopharyngeal closure. The team also recommended that Jared be seen yearly to assess his growth and velopharyngeal function. Once the adenoids have completely shrunk, Jared can be evaluated for pharyngeal wall augmentation.

(*As part of the cleft palate team's full recommendations, I also recommend that Jared discontinue speech therapy to address resonance. I will follow up with his local SLP to provide her with information regarding the problem with resonance therapy when a velopharyngeal mechanism is not structurally or functionally adequate and regarding the lack of evidence for use of NSOMEs. The local ENT likely did not have the appropriate equipment to diagnose the minor velopharyngeal insufficiency. It is important that SLPs are empowered to continue to refer clients who appear to*

have speech issues potentially related to velopharyngeal insufficiency, and not to continue with futile therapy.

I further recommend that Jared be seen by his local ENT every 3 months to monitor his vocal edema. If the vocal folds do not look normal in 6 months and/or if they get worse at any point, he should be seen for voice therapy. In this case, he may need to unlearn some bad habits of hyperfunctional voice use.)

By ENT report, after 3 months, Jared's vocal folds appeared normal. Jared returned to be evaluated by the cleft palate team once a year for 3 years. After the first year, no change was needed in his obturator. His resonance was normal. After the second year, he was again exhibiting mild hypernasality. The prosthodontist increased the size of the obturator bulb slightly to accommodate additional shrinkage of Jared's adenoids. After the third year, when Jared was 14 years old, his adenoids had completely atrophied. He underwent surgery for pharyngeal wall augmentation. When Jared returned for a follow-up at 15 years of age, his resonance and voice were normal. Upon examination, his velopharyngeal mechanism appeared to be functioning adequately for speech.

Case Study 2: Samuel

Samuel was born with a bilateral complete cleft of the secondary palate. At 9 months of age, he underwent surgery to repair the cleft. When Samuel was 2 years old, his family moved. He did not begin to speak until he was 2.5 years old. When Samuel began to produce words, he left out many of the sounds. Samuel's parents realized that he was not producing as many sounds or words as he should, but they attributed it to lasting trauma from his early surgery. His parents assumed Samuel would eventually learn all his sounds. At age 4, Samuel entered a preschool. Samuel's teacher could not understand him and suggested that Samuel's parents take him to see an SLP. A local SLP assessed Samuel and diagnosed a severe articulation disorder. She noted that Samuel omitted all stop, fricative, and affricate consonants. However, she noted accurate production of vowels as well as liquid, glide, and nasal consonants. She immediately began therapy to address Samuel's numerous sound omissions.

Therapy focused on placement of the articulators to produce sounds. Though Samuel was able to imitate articulator placement for sound production, he appeared to struggle when attempting to produce the sounds. Because the preschool teacher and Samuel's preschool classmates could not understand him, and because Samuel seemed frustrated by this, his parents withdrew him from preschool. Samuel continued to receive speech therapy three times a week for six months. At the end of six months, Samuel was still omitting stops, fricatives, and affricates in his speech. Furthermore, his voice was now taking on a harsh, rough quality. The SLP suggested that Samuel's parents have him evaluated by an otolaryngologist to determine whether or not he had vocal nodules.

The otolaryngologist did observe small bilateral vocal nodules on Samuel's vocal folds, but suggested the parents have Samuel evaluated by a cleft palate team. The parents insisted that Samuel's cleft palate had already been repaired. However, they took Samuel to the nearest city's cleft palate team. Following a complete evaluation by the team, it was determined that Samuel had velopharyngeal insufficiency due to a short velum. Though Samuel's speech was judged to be mildly hypernasal, the main characteristic of his speech was inability to produce high-pressure consonants due to leakage of air into the nasal cavity. It was assumed that Samuel had developed a secondary voice disorder due to hyperfunctional use of the laryngeal muscles in attempting to produce high-pressure sounds in therapy. It was recommended that Samuel undergo secondary surgery to create a pharyngeal flap. However, the cleft palate team recommended that the family postpone secondary surgery until additional midfacial growth had occurred. In the meantime, Samuel was fitted for a speech bulb obturator.

On Samuel's 5th birthday, he was seen by the cleft palate team prosthodontist to be fitted for the speech bulb obturator. During fitting, the prosthodontist modified size and placement of the acrylic bulb as the cleft palate team SLP listened to Samuel's speech to judge nasality. When nasality was judged to be normal, the speech bulb obturator was completed. Samuel quickly adjusted to the new appliance. His speech was no longer mildly hypernasal and he gradually began to "acquire" stops, fricatives and affricates. When Samuel was 9 years old, he underwent surgery to create a permanent pharyngeal flap. At that point his speech was normal.

Review Questions

1. How were Samuel's sound errors similar to, and different from, articulation and/or phonological disorders more commonly exhibited by children?

2. Would earlier intervention and assessment by an SLP or a cleft palate team have helped Samuel's development? In what potential ways? Ideally, at what age should Samuel have been assessed?

3. What might Samuel's lack of progress in therapy have indicated to the SLP?

4. How do the SLP and prosthodontist work together during the fitting of the speech bulb obturator to achieve optimal results?

5. Why was it prudent to delay secondary surgery for Samuel's velopharyngeal insufficiency?

Case Study 3: Gretchen

Gretchen was a 4-year-old girl whose parents brought her to an SLP for an articulation evaluation. Gretchen's parents reported that she often produced strange gargling and spitting sounds when she spoke. The SLP discovered that Gretchen had been born with a cleft palate, but this had been repaired when Gretchen was 9 months old. During the speech evaluation the SLP noted that Gretchen produced pharyngeal stops as substitutes for bilabial and lingua-alveolar stops, and glottal stops as substitutes for lingua-velar stops. Likewise, Gretchen produced pharyngeal fricatives as substitutes for labiodental, inter-dental, and lingua-alveolar fricatives, and glottal fricatives as substitutes for lingua-palatal fricatives. Additionally, Gretchen substituted glottal affricates for the lingua-palatal affricates. The SLP noted normal resonance. However, due to Gretchen's history and presenting articulation characteristics, the SLP referred her

to an otolaryngologist for an evaluation. Following an examination, the otolaryngologist reported that Gretchen's velopharyngeal mechanism appeared to be functioning normally. Therefore, the SLP recommended articulation therapy.

In therapy, the SLP worked on placement of stop consonants. The SLP had a difficult time getting Gretchen to change place of articulation. When Gretchen did use a more front place of articulation, it appeared difficult for her to make an audible stop consonant sound. Due to Gretchen's history of cleft palate, as well as her difficulty with therapy, after six months the SLP referred Gretchen to a cleft palate team. Gretchen underwent several tests and examinations. Her evaluation included a videotaped x-ray image of movement of the velopharyngeal mechanism during speech (a procedure called videoflouroscopy) and measurement of oral and nasal airflow during speech to get an idea of size of velopharyngeal port opening (a procedure called pressure-flow technique). The cleft palate team concluded that Gretchen had minor velopharyngeal dysfunction due to a slightly short velum. Velopharyngeal dysfunction was only evident during attempts to accurately produce high-pressure consonants. When Gretchen attempted accurate production of these sounds, the velopharyngeal mechanism required the tightest closure, and a small amount of air leakage into the nasal cavity was evident. The cleft palate team advised Gretchen and her parents of their finding and recommended pharyngeal wall augmentation. After more testing to determine exact injection site, this procedure was performed. Following pharyngeal wall augmentation, Gretchen still produced pharyngeal and glottal stops, fricatives, and affricates. She was referred back to her SLP. This time, with a fully functional velopharyngeal mechanism, Gretchen was successful in therapy. She was dismissed from therapy after three months.

Review Questions

1. How were Gretchen's sound productions different from articulation disorders more typically exhibited by children? Were there any similarities?

2. Why did Gretchen's velopharyngeal dysfunction affect articulation, but not resonance?

3. If Gretchen had continued speech therapy prior to pharyngeal wall augmentation, could she have been successful? Might there have been any negative effects of the continued therapy?

4. Why do you think the cleft palate team recommended pharyngeal wall augmentation rather than a pharyngeal flap?

5. How does the surgeon determine the injection site for the augmentation?

Chapter Review Questions

1. How do the structures referred to in this chapter as *primary palate* and *secondary palate* compare to the structures commonly referred to as "hard palate" and "soft palate"? Why are the terms *primary palate* and *secondary palate* preferable when discussing clefts?

2. Why do you think the multifactorial model of inheritance is the most popular theory to explain clefts?

3. Suppose you are involved in a debate about best age for primary surgery to correct a palatal cleft. What age do

you choose and why? Suppose you must argue for surgery during the first three months of life. What will be your main points? Next, suppose you must argue for postponing surgery. What will be your main points now?

4. Secondary surgery for individuals with a history of cleft lip is performed for a different reason than secondary surgery for individuals with a history of cleft palate. Compare and contrast the two types of secondary surgery.

5. Describe different options for secondary management of velopharyngeal dysfunction. For whom, and at what age, are the various surgical options best? For whom, and at what age, are the various prosthetic options best? For whom, and at what age, is speech therapy best?

6. Discuss how it is possible for an individual with velopharyngeal dysfunction to be both hypernasal and hyponasal.

7. Explain why individuals with a history of cleft palate often produce a lateralized /s/.

8. Nasal emission and weak pressure consonants are often described as "passive" articulation errors whereas compensatory articulation is often described as an "active" articulation strategy. Why are these terms used? Is a "passive" error or an "active" strategy preferable? (Consider such factors as intelligibility, habit formation, need for speech therapy, etc.)

9. Is it possible to assess resonance and articulation in a child who is producing only one-word utterances? If so, what will be your strategy? Provide examples of stimulus items.

10. Suppose you are a speech-language pathologist and an individual with a history of a cleft palate is referred to you. The individual presents with hypernasality, audible nasal emission of high-pressure consonants, and a hoarse voice. What might be the cause of the voice disorder? How will you differentially diagnose the resonance disorder from the voice disorder?

References

American Cleft Palate-Craniofacial Association. (2006). *Speech samples*. Retrieved June 5, 2013, from http://www.acpa-cpf.org/education/educational_resources/speech_samples/

American Cleft Palate-Craniofacial Association. (2009). *Parameters for evaluation and treatment of patients with cleft lip/palate or other craniofacial anomalies*. Retrieved June 17, 2013, from http://www.acpa-cpf.org/uploads/site/Parameters_ Rev_2009.pdf

Aniansson, G., Svensson, H., Becker, M., & Ingvarsson, L. (2002). Otitis media and feeding with breast milk of children with cleft palate. *Scandinavian Journal of Plastic and Reconstructive Surgery and Hand Surgery, 36*, 9–15.

Argamaso, R. V., Shprintzen, R. J., Strauch, B., Lewin, M., Daniller, A., Ship, A., . . . Croft, C. (1980). The role of lateral pharyngeal wall movement in pharyngeal flap surgery. *Plastic and Reconstructive Surgery, 66*, 214–219.

Austin, A. A., Druschel, C. M., Tyler, M. C., Romitti, P. A., West, I. I., Damiano, P. C., . . . Burnett, W. (2010). Interdisciplinary craniofacial teams compared with individual providers: Is orofacial cleft care more comprehensive and do parents perceive better outcomes? *The Cleft Palate–Craniofacial Journal, 47*, 1–8.

Bardach, J. (1994). Unilateral cleft lip. In M. M. Cohen (Ed.), *Mastery of plastic and reconstructive surgery* (Vol. 1, pp. 548–565). Boston, MA: Little Brown.

Bardach, J., & Salyer, K. (1987). *Surgical techniques in cleft lip and palate*. Chicago, IL: Mosby Yearbook.

Barden, C., Ford, M., Jensen, A. G., Rogers-Salyer, M., & Salyer, K. E. (1989). Effects of craniofacial deformity in infancy on the quality of mother-infant interactions. *Child Development, 60*, 819–824.

Berger, Z. E., & Dalton, L. J. (2011). Coping with a cleft II: Factors associated with psychosocial adjustment of adolescents with a cleft lip and palate and their parents. *The Cleft Palate–Craniofacial Journal, 48*, 82–90.

Bille, C., Knudsen, L. B., & Christensen, K. (2005). Changing lifestyles and oral clefts occurrence in Denmark. *The Cleft Palate–Craniofacial Journal, 42*, 255–259.

Brauer, R. O., & Cronin, T. D. (1983). The Tennison lip repair revisited. *Plastic and Reconstructive Surgery, 71*, 633–642.

Bressman, T., Radovanovic, B., Kulkarni, G. V., Klaiman, P., & Fisher, D. (2011). An ultrasonic investigation of cleft-type compensatory articulations of voiceless velar stops. *Clinical Linguistics and Phonetics, 25*, 1028–1033.

Brigger, M. T., Ashland, J. E., & Hartnich, C. J. (2010). Injection pharyngoplasty with calcium hydroxylapatite for velopharyngeal insufficiency: Patient selection and technique. *Archives of Otolaryngology–Head & Neck Surgery, 136*, 666–670.

Broder, H., Smith, F. B., & Strauss, R. (2001). Developing a behavior rating scale for comparing teachers' ratings of children with and without craniofacial anomalies. *The Cleft Palate–Craniofacial Journal, 38*, 560–565.

Broder, H. L., Richman, L. C., & Matheson, P. B. (1998). Learning disability, school achievement, and grade retention among children with cleft: A two-center study. *The Cleft Palate–Craniofacial Journal, 35*, 127–131.

Broder, H. L., & Strauss, R. P. (1989). Self-concept of early primary school age children with visible or invisible defects. *Cleft Palate Journal, 26*, 114–117.

Burdi, A. R., & Silvey, R. G. (1969). Sexual differences in closure of the human palatal shelves. *Cleft Palate Journal, 6*, 1–7.

Bzoch, K. R. (1979). Measurement and assessment of categorical aspects of cleft palate speech. In K. R. Bzoch (Ed.), *Communicative disorders related to cleft lip and palate*. Boston, MA: Little Brown.

Calzolari, E., Milan, M., Cavazzuti, G. B., Cocchi, G., Gandini, E., Magnani, C., . . . Volpato, S. (1988). Epidemiological and genetic study of

200 cases of oral cleft in the Emilia Romagna region of Northern Italy. *Teratology, 38,* 559–564.

Cantarella, G., Mazzola, R. F., Mantovani, M., Baracca, G., & Pignataro, L. (2011). Treatment of velopharyngeal insufficiency by pharyngeal and velar fat injections. *Otolaryngology–Head & Neck Surgery, 145,* 401–403.

Capone, R. B., & Sykes, J. M. (2007). The cleft and craniofacial team: The whole is greater than the sum of its parts. *Facial Plastic Surgery, 23,* 83–86.

Carmichael, S. L., Shaw, G. M., Ma, C., Werler, M. M., Rasmussen, S. A., & Lammer, E. J. (2007). Maternal corticosteroid use and orofacial clefts. *American Journal of Obstetrics & Gynecology, 197,* 683–684.

Castilla, E. E., Orioli. I. M., Lopez-Camelo, J. S., Dutra Mda, G., & Nazer-Herrera, J. (2003). Preliminary data on changes in neural tube defect prevalence rates after folic acid fortification in South America. *American Journal of Medical Genetics Part A, 123,* 123–128.

Chow, E. W. C., Bassett, A. S., & Weksberg, R. (1994). Velo-cardio-facial syndrome and psychotic disorders: Implications for psychiatric genetics. *American Journal of Medical Genetics, 54,* 107–112.

Coy, K., Speltz, M. L., & Jones, K. (2002). Facial appearance and attachment in infants with orofacial clefts: A replication. *The Cleft Palate–Craniofacial Journal, 39,* 66–72.

Denny, A. D., Marks, S. M., & Oliff-Carneol, S. (1993). Correction of velopharyngeal insufficiency by pharyngeal augmentation using autologous cartilage: A preliminary report. *The Cleft Palate–Craniofacial Journal, 30,* 46–54.

Dixon, M. J., Marazita, M. L., Beaty, T. H., & Murray, J. C. (2011). Cleft lip and palate: Understanding genetic and environmental influences. *Nature Reviews Genetics, 12,* 167–178.

Dzioba, A., Husein, M., Dworschak-Stokan, A., & Doyle, P. C. (2012). An evaluation of communication apprehension in adolescents with velopharyngeal inadequacy. *The Cleft Palate–Craniofacial Journal, 49,* 17–24.

Edwards, M. J., Agho, K., Attia, J., Diaz, P., Hayes, T., Illingworth, A., . . . Roddick, L. G. (2003). Case-control study of cleft lip or palate after maternal use of topical corticosteroids during pregnancy. *American Journal of Medical Genetics Part A, 120,* 459–463.

Eliez, S., Blasey, C. M., Schmitt, E. J., White, C. D., Hu, D., & Reiss, A. L. (2001). Velocardiofacial syndrome: Are structural changes in the temporal and mesial temporal regions related to schizophrenia? *American Journal of Psychiatry, 158*(3), 447–453.

Furlow, L., Jr. (1986). Cleft palate repair by double opposing Z-plasty. *Plastic and Reconstructive Surgery, 78*(6), 724–738.

Furlow, L. T., Jr. (1990). Flaps for cleft lip and palate surgery. *Clinics in Plastic Surgery, 17,* 633–644.

Furlow, L. T., Jr. (2009). Correction of velopharyngeal insufficiency by a double-opposing Z-plasty. In J. E. Lossee & R. E. Kirschner (Eds.), *Comprehensive cleft care* (pp. 641–647). New York, NY: McGraw-Hill.

Furlow, L. T., Jr., Williams, W. N., Eisenbach, C. R. D., & Bzoch, K. R. (1982). A long-term study on treating velopharyngeal insufficiency by Teflon injection. *Cleft Palate Journal, 19,* 47–56.

Gangopadhyay, N., Mendonca, D. A., & Woo, A. S. (2012). Pierre Robin sequence. *Seminars in Plastic Surgery, 26,* 76–82.

Grewal, J., Carmichael, S. L., Ma, C., Lammer, E. J., & Shaw, G. M. (2008). Maternal periconceptual smoking and alcohol consumption and risk for select congenital anomalies. *Birth Defects Research Part A: Clinical and Molecular Teratology, 82,* 519–526.

Grollemund, B., Galliani, E., Soupre, V., Vazquez, M. P., Guedeney, A., & Danion, A. (2010). The impact of cleft lip and palate on the parent-child relationships. *Archives de Pediatrie, 17,* 1380–1385.

Hamming, K. K., Finkelstein, M., & Sidman, J. D. (2009). Hoarseness in children with cleft palate. *Otolaryngology–Head and Neck Surgery, 140,* 902–906.

Harding, A., & Grunwell, P. (1998). Active versus passive cleft-type speech characteristics. *International Journal of Language and Communication Disorders, 33*(3), 329–352.

Hashmi, S. S., Waller, D. K., Langlois, P., Canfield, M., & Hecht, J. T. (2005). Prevalence of nonsyndromic oral clefts in Texas: 1995–1999. *American Journal of Medical Genetics Part A, 134,* 368–372.

Heineman-de Boer, J. A., Van Haelst, M. J., Cordia-de Haan, M., & Beemer, F. A. (1999). Behavior problems and personality aspects of 40 children with velo-cardio-facial syndrome. *Genetic Counseling, 10*(1), 89–93.

Izumi, K., Konczal, L. L., Mitchell, A. L., & Jones, M. C. (2012). Underlying genetic diagnosis of

Pierre Robin sequence: Retrospective chart review at two children's hospitals and a systematic literature review. *Journal of Pediatrics, 160,* 645–650.

Jackson, I. T. (1985). Sphincter pharyngoplasty. *Clinics in Plastic Surgery, 12*(4), 711–717.

Jakobsen, L. P., Knudsen, M. A., Lespinasse, J., Garcia Ayuso, C., Ramos, C., Fryns, J.P., . . . Tommerup, N. (2006). The genetic basis of the Pierre Robin Sequence. *The Cleft Palate–Craniofacial Journal, 43,* 155–159.

Jensen, B. L., Kreigorg, S., Dahl, E., & Fogh-Anderson, P. (1988). Cleft lip and palate in Denmark, 1976–1981: Epidemiology, variability, and early somatic development. *Cleft Palate Journal, 25*(3), 258–269.

Jia, Z. L., Shi, B., Chen, C. H., Shi, Y., Wu, J., & Xu, X. (2011). Maternal malnutrition, environmental exposure during pregnancy and the risk of non-syndromic orofacial clefts. *Oral Disorders, 17,* 584–589.

Johansson, B., & Ringsberg, K. C. (2004). Parents' experiences of having a child with cleft lip and palate. *Journal of Advanced Nursing, 47,* 165–173.

Jones, K. L. (1986). Fetal alcohol syndrome. *Pediatric Development, 8*(4), 122–126.

Jones, K. L., & Smith, D. W. (1973). Recognition of the fetal alcohol syndrome in early infancy. *Lancet, 2*(7836), 999–1001.

Kapp-Simon, K. A. (1986). Self-concept of primary-school-age children with cleft lip, cleft palate, or both. *Cleft Palate Journal, 23,* 24–27.

Karayiorgou, M., Morris, M. A., Morrow, B., Shprintzen, R. J., Goldberg, R. B., Borrow, J., . . . Housman, D. E. (1995). Schizophrenia susceptibility associated with interstitial deletions of chromosome 22q11. *Proceedings of the National Academy of Sciences of the United States of America, 92,* 7612–7615.

Karnell, M. P. (2011). Instrumental assessment of velopharyngeal closure for speech. *Seminars in Speech and Language, 32,* 168–178.

Kernahan, D. A., & Stark, R. B. (1958). A new classification system for cleft lip and cleft palate. *Plastic and Reconstructive Surgery, 22,* 435.

Knapke, S. C., Bender, P., Prows, C., Schultz, J. R., & Saal, H. M. (2010). Parental perspectives of children born with cleft lip and/or palate: A qualitative assessment of suggestions for healthcare improvements and interventions. *The Cleft Palate–Craniofacial Journal, 47,* 143–150.

Knezevic, P., Grgurevic, L., Uglesic, B., & Grgurevic, J. (2012). Modified Millard's technique in operations for unilateral cleft lip. *Journal of Plastic Surgery and Hand Surgery, 46,* 326–329.

Kohli, S. S., & Kohli, V. S. (2012). A comprehensive view of the genetic basis of cleft lip and palate. *Journal of Oral and Maxillofacial Pathology, 16,* 64–72.

Kummer, A. W. (2014). *Cleft palate & craniofacial anomalies: The effects on speech and resonance* (3rd ed.). Clifton Park, NY: Delmar Learning.

Lazarus, D. D., Hudson, D. A., van Zyl, J. E., Fleming, A. N., & Fernandes, D. (1998). Repair of unilateral cleft lip: A comparison of five techniques. *Annals of Plastic Surgery, 41,* 587–594.

Lypka, M., Bidros, R., Rizvi, M., Gaon, M., Rubenstein, A., Fox, D., . . . Cronin, E. (2010). Posterior pharyngeal augmentation in the treatment of velopharyngeal insufficiency: A 40-year experience. *Annals of Plastic Surgery, 65,* 48–51.

Maresova, K., Veleminska, J., & Mullerova, Z. (2004). The development of intracranial relations in patients with complete unilateral cleft lip and palate in relation to surgery method and gender aspect. *Acta Chirurgiae Plasticae, 46,* 89–94.

Marsh, J. L. (2009). Sphincter pharyngoplasty. In J. E. Lossee & R. E. Kirschner (Eds.), *Comprehensive cleft care* (pp. 665–671). New York, NY: McGraw-Hill.

McWilliams, B. J., Morris, H. L., & Shelton, R. L. (1990). *Cleft palate speech* (2nd ed.). Philadelphia, PA: B. C. Decker.

Meazzini, M. C., Tortora, C., Morabito, A., Garattini, G., & Brusati, R. (2011). Factors that affect variability in impairment of maxillary growth in patients with cleft lip and palate treated using the same surgical protocol. *Journal of Plastic Surgery and Hand Surgery, 45,* 188–193.

Millard, D. R. (1958). A radical rotation in single harelip. *American Journal of Surgery, 95,* 318–322.

Millard, D. R. (1976). *Cleft craft: The evolution of its surgeries. Vol. I: The unilateral deformity.* Boston, MA: Little Brown.

Millard, D. R. (1977). *Cleft craft: The evolution of its surgeries. Vol. II: The bilateral deformity.* Boston, MA: Little Brown.

Millard, T., & Richman, L. C. (2001). Different cleft conditions, facial appearance, and speech:

Relationship to psychological variables. *The Cleft Palate–Craniofacial Journal, 38,* 68–75.

Munger, R. G., Romitti, P. A., Daack-Hirsh, S., Burns, T. L., Murray, J. C., & Hanson, J. (1996). Maternal alcohol use and risk of orofacial cleft birth defects. *Teratology, 54,* 27–33.

Munger, R. G., Sauberlich, H. E., Corcoran, C., Nepomuceno, B., Daack-Hirsh, S., & Solon, F. S. (2004). Maternal vitamin B-6 and folate status and risk of oral cleft birth defects in the Philippines. *Birth Defects Research, 70,* 464–471.

Murthy, J., Sendhilnathan, S., & Hussain, S. A. (2010). Speech outcome following late primary palate repair. *The Cleft Palate–Craniofacial Journal, 47,* 156–161.

Nash, K., Sheard, E., Rovet, J., & Koren, G. (2008). Understanding fetal alcohol spectrum disorders (FASDs): Toward identification of a behavioral phenotype. *The Scientific World Journal, 8,* 873–882.

Noordhoff, M. S. (1994). Bilateral cleft lip. In M. Cohen (Ed.), *Mastery of plastic and reconstructive surgery* (Vol. 1). Boston, MA: Little Brown.

Orticochea, M. (1968). Construction of a dynamic muscle sphincter in cleft palates. *Plastic and Reconstructive Surgery, 41,* 323–327.

Orticochea, M. (1997). Physiopathology of the dynamic muscular sphincter of the pharynx. *Plastic and Reconstructive Surgery, 100*(7), 1918–1923.

Paradise, J. L., Elster, B. A., & Tan, L. (1994). Evidence in infants with cleft palate that breast milk protects against otitis media. *Pediatrics, 94,* 853–860.

Peterson-Falzone, S. J., Hardin-Jones, M. A., & Karnell, M. P. (2009). *Cleft palate speech* (4th ed.). St. Louis, MO: Mosby.

Peterson-Falzone, S. L., Trost-Cardamone, J. E., Karnell, M. P., & Hardin-Jones, M. A. (2006). *The clinician's guide to treating cleft palate speech.* St. Louis, MO: Mosby.

Pope, A. W., Tillman, K., & Snyder, H. T. (2005). Parenting stress in infancy and psychosocial adjustment in toddlerhood: A longitudinal study of children with craniofacial anomalies. *The Cleft Palate–Craniofacial Journal, 42,* 556–559.

Pradat, P., Robert-Gnansia, E., DiTanna, G. L., Rosano, A., Lisi, A., & Mastroiacovo, P. (2003). First trimester exposure to corticosteroids and oral clefts. *Birth Defects Research Part A: Clinical and Moledular Teratology, 67,* 968–970.

Priya, V. K., Reddy, J. S., Ramakrishna, Y., & Reddy, C. P. (2011). *Journal of Indian Society of Pedodontics and Preventive Dentistry, 29,* 229–234.

Pulver, A. E., Nestadt, G., Goldberg, R., Shprintzen, R. J., Lamacz, J., Wolyniec, P. S., . . . Kucherlapati, R. (1994). Psychotic illness in patients diagnosed with velo-cardio-facial syndrome and their relatives. *Journal of Nervous and Mental Disease, 182,* 476–478.

Randall, P. (1959). A triangular flap operation for the primary repair of unilateral clefts of the lip. *Plastic and Reconstructive Surgery, 23,* 331–347.

Randall, P. (1990). Long-term results with the triangular flap technique for unilateral cleft lip repair. In J. Bardach & H. L. Morris (Eds.), *Multidisciplinary management of cleft lip and palate* (pp. 173–183). Philadelphia, PA: W.B. Saunders.

Ranta, R., & Rintala, A. (1989). Unusual alveolar clefts: Report of cases. *Journal of Dentistry for Children, 56,* 363–365.

Ray, J. G., Meier, C., Vermeulen, M. J., Wyatt, P. R., & Cole, D. E. (2003). Association between folic acid food fortication and congenital orofacial clefts. *Journal of Pediatrics, 143,* 805–807.

Reiter, R., Brosch, S., Ludeke, M., Fischbein, E., Haase, S., Pickhard, A., . . . Maier, C. (2012). Genetic and environmental risk factors for submucous cleft palate. *European Journal of Oral Sciences, 120,* 97–103.

Remacle, M., Bertrand, B., Eloy, P., & Marbaix, E. (1990). The use of injectable collagen to correct velopharyngeal insufficiency. *Laryngoscope, 100,* 269–274.

Richman, L. C., & Eliason, M. J. (1982). Psychological characteristics of children with cleft lip and palate: Intellectual, achievement, behavioral, and personality variables. *Cleft Palate Journal, 19,* 249–257.

Richman, L. C., & Millard, T. L. (1997). Cleft lip and palate: Longitudinal behavior and relationships of cleft conditions to behavior and achievement. *Journal of Pediatric Psychology, 22,* 487–494.

Robin, N. H., Opitz, J. M., & Muenke, M. (1996). Opitz G/BBB syndrome: Clinical comparisons of families linked to Xp22 and 22q, and a review of the literature. *American Journal of Medical Genetics, 62*(3), 305–317.

Robison, J. G., Todd, D., & Otteson, T. D. (2011). Prevalence of hoarseness in the cleft palate population. *Archives of Otolaryngology–Head and Neck Surgery, 137,* 74–77.

Rosenberg, J. M., Kapp-Simon, K. A., Starr, J. R., Cradock, M., & Speltz, M. L. (2011). Mothers' and fathers' reports of stress in families of infants with and without single-suture craniosynostosis. *The Cleft Palate–Craniofacial Journal, 48,* 509–518.

Rossleigh, M., Purcell, A., McGlynn, M., Parkin, M., & Shield, K. (2013). Parental perceptions of posterior pharyngeal wall augmentation using autologous fat for treating velopharyngeal dysfunction. *International Journal of Speech Language Pathology, 15,* 268–278.

Saperstein, E. L., Kennedy, D. L., Mulliken, J. B., & Padwa, B. L. (2012). Facial growth in children with complete cleft of the primary palate and intact secondary palate. *Journal of Oral Maxillofacial Surgery, 70,* 66–71.

Shaw, G. M., Croen, L. A., & Curry, C. J. (1991). Isolated oral cleft malformations: Associations with maternal and infant characteristics in a California population. *Teratology, 43,* 225–228.

Shaw, G. M., & Lammer, E. J. (1999). Maternal periconceptional alcohol consumption and risk for orofacial clefts. *Journal of Pediatrics, 134,* 298–303.

Sheer, F. J., Swarts, J. D., & Ghadiali, S. N. (2010). Finite element analysis of eustachian tube function in cleft palate infants based on histological reconstructions. *The Cleft Palate–Craniofacial Journal, 47,* 600–610.

Shi, M., Wehby, G. L., & Murray, J. C. (2008). Review on genetic variants and maternal smoking in the etiology of oral clefts and other birth defects. *Birth Defects Research Part C: Embryo Today, 84,* 16–29.

Slifer, K. J., Amari, A., Diver, T., Hilley, L., Beek, M., Kane, A., . . . McDonnell, S. (2004). Social interaction patterns of children and adolescents with and without oral clefts during a videotaped analogue social encounter. *The Cleft Palate–Craniofacial Journal, 41,* 175–184.

Slifer, K. J., Beek, M., Amari, S., Diver, T., Hilley, L., Kane, A., . . . McDonnell, S. (2003). Self-concept and satisfaction with physical appearance in youth with and without oral clefts. *Children's Health Care, 32,* 81–101.

Snead, M. P., McNinch, A. M., Poulson, A. V., Bearcroft, P., Silverman, B., Gomersall, P., . . . Richards, A. J. (2011). Stickler syndrome, ocular-only variants and a key diagnostic role

for the ophthalmologist. *Eye (London), 25,* 1389–1400.

Stal, S., Brown, R. H., Higuera, S., Hollier, L. H., Jr., Byrd, H. S., Cutting, C. B., . . . Mulliken, J. B. (2009). Fifty years of the Millard rotation-advancement: Looking back and moving forward. *Plastic and Reconstructive Surgery, 123,* 1364–1377.

Streissguth, A. P., Aase, J. M., Clarren, S. K., Randels, S. P., LaDue, R. A., & Smith, D. F. (1991). Fetal alcohol syndrome in adolescents and adults [see Comments]. *Journal of the American Medical Association, 265*(15), 1961–1967.

Surgeon General's Report. (1987, June). *Children with special needs.* Washington, DC: Office of Maternal and Child Health, U.S. Department of Health and Human Services, Public Health Service.

Templin, M. C., & Darley, F. L. (1960). *The Templin-Darley tests of articulation* (2nd ed.). Iowa City, IA: Bureau of Educational Research and Service, University of Iowa.

Tennison, C. W. (1952). Repair of unilateral cleft lip by the stencil method. *Plastic and Reconstructive Surgery, 9,* 115–120.

Tolarova, M., & Harris, J. (1995). Reduced recurrence of orofacial clefts after periconceptional supplementation with high-dose folic acid and multivitamins. *Teratology, 51,* 71–78.

Trier, W. (1985). Repair of unilateral cleft lip: The rotation-advancement operation. *Clinics in Plastic Surgery, 12,* 573–594.

Trier, W., & Dreyer, T. (1984). Primary von Langenbeck palatoplasty with levator reconstruction: Rationales and technique. *Cleft Palate Journal, 21*(4), 254–262.

Trindade-Suedam, I. K., da Silva Filho, O. G., Carvalho, R. M., de Souza Faco, R. A., Calvo, A. M., Ozawa, T. O., . . . Trindade, I. E. (2012). Timing of alveolar bone grafting determines different outcomes in patients with unilateral cleft palate. *Journal of Craniofacial Surgery, 23,* 1283–1286.

Ulkur, E., Karagoz, H., Uygur, F., Celikoz, B., Cincik, H., Mutlu, H., . . . Ciyiltepe, M. (2008). Use of porous polyethylene implant for augmentation of the posterior pharynx in young adult patients with borderline velopharyngeal insufficiency. *Journal of Craniofacial Surgery, 19,* 573–579.

van Staden, F., & Gerhardt, C. (1995). Mothers of children with facial cleft deformities: Reactions and effects. *South American Journal of Psychology, 25*(1), 39–46.

Vargervik, K., Oberoi, S., & Hoffman, W. Y. (2009). Team care for the patient with cleft: UCSF protocols and outcomes. *Journal of Craniofacial Surgery, 20,* 1668–1671.

Wehby, G. L., Felix, T. M., Goco, N., Richieri-Costa, A., Chakraborty, H., Souza, J., . . . Murray, J. (2013). High dosage folic acid supplementation, oral cleft recurrence and fetal growth. *International Journal of Environmental Research and Public Health, 10,* 590–605.

Wolford, L. M., Oelschlaeger, M., & Deal, R. (1989). Proplast as a pharyngeal wall implant to correct velopharyngeal insufficiency. *Cleft Palate Journal, 26,* 119–128.

Xu, X., Zheng, Q., Lu, D., Huang, N., Li, J., Li, S., . . . Shi, B. (2012). Timing of palate repair affecting growth in complete unilateral cleft lip and palate. *Journal of Cranio-Maxillofacial Surgery, 40,* 358–362.

PART III

Neurogenic Disorders

CHAPTER 6

Traumatic Brain Injury

Lisa Schoenbrodt

Chapter Objectives

Upon completing this chapter, the reader should be able to:

1. Identify and define terms relative to brain injury
2. List primary and secondary injuries resulting from traumatic brain injury
3. Identify factors affecting the outcome of traumatic brain injury
4. Describe characteristics associated with traumatic brain injury
5. Describe appropriate assessments and modifications to be used during evaluation
6. Provide intervention strategies that are important for communication
7. Describe educational strategies for integration into the classroom

Introduction

Traumatic brain injury (TBI) is a neurogenic disorder that is considered to be of relatively low incidence in the pediatric population. Even so, TBI is among the most frequent injuries and causes of "functional morbidity" in children and adoles-

cents (Vu, Babikian, & Asarnow, 2011). However, with recent changes in medical delivery and patients leaving acute care centers more quickly, children with TBI are returning to their schools and communities faster than in the past decade. As many as 29% of students identified with TBI in schools receive services for remediation (Arroyos-Jurado, Paulsen, Ehly, & Max, 2006). Children with TBI present with a unique variety of speech and language as well as cognitive and motoric issues. For this reason, speech-language pathologists (SLPs) and others working with communication disorders need to be aware of all aspects of the injury in order to provide effective assessment and treatment. This chapter discusses the organic etiologies of the disorder, definitions, and characteristics, as well as effective assessment and intervention techniques and implications for educational planning.

Traumatic brain injury is the primary cause of death and disability in children today. Although accidental dropping and physical abuse are the primary causes of TBI in infants, the major causes for toddlers are serious falls, vehicular accidents, pedestrian accidents, and physical abuse. In elementary school-age children, bicycle accidents and recreational sports injuries are the main cause of TBI. Finally, adolescents are the most prevalent age group to suffer a TBI, most commonly due to vehicular accidents, sports-related injuries, and assault (Centers for Disease Control and Prevention, 2011; NIH, 2011).

According to the Centers for Disease Prevention and Control (2011), approximately 1.7 million cases of TBI are reported in the United States annually. Of that group, 52,000 people die and 80,000 more leave the hospital with a disability secondary to a TBI. Today an estimated 5.3 million people live with disabilities caused by a TBI. The most recent statistics indicate that people over age 75 have the highest rate of TBI, followed closely by adolescents and finally toddlers. Males between the ages of birth and 4 have the highest reported rates of TBI-related emergency room visits, hospitalizations, and deaths combined (Centers for Disease Control and Prevention, 2011).

Epidemiological studies show that age and gender play an important role in predicting at-risk groups for TBI (Centers for Disease Control and Prevention, 2011). Boys are more likely than girls to sustain a TBI, and adolescents are at the highest risk for brain injury in the pediatric population followed by preschoolers. In addition, children who have sustained a previous head injury are more likely to sustain another one. Finally, on average, 2,685 children die annually from TBI, and more than 30,000 children per year will survive a TBI having lifelong deficits, consequences, and effects (Fowler & McCabe, 2011).

Terminology and Definitions Related to Brain Injury

It is important to understand the terms and definitions used to describe brain inju-

ries, and this section defines these terms as they relate to brain injury in children.

When the head is struck by an object or is abruptly stopped, the acceleration and deceleration can cause significant injury to the brain. Head injury typically refers to traumatic damage to the head that may fracture the bones of the skull or face and may or may not include injury to the brain. Traumatic brain injury is defined by the Brain Injury Association and is included in the 1990 reauthorization of PL 94-142, now PL 101-476, the Individuals with Disabilities Education Act (IDEA). According to the Individuals with Disabilities Act (2002), TBI is defined as an acquired brain injury caused by an external physical force, resulting in total or partial functional disability, or psychosocial impairment, or both, which adversely affects a child's educational performance. The term applies to open or closed head injuries resulting in impairments in one or more areas, including cognition; language; memory; attention; reasoning; abstract thinking; problem solving; sensory, perceptual, and motor abilities; psychosocial behavior; physical functions; information processing; and speech. The term does not apply to congenital or degenerative brain injuries induced by birth trauma.

Further definitions by the Center for Disease Control (2011) and National Institutes of Health (2011) further expand this definition to include indicators for severity (mild, moderate, severe). The severity is based upon the extent of the trauma to the brain. Mild symptoms include those that are consistent with concussion such as headache, confusion, dizziness, fatigue, trouble with thinking, attention, or behavior changes accompanied by brief or no loss of consciousness. Moderate or severe TBI is defined as above but also including loss of consciousness, seizures, motor weakness, confusion, and significant headache. The CDC reports that the majority of the cases of TBI reported each year are forms of mild TBI.

Head injuries occur primarily in two forms: closed head injury and open head injury. A closed head injury (CHI) is one where there is no penetration or opening from the outside through the dura mater. In a closed head injury, the damage is more diffuse and due to increased intracranial pressure and edema. Damage can occur anywhere in the brain and may cause variable behavior and learning problems. In an open head injury (OHI), the skull is penetrated (e.g., a gunshot wound), and the damage is localized to the site of penetration. Typically, these injuries are from bullets or sharp objects, but can also be from a skull fracture originating from a laceration from significant blunt force (Porter & Kaplan, 2011).

The term traumatic brain injury indicates that there is evidence of brain involvement that is demonstrated by (a) an altered level of consciousness (lethargy, confusion, and coma) or (b) neurological signs, for example, localized weakness that indicates that the brain was injured (Christensen, 2001). The damage can be focal (confined to one area of the brain) or diffuse (involving more than one area of the brain) (NINDS).

Primary or Immediate Injuries

Primary injuries occur at the time of the trauma, and are due to the direct movement of the brain inside the skull. The movement results in the slamming and rubbing of the brain, which may cause contusions, or bruises. The location of the contusions depends on the site and the circumstances of the injury. For example, if the skull is hit with a blunt object, the contusion will be in the cortex at the point of contact. In addition, there may be another bruise on the opposite side of the brain, approximately 180 degrees from the initial bruise. These contusions are frequently referred to as coup (the French word for hit) and contrecoup (opposite the hit) contusions (Blumenstein, Patterson, & Delis, 1995; Fowler & McCabe, 2011; Porter & Kaplan, 2011). According to the Brain Injury Association (2011), injury occurs as a result of the unmoving brain being delayed in the movement of the skull, thus causing brain structures to tear.

A severe CHI involves greater speed and energy, and the head is often moving at the time of the injury. CHI contusions occur when the head is suddenly stopped but the brain keeps moving forward until it stops on impact, hitting the inside of the skull. The brain then collides with the bony protrusions around the frontal and possibly the temporal lobes, resulting in a more severe injury (Christensen, 2001).

Primary injury can also result from shearing and rotation of the axons, known as diffuse axonal injury (DAI), which occurs diffusely throughout the brain rather than in one localized area. DAI is often referred to as a shearing injury. The axons in the brain are particularly susceptible to the rotation of the brain at the time of injury. As the head and brain accelerate, these structures spin violently and then come to a quick stop. As a result, the brain twists on itself, stretching the axons so far as to physically pull them apart. The separation creates an immediate loss of neuron function followed by the death of that neuron (Blosser & DePompei, 2003; Jankowitz & Adelson, 2006; Kaufman & Dacey, 1994). DAI is common in acceleration injuries and may be responsible for many cognitive and behavioral impairments that occur following trauma (Brookshire, 2007).

Secondary or Delayed Injuries

Primary injuries cannot be modified, as they are the direct result of a traumatic incident. Secondary injuries, however, can be prevented or minimized during the acute treatment stage. Several types of secondary injuries may occur, including: (a) bleeding (hemorrhage), (b) herniation syndrome, and (c) edema or swelling.

Bleeding

Bleeding can occur over and within the brain tissue as a result of torn or disrupted vessels. Bleeding within the brain is referred to as an intracerebral hemorrhage; a bleed into the ventricles is known as an intraventricular hemorrhage (IVH); and bleeding into the spaces of the brain is referred to as (a) an epidural hematoma (between the skull and the dura), (b) a subdural hematoma (under the dura), or (c) a subarachnoid hemorrhage (under the arachnoid layer of the meninges and into the cerebrospinal fluid) (Brookshire, 2007; Bruce et al., 1979; Christensen, 2001; Jankowitz & Adelson, 2006; Kaufman & Dacey, 1994; Porter & Kaplan, 2011). The outcome of a bleed varies with respect to the amount of blood lost, how fast the blood accumulates, and the location of the bleeding. Because there is little "extra" space available in the skull, any additional blood that occupies space means that intracranial pressure may increase within that area or that more room may have to be made for excess blood. If the accumulation of blood or the hemorrhage occurs slowly, then the brain has time to adjust by either eliminating some of the cerebrospinal fluid or decreasing the amount of blood in the blood vessels. If

the blood loss or hemorrhage is rapid, the pressure on the brain increases; this is known as increased intracranial pressure (ICP). ICP can result in insufficient circulation of blood flow to the brain, causing further injury due to the lack of oxygen to the brain, otherwise known as hypoxic ischemic injury (Brookshire, 2007; Bruce et al., 1979; Christensen, 2001; Jankowitz & Adelson, 2006; Kaufman & Dacey, 1994; Porter & Kaplan, 2011).

Herniation Syndrome

A second type of delayed injury is herniation syndrome, which occurs if a localized mass or area of swelling pushes on and deforms the shape of the brain. When the brain attempts to squeeze itself into another area within the intracranial space, high pressure on that area of the brain and the surrounding blood vessels occurs. Herniation may result in further localized brain injury and stroke (Porter & Kaplan, 2011).

Edema

Edema, or swelling of the brain, is due to fluid leakage. Edema can cause increased ICP and can either be localized to the area of impact or diffuse. Swelling of the brain is more common in children than adults and may cause deficits similar to those caused by bleeding in the brain.

Severe cases of edema can be monitored through an intracranial pressure monitor that is surgically implanted inside the head. This monitor effectively records information about internal pressures, which allows the early detection of potential problems (Jankowitz & Adelson, 2006; Martin & Falcone, 2008). Both primary and secondary injuries are indicators of the degree of an injury's severity and of the variables related to the outcome of a TBI.

Severity of Injury

The severity of a brain injury is categorized as mild, moderate, or severe. The outcome of a TBI is predicted by several factors, including: (a) degree and length of coma, (b) findings on imaging, (c) duration of posttraumatic amnesia, (d) evaluation of the child's premorbid level of health, (e) preexisting learning or educational problems, and (f) amount of family support. Overall research has demonstrated that there are long-term deficits in children and adolescents who are severely injured, whereas children with mild to moderate injuries show greater recovery. Severity measures have also been shown to be a strong predictor of intellectual change 6 to 8 years following injury. Arroyos-Jurado et al. (2006) found that children who were diagnosed with mild to moderate TBI showed little change on performance on intelligence tests measure from initial injury to 6 to 8 years postinjury. The group diagnosed with severe TBI showed a significant decline in scores over time.

Degree and Length of Coma

The Glasgow Coma Scale (GCS) (Jennett & Teasdale, 1981) is commonly used in assessing degree and length of coma. The GCS measures eye opening, as well as motor and verbal responses, on a scale from 0 to 15 (Table 6–1). This scale is typically used in the hospital as a means of evaluating the degree and severity of the

Table 6–1. Glasgow Coma Scale

Eye Opening	
spontaneous	E4
to speech	3
to pain	2
nil	1
Best Motor Response	
obeys	M6
localizes	5
withdraws	4
abnormal flexion	3
extensor response	2
nil	1
Verbal Response	
oriented	V5
confused conversation	4
inappropriate words	3
incomprehensible sounds	2
nil	1
Coma Score (E + M + V) = 3 to 15	

Source: From Jennett, B., & Teasdale, G. (1981). *Management of head injuries* (p. 78). Philadelphia, PA: F.A. Davis Company. Reprinted with permission.

TBI. A mild head injury is defined as a GCS of 13 or better with either no loss of consciousness or loss of consciousness for less than 20 minutes. A moderate head injury is defined as a GCS of 8 to 12 with loss of consciousness for more than 20 minutes and an accompanying fracture with contusions. A severe head injury is defined as a GCS of 7 or less accompanied by intracranial hematoma, fracture with neurological deficit, bruising, or contusion of brain tissue. Although the GCS is often used, it is reported to be difficult to use with a pediatric population and therefore, often is not reported (Martin & Falcone, 2008). An alternate tool that may be used is the Relative Head Injury Severity Scale (Cuff et al., as cited in Martin & Falcone, 2008). This scale categorizes TBI as mild, moderate, and severe based on the presence or absence of injury, location of the injury or fracture, and length and duration of loss of consciousness. This scale was tested for reliability and validity and was highly correlated with the GCS, indicating it may be a viable alternative to use.

Coma is defined as a period of unresponsiveness or unconsciousness where the child is not aware and is unarousable. In general, patients do not respond to stimuli like pain and light and do not have sleep-wake cycles (NIH, 2011). In a rehabilitation setting, a coma is considered to have ended when the child begins to follow simple commands, which indicates that the child is able to have some interaction with the environment and correlates to long-term outcome (Christensen, 2001; Suskauer et al., 2011). Another classification system similar to GCS is the International Classification of Diseases, which categorizes TBI as (a) mild (less than 1 hour of coma with momentary or no loss of consciousness), (b) moderate (1–24 hours of coma), or (c) severe (24 or more hours of coma) (Keenan & Bratton, 2006).

Findings on Imaging

Imaging using computed tomography (CT) scans of the head have become another tool used in predicting severity and outcomes of TBI (Martin & Falcone, 2008). This type of imaging allows physicians to analyze structure and functions of the brain following injury. Specifically,

they can provide information on the type, location, severity of intracranial injuries, location of skull fractures, and other injuries (Jankowitz & Anderson, 2006; Martin & Falcone, 2008; Suskauer & Huisman, 2009). The use of CT scans, however, does lead to increased risk of radiation exposure, and so is not always routinely used. All that being said, research has shown that there is a strong correlation in outcome between findings on CT scans with scores on the Glasgow Coma Scale; they are considered a valuable tool in the diagnostic process (Claret et al., 2007). CT scans have been shown to be particularly effective in providing information in the acute setting, but are limited in evaluating the extent of injury particularly in diffuse axonal injury (DAI). Magnetic Resonance Imaging (MRI) has a higher sensitivity in identifying DAI (Suskauer & Huisman, 2009). MRIs are able to provide more detailed information on not only global outcome, but also neuropsychological and psychiatric outcomes. Ideally, both types of scans would be used.

Posttraumatic Amnesia

A second indicator for outcome is posttraumatic amnesia (PTA). PTA is defined as a period of amnesia or memory disturbance occurring after the trauma and is characterized by confusion, disorientation, and agitation. Children can recall many old memories that were in long-term storage prior to the accident; however, memory of new information is impaired, causing disorientation and confusion with regard to daily events (Dikman et al., 2009).

PTA provides a good indication of how severely memory and cognition will be affected over the long term. This fact is particularly true for children who experienced no coma or one of very short duration. PTA severity is classified as (a) mild—less than 1 hour, (b) moderate—1 to 24 hours of PTA, (c) severe—1 to 7 days of PTA, or (d) very severe—more than 7 days of PTA. PTA ends when the child can continuously lay down new memories (Brookshire, 2007; CDC, 2011; NIH, 2011).

Premorbid Level of Health

The child's premorbid level of health is also an indicator of outcome. This indicator references the status of the child's physical and mental health prior to the accident. Studies suggest that children who have had a previous TBI are more likely to sustain a second. In addition, children diagnosed with other health concerns such as attention deficit disorder or seizure disorder may have a less optimal outcome than children who have no history of health problems (Anderson & Catroppa, 2007; Arroyos-Jurado et al., 2006; Bazarian, Cernak, Noble-Haesslein, Potolicchio, & Temkin, 2009; Ylvisaker & DeBonis, 2000). In fact, the Brain Injury Association (2011) reports that after one injury, children are three times more susceptible to incurring another injury, and after a second injury, the chances for a third injury increase to eight.

Preexisting Learning or Behavioral Problems

Just as premorbid health can help predict the outcome of a TBI, so can any previously existing learning or educational deficits. Studies showed that children diagnosed with attention deficit disorder have a greater likelihood of incurring a TBI than their peers without attention

deficit disorder (ADHD). Slomine et al. (2005) reported that there are more problems in behavior and overall functioning in children who have TBI and ADHD. Persistent difficulties with memory and organization in children with ADHD were further exacerbated with a resulting TBI. Based on this information, it is critical that preexisting learning disabilities be considered when the child is formally assessed for educational placement following a TBI (Keenan & Bratton, 2006).

Amount of Family Support

Another area for consideration that is related to the above information is the amount of familial support that is available to the child following injury. Research shows that parent stress and adverse environmental factors in the home (such as low SES) can contribute to a poorer outcome (Taylor et al., 2008). Other findings point to the educational level of the mother as an indicator of success; those children with TBI whose mothers had a higher educational level were shown to have a better outcome (Gale & Prigatano, 2010). Another study points to these vulnerabilities in consideration of social outcomes following TBI, which point to persistent problems following injury (Yeates et al., 2004). Based on this information, this area is critical when considering assessment and intervention.

Age

One additional factor in evaluating outcome of TBI that is well worth mentioning is the age at the time of injury. One common myth about TBI holds that the younger the child at the time of injury, the better the outcome. In fact, the opposite is true. Children who sustain a TBI before age 9 display greater long-term cognitive deficits overall, including a reduction in intelligence scores and increased difficulties in reading. The reason for this outcome is again related to the brain: the immature skull is thinner and thus more easily damaged by trauma. The immature brain also has limited protective covering, and there is incomplete myelination of the neurons of the brain. Young children have a greater risk of increased intracranial pressure, diffuse swelling, and secondary brain injuries (Arroyos-Jurado et al., 2006; Chapman & McKinnon, 2000).

Another factor related to age is that the younger the child, the greater the likelihood of long-term cognitive impairment due to the lack of formal learning that has occurred. Preschool children have not experienced as much formal school learning as elementary school children; therefore, they do not have as much stored information simply because of their younger age. The pediatric TBI population is also unique in that there is the potential for delayed onset of deficits. Evidence suggests that children who sustained a TBI before age 2 could be at increased risk for the later onset of seizures (Lajiness, Erodi, & Bigler, 2010).

In addition, studies of children with moderate to severe injuries showed that those less than 6 years of age when acquiring an injury have greater deficits in executive control including working memory when compared to older children. Furthermore, research has shown that children with more severe injuries have growth curves that decline over time as opposed to showing continuous improvement. Children with mild injuries had growth curves that showed improvement over time (Keenan & Bratton, 2006).

Children injured during elementary school years, ages 6 to 12, have difficulty with new learning and will rely predominantly on memorization and rote learning of concepts, and fail to get the main idea or theme of what is being taught in school. In addition, deficits in memory will affect the way the child retains and stores information, which greatly impacts the ability to read and acquire underlying mathematical concepts (Brenner et al., 2007). Overall, although better survival rates have been reported in children as compared to adults with TBI, long-term consequences are typically more devastating due to age and the compromised developmental potential (Lajines-O'Neil, Erodi, & Bigler, 2010).

Neurological Deficits Secondary to TBI

Additional medical difficulties that occur after TBI include various types of neurological problems, such as postconcussion syndrome, headaches, seizures, and motor impairments.

Postconcussion Syndrome

Concussion is defined by the "Consensus Statement on Concussion in Sport" (McCrory et al., 2009) as a "complex pathophysiological process affecting the brain, induced by trauma biochemical forces" (p. i76). This statement further asserts that concussion may be caused by a "direct blow to the head, face, neck or elsewhere on the body with an impulsive force transmitted to the head. Concussion typically results in the rapid onset of short-lived impairment of neurological function that resolves spontaneously" (p. 176). Finally the report indicates that there may be no abnormal findings on imaging scans.

Gioia, Isquith, Schneider, and Vaughn (2009) reported that of the 1.5 cases of TBI reported, 90% of those were estimated to be due to concussion. A concussion may or may not include a brief loss of consciousness, and may be followed by a short period of change in mental status without any focal neurological signs, known as postconcussion syndrome (P-CS). In addition, there may be some signs of amnesia, confusion, poor coordination, and some difficulty with remembering information (Gioia, Isquith, Schneider, & Vaughn, 2009). Symptoms of this syndrome include: (a) headache, (b) fatigue, (c) memory loss (for new information), (d) depression, (e) impaired concentration, (f) increased sensitivity to sound, (g) emotional lability (frequently changing emotions), and (h) disinhibition (acting on inappropriate thoughts or actions) (Christensen, 2001; Gioia et al., 2009). Symptoms are generally worse directly after the injury. These symptoms may resolve spontaneously after weeks or months, though in a small percentage of children, some persist. It is extremely important that educators recognize these symptoms as indicators of P-CS syndrome and not as signs of laziness or a lack of motivation (Dikman et al., 2009; McCrea, 2008).

Headaches

Headaches occur more frequently following a mild TBI than after more severe injuries. There are many types of headaches that can occur following a TBI, including: (a) those related directly to the head trauma, (b) those related to tension, (c) head and neck pain resulting from whiplash, and (d) migraines that result from TBI. Tension headaches are frequently triggered by the stress and/or pressure related to the social and academic challenges faced upon return to the home and school community. Although not as intense as migraines, tension headaches still produce a dull ache and may interfere with day-to-day functioning. Migraines occur frequently in children and may be triggered or worsened by trauma. If such headaches cause significant impairment in functioning, appropriate medical intervention may be necessary (Dikman et al., 2009).

Seizures

Seizures occur when there is excessive or disorderly firing of the neurons, which leads to changes in neurological functioning and disruption in the normal functioning of the brain. The level of alertness, abnormal sensations, and unusual movements are indicators of this abrupt change in functioning. Early posttraumatic seizures (EPTS) are not uncommon and usually occur in the first 7 days following the trauma; with most occurring within the first twelve hours after injury (Liesemer, Bratton, Zebrack, Brockmeyer, & Statler, 2011). Late seizures (those occurring more than 1 week after the TBI) are more positively correlated with the chance of developing posttraumatic epilepsy—which is between 5% and 7%, particularly if the child has incurred a mild head injury. The chance of developing epilepsy increases to 11%, however, if the TBI is severe. Risk factors reported to coincide with developing posttraumatic seizures include focal injuries, such as hematoma (bleeding or the development of blood clots), wounds that involve the penetration of the dura, and factors such as prolonged coma or PTA (Bazarian et al., 2009; Chapman & McKinnon, 2000; Christensen, 2001; Liesemer et al., 2011).

A recent study by Liesemer et al. (2011) found that there was no significant difference in gender, ethnicity, or past medical history in evaluation of patients with or without early posttraumatic seizures. However, overall patients with early posttraumatic seizures were younger, with 53% being below the age of 2. The study further found that children with ETPS were more likely to have injuries secondary to nonaccidental trauma, specifically abuse.

Motor Impairment

As with seizures, a small percentage of children who sustain a TBI may develop long-term motor problems. Types of motor impairments that may occur include weakness; lack of ability to plan and control movements; abnormal muscle tone; inability to sit or stand or to maintain posture and balance; tremors; and lack of overall coordination.

A particularly important category of motor impairment includes any that affect the child's ability to swallow, which can impact nutrition. Morgan, Mageandran, and Mei (2009) reported that swallowing difficulties can include reduced lip closure, delayed swallow initiation, wet voice, and coughing. Swallowing difficulties are more common in severe TBI and may occur during both the oral and pharyngeal stages of swallowing. Dysphagia incidence following severe TBI was reported at 68%, 15% after moderate TBI, and 1% following mild TBI (Morgan, Ward, Murdroch, Kennedy, & Murison, 2003).

Morgan et al. (2009) found that overall there is a low incidence of dysphagia in the pediatric TBI population, but that the greatest proportion of problems occurs with those with more severe injuries. Although the authors do not recommend screening all children with TBI for swallowing impairments, they do suggest that during the inpatient phase severe cases should be referred to the speech-language pathologist for evaluation. Deficits that have been noted for evaluation included abnormal tongue reflexes, poor jaw stability, labored or impaired chewing, and reduced efficiency in preparing food for swallow (Morgan, Ward, & Murdroch, 2004). The oral phase involves moving food around in the mouth, chewing, preparing the food for swallowing, and gathering the food into a bolus. During the pharyngeal phase, muscles move the bolus from the mouth through the pharynx, past the larynx, and into the esophagus. The entire process requires fine motor coordination.

If the child exhibits difficulty with either of these phases, she or he may eat inefficiently or be unable to prepare the food properly for swallowing. Eating or drinking may become a slow, laborious, and sometimes life-threatening process. Choking may occur, and the possibility of aspiration pneumonia (infection or wheezing caused by passing too much food into the lungs) exists.

Characteristics of Children with Brain Injury

A TBI, even in its mildest form, can result in alterations in thinking and behavior. Cognitive changes produce the most disruption to the child and the family in their attempt to return to a typical life and are often more debilitating than disruptions in motor behavior. The following section offers greater detail regarding the characteristics or deficits of children following TBI, specifically in the areas of cognition, perceptual or sensory (visual) deficits, behavior, and communication (Schrief & Thomas, 2011).

Monitoring Cognitive Recovery

Problems in cognition can take a variety of forms. Overall general intellectual ability is assessed through the use of intelligence testing. A common assessment tool that is used for children is the Wechsler Intelligence Scale for Children-Fourth Edition (WISC-IV). Through a series of subtests, the assessment provides summative data resulting in index scores in the areas of Verbal Comprehension, Perceptual Reasoning, Working Memory, and Processing Speed (Donders & Janke, 2008). Although intelligence testing may give some "hard" data as to the level at which the child is functioning, one should employ caution in interpreting these data following a TBI.

The results from IQ testing only describe how the child is functioning at the time of testing. Change or variability in performance is one of the hallmarks of TBI, and can occur within the first year after the injury and beyond. In addition, IQ tests are standardized on children of the same age who have not sustained a TBI. Therefore, the examiner is cautioned that information may not be a reliable

predictor as to how children who have sustained a TBI will perform in the real world (Chesire, Buckley, & Canto, 2011). In general, studies evaluating the long-term effects on academic functioning found that poorer outcomes were related to decreased performance on neuropsychological measure (Ewing-Cobb et al., 2004). Donders and Janke (2008) evaluated the criterion validity of the WISC-IV following TBI. Their results found that of the four index scores, the processing speed index was the only one that had acceptable validity in evaluating children with mild to severe injuries and cautioned that additional measures should be used to supplement this assessment. In addition to deficits in overall general intelligence, TBIs can also result in problems in memory and new learning. Difficulties in these two areas, along with previously discussed variability of performance, are critical to understanding children with TBI (Arroyos-Jurado et al., 2006; Ewing-Cobb et al., 2004; Trudeau, Poulin-Dubois, & Joanette, 2000).

One recovery scale that measures cognitive functioning that may be used in conjunction with IQ testing is the Ranchos Los Amigos Scale of Cognitive Functioning (Hagan & Malkmus, 1979). This scale gives a general description of cognitive behaviors to be expected at each stage of recovery. It is important to note that patients in recovery may remain in one stage for a long period of time, be in more than one stage at a time, or move rapidly through all stages (Blosser & DePompei, 2003; Galvin, Fraude, & Imms, 2009). Malkmus revised the scale in 1982 to include cognitive-communicative descriptions for recovery levels (Table 6–2). This scale is more widely used for persons age 14 and over than for younger patients.

Table 6–2. Rancho Scale of Cognition and Language, Levels of Cognitive Functioning, and Associated Linguistic Behaviors

Level I. No Response	
General Behaviors	**Linguistic Behaviors**
Patient appears to be in a deep sleep and is completely unresponsive to any stimuli presented.	Receptive: No evidence of processing of linguistic input. Expressive: Absence of verbal and gestural expression.

Level II. Generalized Response	
General Behaviors	
Patient reacts inconsistently and nonpurposefully to stimuli in a nonspecific manner. Responses are limited in nature and are often the same regardless of stimulus presented. Responses may be physiological changes, gross body movements, and vocalization. Responses are likely to be delayed. The earlier response is to deep pain.	

Level III. Localized Response	
General Behaviors	**Linguistic Behaviors**
Patient reacts specifically but inconsistently to stimuli. Responses are directly related to the type of stimulus presented, as in turning head toward a sound or focusing on an object presented. The patient may withdraw an extremity and vocalize when presented with a painful stimulus. He or she may follow simple commands in an inconsistent, delayed manner, such as closing eyes, squeezing or extending an extremity. Once external stimuli are removed, the patient may lie quietly. He or she may also show a vague awareness of self and body by responding to discomfort such as pulling at the nasogastric tube or catheter or resisting restraints. He or she may show a bias toward responding to some persons, especially family and friends, but not to others.	As the patient progresses through this phase, linguistic behaviors emerge. Receptive: Progresses from localizing to processing, retaining and following simple commands that elicit automatic responses: inconsistent and delayed. May demonstrate limited graphic processing. Expressive: Emergence of automatic verbal and gestural responses. Negative head nods, requiring less head control, before positive. Single-word expressions or several words used as "holophrastic" responses. Expression is dependent on elicitation by an external stimulus.

Table 6–2. *continued*

Level IV. Confused-Agitated

General Behaviors

Patient is in a heightened state of activity with severely decreased ability to process information. He or she is detached from the present and responds primarily to his or her own internal confusion. Behavior is frequently bizarre and nonpurposeful relative to the immediate environment. He or she may cry out or scream out of proportion to stimuli even after removal, may show aggressive behavior, attempt to remove restraints or tube or crawl out of bed in a purposeful manner. He or she does not discriminate among persons nor objects and is unable to cooperate directly with treatment efforts. Verbalization is frequently incoherent or inappropriate to the environment. Confabulation may be present; patient may be hostile. Gross attention to environment is very brief and selective attention often nonexistent. Being unaware for present events, patient lacks short-term recall and may be reacting to past events. He or she is unable to perform self-care activities without maximum assistance. If not disabled physically, he or she may perform automatic motor activities such as sitting, reaching, and ambulating as part of the agitated state but not as a purposeful act nor on request, necessarily.

Linguistic Behaviors

Severe disruption of frontal-temporal lobes, and resultant confusion, becomes apparent.

Receptive: Marked disruption of integrity of auditory mechanism, with severe decreases in ability to maintain temporal order of phonemic events rate of processing and ability to attend to, retain, categorize, and associate information. Graphic processing is equally affected. Compounded by disinhibition and inability to inhibit response to internal stimuli.

Expressive: Marked disruption of phonological, semantic, syntactic, and suprasegmental features. Characterized by disinhibition, incoherence; bizarre and unrelated to environment. Frequently, literal, verbal and neologistic parphasias are present, with disturbance of logico-sequential features and incompleteness of expression. Prosodic features are disturbed secondary to inability to cognitively monitor and adjust rate, pitch, vocal intensity, and so forth.

Level V. Confused-Inappropriate

General Behaviors

Patient appears alert and is able to respond to simple commands fairly consistently. However, with increased complexity of commands or lack of any external structure, responses are nonpurposeful, random or, at best, fragmented toward any desired goal. He or she may show agitated behavior but not on an internal basis, as in Level IV; rather as a result of external stimuli and usually out of proportion to the stimulus.

Linguistic Behaviors

Marked by presence of linguistic fluctuations according to degree of external structure present and familiarity-predictability of linguistic events.

Receptive: Processing improved, with increased ability to retain temporal order of phonemic events, but persistence of semantic and syntactic confusions. Length of retained input is limited to phrases or short sentences.

continues

Table 6–2. *continued*

Level V. Confused-Inappropriate *continued*	
General Behaviors	**Linguistic Behaviors**
The patient has gross attention to the environment, is highly distractible and lacks ability to focus attention to a specific task without frequent redirection. With structure he or she may be able to converse on a social-automatic level for short periods of time. Verbalization is often inappropriate; confabulation may be triggered by present events. Memory is severely impaired, with confusion of past and present in reaction to ongoing activity. Patient lacks initiation of functional tasks and often shows inappropriate use of objects without external direction. He or she may be able to perform previously learned tasks when structured, but is unable to learn new information. He or she responds best to self, body, comfort and, often, family members. The patient usually can perform self-care activities with assistance and may accomplish feeding with supervision. Management on the unit is often a problem if the patient is physically mobile as he or she may wander off, either randomly or with vague intention of "going home."	Rate, accuracy and quality remain significantly reduced, with auditory processing better than graphic. Expressive: Disruption of phonological, semantic, syntactic and prosodic features persists. Characterized by disturbance of logico-sequential features: irrelevances, incompleteness, tangential circumlocutious and confabulatory expression. Decrease in literal paraphrasias: neologisms and/or verbal paraphasias persist. Length of utterance may be decreased or increased, depending on inhibition-disinhibition factors. Expressive responses are stimulus-bound. Word retrieval deficits become apparent, as characterized by delay, generalization, description, semantic association and/or circumlocution. Disruption of syntactic features evidence beyond concrete level of expression or with increase in length of output. Graphic expression is severely limited; gestural expression is limited and incomplete.

Level VI: Confused-Appropriate	
General Behaviors	**Linguistic Behaviors**
Patient shows goal-directed behavior, but is dependent on external input for direction. Response to discomfort is appropriate and he or she is able to tolerate unpleasant stimuli, for example, NG tube, when need is explained. He or she follows simple directions consistently and shows carryover for tasks learned; for example, self-care. He or she is at least supervised with old learning, unable to maximally assisted for new learning with little or no carry over. Responses may be incorrect due to memory problems but are appropriate to the situation.	Receptive: Processing remains delayed, with difficulty retaining, analyzing-synthesizing input: Processing of auditory input improves to compound sentence level; graphic stimuli processed at short sentence level. Self-monitoring capacity emerges. Expressive: Expression reflects internal confusion-disorganization, but is appropriate to situation or idea. Information retrieval and expression reflects significantly reduced new learning and displacement of temporal and situational contexts.

Table 6–2. *continued*

Level VI: Confused-Appropriate *continued*

General Behaviors

They may be delayed to immediate and he or she shows decreased ability to process information with little or no anticipation or prediction of events. Past memories show more depth and detail than recent memory. The patient may show beginning awareness of the situation by realizing he or she doesn't know an answer. He or she no longer wanders and is inconsistently oriented to time and place. Selective attention to tasks may be impaired, especially with difficult tasks and in unstructured settings, but is now functional for common daily activities. The patient may show vague recognition of some staff and has increased awareness of self, family, and basic needs.

Linguistic Behaviors

Social automatic expression is essentially intact; expression remains stimulus-bound. Tangential, irrelevant responses are diminished in familiar, predictable situations; re-emerge in open-ended communicative situations requiring referential language. Confabulatory responses and neologisms extinguish. Literal paraphasia persists only if specific apraxia is present. Word retrieval errors occur in referential language but seldom in confrontation naming. Length of utterance remains reduced unless marked disinhibition is present, resulting in inability to channel flow of ideas-expression. Limited graphic expression emerges. Gestural expression increases. Prosodic features reflect "voice of confusion": equal stress, monopitch and monoloudness.

Level VII. Automatic-Appropriate

General Behaviors

Patient appears appropriate and oriented within hospital and home settings, goes through daily routine automatically but robot-like, with minimal to absent confusion and has shallow recall for what he or she has been doing. He or she shows increased awareness of self, and other individuals. The patient has superficial awareness of but lacks insight into his or her condition; decreased judgment and problem solving; lacks realistic planning for the future. He or she shows carryover for new learning at a decreased rate. The patient requires at least minimal supervision for learning and safety purposes. He or she is independent in self-care activities and supervised in home and community skills for safety. With structure, he or she is able to initiate tasks or social and recreational activities in which there is now interest.

Linguistic Behaviors

Majority of linguistic behaviors appear "normal" within familiar, predictable, structured environments, but persistent deficits are apparent in open-ended communication and less structured settings.

Receptive: Difficulty processing linguistic stimuli of increasing length, and complexity particularly with competing stimuli. Retention improves to short paragraph level, but difficulty discerning salient features, organizing/integrating input, and absence of detail persists.

Expressive: Automatic level of language is apparent in referential communication, verbal reasoning; primarily self-oriented and concrete. Tangential expression and irrelevancies evidenced in abstract linguistic attempts. Word retrieval errors persist, with reduced frequency.

continues

Table 6–2. *continued*

Level VII. Automatic-Appropriate *continued*	
General Behaviors	**Linguistic Behaviors**
His or her judgment remains impaired. Prevocational evaluation and counseling may be indicated.	Length of utterance and gestural expression approximate normal. Graphic expression increases to short paragraphs; syntactic disorganization, simplistic, with irrelevancies. Prosodic features remain aberrant.
Level VIII. Purposeful-Appropriate	
General Behaviors	**Linguistic Behaviors**
Patient is alert and oriented, and is able to recall and integrate past and recent events and is aware of and responsive to his culture. He or she shows carryover for new learning if acceptable to him or her and his other life role and needs no supervision once activities are learned. Within his or her physical capabilities, the patient is independent in home and community, skills. Vocational rehabilitation, to determine ability to return as a contributor to society, perhaps in a new capacity, is indicated. He or she may continue to show decreases, relative to premorbid abilities in quality and rate of processing, abstract reasoning, tolerance for stress and judgment in emergencies or unusual circumstances. His social, emotional and intellectual capacities may continue to be at a decreased level for him, but functional within society	Language capacities may fall within normal limits. Otherwise, problems persist in competitive situations and in response to fatigue, stress and emotionality reducing effectiveness, efficiency and quality of performance.

Note. Adapted from Malkmus, D. (1982). *Cognition and language, models and techniques of cognitive rehabilitation.* Second Annual International Symposium, Indianapolis, Indiana.

A revision to this scale was made in 1998 by Hagen. The Expanded Rancho Levels of Cognitive Function adds two new levels to the original eight. The purpose of this addition was to provide better descriptive information of the later phases of recovery. Interestingly, the Rancho Los Amigos Center continues to use the earlier edition as there is currently no information on validity and reliability regarding the additional two levels. In addition, the center asserts that there may be confusion when some but not all of the descriptors are met at one level, and perhaps some at another, leaving the evaluator to make a subjective decision as to which level is most appropriate. They continue to note that at these later levels, other standardized assessments will provide more accurate information for rehabilitation (http://www.rancho.org, January 17, 2012).

While the Ranchos Los Amigos Cognitive Scale (RLAS) is most commonly used in describing cognitive function, there are other measures that can also be used at various points following TBI. The Cognitive and Linguistic Scale (CALS) (Slomine et al., 2008) was developed to assess recovery of cognitive and linguistic functioning in inpatient rehabilitation following TBI in children. This scale was developed to assess strengths and weaknesses in order to provide information for treatment and discharge. Members of an interdisciplinary team treating the child administer the scale. There are 20 items on this scale that assess: "arousal, responsivity, emotional regulation, inhibition, attention, response time, orientation, memory, simple and complex receptive language, simple and complex expressive language, initiation, pragmatics, simple and complex problem solving, visuoperceptual ability, visuospatial ability self-monitoring, and cognitive safety" (Slomine et al., 2008, p. 288). The authors conducted a study evaluating the psychometric properties of the scale and found that there was good reliability and validity for use of this tool with the target population of children with TBI. Results also showed that the CALS was better at providing information about even slight changes in functioning when compared to the Functional Independence Measure for Children (WeeFIM), which measures overall functional independence in children.

Another evaluation tool that measures the impact of health conditions with children is the Pediatric Quality of Life Inventory (PedsQL) (McCarthy et al., 2005). This tool looks at "health related quality of life in the core dimensions of physical, mental, and social health, as well as role (school) function" (p. 1901). This tool is specifically developed for use with children and is easily administered. The PedsQL has been shown to have good reliability and validity in measuring health among children having a TBI.

The Pediatric Test of Brain Injury (Hotz, Helm-Estabrooks, Nelson, & Plante, 2009) was developed to assess skills related to academic performance at multiple points in the rehabilitation process. It can be used in the acute phases of recovery to give overall prognostic indicators, but also in latter stages to provide information critical for transition to the academic setting. This instrument is also designed for use with children ages 6 to 16 years of age and assesses memory, language, literacy, and processing, and is considered a standardized criterion referenced test. The PTBI has been shown to be effective in documenting changes during recovery, and in providing specific recommendations for curriculum-based language assessment and intervention.

Yet another battery that should be mentioned is the Pediatric Concussion Battery, which includes several symptom scales including: the Acute Concussion Evaluation (Gioia et al., 2009), and the Post-Concussion Symptom Inventory, and the Pediatric Immediate Post-Concussion Assessment and Cognitive Testing (ImPACT) (Lovell, Collins, & Maroon, 2002). These instruments were specifically designed for individuals with concussion. Because mild TBI is most commonly "unseen" or "silent" due to the fact that oftentimes there is no admission to a hospital, these tools are essential in providing information about cognitive deficits that may be subtle and would otherwise go undocumented (Howard & Shapiro, 2011).

Memory

Whereas TBI in school age children is associated with overall cognitive impairments, measures of memory and attention are particularly pronounced (Taylor et al., 2008).

Learning of any kind, particularly academic learning, involves memory, which is thus an important indicator of learning ability. Although TBI often disrupts memory of new information, memory of old information (information that is well learned) is preserved even following a severe TBI. This preservation of old information can be misleading when testing prior to the child's return to school. Academic, speech and language, and intelligence testing may show scores that indicate that the child has lost few academic skills following the TBI. For the "novice" in TBI, one might assume that the child can go back to the same classroom and return to "normal." In fact, the assessments have tapped into the child's old memory of overlearned material. These assessments do not always evaluate new learning, which needs to be assessed before a child returns to the classroom setting.

New learning is the result of information stored in short-term memory, which is not permanent. Short-term memory lasts for a few seconds at a time but can be extended with continuous rehearsal of information. Short-term memory can be disrupted if any distraction occurs before the information is transferred into long-term memory for permanent storage. Short-term memory can be very unstable following TBI. In the school setting, memory deficits can be manifest as difficulty with recalling events from earlier in the day or previous days. The child may not complete assignments simply because he or she did not remember, not because he

or she is showing noncompliant behavior. Difficulty retrieving information in an organized manner may also be symptomatic of a memory deficit. In this situation, the child may need information repeated again and again in order to store it in short-term memory (Boudreau & Smith, 2011).

While short-term memory is important in language learning and use, both long-term and working memory play an important role as well. Long-term memory is that which serves as long-term storage for information and must "be brought to a conscious level in order to complete a given task" (Boudreau & Smith, 2011, p. 153). Long-term memory is important for learning and retaining new information.

More recent research focuses on working memory, particularly in relation to higher-level language and cognitive skills. Working memory allows a finite amount of information to be stored temporarily during processing (Montgomery, Magimairj, & Finney, 2010). Boudreau and Smith (2011) give examples of working memory as acting on multistep directions that "build" on each other, or by following the events of several themes or characters in a story, or writing verbatim information that was heard as in note-taking. In each instance, information must be held while the direction is complete. The aforementioned is a model that was developed by Baddeley (1990) and states that working memory has two systems that include a phonological buffer that involves rehearsal of information until it is stored, as well as a short-term storage unit that processes the phonological information. If there is a break in the system and the demands are too great, difficulties in processing and storage will occur.

Children with language impairments have been documented to have deficits in working memory, particularly in processing information. These problems are related not only to processing issues in general, but also to difficulty in executive functions and inhibition (Isaki, Spaulding, & Plante, 2008; Mandalis, Kinsella, Ong, & Anderson, 2007). As a result, it is important for clinicians to assess working memory specifically during the evaluation process (Lajiness-O'Neil, Erodi, & Bigler, 2010).

Attention

Attention problems are another persistent symptom following TBI. Attention is a prerequisite to all other cognitive activity. In order for someone to perceive, remember, or manipulate information, one must attend to it on some level. Location and different types of brain injury may result in different attention problems. The most basic of these dysfunctions is coma, which results from injury to the brain stem. Injury to the sensory input unit (the temporal, parietal, and/or occipital lobes) may manifest as omissions and/or errors in processing and integrating incoming signals (Galvin et al., 2009). Difficulty managing, allocating, and directing attention in a purposeful, productive manner results from an injury to the frontal lobe (Brady, 2001; Catroppa & Anderson, 2005). Specific types of attention include sustained, selective, alternating, and divided attention.

Sustained Attention

Sustained attention, often referred to as attention span or concentration, involves the ability to respond consistently for the amount of time needed to complete a task. The length of time of response and consistency of response to be maintained over time are important aspects of sustained attention. Problems with sustained attention appear more often in the early stages of recovery. Children have difficulties with previously nondemanding tasks, such as watching a television program (Brady, 2001).

Selective Attention

Selective attention involves the ability to focus on "relevant stimuli in the presence of a distraction—and is often referred to as freedom from distractibility" (Brady, 2001, p. 153). Deficits can result in difficulty focusing attention and filtering out distractions. After sustaining a TBI, the child may not follow instructions in class or pay attention to the lesson because he or she is unable to filter out distractions, whether in the surrounding environment or internal feelings or thoughts. Problems in selective attention can cause numerous difficulties for a child in a "normal" environment with many competing noises (Catroppa & Anderson, 2005).

Alternating or Shifting Attention

A difficulty with alternating attention means the child encounters problems when shifting focus from one task to another. Children with TBI may have difficulty transitioning from one activity or task to the next, for example, moving from topic to topic in a conversation or even going from class to class. If teachers give advance warning of a change in events or specific directions for beginning a new task, the child may have better success in alternating attention. Problems in alternating attention may not always be apparent in younger children with TBI because alternating attention involves cognitive processes that are more complex and may not be evident until children begin school.

Divided Attention

Children with divided attention deficits exhibit difficulties in attending to many tasks or multiple components of a task. Examples of behavior requiring divided attention include the ability to talk on the phone while typing on the computer, or more typically, doing homework while watching television. This type of attention is not generally seen in younger children with TBI and may appear later as a residual effect of the TBI (Anderson & Catroppa, 2007; Brady, 2001; Catroppa & Anderson, 2005; Savage & Wolcott, 1999).

Memory and attention problems may be "invisible" because they are not as obvious as other physical or behavioral issues, and may not be detected as quickly. However, both are critical in the functioning of the student returning to the classroom. These deficits may confuse teachers and caregivers leading to unrealistic expectations or a misinterpretation of laziness (Schrieff, Donald, & Thomas, 2011).

Executive Functioning

Executive function involves a cluster of cognitive processes necessary for organized, goal-directed behavior. Executive functioning involves the ability to think about and plan responses. Executive function deficits are very common following TBI and can involve any of the following (Ciccia, Meulenbrook, & Turkstra, 2009; DePompei, 2010; Solmine et al., 2002;

Schrieff, Donald, & Thomas, 2011; Ylvisaker, Turkstra, & Coelho, 2005; Ylvisaker & DeBonis, 2000):

- Difficulty setting goals
- Difficulty planning tasks
- Difficulty in self-monitoring
- Difficulty in self-evaluation
- Inability to evaluate individual strengths and needs realistically
- Problems in initiation
- Difficulty controlling and suppressing behavior

The responses of the executive system are related to deficits in the area of the frontal lobes. Because a TBI almost always affects the frontal lobes, deficits in executive functioning are expected. One executive function that is controlled by the frontal lobes is inhibition, which involves the ability to control or suppress impulsive, automatic responses to a stimulus, whether external, such as a comment or gesture from a person, or internal, such as feelings of fear or aggression. For example, a child who is teased has the ability to inhibit the initial response of reacting to the teasing, by thinking of the various consequences of his or her actions before reacting. The child with TBI may have deficits in executive functioning, and may not be able to inhibit the initial response, thus facing far greater consequences of his or her actions.

Impaired planning ability, another deficit, also has an impact on post-TBI functioning. Symptoms of impaired planning vary and range from solving problems in an unrealistic manner to difficulty with organization of steps in order to perform a task to perseveration on a thought or activity. The child may encounter difficulty in self-evaluation of a task. It is also possible that the child may have difficulty performing the task because she or he cannot interpret abstract language and may be too literal in comprehension. Problems in handling abstraction and poor judgment are also implicated in the executive system following TBI.

Impaired abstraction means the child is unable to generalize thinking to other situations, a behavior often referred to as "stimulus-bound," because the brain recognizes and reacts to the actual objects in that particular environment. More subtle difficulties may include the inability to differentiate between variations in facial expression. The child may misinterpret a facial expression of someone who is showing concern, reading the expression as anger or disappointment instead. These abstraction difficulties also affect the ability to comprehend and interpret abstract language. The child with TBI has difficulty interpreting abstract language such as idioms and metaphors, therefore making it more difficult for the child to continue to "fit in" and not look awkward with peers. Poor judgment is another characteristic that is frequently evident following TBI. The child may be unaware of his or her problems, or may deny having difficulties (Ciccia et al., 2009). Children may have social cognition deficits in recognizing emotions and have impaired Theory of Mind. Theory of Mind, as defined by Premack & Woodruff (1978) (as cited in Ciccia et al., 2009) involves the ability to make inferences about the emotions of others and then to act upon that information. Decision- making often is impaired and may cause safety issues at both home and school. For example, a child who was typically capable of preparing an afternoon snack, like popcorn in the microwave, may forget to put the popcorn in the microwave and turn it on anyway, thus causing danger to himself or her-

self and damaging the appliance as well. Performance monitoring is related to this area. Deficits in monitoring may involve the child making an error and not being concerned about the consequence of that error. This behavior can lead to problems with goal setting (Ornstein et al., 2009).

The final aspect of the executive system to be discussed is initiation and goal setting behavior, the lack of which is underscore. Deficits in this area need to be monitored as they may require intervention well into adulthood (Beachamp et al., 2011). Many times following TBI, children appear unmotivated or disengaged and teachers may categorize them as lazy or as exhibiting behavior problems. Such children require continual prompting in order to get up and get dressed, start assignments in school, and engage in or initiate conversation (Schrief, Donald, & Thomas, 2011; Sesma, Slomine, Ding, & McCarthy, 2008; Slomine et al., 2002). It is important to emphasize to teachers and caregivers that the behaviors that result from a lack of initiation are organically and not behaviorally based.

Perceptual and/or Sensory Deficits

Sensory processing refers to the child's ability to receive, integrate, and respond to information from the environment (Galvin et al., 2009). The ability to adapt and respond to sensory information is critical in the development of cognitive and social skills. Sight, sound, touch, taste, and smell can be lost or damaged following a TBI. The child may become more sensitive to touch or be unable to see objects in a different part of the visual field. The child may encounter difficulty perceiving spatial orientation of objects, or difficulty with depth perception. The child with TBI may also have problems scanning and visually searching information in an organized way, which can affect reading comprehension.

Visual processing is particularly critical to self-care, work, play, and school academics. The visual system is widely distributed throughout the brain; therefore, disruptions of the visual system are not uncommon following a TBI, although they may not be immediately apparent. When damage to the visual system involves cranial nerve dysfunction (from swelling and bleeding, or other sources of pressure), numerous problems can occur, including:

- Ptosis: the drooping of the eyelid
- Dilation of the pupil: the inability of the pupil to get smaller in response to light
- Strabismus: a condition in which both eyes cannot focus on the same point due to the fact that one eye deviates upward, outward, and/or inward, resulting in double vision
- Inability of both eyes to focus on the side opposite the injury, resulting in a fixed gaze to one side or the other

Most of these problems will resolve as the swelling subsides. Other less transitory deficits include visual-perceptual problems.

Visual-Perceptual Problems

If damage occurs to the right side of the brain, unilateral visual neglect, which refers to inattention to or failure to respond to anything that is in the opposite field of view, may occur. Neglect is a failure of attention due to loss of spatial awareness and may occur even though the child has intact vision. Children experiencing neglect are not aware that they are not attending to that part of the environment. The problems may be subtle, in that the child may start in the middle of the page when writing, may not return to the left margin when reading, or may complete only the right half of the page of a worksheet. Most forms of neglect improve over time; however, some of the more subtle signs may persist but can be compensated for through various techniques, such as placing items in a vertical rather than horizontal array.

Another type of visual-perceptual problem involves deficits in interpreting spatial information. Many activities, particularly in the classroom, rely on the interpretation of spatial information. Following directions, for example, involves the interpretation of words with visual-spatial meanings. Words such as "over," "under," "behind," and "inside," may become confusing, particularly to a child who is hearing instructions from the teacher in the classroom. In this case, the child, who may be overwhelmed by too many pictures and displays on the walls and overly stimulated by the amount of noise in the classroom, will experience difficulty following a spoken direction like, "Take out your book, put it on top of your desk, put your paper inside your book, and put your pencil beside the book." By the time the child processes this information, the class has already moved on to another activity. The child with TBI may also experience difficulty manipulating graphs, charts, and other visual displays in the classroom. Processing problems may even make it difficult for the child to locate the classroom or her or his house. Reading a map and telling time may also be skills that are impaired as these tasks require the comprehension and manipulation of space. Problems interpreting spatial information also have an effect on visual-motor integration, or the ability to convert information received through the eyes mentally into a plan for motor output (Galvin et al., 2009).

Visual-motor integration is important in moving the body through visual space, such as walking, but is also important in activities such as copying, writing, and drawing. Difficulties with visual-motor integration can certainly impair motor speed and motor planning, both important skills for functioning in school. Deficits in physical capabilities and cognition, as well as the organic nature of some neurological insult, may lead to behavior problems.

Behavior

The interpretation and control of feelings involves cognitive abilities and emotional regulation. Many behavioral manifestations may occur following TBI, including:

- Impulsivity
- Disinhibition
- Poor judgment
- Dependency
- Aggression
- Apathy or indifference
- Lack of goal direction
- Depression
- Emotional lability
- Social withdrawal
- Denial

Behaviors such as agitation, frustration, impulsivity, depression, and disinhibition are the most common. An individual's ability to cope with these problems depends upon both the extent of neurological damage and the presence of any premorbid psychological conditions, such as moodiness or depression (Fowler & McCabe, 2011).

Survivors of brain injury often experience frustration during the rehabilitation process for a variety of reasons. They may be unable to perform tasks that were easy prior to the trauma, or they do not understand the words and actions of others, or they are disoriented in their surroundings and thus do not understand where they are or why. All these feelings of confusion or frustration may cause children to become verbally and physically aggressive to those around them. This agitation is not directed toward any one person, which is difficult for most family members to understand. The behaviors displayed are simply a way of coping with all the difficulties and demands that they are experiencing.

When the brain is injured, the child may lose the ability to monitor behavior in a socially acceptable way. The child may be uninhibited or impulsive, and may act out of character. Adolescents may act inappropriately on sexual impulses. Others may demonstrate social immaturity by making inappropriate comments and noises. This type of behavior can be very embarrassing for family members.

Going out to dinner in a restaurant may end in extreme frustration and embarrassment when the child with TBI curses loudly at the table and makes burping noises throughout dinner. Coping with this problem not only requires a great deal of patience from teachers and family members, but also prompting and cueing in order to help the child regulate her or his behavior. This impaired self-awareness can also have a negative impact on rehabilitation efforts because the child may not perceive there are any problems and resist treatment for remediation. Research has shown that following TBI, patients rated themselves as significantly more competent than did therapists in social and emotional function, activities of daily living, and on cognitive tasks (Hart, Sherer, Whyte, Polansky, & Novack, 2004).

Perhaps due to the impaired self-awareness, children may appear self-centered and demanding. Oftentimes, friends and family members may withdraw from them, which complicates issues of self-esteem, a loss of which is common in children with brain injuries. Children may see themselves as defective following the injury. For example, the straight A high school athlete who was counting on a scholarship to a top-notch university must face the fact that not only may he be unable to play sports again, but he may not be able to handle his course load any longer and may not be going to the school of his dreams. This loss often seems insurmountable and these feelings can result in depression and thoughts of suicide. In addition, studies support that family environment and injury severity are critical in predicting outcome in this area (Lajiness-O'Neil, Erdodi, & Bigler, 2010; Schrieff, Donald, & Thomas, 2011).

Communication

Children who have sustained a TBI can face many problems with communication—the giving and receiving of information. These difficulties may be only temporary and improve over time, but can be permanent. Communication problems often persist for years, depending on the severity of the TBI. Communication involves listening, speaking, reading, and writing to express ideas (DePompei, 2010; Savage,

DePompei, Tyler, & Lash, 2005; Sullivan & Riccio, 2010).

Expressive Speech Problems

Effective speech requires coordination of structures involved in phonation and articulation. A brain injury may affect these areas. Overall, however, speech problems are less common than language problems in children with TBI (Blosser & DePompei, 2003; DePompei, 2010).

Following TBI, children may experience dysarthric or dysfluent speech in the initial phases of recovery. Dysarthric speech is slow and labored, sometimes accompanied by imprecise articulation. Dysfluent speech, otherwise known as stuttering, is characterized by repetition of sounds, syllables, words, or phrases, which impairs the overall flow of speech. Both conditions make intelligibility of speech difficult. Other speech problems that can result from a brain injury include:

■ Speech sound production difficulties: include dysarthria, apraxia, or dyspraxia. In apraxia, a child is unable to plan and execute the movements necessary to produce sounds or words. A study by Morgan et al. (2009) found that children with severe TBI exhibited speech deficits in respiration, phonation, resonance, articulation, and prosody. They further reported that these characteristics were pronounced in the acute phase of recovery, and that these symptoms more often than not, resolved on their own. Their results showed that of the incidence of children with severe injury was estimated at 20%, which is relatively low, indicating that there is not a need for screening of all cases referred in the acute phase of rehabilitation.

- Vocal problems: include problems with resonance involving the way in which the air vibrates within the oral and nasal cavities, which can result in a child's voice sounding too nasal. Problems with voice quality can result in a hoarse, breathy, or other atypical voice quality (Vitorino, 2009).

Language Problems

Language problems are more common than speech problems in children with TBI. These problems can range from mild to severe and may be temporary or permanent. One reason that children with TBI have language problems is that language abilities are closely linked to cognitive functions. In particular, language abilities involve the use of words and sentences to convey ideas (DePompei, 2010; Savage et al., 2005). In the area of language, receptive, expressive, or pragmatic areas may be affected. Two more recent areas to be researched include discourse and literacy (Sullivan & Ricciom, 2010). Receptive language deficits may include: problems with comprehension of vocabulary (particularly figurative language including words with multiple meanings), difficulty with reading comprehension, problems with recall of information, and problems following directions or restating what directions (Lewis & Murdoch, 2011; Savage et al., 2005; Vu et al., 2011).

Expressive language abilities affected may include: difficulty acquiring new vocabulary (particularly that which is abstract, including figurative language), tangential speech (talking about unrelated topics), problems composing written sentences, word retrieval deficits (not using the exact name of the desired "thing"), and problems with spelling.

Pragmatic language or the use of language to engage in social exchanges or the ability to be able to express intent may also be impaired. Deficits include: problems with initiation, turn taking, maintaining, and terminating conversations, using socially inappropriate words, inability to understand proxemics, or facial expressions.

Conversational skills are part of the subset of pragmatic skills, involving the social use of language. Again, depending on the severity of the injury, children will display a variety of pragmatic problems, conversational skills and friendship-making skills being two of the more obvious problem areas. Pragmatic skill deficiencies can overlap with behavioral problems such as disinhibition. As stated earlier, post-TBI children frequently have difficulty "turning on and off" inappropriate comments and gestures due to the injury. Though the child is doing his or her best to fit in, inappropriate comments may be incorporated into language use, thereby alienating friends. This cycle can spin out of control, leading to depression and other problems. Equally as frustrating is the child who has difficulty expressing basic wants and needs, due to deficits in speech production or in the ability to use language. This child may need a communication board or a communication device in order to better express her or himself (Schoenbrodt, 2001).

In addition, children may have many difficulties with conversational speech. Their conversations may be tangential, meaning that they talk around the topic and switch topics frequently, leaving fragments or tangents of unfinished conversation. Conversational speech may also be characterized by irrelevant information, and often is confabulatory, or made up (the information provided is not real or true). Although conversational skills will improve, many of the above characteristics may continue and much cueing and prompting may be necessary for the child to become an effective communicator.

Another area in communication that may be compromised is discourse processing. Discourse processing has been assessed more recently in the pediatric population with TBI. These processes rely on underlying skills needed to be effective in communicating using context clues in the environment. Much research in this area has shown that children with TBI have difficulty: getting the main idea of stories, summarizing the "gist" of the story, interpreting figurative language such as idioms and metaphors, and interpreting humor (Chapman et al., 2005; Ewing-Cobbs & Barnes, 2002; Hay & Moran, 2005).

The final characteristic in this area to be introduced is reading. Research indicates that the younger the child is at time of injury, the more impaired reading skills, such as word decoding, may be. The critical piece is the timing of the injury. If children are injured when literacy skills are developing, the outcome for development is worse. Studies have shown that, in general, children with TBI have deficits in decoding, processing speed, and comprehension (Ewing-Cobbs & Barnes, 2002; Hanten et al., 2004; Sullivan & Riccio, 2011).

Cognitive-Communication

Cognitive communication involves the ability to use language and other skills such as the following:

- Attention
- Memory

- Conceptual organization
- Speed of processing
- Analysis and synthesis of environmental cues and conversation (DePompei, 2010; Savage et al., 2005)

Gamino, Chapman, and Cook (2009) found that adolescents with TBI experience greater problems in teenage years. They noted that adolescents have "impaired strategic learning," which involves the ability to organize and condense information from text, conversation, and so forth, to get the main idea. This type of learning is positively correlated with executive control and academic success because it involves the organization and synthesis of information to generalize to other areas. The results of their study showed that there is a "stall" in these skills, which can occur years after the initial occurrence of the TBI, indicating that children need to be followed throughout their academic careers for possible residual effects of the TBI (Beachamp et al., 2011; De Pompei, 2010).

The combination of all of the characteristics of TBI—physical, emotional, cognitive, communication, and sensory—and the variability of the severity of the injury create a need for continuous evaluation and reevaluation of deficit areas. Individuals providing assessment need to be knowledgeable about the sequelae that result from the injury.

Assessment

Every child with TBI is unique. Cognitive, psychomotor, and psychosocial profiles are unpredictable and cannot be generalized from one child to the next. Variability is one of the hallmarks of TBI and can be seen throughout all stages of recovery. This is the reason why continuous evaluation is critical. When conducting assessments, the evaluator must keep in mind the child's premorbid level of functioning as a mechanism for comparison in determining educational placement and the level of support services needed (Schoenbrodt, 2001; Schoenbrodt & Smith, 1995; Sullivan & Riccio, 2010).

An interdisciplinary or team approach to evaluation and coordination of services is important for many reasons:

1. If each specialist and each classroom teacher evaluates and develops goals and objectives independently, a fragmented program may evolve that can cause even more confusion for the child.
2. If each evaluator operates independently, valuable crossover of goals, objectives, and ideas for intervention is lost, decreasing the chances of generalization of skills to all environments.
3. Although each evaluator is responsible for his or her area of expertise (e.g., the speech-language pathologist administers speech and language testing), the team of evaluators decides which assessments should be administered based on the child's individual profile. If evaluators operate independently, skills testing may overlap, artificially increasing the time needed to evaluate the child fully and increasing the risk that the results will be skewed by fatigue (to be discussed later).

Research supports the fact that severe TBI in early childhood can have long-lasting effects in cognitive impairment and academic skills. This means that these children with TBI can show new deficits later on that may be due to increasing cognitive demands in the environment (Hay & Moran, 2005). For example, as children progress into adolescence, the need to understand and use figurative language in a variety of settings increases. This "new" demand may be indicative of a deficit in this area that was not visible in earlier years because the skills were not required in earlier. Given that language development continues into adolescence, it would seem logical that children with TBI would likely exhibit deficits in these areas. In fact, the opposite has been shown to be true. Studies show that memory, spatial relations, and executive functions may be more impacted than general speech and language skills (Taylor et al., 2008). Only children who suffered severe TBI had persistent problems across language areas (Hay & Moran, 2005). One reason for this discrepancy goes back to earlier statements about variability of performance and the fact that many children will not "show" deficits in scores on standardized tests. For this reason, it is important to utilize both standardized and nonstandardized measures.

Speech and Language Evaluation

Two types of speech and language assessments should be used when evaluating a child with TBI: formal (or standardized) assessments and informal (or naturalistic) assessments. Standardized testing is necessary to document comparable scores and to establish eligibility for educational and support services. Because few formalized assessments have been normed on children with TBI, clinicians should combine formal assessments with careful observation of language and communication in a variety of settings and contexts (Sullivan & Riccio, 2010; Ylvisaker, Urbanczyk, & Feeney, 1992). A comprehensive, interdisciplinary formal assessment battery should evaluate functioning in the following areas: intellectual, executive function, problem solving, attention, concentration, memory, speech, language, perceptual-motor, and academic abilities (Chesire et al., 2011). In a speech and language battery, tests should specifically sample behaviors in:

- Language (syntax, semantics, pragmatics)
- Speech (articulation, fluency, voice quality)
- Word finding
- Memory
- Discourse
- Written language
- Reading

When considering assessment and intervention, clinicians should "consider existing functions that are affected by the injury as well as the functions that are dependent on the development of injured regions in the future" (Sohlberg & Mateer, 2001, p. 261).

There are many standardized assessments that can be used to tap into language areas at different levels. A comprehensive language evaluation that evaluates all areas such as the Clinical Evaluation of Language Fundamentals (CELF-5; Semel, Wiig, & Secord, 2013) and the Comprehensive Assessment of Spoken Language (CASL, 1999) can be used. To assess receptive vocabulary, the Peabody Picture Vocabulary Test-Fourth Edition (PPVT-4; Dunn & Dunn, 2007) can be used. In evaluating expressive vocabulary, the Expres-

sive Vocabulary Test-EVT-2 (Williams, 2007), or the Expressive One Word Picture Vocabulary Test (EOWPVT; Gardner, 2000) can be used. The Test of Language Competence Expanded edition (TLC-E; Wiig & Secord, 1989) is valuable in assessing figurative language such as metaphors and idioms. In measuring memory, the subtests of the CELF-5 assess functional working memory, and the Comprehensive Test of Phonological Processing (CTOPP; Wagner, Torgesen, & Rashotte, 1999) measures working memory as well as phonological working or short-term memory (Boudreau & Costanza-Smith, 2011). Assessment of pragmatic skills includes discourse processes and social communication skills. These skills can be assessed using The Test of Pragmatic Language (TOPL-2; Phelps-Terasaki & Phelps-Gunn, 2007) and the Test of Narrative Language (TNL, 2004). According to Sullivan and Riccio (2011) reading and writing can be assessed through the Woodcock-Johnson III Tests of Achievement (Woodcock, McGrew, & Mather, 2001).

During the evaluation, the examiner should document the occurrence of any of the following characteristics:

- Level of attention
- Tolerance of stress (time constraints, noise, frustration)
- Degree of cueing and prompting necessary
- Use of compensatory strategies
- Processing time
- Delayed response or slowed performance
- Anxiety
- Fear of failure
- Fatigue

If any of the above characteristics are noted, modifications may be necessary during the testing session. For example, fatigue is common in children with TBI, thus assessments may need to be broken down into several testing sessions. Likewise, if children evidence visual field deficits, printed material may need to be enlarged or presented to the nonaffected side. Many researchers have suggested additional modifications. Blosser and DePompei (2003, p. 103) compiled the following list of testing modifications:

1. Allowing untimed testing
2. Dividing testing into several sessions to prevent fatigue or loss of attention
3. Lengthening the test time to determine if attention to task decreases or if a child can persevere
4. Introducing auditory or visual distractions, such as testing in a classroom, cafeteria, or busy physical therapy area
5. Reducing distractions in a one-on-one quiet environment to determine maximum performance potentials
6. Enlarging printed materials or placing fewer items on each page
7. Permitting different types of response modes, such as gesturing or writing, rather than relying strictly on verbal responses
8. Restating test directions by using simpler directions or by making directions more lengthy and complex
9. Using pictures or printed cards to reinforce an understanding of test procedures
10. Repeating and cueing to determine if multiple bits of information will stimulate recall
11. Selecting various subtests of different tests according to the needs of the individual
12. Observing pragmatic language skills during testing to sense appropriate use of problem solving, questioning, turn-taking, and self-monitoring

Although modifications in testing may be necessary, the SLP must adhere to all instructions and time constraints outlined in the standardized assessment. Adhering to these rules is necessary to ensure that the results are reliable and valid. Failure to institute some modifications, however, may result in the loss or misinterpretation of the child's performance. For example, if a test item is supposed to be answered in 20 seconds, a potential modification may be for the SLP to mark the item as incorrect if the child does not respond within the time constraints, but then allow the child a longer period of time in which to answer. The child may need additional time to process the information to give a correct response. Without modification, the evaluator might conclude that the child does not have the knowledge to complete the test, when in reality, he or she simply needs more processing time (Carney & Schoenbrodt, 1994; Chesire, Buckley, & Canto, 2011; Schoenbrodt, 2001; Schoenbrodt & Smith, 1995).

Interpretation of Standardized Tests

Though standardized testing is important in the evaluation process, the clinician must remember that most instruments have not been normed on the population with TBI. Therefore, interpretation of scores should provide insight into the strengths and weaknesses of the student but should not be considered definitive. Information obtained on a formal assessment can be deceiving. A student may obtain an "average" score on the administered assessment but be unable to function appropriately at home or in the school environment. Conversely, a child may function below average on many assessments, but be able to function adequately in daily life activities. In general, the results obtained from the standardized testing battery should be interpreted cautiously. For this reason naturalistic or informal assessments are an essential portion of the overall evaluation of communication of the child with TBI (Chesire et al., 2011; Ciccia et al., 2009; Sullivan & Riccio, 2010).

Informal Assessment

Naturalistic assessments are carried out in the child's natural environment and are not standardized. These assessments can provide important information about the child's language functioning that may not be apparent with standardized tests. Informal assessment can take many forms, including interviews, questionnaires, behavioral observations, curriculum-based language assessments, expository and narrative discourse samples.

Interviews and Questionnaires

Interviews and questionnaires can provide the SLP with more in-depth information from parents and teachers about communication problems that may be occurring at home or in the classroom (Blosser & DePompei, 2003; Savage et al., 2005). Possible questions include:

1. How do communication problems affect the child's ability to indicate wants and needs?
2. How well is the child able to hold appropriate conversations with family members or peers?
3. Is the child able to express the need for clarification or repetition of assignments?

Behavioral Observations

Both the SLP and the classroom teacher should observe the child in a variety of settings and contexts, such as the gymnasium, cafeteria, playground, and classroom. An observation in the cafeteria, for example, yields information regarding the child's ability to process information in a noisy environment, to communicate under time constraints (ordering food in the lunch line), to communicate effectively in conversation, to find required vocabulary, and so on. Standardized assessments cannot adequately provide such valuable information (Chesire et al., 2011).

Curriculum-Based Language Assessment

Curriculum-based language assessment (CBLA) is another form of informal assessment. CBLA assesses:

- The types of language skills and strategies the child has for processing the language of the curriculum or classroom content areas (math, social studies, science)
- The resources the child is using to handle the class curriculum
- The skills the child has in place to process classroom information more efficiently
- Any modifications that could be made in the curriculum or its presentation to make it more accessible to the child

In CBLA, the child's schoolwork is reviewed with the understanding that it is only the end product and does not give insight into the process the child uses to complete the work. For example, a review of the child's science quiz may uncover an obvious pattern of errors, but fail to offer insight into why the child is having difficulty or how she or he solved the problem.

The child should be observed in different classroom environments at various times of the day in order to record the potentially problematic language and communication demands in the curriculum. The diagnostic information obtained from CBLA can identify the language demands of the curriculum and how well the child handles them. CBLA is the best way of gathering functional information for use in developing meaningful instructional goals for the child.

For instance, the SLP may observe that the teacher frequently gives directions to the class orally but does not write them on the board. If the child with TBI has difficulty processing language, he or she may never be able to write down the information, let alone comprehend what was said. Goals for intervention would then include working on methods to teach the child how to focus on important pieces of oral information instead of being concerned with everything that is said. The SLP may teach the child to listen for key words like "turn to page . . . " or "your assignment is . . . " In addition, the clinician may talk to the teacher and the child about modifications that may be needed in the classroom, such as tape recording directions so that the child can listen to them as many times as needed (Ciccia et al., 2009).

Narrative Language Samples

Another form of naturalistic assessment is narrative assessment—evaluating a child's ability to tell or retell a story. These types of evaluations are important because being able to produce and understand narratives is vital to both academic success (reading and writing) and to participation in conversations. Studies of children with TBI have consistently shown deficits in this area, which supports the need for assessment (Chapman, 1995; Chapman, Levin, & Lawyer, 1999; Chapman et al., 2004; Hay & Moran, 2005).

Several methods can be used to obtain narrative samples:

1. Having the child relate a personal experience
2. Having the child create a fictional story from pictures or from a given story stem, such as, "One night in a dark and scary woods . . ."
3. Having the child retell a story after hearing the story presented orally or after viewing a videotape
4. Having the child relate a narrative about routine events in daily life (e.g., getting ready for school)

In general, it is more difficult for children to create a novel story than to retell a story or tell about an everyday event. For this reason, it is important that as many narrative samples as possible be obtained in each of the above four areas.

Once the narrative samples are obtained, they are analyzed for story grammar elements (Stein & Glenn, 1979, 1982), including introduction of the characters, a theme or plot, and a closing or resolution. The samples are also analyzed for narrative style and cohesiveness, that is, does the story make sense and flow from one thought to the next? Narratives are further analyzed for total number of words, total number of thematic units (T-units), and sentence complexity. In addition, mean length of utterance and type token ratios (the calculation of the variety of words that are used) can be obtained from the samples.

Expository Discourse

Expository discourse has become a recent focus in assessment and intervention (Hay & Moran, 2005; Horn, 2010). Expository discourse is what is used in school for instruction, including lectures, and texts that call on the student to show his or her knowledge about a topic or content area. As opposed to narrative discourse, which focuses on using stories, or fables for retell, expository discourse uses text that is instructive. For example, Hay and Moran (2005) assessed narrative and expository discourse in children with TBI. They used fables as the stimulus for narrative discourse retelling and two "procedural" discourse passages for the expository retelling. In their study, they found that children with TBI performed poorly on both discourse measures as compared to peers. In addition, the authors found that the children with TBI performed worse on expository versus narrative measures. They performed further analyses, which confirmed that deficits in working memory were highly correlated with difficulties in storing and processing information to be retold.

These findings are critical in developing assessment and treatment for school age children, (and particularly adolescents) as expository discourse is what is primarily used for instruction and measurement of skills in the academic setting.

The information collected through each of these types of informal evaluation reveals a great deal about the child's communication needs at school and in less formal settings (playground, lunchroom, with peers) and should be evaluated along with the information collected through standardized tests for a complete evaluation of the post-TBI child. Continuing brain development can also make it difficult to predict success from test scores, because brain function may or may not continue to improve. Furthermore, there is no way to know how quickly improvement will occur. The combination of both informal and formal evaluations therefore yields a better descriptor of communication competence than either assessment alone and this helps to develop more effective intervention plans.

Intervention

Traumatic brain injury presents a number of deficits that require intervention. As with any population, the most suitable interventions are those that are evidence-based. Many states are now mandating that efficacy studies be conducted regarding intervention. As with assessment, intervention should be interdisciplinary in order to promote carryover and generalization to all environments. Effective intervention for speech and language involves forging a collaboration between teachers and specialists who are working with the child. The goals of speech-language intervention will depend on a number of factors, including: (a) chronological age; (b) the developmental age or stage at which the child is functioning; (c) the extent of damage from the TBI; (d) the degree of current functioning at home, at school, and in the community; and (e) the amount of family support available. Studies have shown that children with mild TBI have the best outcome; however, many of these children may be misidentified, or more likely under identified for requiring services at school. Children with moderate TBI showed variable outcomes depending on the time since injury. Children with moderate to severe TBI make the most gains within the first two years post injury, but children with severe deficits continue to make gains after this point. These wide variations suggest that recovery is ongoing and not all children follow the same pattern of recovery. Frequent assessment of skills, both formal and informal, is needed during the intervention phase (Lajiness-O'Neil, Erodi, & Bigler, 2010; Vu et al., 2011). Overall, intervention should focus on helping the child function in various environments. Rather than teaching or re-teaching skills through drills, it is more helpful to teach skills in a meaningful way that will encourage transfer of skills to all settings (Galvin et al., 2009; Savage et al., 2005; Vu et al., 2011).

Motor Speech Disorders Intervention

Problems with motor speech disorders may involve phonation, respiration, articulation, and resonance. For children with motor speech disorders, oral motor therapy, phonation exercises, and articulation therapy may be implicated. In most instances, speech production problems are resolved without direct intervention (Blosser & DePompei, 2003; Morgan, Mageandran, & Mei, 2009). If motor speech problems persist and production or intelligibility is impaired, alternative or augmentative forms of communication may be explored, such as electronic communication boards, sign language, picture communication boards, and other means.

Language Disorders Intervention

Language disorders are more common than speech disorders in children with TBI. For children with language disorders, therapy may focus on one or more of the following areas.

Vocabulary

The development of vocabulary is crucial for both comprehension and speaking. Children need to develop vocabulary that is meaningful in a variety of settings, including home, school, work, extracurricular activities, and social activities. The child needs to learn not only classroom vocabulary, but also common slang expressions used in conversational speech. Visualization techniques are helpful as well as the use of categorization to aid in word retrieval. Word webs are also effective in helping children to expand ideas and increase word vocabulary (Savage et al., 2005).

Expository Discourse Intervention

Older children and adolescents with TBI have problems with summarizing or getting the "gist" of material that is presented, such as texts, lecture, or conversation, which may be due to impairments in strategic learning. Gamino et al. (2009) found that adolescents with TBI were able to recall factual details but not able to reconstruct an elaborate summary of information presented.

In intervention, the student's text in content areas can be analyzed for the demands of the curriculum. The first step is to identify content from the curriculum that facilitates generalization, such as science and social studies. In evaluating the text, look at how the vocabulary is introduced, how the text is organized, and how much vocabulary is abstract or specific to the content area. In addition, evaluate how cohesive the text is in connecting information across headings or themes. All these things will determine who much facilitation is needed in understanding the text. After the text has been analyzed, the SLP can teach vocabulary that can be generalized across content areas. Strategies can be taught to find alternate sources that are useful in helping with comprehension other than the text itself. Linking important elements to each other, teaching skills for prereading, during reading, and after reading will keep the student actively engaged in learning. Finally, teaching self-evaluation skills is important for the student to be able to gauge comprehension and self-advocate where further intervention is needed.

Pragmatic Skills

Pragmatic skills for language usage are often deficit areas for children with TBI. Conversational and social skills are best taught in settings with peers. In the beginning of therapy, a quiet therapy room with a small group of peers may prove the best setting in which to teach conversational skills. In order for the child to transfer these skills successfully to more natural environments, however, intervention needs to move out of the therapy room into the cafeteria, playground, restaurant, or job setting. By monitoring the child's communication in a variety of settings, the SLP can help the child evaluate where communication breakdowns occur. Therapy can then continue to incorporate problem-solving cognitive skills so the child acquires the ability to think about language and use effective communication (Sullivan & Riccio, 2010).

Cueing or prompting in conversational speech may be effective in decreasing circumlocution (talking around a topic without getting to the point). For example, the SLP might put her finger on her chin to signal to the child that he is off-topic. This cue may be enough for the child to stop and think about what he is saying and get back on topic. This cueing system should then be taught to peers, teachers, and family members to help the child communicate more effectively in conversation.

Humor

The child with TBI may also need help in understanding and using humor appropriately. If the child cannot understand humor, she or he will not "get" jokes and will have trouble fitting in with peers. He or she may also fail to recognize sarcasm. Understanding and using humor involves abstract language and is a higher-level skill. Cartoons, comic strips, and books of jokes and riddles can also be used. The list of possible interventions outlined in this section is clearly not all-inclusive. The type and degree of intervention necessary depends upon the severity of the injury and the residual outcomes.

Organizational Skills

Organizational skills should also be taught to facilitate language learning. Examples of such skills include:

- Classification
- Categorization
- Association
- Sequencing

Memory

Intervention for memory should include observing and examining the demands of working memory in classroom discourse and assignments (Boudreau & Costanza-Smith, 2011). Collaboration with teachers is important in determining things like: Are the instructions too lengthy? Are students required to write sentences to dictation, and what amount? How complex are the instructional materials being used? Answers to these questions can provide information as to how the classroom environment can be modified to meet the needs of the child with TBI wherever he or she is in the course of recovery. The (SLP) can also provide the teacher with strategies and supports to enhance memory. The use of visual organizers, or helping the teacher to adjust how much information is presented orally, and combine that with visual supports, are methods that can be suggested. Teachers and clinicians can always work together in preteaching key concepts for academic subjects. All these strategies will help with reinforcing working memory in the classroom. Strategies specific to the child include the use of rehearsal strategies (Boudreau & Costanza-Smith, 2011). Rehearsal of information can include chunking words together and has been shown to be effective particularly in older children (over 7) and adolescents (Minear & Shah, 2006). Another strategy may be the use of personal digital assistants (PDAs) and smartphones to enhance memory following brain injury (DePompei et al., 2008). One study evaluated the use of these devices in children with TBI who had memory and organization problems. Their results showed that students were highly motivated to use these tools and as a result were effective in assisting with memory and providing organizational independence (DePompei et al., 2008).

School Re-Entry

Contributed by Joan Carney

Children and adolescents who have sustained mild TBI or concussions will often return to school gradually upon the recommendation of their physician. The Acute Concussion Evaluation (ACE) was developed by Gioia and Collins (2006). This tool provides the school with a plan for gradual return to school and outlines areas that will need to be monitored. Impairments in these cases are usually transient and with cognitive rest this gradual school re-entry is typically successful. Those children with TBI who have been hospitalized in acute care and/or rehabilitation will require more thoughtful school re-entry to address the new impairments to motor, language, cognition or emotional-regulation that may now be present (Carney & Porter, 2009).

As part of either the child's rehabilitation or educational team, the speech-language pathologist should play an active role in coordinating the child's transition from the rehabilitation center to the school. SLPs have knowledge of the neurological deficits and educational needs following TBI that may provide them a stronger foundation than others on the interdisciplinary school team, to act in the role of case manager (Blosser & De Pompei, 2003; Russell, 1993).

Whoever provides the case management role, early and ongoing communication should be a major component.

The school and rehabilitation facility should have two-way communication throughout the process to facilitate optimal school re-entry. It will be important for the rehabilitation professionals to have knowledge of the child's pretraumatic functioning in the school setting and it is important for the school professionals to have ongoing information about the rate of the child's improvement and anticipated needs upon return to school. Timing of school meetings to facilitate smooth school re-entry, without a lapse in services, will also require close coordination as the typical timeline for obtaining special services in the school setting will need to be expedited.

Children who have sustained significant TBI, with their newfound impairments, will likely require special education and related services for successful school re-entry. They have a federally protected right to such services when, due to a disability, they need them to benefit from education. Special education, not necessarily a special classroom, but a program designed by an interdisciplinary school team, should provide the support to make the child with TBI successful as he or she returns to school and for as long as those services are needed. As mandated by law, each student's program must be individualized to meet the specific needs of that child and his or her unique constellation of impairments.

Federal legislation is the basis for each state's law governing special education and other support services for students with disabilities. States can reinterpret the federal statute as long as they do not relax any of the provisions. Within states, local jurisdictions then develop guidelines and procedures. This evolution of the federal law has resulted in particular procedures for obtaining special education and related services varying slightly from one school system to the next. However, they do follow the same series of steps but the whole process can take several months. This situation can be problematic for a child or adolescent with TBI. A possible scenario could mean that the child will be medically stable to return to school but that the proper services will not be in place to allow success thus making it crucial to have early contact with the school to begin the process and expedite the procedures. The family, the physician, or therapist should initiate this contact as soon as possible so that school personnel can begin to consider appropriate options for the returning student.

The process to obtain special education and related services includes referral for services, screenings and assessments, eligibility determination, development of the Individual Education Plan (IEP) or Individual Family Service Plan (IFSP), implementation of the plan, review, and re-evaluation.

Assessment

In the case of the child with recent TBI, a series of pertinent assessments are likely to have been done for medical or rehabilitative treatment. Appropriate domains for evaluation by the speech-language pathologist have been previously discussed. If the child is being treated in a pediatric facility, rehabilitation therapists are likely to know what is important to include in an assessment to be used in school planning. Impairments that might warrant outpatient rehabilitation therapy may not impact on the student's access to education and thus may not warrant a related service or therapy in the school context. Goals for treatment in the two settings, that is outpatient versus educational, should be clearly delineated for the purposes of discharge planning and school re-entry.

It is helpful when the child or adolescent with TBI is treated in a comprehensive pediatric rehabilitation program that can provide the school with all of the pertinent evaluations needed to determine eligibility and appropriate programming. An educator is not usually part of a rehabilitation team and an educational assessment is always required to determine special education eligibility because the school team needs to assess whether the impairments affect educational performance. In those cases an educational evaluator from the school system can be invited to perform the assessment while the child is still undergoing rehabilitation. Because recovery from TBI is ongoing in the first few years, timing of the evaluations needs to be considered. The evaluations used for school planning need to be completed near the time when the child will return to school so that the information will be current.

Eligibility

The school team reviews the assessments at an interdisciplinary team meeting to determine if the student meets the conditions to be eligible for special education and related services under the defined federal eligibility codes. "Traumatic Brain Injury" (TBI) is an eligibility category appropriate to some children with TBI; however, under IDEA TBI is narrowly defined as injury caused by external force. In the case of a tumor or disease process that causes injury to the brain it may not be used. In those cases the category 'Other Health Impaired" is often employed.

Individual Educational Program

The individual educational program (IEP) documents the student's special education and related services. Although TBI is prevalent, in each individual school it is of low incidence and the school team may consider students with similar impairments that they have programmed for successfully. Although this approach may be effective, due to the nature of TBI, it is important that the team also keep the differences between TBI and developmental disabilities in mind.

One major difference is that the child's learning and communication deficits were acquired as a result of a traumatic injury. In many cases, the child had no learning difficulties prior to the trauma. Table 6–3 lists some similarities and differences between children with TBI and those with learning disabilities.

The IEP should address all of the impairments that could affect both nonacademic school participation, such as deficits in orientation, and academic success, such as memory or language processing. Carefully crafted goals will assist in success of the school re-entry.

A therapist who has been treating the child with TBI during the rehabilitation phase can be quite helpful during the school re-entry process. Parents may have had no experience with the special education process and could benefit from experienced assistance. In addition, the receiving school can benefit from direct consultation with the rehabilitation therapists.

The SLP may share pertinent information with the child's teachers so that they will be able to develop an awareness of the child's strengths and weaknesses and be able to program for the child optimally in the classroom. Strategies the child was

Table 6–3. Similarities and Differences in Characteristics of Children with Traumatic Brain Injury (TBI) and Children with Learning Disabilities (LD)

Children with TBI	Children with LD
Acquired. Sudden onset.	Congenital defect. Usually early onset.
Documented history of coma in many cases.	No coma.
Cause attributed to event such as motor vehicle accident, gunshot wound, and so forth.	Cause not clear.
Documented posttraumatic amnesia (PTA) affecting memory.	Memory deficits not related to PTA.
Noticeable differences in premorbid skills and posttrauma abilities.	No pre/post effect.
New learning difficult, can remember old skills.	Learning may be slow with continued progress in new learning.
Range of deficits from mild to severe.	Range of deficits from mild to severe.
Poor social/pragmatic skills secondary to injury.	Poor social/pragmatic skills secondary to language impairment.
Inability to comprehend posttraumatic deficits.	Good comprehension of learning strengths and weaknesses.
Seizure medications given for traumatically induced seizures.	No antiseizure medication.
Marked impairment of progress initially indicating a need for frequent monitoring of progress. At the school level, annual review and dismissal meetings should be held monthly until progress stabilizes.	Slow, steady progress. Monitoring of progress may take place at the school level one or two times a year to document gains.
Once in school change of classroom placement may be needed if progress occurs.	Relatively stable. Classroom placement remains constant.
Needs modification in testing due to impairments (fatigue, distractibility, etc.) secondary to TBI.	Needs modification in testing due to impairments (distractibility, language deficits, etc.) of the LD.
Family may not accept child's school placement and needs due to problems coping with the deficits presented secondary to the sudden trauma.	Family generally understands strengths and weaknesses of child as well as the LD because onset was early and gradual.

taught during rehabilitation to accommodate for their current impairments can be carried over to the school setting. Requirements for class assignments may also need to be modified and suggestions can be made for this as well.

Upon return to school the SLP might serve several important roles: (a) to provide information to the educators managing the student in the classroom; (b) to monitor the progress of the student, which may be variable due to the constantly changing nature of postinjury medical, behavioral, and cognitive deficits; (c) to assist in making updates to the IEP and enacting changes in placement due to these variables; and (d) to act as a liaison for the student when the family is under emotional stress and may lack the knowledge necessary to act as an advocate for their child (Schoenbrodt, 2001; Schoenbrodt & Smith, 1995).

Family Issues

The family of the child with TBI plays an important role in facilitating the child's integration into the school and the community. As a result of the trauma, the family also experiences major alterations of roles, rules, and internal responsibilities in its adjustments to the affected family member. The impact on the family of the child with the TBI begins with the telephone call that informs them of the injury and continues through the rehabilitation process and a lifetime of outpatient care (DePompei, 2010; Roscigno & Swanson, 2011; Savage et al., 2005). Many studies document that TBI affects all aspects of family life and that major changes in structure and organization are inevitable (Lajiness-O'Neil, Erodi, & Bigler, 2010;

Roscigno & Swanson, 2011; Schrief, Donald, & Thomas, 2011).

The stress resulting from the changes in routine, social status, family health, and patient behaviors has a major impact on a family's ability to adjust to the child with TBI. In addition, the family of the person with the TBI has particular difficulty with the mourning process. Unlike the death of a family member, TBI means that the individual with TBI remains with the family, often in the same physical state but in an altered cognitive state.

The family must mourn the characteristics of the child that were lost while learning to respond to the differences in the person, a step that is crucial to the outcome of the child with the TBI. The family often is faced with overwhelming economic burdens in providing the required long-term care. The family of a younger child with TBI is faced with the concern that they will be "parenting" forever. On the other hand, the family of an adolescent is faced with handling a child who was once independent who is now dependent again. This situation is further complicated when the adolescent is aware of prior independence and feels "babied" by parents when he or she is fully aware of prior boundaries.

The functional family eventually draws internal and external support to respond to new needs of the family member and maintains hope for the future. A dysfunctional family is unable to focus on any factor other than the trauma and tends to concentrate on the individual's weaknesses rather than strengths. Research continues to show that family variables, including the ability to handle stress and access to resources, are vital in predicting long-term outcome (Keenan & Bratton, 2006; Lajiness-O'Neil et al., 2010; Schrief, Donald, & Thomas, 2011; Taylor et al., 2008). Because of these outcomes, developing family-centered programs has become a priority for health care in the United States (Institute of Medicine, 2001). In order to formulate effective programs, input from families is needed. Roscigno and Swanson (2011) designed a study evaluating parents' experiences following the TBI of their child. They conducted interviews and found that there were four overall themes that were apparent. These themes included: "grateful to still have my child, grieving for the child I knew, running on nerves, and grappling to get what my child and family need" (Roscigno & Swanson, 2011, p. 1416). Parents also reported frustration in getting conflicting and confusing information from professionals in all stages of recovery, from acute care through school placement. They found that jargon that was unfamiliar was often used and not explained, and that physicians often attempted to squash their hopes, which was counterproductive to the family working together as a unit. Finally, parents reported great difficulties in working with insurance carriers, which was a deterrent in finding adequate resources for their child and themselves. This situation created problems for families finding community support. These resources would have helped in lessening the stress the families were facing. Clearly, there is a need to continue to include families in the communication phases of rehabilitation for their child. Interventions at all levels need to include families for the best outcome in all domains for the child with a TBI.

Conclusion

The neurological and cognitive sequelae that result from TBI vary greatly in terms of severity across the population. For this reason, a child with TBI must be considered unique and be treated on an individual basis.

Communication is essential in all aspects of life, thus communication needs should be identified and monitored continuously throughout the acute care stage as well as through the child's reentry to a school or possibly work setting. Goals for successful communication should also be monitored and frequently revised to match the child's needs in the environment. Plans for intervention should take into consideration functioning in all areas, including cognitive, motor, and behavioral. The ultimate goal should be to enable the child to function effectively at home, in school, and in the community.

Case Study 1

The following case study shows the thinking of the speech-language pathologist throughout the assessment process. The commentary is noted in the italicized text.

Janice, a 6-year, 1-month-old girl suffered a traumatic brain injury when she fell out of a 3rd-story window. She was initially taken to a Children's Medical Center for immediate care. Results at that time indicated a CT scan that was positive for intraparenchymal hemorrhages, parietal intraventricular hemorrhage, and a vertex skull fracture. Janice was unresponsive when the ambulance arrived. When she was admitted to the medical center, she had a Glasgow Coma Score of 3–4. In addition, she had a broken arm and liver/spleen lacerations. An initial speech and language evaluation was conducted following admission to an inpatient rehabilitation center. At that time, no formal testing was administered. Based on clinical observation and parent report, at that time Janice was functioning at a Rancho level VI–VII and demonstrated a mixed receptive and expressive language disorder, dysarthria, cognitive-communication deficits, oral motor deficits, and suspected dysphagia.

This child had findings on her imaging, and bleeding within the parietal lobe. She had fallen head first from a window onto the pavement below. She had additional injuries besides the brain injury that also required treatment. The SLP at the acute care facility indicated that she quickly was alert and responsive and was oriented to people, place, and time. She remained in the acute care setting for 17 days before being transferred to the inpatient facility specializing in brain injury rehabilitation. There was no formal or standardized testing completed until she was admitted. At the time of transfer, she was functioning at a Rancho level VI–VII, which means she was between confused and appropriate and automatic and appropriate. At level VI, she may be confused due to memory and thinking problems and people may have to repeat things often. She can pay attention for 30 minutes but is easily distracted particularly if there is a lot of noise or other activity going on at the same time. At level VII, she is able to follow routines, like bathing, getting dressed by herself, but will have trouble in novel situations. She still has problems concentrating and will require supervision because she lacks good judgment and safety awareness. In Janice's case, she also is still recovering from physical injuries as well. At the time of admission, she also demonstrated slow and labored speech and had some swallowing problems, in addition to problems both understanding and expressing herself.

Janice lives with her parents, older sister, and grandmother. Janice's primary language is Gujrati, and she speaks English as a second language. She was attending kindergarten at the time of injury and should continue in first grade in public school next year. It was reported that

premorbid educational skills were above average.

Janice has a very supportive family. Both her parents work and Janice and her sister remain in the care of their grandmother during the day. The first language is spoken at home and her parents are somewhat but not totally fluent in English. Her grandmother only speaks the first language and her sister is fluent in both. Communication is sometimes difficult with the family because they rely on the older sister (age 11) to translate. Regardless, her family is very supportive and anxious to participate in the recovery process. Janice's kindergarten teacher reports that she was well above level and was reading fluently before the injury.

Initial Evaluation Results

The first formal evaluation was conducted two weeks following admission.

The CASL was administered on two dates. Core and supplementary tests were used. The core composite gives a global measure of language performance. Janice obtained a standard score of 93 on the core composite, with a percentile rank of 32, indicating oral language functioning in the average range.

The comprehension of basic concepts test measures the ability to comprehend words representing basic concepts. These words include nouns, pronouns, prepositions, and adjectives including those for size, shape, quality, and quantity, distance, direction, and position. Janice obtained a standard score of 98, a percentile of 45 indicating performance in the average range.

The antonyms test is designed to measure the ability to identify words that are opposite in meaning. Janice must retrieve and produce a single word when its opposite is given as a stimulus. Janice obtained an 84, and a percentile rank of 14, and functioning in the below average range.

Janice struggled with word retrieval and in overall comprehension of the stimulus word. As difficulty increased, she became frustrated and distracted with the task.

The sentence completion test is a measure of word retrieval, knowledge, and expression within a linguistic context. The format assesses the ability to retrieve and express and appropriate word that fits the meaning of a spoken sentence. To succeed, Janice had to comprehend the vocabulary and syntax of the sentence in addition to having solid world knowledge to generate an acceptable response. Janice obtained a standard score of 102, with a percentile of 55, and functioning in the average range.

The syntax construction test assesses the ability to generate sentences using a variety of morphosyntactic rules. Janice obtained a 94 and a percentile of 34 indicating average performance.

The paragraph comprehension of syntax test measures comprehension by means of a series of spoken narratives. It assesses the ability to derive meaning from syntactic structures. Janice answered a series of questions by choosing the appropriate answer by pointing to a picture in response to the question. Janice obtained a 101 and a percentile of 53 indicating average performance.

The final subtest administered was the pragmatic judgment test, which measures the awareness of the appropriateness of language in relation to the situation in which it is used and the ability to modify language to the situation. Janice obtained a standard score of 101 with a percentile of 53 indicating average performance. It should be noted that Janice missed items at a lower level and then continued to perform above level to finally achieve a ceiling indicating inconsistent performance that is congruent with individuals having TBI.

Informal evaluation of language skills indicates deficits in word retrieval, following directions, answering questions, and naming in discrete categories, which is consistent with formal testing. Conversational speech was tangential and frequently Janice had to be redirected to the focus of the conversation.

Speech/voice/fluency: All areas were noted to be within acceptable limits. Dysarthria of speech was no longer noted.

Oral-motor/swallowing: Appears to be adequate at this time

Hearing: Was not evaluated during this evaluation formally, but appears to be adequate.

Summary

- Impairments—Receptive and expressive language; cognitive communication, pragmatics

The SLP chose to use several evaluations including the Comprehensive Assessment of Spoken Language (CASL), a comprehensive language evaluation, as well as informal evaluation of performance using activities that were academically based and assessed things like following directions and answering questions. This was done using stories to answer questions and to retell a story, and prompts to follow directions, such as touch your head and then your foot. Janice was cooperative and eager to please the clinician. She tired quickly and needed frequent breaks. Testing needed to be conducted on two different occasions due to fatigue. Janice was also distractible and needed to be redirected if there was any ambient noise in the environment. Janice also had difficulty with problem-solving, which is consistent with cognitive communication disorders.

There was no evidence of dysarthria or dysphagia at the time of the evaluation. Articulation was typical for her age. The other findings on the formal assessment are somewhat typical in that given Janice's above average premorbid skills, she performed at least at the average range on most subtests. She did demonstrate difficulty with word retrieval or word finding and required extra time to process information to remember the word. What is important to note is that given extra time she was able to retrieve the information. In a school environment, she will require modifications so that she can be successful. Her literacy skills were also informally assessed and there were noticeable gaps in the skills that she had prior to the injury. Janice was also quite aware that there are things that she had been able to do academically and was struggling with now. She became frustrated with tasks that she knew were easy for her before and tried to manipulate the situation so that she could avoid certain tasks. Janice should have extensive therapy to get her ready for school next year. Contact has been made with her home school that she attends. Unfortunately, because it is summer, none of the teachers who knew her are available for consultation, only the administration at the school. An initial IEP meeting has been scheduled to make recommendations for speech and language therapy and special education services, as well as a consultation for physical and occupational therapy. Speech language therapy will continue through the rehabilitation center until the school year begins. An additional evaluation will be performed immediately before transition to the school. Immediate goals for speech language therapy include the following.

Recommendations/Goals

It is highly recommended that Janice receive speech-language services at least two times per week. The following goals should be addressed during therapy.

Maximize Receptive and Expressive Language Abilities

1. To follow commands of increasing length and complexity.
2. To listen to narratives and answer comprehension questions including narrative and story grammar questions.
3. To answer WH questions.
4. To answer inferential and factual questions.
5. To identify and label simple and complex categories appropriate to her age.
6. To divergently name items in concrete categories.

Maximize Cognitive Communication Abilities

1. To recall new information after a delay of 20 minutes or more.
2. To identify solutions to problems.
3. To complete basic reasoning tasks.

Maximize Pragmatic Skills

1. To increase ability to stay on topic for a 5-minute conversation.
2. To maintain attention and focus to conversation for 5 minutes or more.
3. To use turn-taking skills appropriately for 5 minutes or more in conversation.

Review Questions

1. What is the significance of primary and secondary injuries on the outcome of a child with TBI?

2. Describe the indicators that determine the impact of TBI.

3. Why is age a factor in determining outcome?

4. What has research shown about the characteristics of the family that can impact the outcome of children with TBI? Why are these results important in rehabilitation?

5. What specific assessments are used in determining cognitive recovery? What are important factors to consider about neurological and academic testing?

6. Define working memory. How would deficits in working memory be expressed in the classroom? What strategies can the SLP use to enhance working memory?

7. Explain how discourse is assessed and intervened.

8. Why is it important to have ongoing communication with the child's school? Provide specific ideas for enhancing this communication.

9. What type of assessment information would be particularly important in determining goals for school re-entry (think beyond speech and language skills).

10. Explain the role of the SLP as part of the interdisciplinary team and case manager. Provide specific ways that the SLP can help the family during the rehabilitation process from acute care to school re-entry.

Case Study 2: Nina's Case History

Nina is a 9-year, 10-month-old girl who was referred for a complete interdisciplinary assessment subsequent to a severe traumatic brain injury sustained while she was a passenger restrained in the backseat of a car. The current assessments were requested to aid in the transition from the rehabilitation center to the school.

Nina currently resides with her mother, father, and older brother. There is no reported family history of psychiatric illness or learning disabilities. According to parental reports, there were no problems with the pregnancy or labor. Nina was delivered at a weight of 8 pounds, 11 ounces. Early developmental milestones were reported within normal limits. Nina is very active in the neighborhood, and has many friends.

Nina was attending third grade in elementary school at the time of the injury. A review of her records indicated above average performance on report cards and the Comprehensive Test of Basic Skills (CTBS) given at the school. Nina's mother reported that she was diagnosed with ADHD one year ago and was taking medication prior to this injury. School records and teacher reports indicate that Nina had difficulty staying on task, following directions, avoiding careless mistakes, sustaining attention, and controlling her emotions.

Nina was injured as a restrained backseat passenger. According to medical records, the car she was riding in was hit on the right rear passenger side. Nina lost consciousness at the scene of the accident. She was stabilized at a local hospital and was intubated and resuscitated. She was transferred to a trauma center, where a Glasgow Coma Scale score of 5 (intubated) was reported upon admission.

According to medical records, Nina had a massive injury to the right side of the face and experienced a great deal of blood loss. Her left pupil was small and reactive, whereas the right pupil was unable to be assessed. A head CT scan revealed two large areas of hemorrhagic contusions. Blood and air were seen within the contusions as well as in the left temporal lobe. There were also extensive temporal bone fractures with disruptions of the inner ear structures bilaterally. Coma duration was noted as 7 weeks. An end of PTA was noted 2 months after admission, indicating a duration of 6 to 7 weeks between the termination of coma and the termination of posttraumatic amnesia. Conductive hearing loss was identified in the left ear as well as complete hearing loss in the right ear.

Premorbid intellectual skills were judged to be within the average range. Current neuropsychological testing revealed a discrepancy between verbal and performance on the WISC-R, suggesting that nonverbal intellectual skills are currently stronger than language-based problem-solving abilities.

Formal and informal speech and language evaluation revealed receptive and expressive language skills to be in the below average to well below average level for concepts and directions, word classes, semantic relationships, paragraph comprehension, formulating sentences, recalling sentences, and assembling sentences. During the testing, it was observed that Nina required increased time to process information when responding to a question. When Nina was provided with additional time to respond, as well as with visual, auditory, and phonemic cues to elicit words, this increased her ability to answer questions. Word-finding deficits, processing deficits, attention deficits, and hearing loss will significantly impact her ability to perform within academic and social environments.

An informal speech and oral motor evaluation revealed mild oral motor deficits secondary to a TBI. Nina presented with slightly decreased strength and mobility of her tongue. Despite mild weakness, oral motor skills appeared to be adequate for speech and eating. Nina tolerated a regular diet with thin liquids.

Results of the interdisciplinary evaluation team revealed that Nina requires direct speech language therapy upon reentry to school, as well as significant modifications to the classroom. As Nina's language skills are changing frequently, it is recommended that she be reevaluated weekly for the first month and then monthly for at least the next year.

Review Questions

1. How would Nina's premorbid characteristics influence her outcome?

2. What specific intervention goals will Nina require for speech and language?

3. What other factors should be considered when Nina returns to school?

4. Design an assessment battery to evaluate ongoing speech and language skills one- month post return to school.

5. What recommendations should be given to the family?

Case Study 3: Ron's Case History

Ron is a 6-year, 10-month-old student who was referred for an interdisciplinary assessment following a CHI secondary to a motor vehicle accident. Ron was comatose for four days and received surgery for a subdural hematoma. He remained in a rehabilitation center for one month following the injury. At that time, he was evaluated and weaknesses were demonstrated in attending, following directions, vocabulary, word retrieval, and verbal expression skills.

The current evaluation is being conducted prior to his return to school. Behaviorally, Ron accompanied the examiner willingly and engaged in conversation easily. He was somewhat silly, and inappropriate giggling was noted. His attention to tasks was varied. As tasks became more difficult, off-task behavior was noted. Frequent redirection and breaks were needed in order to complete the testing. In addition, Ron demonstrated slow processing and frequently asked for repetition and/or clarification of oral directions and information. His expressive vocabulary was characterized by frequent restarts, word retrieval, sequencing, and organizational difficulties. Spontaneous conversation was tangential, requiring the listener to clarify and question what was said continually.

Formal and informal evaluations were conducted to evaluate speech and language functioning. The results of the evaluation showed that Ron demonstrates a speech or language impairment characterized by moderate deficits in auditory processing, language content, language structure, and language usage. Overall language skills were in the below average range, with individual scores ranging from average to significantly below average. An individual strength was noted in his ability to perceive relationships between words. Weaknesses were noted in knowledge of antonyms, knowledge of form and meaning of grammatical morphemes, knowledge of synonyms, word knowledge in linguistic context, comprehension of intended meaning, ability to initiate and maintain conversation, and knowledge of form and meaning of grammatical morphemes and comprehension of syntax in spoken narratives.

The results of the evaluation showed that Ron's speech and language impairment significantly impact his performance throughout the school day. The impairment affects his ability to comprehend oral information and lectures, follow directions, answer questions, understand, integrate, and use curriculum vocabulary, express thoughts and ideas in a clear, concise manner, and interact with peers and adults within an educational environment.

As a result of the evaluation, the interdisciplinary team recommended speech and language therapy to focus on remediation of weaknesses and modifications in his academic program, including reducing rate, length, and complexity of oral directions and input; repeating and clarifying directions; preteaching vocabulary and concepts; providing listening, memory, organization, and retrieval strategies; and providing opportunities for participating in social skills groups with peers. Ron's family is encouraged to help with these modifications in his home environment. The assessment team at his school should reevaluate his progress in 30 days to be sure recommendations and modifications are in place.

Review Questions

1. What is important to consider in Ron's assessment behaviors?

2. Explain the speech and language deficits and how these would impact his performance in and out of school?

3. What recommendations would you give the teacher to aid communication in the classroom?

4. How (specifically) would modifications be implemented at home?

5. When should Ron be re-evaluated and in what areas?

References

Anderson, V., & Catroppa, C. (2007). Memory outcome at 5 years post-childhood traumatic brain injury. *Brain Injury, 21*(13–14), 1399–1409. doi:10.1080/02699050701785070

Arroyos-Jurado, E., Paulsen, J., Ehly, S., & Max, J. (2006). Traumatic brain injury in children and adolescents: Academic and intellectual outcomes following injury. *Exceptionality, 14*(3), 125–140. Retrieved from http://search.proquest.com/docview/62102898?accountid=12164;http://dx.doi.org/10.1207/d15327035ex1403

Baddeley, A. (1990). The development of the concept of working memory: Implications and contributions of neuropsychology. In G. Vallar & T. Shallice (Eds.), *Neuropsychological impairments of short-term memory* (pp. 54–73). New York, NY: Cambridge University Press.

Bazarian, J., Cernak, I., Noble-Haeusslein, L., Potolicchio, S., & Temkin, N. (2009). Long-term neurologic outcomes after traumatic brain injury. *The Journal of Head Trauma Rehabilitation, 24*(6) 439–451. Retrieved from http://search.proquest.com/docview/74278435?accountid=12164

Beachamp, M., Catroppa, C., Godfrey, C., Morse, S., Rosenfeld, J., & Anderson, V. (2011). Selective changes in executive functioning ten years after severe childhood traumatic brain injury. *Developmental Psychology, 36*(5), 578–595.

Blosser, J., & DePompei, R. (2003). *Pediatric traumatic brain injury* (2nd ed.). Clifton Park, NY: Delmar Learning.

Blumenstein, E., Patterson, C. M., & Delis, D. (1995). Verbal learning and memory following pediatric closed-head injury. *Journal of International Neuropsychological Society, 11*(1), 84–98. doi:http://dx.doi.org/10.1017/S1355617700000138

Boudreau, D., & Costanza-Smith, A. (2011). Assessment and treatment of working memory deficits in school-age children: The role of the speech-language pathologist. *Language, Speech, and Hearing Services in Schools, 42*, 152–166. doi:10.1044/0161-1461(2010/09-0088)

Brady, K. (2001). How TBI affects learning and thinking. In L. Schoenbrodt (Ed.), *Children with traumatic brain injury: A parent's guide* (pp. 133–176). Bethesda, MD: Woodbine House.

Brain Injury Association. *Brain injury fact sheet.* Retrieved from http://www.biausa.org/Images/PDFs/Fact SheetBrainInjury.pdf

Brenner, L., Dise-Lewis, J., Bartles, S., O'Brien, S., Godleski, M., & Selinger, M. (2007). *Journal of Head Trauma Rehabilitation, 22*(1), 56–64. Retrieved from http://www.headtrauma rehab.com

Brookshire, R. (2007). *Introduction to neurogenic communication disorders* (7th ed.). St. Louis, MO: Mosby.

Bruce, D., Raphaely, R., Goldberg, A., Zimmerman, R., Bilaniuk, L., Schut, L., . . . Kuhl, D. (1979). Pathophysiology, treatment, and outcome following severe head injury in children. *Child's Brain, 5*, 174–191.

Carney, J., & Porter, P. (2009). School reentry for children with acquired central nervous systems injuries. *Developmental Disabilities Research Reviews, 15*(2), 152–158. doi:10.1002/ddrr.57

Carney, J., & Schoenbrodt, L. (1994). Educational implications of traumatic brain injury. *Pediatric Annals, 23*(1), 47–52.

Carney, N., Chestnut, R., Maynardt, H., Mann, N., Patterson, P., & Helfend, M. (2000). Effect of cognitive rehabilitation on outcomes for persons with traumatic brain injury: A systematic review. *Journal of Head Trauma Rehabilitation, 14*(3), 277–307.

Carrow-Woolfolk, E. (1999). *Comprehensive assessment of spoken language.* Torrance, CA: WEPS.

Catroppa, C., & Anderson, V. (2005). A prospective study of the recovery of attention from acute to 2 years following pediatric traumatic brain injury. *Journal of the International Neuropsychological Society, 11*, 84–98. doi:10.1017/S13556177050101

Centers for Disease Control and Prevention. (2011). *What to expect after a concussion. A part of the CDC's "Heads Up" Series.* Retrieved from http://www.cdc.gov/concussion/pdf/TBI_Patient_Instructions-a.pdf

Chapman, S. (1995). Discourse as an outcome measure in pediatric head injured patients. In S. Broman & M. E. Michel (Eds.), *Consequences* of traumatic head injury in children: Variability in short and long term outcomes (pp. 95–116). New York, NY: Oxford University Press.

Chapman, S., Levin, H., & Lawyer, S. (1999). Communication problems resulting from brain injury in children: Special issues of assessment and management. In S. McDonald, L. Togher, & C. Code (Eds.), Communication disorders following traumatic brain injury (pp. 235–270). East Sussex, UK: Psychology Press Ltd.

Chapman, S., & McKinnon, L. (2000). Discussion of developmental plasticity: Factors affecting cognitive outcome after pediatric traumatic brain injury. Journal of Communication Disorders, 33, 333–344.

Chapman, S., Sparks, G., Levin, H., Dennis, M., Roncadin, C., Zhang, L., . . . Song, J. (2004). Discourse macrolevel processing severe pediatric traumatic brain injury. Developmental Neuropsychology, 25(1&2), 37–60.

Chesire, D., Buckley, V., & Canto, A. (2011). Assessment of students with traumatic brain injury. Communiqué, 40(2), 8–10.

Christensen, J. (2001). What is traumatic brain injury? In L. Schoenbrodt (Ed.), Children with traumatic brain injury (pp. 1–23). Bethesda, MD: Woodbine House.

Ciccia, A., Meulenbrook, P., & Turkstra, L. (2009). Adolescent brain and cognitive development. Topics in Language Disorders, 29(3), 249–265.

Claret, T. G., Palomeque, R. A., Cambra, L. F., Catala, T. A., Noguera, J. A., & Costa, C. J. (2007). Severe head injury among children: Computed tomography evaluation as a prognostic factor. Journal of Pediatric Surgery, 42(11), 1903–1906. doi:10.1016/j.jpedsurg.2007.07.020

DePompei, R. (2010). Pediatric traumatic brain injury: Where do we go from here? ASHA Leader, 15(20), 16–20.

DePompei, R., Gillette, Y., Goetz, E., Xenopoulos-Oddsson, A., Bryen, D., & Dowds, M. (2008). Practical applications for use of PDAs and smartphones with children and adolescents who have traumatic brain injury. NeuroRehabilitation, 23, 487–499.

DePompei, R., & Zarski, J. (1989). Families, head injury, and cognitive-communicative impairments: Issues for family counseling. Topics in Language Disorders, 9(2), 78–89.

Dikmen, S., Corrigan, J., Levin, H., Machamer, J., Stiers, W., & Weisskopf, M. (2009). Cognitive outcome following traumatic brain injury. The Journal of Head Trauma Rehabilitation, 24(6), 430–438.

Donders, J., & Janke, K. (2008). Criterion validity of the Wechsler Intelligence Scale for Children-Fourth Edition after pediatric traumatic brain injury. Journal of the International Neuropsychological Society, 14, 651–655. doi:10.1017/S1355617708080752

Dunn, L., & Dunn, L. (2007). Peabody Picture Vocabulary Test-Revised. Circle Pines, MN: American Guidance Services.

Ewings-Cobbs, L., & Barnes, M. (2002). Linguistic outcomes following traumatic brain injury in children. Seminars in Pediatric Neurology, 9, 209–217.

Ewings-Cobbs, L., Barnes, M., Fletcher, J., Levin, H., Swank, P., & Song, J. (2004). Modeling of longitudinal academic achievement scores after pediatric traumatic brain injury. Developmental Neuropsychology, 25(1&2), 107–133.

Feeney, J., & Urbanczyk, A. (1992). Educational programming following acquired brain injury. Paper presented at the Annual Conference on Cognitive Rehabilitation, Richmond, VA.

Fowler, M., & McCabe, P. C. (2011). Traumatic brain injury and personality change. Communiqué, 39(7), 4, 6, 8, 10. Retrieved from http://search.proquest.com/docview/867665184?accountid=12164

Gale, S., & Prigatano, G. (2010). Deep white matter volume loss and social reintegration after traumatic brain injury in children. Journal of Head Trauma Rehabilitation, 25(1), 15–22.

Galvin, J., Froude, E., & Imms, C. (2009). Sensory processing abilities of children who have sustained traumatic brain injuries. The American Journal of Occupational Therapy, 63(6), 701–709.

Gamino, J., Chapman, S., & Cook, L. (2009). Strategic learning in youth with traumatic brain injury: Evidence for stall in higher-order cognition. Topics in Language Disorders, 29(3), 56–63.

Gardner, M. F. (2000). Expressive One Word Picture Vocabulary Test. Novato, CA: Academic Therapy.

Gillam, R., & Pearson, N. (2004). Test of Narrative Language. Austin, TX: Pro-Ed.

Gioia, G., Isquith, P., Schneider, J., & Vaughan, C. (2009). New approaches to assessment and monitoring of concussion in children. Topics in Language Disorders, 29(3), 266–281.

Hagen, C. (1998). The Rancho Levels of Cognitive Functioning–Revised (3rd ed.). Rancho Encinitas, CA: Los Amigos Medical Center.

Hagan, C., & Malkmus, D. (1979, November). *Intervention strategies for language disorders secondary to head injury*. Short course presented at the annual convention of American Speech-Language-Hearing Association, Atlanta, GA.

Hanten, G., Dennis, M., Zhang, L., Barnes, M., Roberson, G., Archibald., J., . . . Levin, H. (2004). Childhood head injury and metacognitive processes in language and memory. *Developmental Neuropsychology, 25*, 85–106.

Hart, T., Sherer, M., Whyte, J., Polansky, M., & Novack, T. (2004). Awareness of behavioral, cognitive, and physical deficits in acute traumatic brain injury. *Archives of Physical Medicine and Rehabilitation, 84*, 1450–1460. doi:10.1016/j.apmr.2004.01.030

Hay, E., & Moran, C. (2005). Discourse formulation in children with closed head injury. *American Journal of Speech-Language Pathology, 14*, 324–336. doi:1058- 0360/05/1404-0324

Horn, D. (2010). Expository intervention with adolescents. *Topics in Language Disorders, 30*(4), 350–367.

Hotz, G., Helm-Estabrooks, N., Wolf Nelson, N., & Plante, E. (2009). The Pediatric Test of Brain Injury: Development and interpretation. *Topics in Language Disorders, 3*, 207–223.

Howard, P., & Shapiro, S. (2011). Diagnosing and treating mild traumatic brain injury in children. *Advanced Emergency Nursing Journal, 33*(4), 274–278.

Isaki, E., Spaulding, T., & Plante, E. (2008). Contributions of language and memory demands to verbal memory performance in language-learning disabilities. *Journal of Communication Disorders, 41*, 512–530.

Jankowitz, B., & Adelson, P. (2006). *Developmental Neuropsychology, 28*, 264–275. doi:10.1159/00094153

Jennett, B., & Teasdale, G. (1981). *Management of severe head injuries*. Philadelphia, PA: F. A. Davis.

Kaufman, B., & Dacey, R. (1994). Acute care management of closed head injury in childhood. *Pediatric Annals, 23*(1), 18–27.

Keenan, H., & Bratton, S. (2006). Epidemiology and outcomes of pediatric traumatic brain injury. *Developmental Neuropsychology, 28*, 256–263. doi:10.1159/000094152

Lajiness-O'Neill, R., Erodi, L., & Bigler, E. (2010). Memory and learning in pediatric traumatic brain injury: A review and examination of moderators of outcome. *Applied Neuropsychology, 17*, 83–92. doi:10.1080/09084281003708837

Lewis, F., & Murdoch, B. (2011). Language function in a child following mild traumatic brain injury: Evidence from pre and post injury testing. *Developmental Neuropsychology, 14*(6), 348–354.

Liesemer, K., Bratton, S., Zebrack, C., Brockmeyer, D., & Statler, K. (2011). Early posttraumatic seizures in moderate to severe pediatric traumatic brain injury: Rates, risk factors, and clinical features. *Journal of Neurotrauma, 28*, 755–762. doi:10.1089/neu.2010.1518

Lovell, M., Collins, M., & Maroon, J. (2002). ImPACT: The best approach to concussion management, user's manual (Version 2.1) [Computer software and manual]. Pittsburgh, PA: ImPACT.

Malkmus, D. (1982, August). *Levels of cognitive functioning and associated linguistic behaviors*. Paper presented at Models and Techniques of Cognitive Rehabilitation, London, UK.

Mandalis, A., Kinsella, G., Ong, B., & Anderson, V. (2007). Working memory and new learning following pediatric traumatic brain injury. *Developmental Neuropsychology, 32*(2), 638–701. doi:10.1080/87565640701376045

Martin, C., & Falcone, R. (2008). Pediatric traumatic brain injury: An update of research to understand and improve outcomes. *Current Opinion in Pediatrics, 20*, 294–299.

McCarthy, M., MacKenzie, E., Durbin, D., Aitken, M., Jaffe, K., Paidas, C., . . . CHAT Study Group. (2005). The Pediatric Quality of Life Inventory: An evaluation of its reliability and validity for children with traumatic brain injury. *Archives of Physical Medicine Rehabilitation, 86*, 1901–1909. doi:10.1016/j.apmr.2005.03.026

McCrea, M. (2008). *Mild traumatic brain injury and postconcussion syndrome*. New York, NY: Oxford University Press.

McCrory, P., Meeuwisse, W., Johnston, K., Dvorak, J., Aubry, M., Molloy, M., . . . Cantu, R. (2009). Consensus statement on concussion in sport. The 3rd International Conference on Sport. *British Journal of Sports Medicine, 43*, i76–i84.

Minear, M., & Shah, P. (2006). Sources of working memory deficits in children and possibilities for remediation. In S. E. Pickering & G. D. Phye (Eds.), *Working memory and education* (pp. 273–297). Mahwah, NJ: Erlbaum.

Montgomery, J., Magimairaj, B., & Finney, M. (2010). Working memory and specific language impairment: An update on the relation and perspectives on assessment and treatment. *American Journal of Speech Language Pathology, 19*, 78–94.

Moreau, T. (2010). Assessment of traumatic brain injury. *Journal of the American Academy of Physician Assistants, 23*(11), 20–23.

Morgan, A., Mageandran, S., & Mei, C. (2009). Incidence and clinical presentation of dysarthria and dysphagia in the acute setting following pediatric traumatic brain injury. *Childcare, Health, and Development, 36*(1), 44–53. doi:10.1111/j.1365-2214.2009.00961.x

Morgan, A., Ward, E., & Murdoch, B. (2004). Clinical progression and outcome of dysphagia following pediatric traumatic brain injury: A prospective study. *Brain Injury, 18*, 359–376.

Morgan, A., Ward, E., Murdoch, B., Kennedy, B., & Murison, R. (2003). Incidence, characteristics and predictive factors for dysphagia after pediatric traumatic brain injury. *Journal of Head Trauma Rehabilitation, 18*, 239–251.

Ornstein, T., Levin, H., Chen, S., Hanten, G., Ewing-Cobbs, L., Dennis, M., . . . Schacher, R. (2009). Performance monitoring in children following traumatic brain injury. *The Journal of Child Psychology and Psychiatry, 50*(4), 506–513. doi:10.1111/j.1469-7610.2008.01997.x

Phelps-Terasaki, D., & Phelps-Gunn, T. (2007). *Test of Pragmatic Language* (2nd ed.). Austin, TX: Pro-Ed.

Porter, R., & Kaplan, J. (2011). *The Merck Manual* (19th ed., pp. 318–322). Whitehouse, NJ: Merck Sharp & Dohme.

Roscigno, C., & Swanson, K. (2011). Parents' experiences following children's moderate to severe traumatic brain injury: A clash of cultures. *Qualitative Health Research, 21*(10), 1413–1426. doi:10.1177/1049732311310988

Russell, N. K. (1993). Educational considerations in traumatic brain injury. *Language, Speech, and Hearing Services in Schools, 24*, 67–75. doi:10.1044/0161-1461.2402.67

Savage, R., DePompei, R., Tyler, J., & Lash, M. (2005). Pediatric traumatic brain injury: A review of pertinent issues. *Pediatric Rehabilitation, 8*(2), 92–103.

Savage, R., & Wolcott, G. (1999). *An educator's manual: What educators need to know about students with brain injury.* Washington, DC: Brain Injury Association.

Schoenbrodt, L. (2001). How TBI affects speech and language. In L. Schoenbrodt (Ed.), *Chil-*

dren with traumatic brain injury (pp. 177–204). Bethesda, MD: Woodbine House.

Schoenbrodt, L., & Smith, R. (1995). *Communication disorders and interventions in low incidence pediatric populations.* Clifton Park, NY: Delmar Learning.

Schrief, L., Donald, K., & Thomas, K. (2011). Cognitive and behavioral outcomes after traumatic brain injury in children. *Continuing Medical Education, 29*(4), 160–161.

Semel, E., Wiig, E. H., & Secord, W. A. (2013). *Clinical Evaluation of Language Fundamentals* (5th ed.). San Antonio, TX: Pearson.

Sesma, H., Slomine, B., Ding, R., & McCarthy, M. (2008). Executive functioning in the first year after pediatric traumatic brain injury. *Pediatrics, 121*, 1686–1695. doi:10.1542/peds .2007-2461

Slomine, B., Eikenberg, J., Salorio, C., Suskaurer, S., Trovato, M., & Christensen, J. (2008). Preliminary evaluation of the cognitive and linguistic scale: A measure to assess recovery in inpatient rehabilitation following pediatric brain injury. *Journal of Head Trauma Rehabilitation, 23*(5), 286–293.

Slomine, B., Salorio, C., Grados, M., Vasa, J., Christensen, J., & Gerring, J. (2005). Differences in attention, executive functioning, and memory in children with and without ADHD after severe traumatic brain injury. *Journal of the International Neuropsychological Society, 11*, 645–653. doi:10.1017/s1355617705050769

Sohlberg, M., & Mateer, C. (2001). *Cognitive rehabilitation: An integrative neuropsychological approach.* New York, NY: Guilford Press.

Stein, N., & Glenn, C. (1979). An analysis of story comprehension in elementary school children. In R. O. Freedle (Ed.), *New directions in discourse processing* (pp. 53–120). Norwood, NJ: Ablex.

Stein, N., & Glenn, C. (1982). Children's concept of time: The development of a story schema. In W. Friedman (Ed.), *The developmental psychology of time* (pp. 255–282). New York, NY: Academic Press.

Sullivan, J., & Riccio, C. (2010). Language functioning and deficits following pediatric traumatic brain injury. *Applied Neuropsychology, 17*, 93–98. doi:10.1080/09084281003708852

Suskauer, S., & Huisman, T. (2009). Neuroimaging in pediatric traumatic brain injury: Current and future predictors of functional outcome. *Developmental Disabilities Research Reviews, 15*, 117–123. doi:10.1002/ddrr.62

Suskauer, S. J., Christensen, J. R., DeMatt, E., Kramer, M., Salorio, C. F., & Slomine, B., & Trovato, M. (2011). Poster 373 predicting outcome for children with traumatic brain injury admitted to inpatient rehabilitation with total functional dependence: Test operating characteristics. *American Academy of Physical Medicine and Rehabilitation, 3*(10, Suppl. 1), S303.

Taylor, H., Swartwout, M., Yeates, K., Chertkoff Walz, N., Stancin, T., & Wade, S. (2008). Traumatic brain injury in young children: Postacute effects on cognitive and school readiness skills. *Journal of the International Neuropsychological Society, 14*, 734–745. doi:10.1017/S1355617708081150

Trudeau, N., Poulin-Dubois, D., & Joanette, Y. (2000). Language development following brain injury in early childhood: A longitudinal case study. *International Journal of Language and Communication Disorders, 35*(2), 227–249.

Vitorino, J. (2009). Laryngeal function: A comparative analysis between children and adults subsequent to traumatic brain injury. *Journal of Head Trauma Rehabilitation, 24*(5), 374–383.

Vu, J., Babikian, T., & Asarnow, R. (2011). Academic and language outcomes in children after traumatic brain injury: A meta-analysis. *Council for Exceptional Children, 77*(3), 262–281.

Wade, S., Michaud, L., & Maines Brown, T. (2006). Putting the pieces together. *Journal of Head Trauma Rehabilitation, 21*(1), 57–67.

Wagner, R. K., Torgesen, J. K., & Rashotte, C. A. (1999). *Comprehensive Test of Phonological Processing.* Austin, TX: Pro-Ed.

Wechsler, D. (2003). *Wechsler Intelligence Scale for Children-Fourth Edition.* San Antonio, TX: Psychological Corporation.

Wiig, E. H., & Secord, W. (1989). *Test of Language Competence–Expanded edition.* San Antonio, TX: Psychological Corporation.

Williams, K. T. (2007). *Expressive Vocabulary Test* (2nd ed.). Minneapolis, MN: Pearson.

Woodcock, R. W., McGrew, K. S., & Mather, N. (2001). *Woodcock-Johnson III Tests of Achievement.* Itsasca, IL: Riverside.

Yeates, K., Swift, E., Taylor, H., Wade, S., Drotar, D., Stancin, T., . . . Minich, N. (2004). Short- and long-term social outcomes following traumatic brain injury. *Journal of the International Neuropsychological Society, 10*, 412–426. doi:10.1017/S1355617704103093

Ylvisaker, M., & DeBonis, D. (2000). Executive function impairment in adolescence: TBI and ADHD. *Topics in Language Disorders, 20*(2), 29–57.

Ylvisaker, M., & Goebbel, E. (1987). *Community re-entry for head injured adults.* Boston, MA: Little Brown.

Ylvisaker, M., Szekeres, S., Henry, K., Sullivan, D., & Wheeler, P. (1987). Topics in cognitive rehabilitation. In M. Ylvisaker (Ed.), *Communication for head injured adults.* Austin, TX: Pro-Ed.

Ylvisaker, M., Turkstra, L., & Coelho, C. (2005). Behavioral and social interventions for individuals with traumatic brain injury: A summary of the research with clinical implications. *Seminars in Speech & Language, 26*(4), 256–267.

Ylvisavaker, M., Urbanczyk, B., & Feeney, T. (1992). Social skills following traumatic brain injury. *Seminars in Speech and Language, 13*, 308–321.

PART IV

Disorders Secondary to Environmental Factors

CHAPTER 7

Fetal Alcohol Spectrum Disorders

Brianne Higgins Roos

Chapter Objectives

Upon completing this chapter, the reader should be able to:

1. Define fetal alcohol spectrum disorders
2. Describe how alcohol affects a fetus
3. Identify factors that lead to a diagnosis of FASD
4. Explain the communication characteristics of children with FASD
5. Describe appropriate communication intervention strategies for children with FASD
6. Understand the "whole child" by integrating parents and teachers into the intervention plan

Introduction

Fetal alcohol syndrome (FAS) is a congenital syndrome caused by maternal consumption of alcohol during pregnancy. Alcohol is a teratogen, or an agent that can cause birth defects, and fetal exposure to alcohol is considered the leading cause of preventable developmental dis-

abilities in the United States. Current estimates of prevalence of fetal alcohol syndrome range from 2 to 7 cases per 1,000 live births in the United States; however the number of children who are exposed to alcohol in utero but are not diagnosed with FAS could be 2% to 5% of the population (May et al., 2009).

FAS is a worldwide health concern that has been documented for centuries. The first published report about the syndrome was in 1973 by Jones and Smith; however, speculation exists about biblical references and whether the ancient Greeks and Romans understood the dangers of prenatal alcohol exposure (Abel, 1999). The historic appreciation for FAS in the Middle East and Europe is now secondary to its modern-day prevalence in countries like Italy and Croatia, as well as on the continent of Africa (Riley, Infante, & Warren, 2011). South Africa has the highest reported rate of FAS in the world, with an estimated 68.0 to 90.2 per 1,000 live births (May et al., 2007). Regardless of the nationality of the child, prenatal alcohol exposure can cause permanent disabilities that will negatively impact the child's ability to learn in school and function in society.

The effects of alcohol on a fetus range in both scope and severity because there are so many variables that surround maternal drinking. The patterns of alcohol use, including the types and quantities of alcohol consumed, and when in the course of the pregnancy the fetus was exposed, all influence the effects on the developing brain of the fetus (Lebel, Roussotte, & Sowell, 2011; Riley et al., 2011). The physical stature, general health, nutrition, and metabolism of the mother also influence the nature of exposure for the fetus (Riley et al., 2011). These variables are challenging for researchers to measure, however the devastating lifelong effects of prenatal alcohol exposure are clear (May & Gossage, 2011). Growth retardation, facial dysmorphology, and central nervous system (CNS) dysfunction are the defining criteria of a child with FAS.

However, not every child who was exposed to alcohol prenatally is diagnosed with FAS. Those who are most profoundly affected by prenatal alcohol may be diagnosed with FAS; however, there are several terms that were used historically to describe people displaying some (but not all) characteristics of FAS, including: fetal alcohol effects (FAE), partial FAS (PFAS), and alcohol-related neurodevelopmental disorder (ARND) (Aase, Jones, & Clarren, 1995; Kodituwakku, 2010). The term fetal alcohol spectrum disorders (FASD) is now used to encompass these descriptions and to more properly and objectively define the spectrum of disorders related to prenatal alcohol exposure (Astley, 2011).

How Alcohol Affects a Fetus

When a pregnant woman ingests alcohol, it passes to her unborn baby. Alcohol is introduced to the womb via the placenta, and affects the developing brain by interrupting neuron inception (i.e., neurogenesis), growth, and movement and can cause neural cell death. Myelination, which facilitates efficient neural transmission, is also negatively affected (Riley et al., 2011). Goodlett, Horn, and Zhou (2005) describe the failure of natural neural development as a "pathogenesis cascade" whose effects are devastating because neurons are the most fundamental component of the brain (p. 395). Neurons facilitate nearly all actions within the body, both volitional and involuntary, and they are supported by glial cells, which are also negatively affected by alcohol exposure (Jones, Leichter, & Lee, 1981; Mukherjee & Hodgen, 1982).

The effects of alcohol on a fetus are not limited to neural impairment. Alcohol reduces umbilical blood flow to the fetus, which causes hypoxia (lack of oxygen) and growth retardation, because nutrition is passed to the fetus via the umbilical cord (Jones et al., 1981; Mukherjee & Hodgen, 1982). Poor fetal nourishment can lead to low birth weight, which is often a characteristic of babies with FASD. Prenatal alcohol exposure also causes a distinctive triad of facial features to develop in some babies. The facial phenotype of FAS includes three characteristics: small palpebral fissures, smooth philtrum, and thin upper lip (Clarren & Smith, 1978). The palpebral fissure is the horizontal opening between the outer (exocanthion) and inner (endocanthion) corners of the eye, which is shorter in people with FAS. The philtrum is the groove between the upper lip and the nose, and that groove is reduced or absent in people with FAS. Just below the philtrum, the upper lip of a person with FAS will be markedly thin (Figure 7–1).

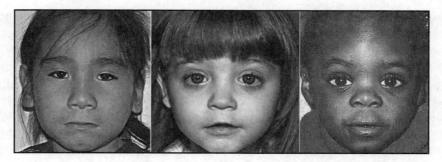

Figure 7–1. Astley's pictures of facial dysmorphology. Copyright 2014, Susan Astley PhD, University of Washington.

Feldman et al. (2012) sought to associate specific facial dysmorphologies in babies with prenatal alcohol exposure, with the time and patterns (i.e., drinks per day, binge episodes, drinks per episode) of alcohol exposure during gestation. They found that alcohol exposure during the second six weeks postconception substantially increases risk of a smooth philtrum, thin vermilion zone, microcephaly, and low birth weight and length. These risks increased even further for every increase of one drink over the average number of daily drinks consumed during those second six weeks postconception. First trimester exposure also negatively affected head circumference (Feldman et al., 2012). Second trimester exposure was associated with smooth philtrum and low birth weight and length, while third trimester exposure was most closely linked with decreased birth length. These observations were made clinically by trained dysmorphologists (Feldman et al., 2012). However, historically, study of the macrostructural neurological effects of fetal alcohol exposure was conducted via autopsy (Lebel, Roussotte, & Sowell, 2011). Current imaging studies such as magnetic resonance imaging (MRI), functional MRI (fMRI), and diffusion tensor imaging (DTI) allow for extensive examination of the structural and functional neurological effects of prenatal alcohol exposure.

Imaging Studies

MRI studies are invaluable for analyzing neurological structures and differences among alcohol-exposed and nonalcohol-exposed people. However, it is important to appreciate the challenges that come with studying the alcohol-exposed population. First, determining the type, amount, and patterns of maternal alcohol use is difficult (Lebel et al., 2011). Secondly, mothers who ingest alcohol during pregnancy often partake in other substances as well, such as marijuana, tobacco, and opiates (Shor, Nulman, Kulaga, & Koren, 2009). Finally, people with fetal alcohol exposure are often diagnosed with other disorders that may affect neurological structure and function, like attention deficit hyperactivity disorder (ADHD) or oppositional defiant disorder (O'Conner & Paley, 2009). Therefore, identifying prenatal alcohol exposure as the etiology of specific neurological differences is difficult, however finer discrimination among research subjects and more detailed diagnostic criteria can alleviate some of the complicating factors.

Several research studies reveal consistent results of MRI studies of the brains of alcohol-exposed and nonalcohol-exposed people. Lebel et al. (2011) completed a review of these studies and reported that small cerebral and cerebellar volumes, as well as reduced white and gray matter, are the predominant consistent findings for alcohol-exposed individuals. The frontal, parietal, and temporal lobes and cerebellum are typically smaller (with the frontal lobe most affected), and the occipital lobe is largely spared (Lebel et al., 2011). The brains of people with FASD typically consist of less white and gray matter, even when adjusted for the smaller brain size (Archibald et al., 2001; Li et al., 2008). The caudate nucleus, hippocampus, and basal ganglia are examples of deep gray matter structures that are reduced in size secondary to prenatal alcohol exposure (Astley, Aylward, et al., 2009; Lebel et al., 2011).

The impacts of a smaller brain and reduced gray matter are significant, and the teratogenic effect of prenatal alcohol exposure on white matter is considerable as well. Myelin is the substance that coats the axons of neurons and is white in color, and one of its primary functions is to facilitate efficient neuronal transmission. Myelination is important for sensory and motor actions, as well as higher-level cognitive functions such as executive functioning, attention, processing time and motor skills.

Myelination of neurons within the cerebrum occurs extensively from the prenatal phase through age 2, at which point the process continues at a slower pace into adulthood (Holland, Haas, Norman, Brant-Zawadzki, & Newton, 1986). Commissural fibers are myelinated first (i.e., prenatally), followed by association and projection fibers (Wozniak & Muetzel, 2011).

The corpus callosum, a major white matter commissural tract that connects the left and right hemispheres of the brain, is also widely reported to be negatively affected by prenatal alcohol exposure (Astley, Aylward, et al., 2009; Dodge et al., 2009; Wozniak et al., 2011; Wozniak & Muetzel, 2011; Wozniak et al., 2009). Effects can range from complete agenesis, or absence, to structural abnormalities (Wozniak et al., 2011). MRI studies reveal macrostructural abnormalities of the corpus callosum, whereas DTI shows microstructural changes by examining the white matter at a microscopic level (Wozniak & Muetzel, 2011). Several studies utilized DTI to look at the corpus callosum specifically, and revealed abnormalities in the posterior portion of the fiber tract, which connects the posterior temporal and inferior parietal regions of the brain (Sowell et al., 2008; Wozniak et al., 2009). One study reports children with FASD have 12% lower interhemispheric functional connectivity via the corpus callosum than their nonexposed peers (Wozniak et al., 2011).

In order to more specifically define the neurological effects of alcohol on the developing brain, Astley, Richards, et al. (2009) conducted a comprehensive magnetic resonance study of three groups of subjects who had varying degrees of FASD, as well as one group of nonalcohol-exposed controls. The first group had a diagnosis of FAS or partial FAS. The second group had a diagnosis of static encephalopathy/alcohol exposed. The third group had a diagnosis of neurobehavioral disorder/alcohol exposed, and the fourth group was a control group with no reported alcohol exposure. All diagnoses were made based on the four-digit scale (Astley, Richards, et al., 2009).

The results of the study found clear neuroimaging distinctions between children in the first three groups, who were within the spectrum of FASD. For example, the frontal lobe and caudate nucleus are much smaller in people who are more severe on the spectrum (i.e., those with facial dysmorphology). Choline concentration, which shows the stability of a cell membrane and myelination, was also lower in the frontal and parietal lobes of people with prenatal exposure (Astley, Richards, et al., 2009). Additionally, fMRI results showed that neuroactivation during a difficult memory task decreased as the subjects' FASD severity increased. Such comprehensive results are important for diagnostic purposes, because the neuropsychological assessment results alone were similar in magnitude of impairment (although different in specific areas of deficit) among the three groups of subjects with FASD. Therefore, magnetic resonance studies could be an important diagnostic tool to specifically define the level of FASD, and ultimately contribute to an accurate diagnosis and appropriate intervention (Astley, Richards, et al., 2009).

Linking Structure and Function

Associating anatomical and physiological differences with functional outcomes is essential to make research clinically relevant. For example, corpus callosum shape appears to be related to motor and executive function deficits in children with FASD (Bookstein, Streissguth, Sampson, Connor, & Barr, 2002), whereas the microstructural abnormalities revealed by DTI appear to correlate with visual-motor difficulties (Sowell et al., 2008). Additionally, cortical thickening was appreciated via MRI in the parietal and posterior temporal regions of the brain, which is associated with poorer language functioning (Sowell et al., 2007).

Once definitive links between structural differences and clinical outcomes are established, imaging can play a greater part in diagnosing FASD. Because the signs of CNS dysfunction associated with prenatal alcohol exposure are not typically detectable until a child enters school, an imaging study earlier in life that reveals structural abnormalities consistent with FASD could prompt a myriad of beneficial services for the child and family. Medical and social support and education, as well as skilled early intervention therapy can help children with FASD and their families learn to adapt to different learning and behavioral styles. However, a diagnosis of FASD must be made prior to the provision of services.

Diagnostic Criteria

Recognizing and diagnosing FASD is an ongoing challenge for families and clinicians alike. Given the multifaceted effects FASD can have on a child, early assessment and diagnosis is critical to be sure the child is provided with appropriate intervention services from an early age. An early diagnosis, followed by specific intervention and coupled with education and family support, can help children with FASD to avoid adverse life outcomes such as trouble in school and with the law, confinement in an inpatient facility such as jail or a psychiatric unit, sexual misconduct, and alcohol and drug problems of their own (Streissguth et al., 2004). Despite the importance of early diagnosis, identifying FASD is not necessarily clear-cut.

Many characteristics of FASD overlap with other disorders like attention deficit hyperactivity disorder (ADHD) and less commonly, oppositional defiant (ODD) and conduct disorders (CD) (Disney, Iacono, McGue, Tully, & Legrand, 2008). Research indicates that although there are many similarities between the behavioral manifestations of FASD and ADHD in particular, they are *not* the same and intervention should not be identical. Although children with FASD present with behaviors that are similar to those exhibited by someone with ADHD, they should not necessarily be treated with the same behavioral and/or pharmaceutical techniques. In order to be sure children receive the appropriate interventions, they must first have the correct diagnosis.

DSM-5

Diagnosing FASD is a multifaceted process because the disorder affects several areas of growth and development to varying degrees in each child, and its etiology is maternal consumption of alcohol during pregnancy, which can be challenging to quantify. However, the importance of diagnosing FASD is clear and recognized by the *Diagnostic and Statistical Manual of Mental Disorders–Fifth Edition* (DSM-5) (American Psychiatric Association, 2013). FASD, which is named Neurobehavioral Disorder Associated with Prenatal Alcohol Exposure (ND-PAE) in the DSM-5, is included as a Condition for Further Study. ND-PAE does not have a diagnostic code in the DSM-5. However there are proposed diagnostic criteria with additional supporting information regarding prevalence, development and course, suicide risk, associated features, functional consequences, differential diagnosis, and comorbidity (American Psychological

Association, 2013). One striking difference between the diagnostic criteria in the DSM-5 and the criteria that are used in clinical practice is the absence of physical characteristics (i.e., growth retardation and facial dysmorphology) as diagnostically relevant factors in the DSM-5.

The physical features of ND-PAE may be the most clearly identifiable signs of the disorder at an early age. Although a child may display these distinctive facial characteristics, the DSM-5 suggests diagnosis is often deferred until a child is at least 3 years old. The DSM-5 focuses on impairment in neurocognitive, self-regulation and adaptive function domains for diagnosis of ND-PAE, and these areas are more easily assessed and recognized in children who are at least preschool, if not school-aged (American Psychological Association, 2013). In addition to the neurobehavioral characteristics, the first proposed diagnostic criterion is "More than minimal exposure to alcohol during gestation, including prior to pregnancy recognition. Confirmation of gestational exposure to alcohol may be obtained from maternal self-report of alcohol use in pregnancy, medical or other records, or clinical observation" (American Psychological Association, 2013, p. 798). Required confirmation of prenatal alcohol exposure is another distinction between the DSM-5 and the widely used 4-Digit Diagnostic Code by Astley (2004). However, in the absence of growth retardation and facial dysmorphology as diagnostic criteria, confirmation of alcohol exposure is essential for differential diagnosis from other neurobehavioral and genetic disorders. The DSM-5 does not discount the importance of the distinctive facial dysmorphology features entirely, because a clinical diagnosis of FAS (which is dependent on the presence of facial dysmorphology to some degree) does fall under the ND-PAE umbrella term (American Psychological Association, 2013).

Inclusion of FASD in the DSM-5 is an acknowledgment of the importance of accurate diagnosis of the disorder, and comes after hard work from advocacy groups such as the National Organization on Fetal Alcohol Syndrome (NOFAS). NOFAS and other groups worked together to communicate the legitimacy of FASD by referencing research that carefully defines its characteristics and effects, as well as how it differs from other disorders. Advocates believe that the absence of FASD in the DSM results in underdiagnosis, and therefore improper treatment (medical and/or behavioral) for children with FASD (Rich, 2012). Additionally, practitioners cannot necessarily be reimbursed for their services without certain billing codes, which are often based on diagnostic criteria listed in the DSM, which could limit availability of services to people with FASD.

The underdiagnosis of FASD causes a domino effect: the lack of diagnosis results in perceived limited prevalence of FASD, and subsequently fewer resources to promote education and social awareness to at-risk populations (Astley & Clarren, 2000). Because people are not necessarily aware of the dangers of drinking alcohol during pregnancy, the incidence of FASD is perpetuated. However, if FASD was diagnosed appropriately, the disorder would be more commonly known and preventative education could become widely funded and available.

Varying diagnostic criteria for FASD have been proposed over the years. Within the past 20 years, The Institute of Medicine (IOM) published guidelines for diagnosis that served as the foundation from which current diagnostic techniques were developed. However, researchers within the field of FASD, specifically out of the University of Washington FAS Diagnostic & Prevention Network (FAS DPN), challenged the level of detail in the IOM report defining both the physical characteristics of FASD (Astley & Clarren, 2000) as well as the neurobehavioral components of the disorder (Astley, 2011). The dysmorphic facial features of a person with FASD are unique to FASD; however, the severity of these features varies significantly and are not necessarily overt enough to confirm a diagnosis (Astley & Clarren, 2000). Emerging neuroimaging research is moving in the direction of identifying specific neurological characteristics unique to FASD, which would help to objectify the diagnostic process (Astley, Olson, et al., 2009). In the interim though, other criteria must exist to make a definitive diagnosis. These other criteria are deficiencies in the areas of growth, central nervous system damage (which can manifest as behavioral/social/learning challenges), and prenatal exposure to alcohol (Astley & Clarren, 2000).

Confirmation of prenatal alcohol exposure can be difficult or impossible to obtain. Many children with FASD do not live with their biological mothers. In addition, their mothers may be unwilling to admit to drinking alcohol while pregnant. If a mother does report alcohol consumption, many subsequent questions are raised. How much did she drink? How often did she drink? What did she drink? The subjectivity of maternal consumption of alcohol during pregnancy is clear, and although this information is important and useful in differential diagnosis, it cannot be relied upon exclusively.

4-Digit Diagnostic Code

In the absence of existing clear and definitive diagnostic criteria, Astley (2004) developed the third edition of a specific, user-friendly 4-Digit Diagnostic Code that is based on the presence and severity of growth deficiency, FAS facial phenotype, central nervous system dysfunction, and prenatal alcohol exposure. Each of the four areas are scored using a four-point Likert scale, where a score of one represents absence of the FASD characteristic and a score of four represents strong presence of the particular characteristic (Astley, 2004). The code and accompanying grid (Table 7–1) were designed for use by a range of specially trained professionals who care for people of all ages with FASD, such as physicians, therapists, and family advocates (Astley, 2004).

Astley (2004) recognized the importance of a diagnostic team approach in assessing people with possible FASD. The effects of FASD are broad, and in order for the most accurate diagnosis to be made, specialists in each of the affected areas should be consulted (Astley, 2011).

Speech-language pathologists may work alongside occupational therapists, whose reports will be taken into consideration along with the input from physicians and possibly psychologists and social workers (Astley, 2011). However, in areas where all of these specialists are not available, the 4-Digit Diagnostic Code can be used by one professional who is trained to administer the battery of subtests (Astley, 2011).

The first area that is assessed using the 4-Digit Diagnostic Code is growth deficiency. This is a straightforward measurement of height and weight, which is analyzed against gender and age-matched norms. If medical history and prior growth measurements are available, these are plotted as well and the practitioner can assess the trend. The growth deficiency is given a score based on whether the person falls ≤3rd percentile, >3rd and ≤10th percentile, or >10th percentile. The score, which is a combination of height- and weight-specific percentiles, is then converted into a number or "rank" of 1 to 4, which is used in the overall 4-Digit Diagnostic Code calculation (Astley, 2004).

Table 7–1. 4-Digit Diagnostic Code Grid

Significant	Severe	Definite	4					4	High risk
Moderate	Moderate	Probable	3					3	Some risk
Mild	Mild	Possible	2					2	Unknown
None	None	Unlikely	1					1	No Risk
Growth Deficiency	FAS Facial Features	CNS Damage	Growth	Face	CNS	Alcohol			Prenatal Alcohol

Note. The FASD 4-Digit Diagnostic Code Grid. Copyright 2014. Susan Astley PhD University of Washington.

Whereas growth deficiency is objective and easily determined using this method, assessing the presence of the facial phenotype of FAS is a more involved process. The presence of a short palpebral fissure, smooth philtrum, and thin upper lip can be evaluated in-person or via digital photo, from which measurements are obtained (Astley & Clarren, 1996). A rank of 4 on the scale is given when all three of the facial anomalies are present (Astley, 2011).

The palpebral fissure is the horizontal opening between the outer (exocanthion) and inner (endocanthion) corners of the eye, which is shorter in people with FAS (Figure 7–2). The measurement is considered abnormal if it is two standard deviations below the norm (Astley, 2011). A short palebral fissure length can be easily recognized and is a visually defining physical characteristic of people with FAS. The presence of a smooth philtrum and thin upper lip are also distinguishing facial anomalies in people with FAS. Interestingly, measurements of the philtrum and upper lip depend significantly on the facial expression of the patient at the time of assessment. In order to be measured for the 4-Digit Code, the patient's lips upper and lower lips should be gently closed and he or she should not be smiling (Astley, 2004). Closing lips tightly and smiling can change measurements so drastically

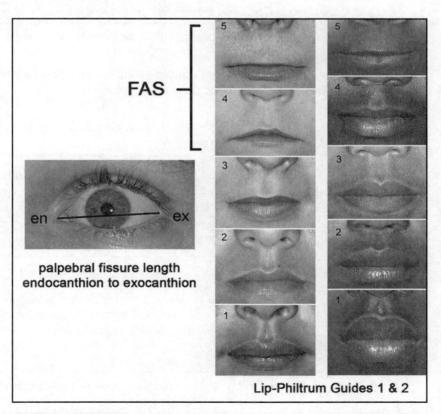

Figure 7–2. Astley's 4-digit diagnostic code grid. Copyright 2014, Susan Astley PhD, University of Washington.

that the patient could be misdiagnosed in the facial anomaly category.

Quantifying and qualifying the presence of central nervous system (CNS) dysfunction, the third of the four areas of assessment within the 4-Digit Code, is not as easy as looking in the mirror or taking measurements. Astley's (2004) description of each rank on the scale of CNS damage is summarized in Table 7–2.

Whether or not a patient is diagnosed with FASD, results from the assessments to determine the level of CNS dysfunction can be used to guide the most appropriate individual treatment plans. In other words, even if children are not assigned a rank of three or four, but they demonstrate difficulty within language and adaptation, that information is clinically valuable regardless of the ultimate diagnosis.

The fourth and final criterion for diagnosis of FASD according to the 4-Digit Code is confirmation of prenatal alcohol exposure. Astley (2004) acknowledges the difficulty of obtaining accurate information within this category. The scale assigns

Table 7–2. Criteria for CNS Ranks 1 Through 4

4-Digit Diagnostic Rank*	Probability of CNS Damage	Confirmatory Findings
4	Definite **Structural and/or Neurological Abnormalities** *Static Encephalopathy*	• Microcephaly: OFC 2 or more SDs below the norm. *and/or* • Significant abnormalities in brain structure of presumed prenatal origin. *and/or* • Evidence of hard neurological findings likely to be of prenatal origin.
3	Probable **Significant Dysfunction** *Static Encephalopathy*	• Significant impairment in three or more domains of brain function such as, but not limited to: cognition, achievement, memory, executive function, motor, language, attention, activity level, neurological "soft" signs.
2	Possible **Mild to Moderate Delay or Dysfunction** *Neurobehavioral Disorder*	• Evidence of delay or dysfunction that suggest the possibility of CNS damage, but data to this point do not permit a Rank 3 classification.
1	Unlikely	• No current evidence of delay or dysfunction likely to reflect CNS damage.

Note. The criteria for CNS Ranks 1 through 4 for the FASD 4-Digit Diagnostic Code. Copyright 2014. Susan Astley PhD University of Washington.

a rank of 4, *high risk* for prenatal alcohol exposure, when alcohol consumption during pregnancy is confirmed and the fetus is considered at high risk according to medical literature (e.g., high alcohol content consumed at least weekly early in pregnancy). A rank of 3, *some risk* for prenatal alcohol exposure, is assigned when alcohol consumption is confirmed, but in amounts less than a rank of 4. If there is *unknown risk* of prenatal alcohol exposure, that is the information is literally unknown or comes from an unreliable source, a rank of 2 is assigned. Finally, if the complete lack of alcohol consumption during pregnancy is confirmed, a rank of 1 is assigned. Given the sensitivity and potential subjectivity of this category, a diagnosis of FAS is still possible even in the absence of confirmed maternal consumption of alcohol during pregnancy.

Results from all four categories are calculated and result in a diagnosis that ranges from "Fetal alcohol syndrome, alcohol exposed" to "No sentinel physical findings or CNS abnormalities detected, no alcohol exposure," and many in between to create the spectrum of disorders abbreviated as FASD (Astley, 2004, p. 47). Just as their places along the FASD spectrum are unique, children with FASD display a range of communication abilities.

Communication Characteristics of Children With FASD

The physical characteristics of children with FAS may be evident at birth or from an early age; however, the extent of speech, language, and cognitive deficits becomes more apparent as a child ages. Literature dating back to 1968 by Lemoine, Harousseau, Borteyru, and Menuet reports that children with FAS exhibit speech and language deficits. More recently, Chasnoff, Wells, Telford, Schmidt, and Messer (2010) examined the differences in neurodevelopmental functioning in children with varying degrees of prenatal alcohol exposure. General intelligence, executive functioning, achievement, memory, adaptive learning skills and behavior were assessed, and children with FAS had significantly worse results than those with less exposure (Chasnoff et al., 2010). Prenatal alcohol exposure does seem to have an effect on communication skills, though the severity varies across domains.

Speech Impairment

The effect of prenatal alcohol exposure on speech has not been examined extensively in the literature, and the few existing studies have small sample sizes. Becker, Warr-Leeper, and Leeper (1990) wrote a widely cited article that compares the speech (i.e., oral motor and articulation) and language skills of eight children with FAS with nonexposed, age-matched peers. Oral motor assessments were conducted, and articulation was judged based on phonological processes and overall severity (Becker et al., 1990). The most notable oral motor characteristics observed in the children with FAS were: presence of class II malocclusion, reduced lingual speed, reduced loudness, and transpositions of vowels within syllables on the verbal apraxia assessment. The articulation assessment revealed impairments in both the FAS and control groups. However, the children with FAS tended to use nasal and labial assimilation more than the nonexposed children (Becker et al., 1990).

Similar to Becker et al. (1990), another study found that 90%, 18 of 20 test subjects, of children with FAS demonstrated disordered speech (Church, Eldis, Blakley, & Bawle, 1997). However, the children presented with a range of different speech deficits, such as dysfluency, cluttering, poor lingual coordination resulting in decreased intelligibility, and hypernasality (usually associated with cleft palate). There does not seem to be a characteristic speech pattern exhibited by children with FASD, rather the uniformity lies in the general presence of some disordered speech. Perhaps the varying speech patterns result from different etiologies, such as craniofacial structural differences, oral motor impairment, cognitive deficits, and hearing loss (Church et al., 1997).

Hearing Impairment

Some research indicates that children with FASD have slow auditory maturation, sensorineural hearing loss, and conductive hearing loss, however hearing deficits are not universal in the FASD population and are more common in children who display dysmorphic facial features (Church et al., 2012; Cohen-Kerem, Bar-Oz, Nulman, Papaioannou, & Koren, 2007; Cone-Wesson, 2005). Children with craniofacial abnormalities are prone to hearing loss, however not all children with FASD have dysmorphic facial features (Cohen-Kerem et al., 2007; Cone-Wesson, 2005). Early hearing screenings are important for all children with FASD, because there are discrepancies in the research about prevalence and types of hearing loss within the population. For example, Church et al. (1997) reported that 77% of their test subjects with FAS (17 of 22) had intermittent conductive hearing loss as a result of recurrent otitis media, and 27% (six of 22) had sensorineural hearing loss (SNHL).

Interestingly, their data indicated that the children with FAS in the absence of a cleft palate were just as likely to have SNHL as those children who did have a cleft palate, which underscores the need for early hearing screenings within the FASD population (Church et al., 1997).

Assessment should also include an examination of central auditory processing in children with FASD. Church et al. (1997) found that 100% of their test subjects demonstrated abnormal central auditory processing skills. The children had difficulty discriminating auditory input, which would be detrimental in a busy, noisy environment such as a chaotic home or classroom. Stephen et al. (2012) also found children across the FASD spectrum demonstrated delayed auditory processing. Because of the widespread prevalence, delayed auditory processing could potentially become one of the diagnostic markers within an FASD assessment (Stephen et al., 2012). Early hearing and auditory processing screenings and appropriate intervention services are indicated for all children with FASD, as hearing loss at a young age can negatively impact speech and language development (Cohen- Kerem et al., 2007).

Language Impairment

Early language use is a predictor of future academic success, and language acquisition is generally delayed in children with FASD (deBeer, Kritzinger, & Zsilavecz, 2010; Rossetti, 2001). Evidence of both delayed and disordered language is present in the literature, however the etiology of the language differences is not entirely clear (Aragon et al., 2008; Coggins, Timler, & Olswang, 2007; Thorne, Coggins, Olson, & Astley, 2007). As with so many characteristics of FASD, a combination of both neurological abnormalities related to prenatal alcohol exposure and the unstable environmental and social factors of life experienced by children with FASD are likely contributing factors. Regardless of the specific cause, identification of the language deficits is critical to initiate appropriate intervention.

Wyper and Rasmussen (2011) sought to discern trends of language deficits in children with FASD. They determined that both expressive and receptive language skills are equally impaired as compared to typically developing children in the control group. That is, children with FASD had the same level of difficulty verbally describing pictures (expressive language) as matching pictures to spoken words (receptive language), and both expressive and receptive language skills were deficient compared to typically developing peers (Wyper & Rasmussen, 2011).

Narrative discourse analysis also points to differences in language skills between children with FASD and their typically developing peers. Narrative discourse analysis provides a means to thoroughly assess longer, potentially complex utterances that are more representative of typical language, versus most standardized tests that use yield brief, discrete responses. The results of a narrative discourse study by Thorne et al. (2007) revealed that children with FASD have more difficulty than their typically developing peers using specific versus ambiguous language, as well as differentiating between new and shared information (Thorne et al., 2007). The use of ambiguous nomimal references is commonly found in the language of children with FASD. Ambiguous nominal references occur when the child's introduction or reference to a particular object, concept, or person is unclear. The correlation between nominal reference errors and FASD is so strong, the analysis of nominal reference errors could become part of the diagnostic process for FASD (Thorne et al., 2007; Thorne & Coggins, 2008).

Children with FASD also have difficulty completing letter fluency tasks, wherein they verbally name as many words as possible that begin with a selected letter in one minute (Aragon et al., 2008; Kodituwakku, Adnams, et al., 2006). The task becomes even more difficult because they must remember and abide by three rules: no proper nouns, no variations of words (e.g., jump, jumping, jumped) and no repeating responses. Alcohol-exposed children had more difficulty following the three rules than their typically developing peers (Aragon et al., 2008).

Letter fluency tasks are a strong indicator of reading success and are often conducted in conjunction with category fluency tasks, where the subject names as many items as possible from a given semantic category (e.g., fruits, clothing, colors) (Aragon et al., 2008). Most children have greater success with category fluency than letter fluency, perhaps because they can use visual strategies to name objects within a category (Rasmussen & Bisanz, 2009). For example, if the category is "ice cream flavors" the child can visualize an ice cream shop and name the flavors "seen" in mind. Children with FASD also tend to do better on category naming, however their letter fluency results are markedly more impaired than their nonalcohol-exposed peers (Aragon et al., 2008; Rasmussen & Bisanz, 2009).

Children with FASD tend to have difficulty with specific areas of language depending on their age. For example, younger children with FASD often have more trouble with expressive and receptive vocabulary and word relationships, however they are not impaired in their ability to understand and use common morphological forms (e.g., plurals, possessives) or in sentence comprehension (Wyper & Rasmussen, 2011). Older children struggle significantly with syntax, morphology, and the ability to identify and correct malapropisms, which are words that are used incorrectly, often in a humorous way (Wyper & Rasmussen, 2011).

The conversational demands of an older child require a strong understanding of how language is used, which includes syntax, morphology and the ability to recognize when words are used correctly and incorrectly. For older children, language is not structured in the same way as classroom language might be for young children, where phrases and demands are more simple and predictable. Rather, social conversations among older students require the ability to process and reply to unstructured information quickly (Wyper & Rasmussen, 2011). The direct relationship between the complexity of a task and the difficulty that alcohol-exposed children have completing the task is a recurring theme in every cognitive-linguistic-social skills domain in children with FASD.

Cognitive Impairment

Just as language demands increase as a child ages, the cognitive skills required of an effective communicator, student, and member of society also become more complex. Kodituwakku (2009) reported that children with FASD were able to perform simple cognitive tasks well; however, there was a clear decline when tasks became more difficult. Kodituwakku (2009) suggested that perhaps children

with FASD employ the same strategies to complete all tasks, but those strategies are not sufficient for more involved problems. This concept is known as the ceiling effect.

The ceiling effect is supported by functional magnetic resonance (fMRI) imaging of children with and without FASD (Astley, Aylward, et al., 2009). Both groups of children were given tasks of varying difficulty to complete while their brains were being imaged. Neuronal activation was observed, and both groups of children responded at approximately the same rate to easier tasks, though the control group's responses were more accurate. The rate of response for children with FASD remained the same on a more difficult task, and accuracy decreased further. The control group demonstrated a slower rate of response on the more difficult task, as well as following their own incorrect responses. This suggests an awareness of self-error and an appropriately increased processing time for harder tasks. Children with FASD did not demonstrate awareness of their deficits or distinguish between easy and difficult tasks. Astley, Aylward, et al. (2009) suggested the results of their study provide objective evidence of both neuronal inefficiency and deficiency in children with FASD, and these neuronal differences negatively affect cognition.

Intellectual Functioning

Cognitive competence is generally measured in terms of intelligence quotient (IQ) testing. IQ tests assess a range of cognitive functioning, including attention, reasoning, language and visual perception and construction (Kodituwakku, 2009). Children with FASD tend to earn scores that are lower than age-matched, culturally matched nonexposed peers across intellectual domains (Aragon et al.,

2008; May et al., 2009). May et al. (2009) provided a review of the literature based on the assessment of first grade students in intelligence, development and behavior. Children with FASD scored lower in verbal and nonverbal intelligence, as well as coding, reading, digit span, and decision making than nonexposed controls. The children with FASD also displayed more behavior problems than the control group (May et al., 2009). Data were collected from studies that used assessments such as the Wechsler Intelligence Scale for Children, Wechsler Adaptive Scales of Intelligence, Wide Range Achievement Test, Vineland Adaptive Behavioral Scales, and the Ravens Coloured Progressive Matrices. Ideally, these tests provided objective data to support the intelligence, development, and behavioral characteristics that the first-grade students with FASD demonstrated at home and at school. The results are uniform in that children with FASD perform more poorly than their nonexposed peers. However, what the static scores do not indicate is that the discrepancy between the children with FASD and their nonexposed peers will likely increase as the children age and the cognitive-linguistic demands placed on them become more complex (Aragon et al., 2008; Kodituwakku, Coriale, et al., 2006). One cognitive domain that is problematic for children with FASD from a young age and becomes amplified as they get older is attention.

Attention

Attention is a cognitive domain that is impaired in children with FASD. There is some overlap in children who have FASD and those with attention deficit hyperactivity disorder (ADHD); however, whereas children with FASD and ADHD

may present with clinical similarities, detailed testing reveals subtle differences in the ways the two groups are impaired (Kodituwakku, 2009).

Focus, sustain, encode, and *shift* are four components of attention described by Mirsky, Anthony, Duncan, Ahern, and Kellam (1996) that are examined by Coles et al. (1997) in children with FASD and ADHD. The *focus* (ability to concentrate on a task) and *sustain* (ability to maintain attention) domains were more difficult for children with ADHD than children with FASD (Coles et al., 1997). However, children with FASD had difficulty with *encode* (holding information in ones memory while performing a mental operation on the information) and *shift* (flexibility to change attention from one task to another). Functionally, having trouble with encoding and shifting means that children with FASD tend to have difficulty processing complex information quickly (Kodituwakku, 2009). In other words, their inattention may be directly connected to slow information processing.

If information is presented too quickly, children with FASD might not comprehend the meaning of the message. For instance, if a teacher provides directions for an in-class project and the children with FASD do not understand the directions, they will not complete the project correctly. Perhaps they will avoid the project all together, or complete it improperly, which could be misinterpreted as lack of interest and disregard for schoolwork. However, the etiology of the problem is likely impaired attention, with particular difficulty encoding and shifting information (Coles et al., 1997).

Attention deficits are reported by mothers, teachers and researchers of children with FASD (Kodituwakku, Coriale, et al., 2006). These deficits correlate with behavioral problems that are identified at home and in the classroom across domains like academic performance, self-care, emotional management, and social interaction (Kodituwakku, Coriale, et al., 2006). As a child ages, academic and social demands become increasingly more complex and require immediate processing and the ability to move quickly from one idea to another. As children with FASD grow older, their attention and behavioral skills do not mature at a rate commensurate with the cognitive demands placed on them by their changing environments (Kodituwakku, Coriale, et al., 2006). In a similar way, memory deficits in children with FASD become more apparent when tasks become more difficult (Aragon et al., 2008).

Memory

There are many different types of memory. Working memory is the ability to temporarily store and use new information at the same time (Stuart, n.d.). There are two components of working memory: or auditory (or verbal) and visual-spatial memory. Auditory working memory is the ability to hear, remember, and use new information quickly. If a teacher says "write your name on the first page of the packet, skip page two and complete page three" students must process the meaning of "write your name on the first page" and execute that task. While doing that, they must also remember to skip the second page and then complete the third page. In order to successfully complete this three-step task, students must be able to hear, process, remember, and act at the same time.

Whereas auditory working memory is based on information that is heard, visual-spatial working memory is based on one's ability to envision things like places, figures, patterns and sequences (Stuart, n.d.). A teacher says, "finish your morning work, then choose a book and come to the carpet for quiet reading time." The student must envision the layout of the classroom to successfully transition from sitting at his desk to the library area to select a book and then to the carpet for reading (Stuart, n.d.). This would be especially difficult at the beginning of the school year in a new classroom setting. If visual-spatial memory is impaired and the children are not able to follow the teacher's directions, they may be labeled as having difficulty paying attention. However, the etiology of the deficit could actually be a memory deficit.

Neuronal activity during spatial and nonspatial working memory tasks is markedly different in children with and without FASD, as evidenced by fMRI assessment (Astley, Aylward, et al., 2009). Children across the spectrum of FASD demonstrate aberrant neuronal activation during these tasks, regardless of whether their brain damage is at the microcellular or gross structural level (Astley, Aylward, et al., 2009). Malisza et al. (2012) conducted fMRI assessments of children with FASD (specifically ARND, not full FAS) and children with ADHD. Both groups completed spatial working memory tasks and their results were impaired in comparison to typically developing (TD) controls. However, the neurological processing varied between the FASD and ADHD groups. White matter structure and function differed in the children with FASD versus both the ADHD and control groups. Children with FASD were noted to have fewer white matter fibers and their white matter has a smaller volume than that of the TD group (Malisza et al., 2012)

Additionally, areas of cortical activation during spatial working memory tasks were distinct for children with FASD. Generally, cortical activation was weaker for the FASD group as compared to the ADHD and TD groups. However, increased activity in the frontal and parietal lobes was noted, and that activity was associated with decreased accuracy on the memory tasks. The FASD group also demonstrated a greater increase in response time for difficult tasks than the ADHD and TD groups, perhaps suggesting the need for increased time for neurological compensation to complete more challenging tasks (Malisza et al., 2012). There was also an appreciable lack of cortical activation in the occipital lobes of the FASD group during both simple and complex tasks. Accuracy was not impacted on the simple task; however, the FASD group's results were significantly worse on the more difficult task that required visual-spatial processing (Malisza et al., 2012). The objective data describing neurological distinctions between children with FASD and children with ADHD support the functional cognitive differences between the two groups at home and in school.

Another comparison between children with FASD and children with ADHD examined memory and verbal language skills (Croker, Vaurio, Riley, & Mattson, 2011). Although both groups were impaired in memory and verbal language compared to the typically developing controls, specific areas of cognitive deficits were distinguished for children with FASD versus ADHD. The study was conducted using the California Verbal Language Test-Children's Version (CVLT-C; Delis et al., 1994, as cited in Crocker, Vaurio, Riley, & Mattson, 2011), among other tests.

The CVLT-C is based on two lists of 15 words from three semantic categories, and the child completes initial learning trials, immediate recall, free and cued delayed recall (20-minute delay) and a delayed (20 minutes) yes/no recognition task using the two lists. Children with FASD demonstrated more difficulty on the initial learning and long-delay free recall tasks than children with ADHD, and both groups performing worse than the control group. However, more specific analysis revealed children with FASD were able to recall information that was previously learned after the long delay. Therefore, while children with FASD do have memory deficits, their lack of initial learning cannot be overlooked. If children are unable to learn information when it is first presented, they will not recall it later. Conversely, children with ADHD appear to learn new information initially, but demonstrate difficulty with recall (Crocker et al., 2011). These results underscore the importance of understanding exactly where the cognitive-linguistic breakdown occurs, so that intervention is focused on the child's specific areas of need. Impairments in both initial learning and memory will affect the broad cognitive domain of executive function (Kodituwakku, 2009).

Executive Function

Kodituwakku (2009) describes executive functioning as "a set of abilities required to attain goals efficiently in nonroutine situations" (p. 219). In order for this to occur, a person must be able to plan one's actions, manage internal and external distractions while executing the plan, change actions if required, and recognize and correct mistakes if necessary (Kodituwakku, 2009). The aforementioned deficits in encoding and shifting attention, memory, and initial learning converge during executive functioning tasks because several cognitive demands are placed on the child with FASD simultaneously.

A card-sorting task was completed by children with FASD and typically developing peers, and revealed the children with FASD had difficulty sorting and describing their own cards and the examiner's cards (Rasmussen & Bisanz, 2009). Impaired card sorting suggested the children with FASD had deficits in several cognitive domains, such as problem solving, flexible thinking, and verbal and spatial concepts.

The challenges of executive functioning occur both at home and in school, according to parents and teachers of children with FASD (Schonfeld, Paley, Frankel, & O'Connor, 2006). The Behavioral Rating Inventory of Executive Functioning (BRIEF) is a survey that assesses a child's abilities in areas such as metacognition, inhibition, shift, emotional control, initiative, working memory, planning, organization of materials, and monitoring (Gioia et al., 2000, as cited in Shonfeld et al., 2006). The results of parent surveys indicated their children with FASD had difficulty with behavior regulation, specifically characterized by the lack of flexibility in different situations. Parents also reported their children with FASD had an inability to regulate their emotions and displayed a general lack of inhibition. On the other hand, teachers reported metacognitive deficits were particularly problematic for their students with FASD. Metacognitive deficits negatively impact students' ability to plan, execute, and self-monitor tasks, which are essential functions in a school setting. Schonfeld et al. (2006) compared the results of the BRIEF to results of the Parent and Teacher forms of the Social Skills Rating System (SSRS) (Gresham & Elliott, 1990, as cited in Shonfeld et al., 2006) to establish a relationship between executive function and social skills in children with FASD.

The SSRS is a survey that measures social skills and behavior in children, as measured by their parents and teachers. The social skills domains include Cooperation, Assertion, Responsibility, and Self-Control. Behavior is broken down into Internalizing and Externalizing Behaviors, as well as Hyperactivity. Schonfeld et al. (2006) reported poor behavioral regulation scores on the parent report of the BRIEF correlated with poor social skills on the SSRS. Similarly, teacher report of impaired metacognition on the BRIEF was predictive of impaired social skills on the SSRS. There appears to be a link between executive function and social skills in children with FASD and the correlation extends across home and school settings (Schonfeld et al., 2006). Interestingly, the degree of executive functioning and social skills impairment was not affected by the severity of the children's diagnosis within the FASD spectrum (e.g., FAS vs. partial FAS), which reinforces that children who do not have full FAS need access to diagnostic and intervention services as well. Children across the spectrum are negatively impacted by deficits in executive functioning, which appear to correlate with impaired social skills.

Social Communication Impairment

Social communication is a broad area that spans both cognition and language. Coggins et al. (2007) reported on the social implications of language impairments in children with FASD and focused specifically on examining the following three areas: language, social cognition, and higher-order executive function.

Language is the way people establish and maintain relationships (Coggins et al., 2007). People use language to both convey and obtain information, and the language deficits experienced by children with FASD negatively impact their ability to participate in basic social exchanges. Although it is clear that children with FASD are often not effective communicators, identifying specific pragmatic deficits is difficult because of the variability of each communicative exchange. Internal variables may include a person's mood, physical well-being, and relationship with the conversational partner. External variables could be location, surroundings, and weather. These overt or subtle changes among communicative interactions should cause communicators to adapt their verbal and nonverbal behaviors quickly and accordingly.

In other words, the communicator has to quickly assess the internal and external variables (initial learning), hold that information in mind and use it to determine the appropriate verbal and nonverbal responses (encoding), understand the conversational partner's reply, and modify the next planned response (shifting). Formulation of an appropriate response is based on combining information about the conversational partner's background knowledge, interests, and opinions with details relevant to the current topic. The communicator must also have an appropriate lexicon to express their understanding of others' feelings and behaviors, and the vocabulary of children with FASD can be lacking (Timler, Olswang, & Coggins, 2005). Children with FASD have difficulty with initial learning, encoding, shifting, memory and vocabulary individually, and effective communication relies on the seamless interaction of attention, memory, executive functioning, and basic pragmatic skills. Consequently, children with FASD tend to be less effective social communicators than their nonexposed peers (Coggins et al., 2007). Children with FASD spent less time in "prosocial/engaged performance and a larger proportion of their time displaying passive/disengaged and irrelevant performances" than their typically developing peers, as explained in a study conducted by Olswang, Svensson, and Astley (2010, p. 1699).

Impaired social cognition and resulting poor social and behavioral skills are significant and wide-reaching deficits for children with FASD (Way & Rojahn, 2012). Maladaptive behaviors like tantrums in young children can transition to disruptive and inappropriate conduct in school, and ultimately to delinquent and unlawful actions as the child with FASD ages (Fast, Conry, & Loock, 1999; Schonfeld, Mattson, & Riley, 2005). Schonfeld et al. (2005) conducted a study that examined moral maturity (i.e., moral judgment and reasoning) and delinquency in children with prenatal alcohol exposure and controls without exposure. The subjects varied in their levels of alcohol exposure and diagnosis along the FASD spectrum (including full FAS) and were given tests to assess moral judgment, cognitive inhibition, delinquency, and conduct. Subjects with prenatal alcohol exposure demonstrated decreased moral judgment and increased delinquency versus the nonexposed controls. A specific correlation between poor moral reasoning regarding "affiliation" and "property and law" was observed in children with FASD. Shonfeld et al. (2005) suggest that early difficulty with socialization (i.e., poor affiliation) and decreased appreciation and respect for property and obeying the law may be precursors of later delinquent behavior. There are a disproportionate number of youth with FASD in the juvenile criminal justice system, as compared to those without an alcohol-related diagnosis (Fast et al., 1999).

Although it is difficult to identify which specific characteristics of children with FASD cause delinquency, poor adaptive behaviors were linked to poor executive functioning in children with FASD and children with ADHD who were not alcohol-exposed (Ware et al., 2012). Both groups scored lower than the typically developing, nonexposed controls, however specific areas of deficit differed for the test groups within the executive functioning assessment, the Delis-Kaplan Executive Function System (Delis et al., 2001, as cited in Ware et al., 2012). The children with FASD had more difficulty with the nonverbal subtests, Design Fluency– Switching and Trail Making Test-Switching, whereas children with ADHD demonstrated difficulty with all executive functioning subtests. Poor adaptive behavior was associated with decreased executive function scores for the test groups with both FASD and ADHD (Ware et al., 2012).

Although the wide range of communication deficits associated with FASD is daunting, early identification can set children with FASD on the right path toward appropriate intervention.

Intervention

Early Intervention

Early intervention (EI) for children with FASD is critical because of the broad range and long-lasting negative effects of prenatal alcohol exposure. The U.S. government recognizes the importance of EI services through several federal regulations, including the Keeping Chil-

dren and Families Safe Act (2003) and the Individuals with Disabilities Education Improvement Act (IDEA) of 2004 (Olson, Jirikowic, Kartin, & Astley, 2007). Once a child is referred and assessed, the resulting diagnosis determines the services that will be provided. A diagnosis of FAS versus FASD may yield different services, depending on the state of residence (Olson et al., 2007). Children with FASD are labeled "at risk" because of imminent future deficits, and they may or may not quality for EI services. Children with FASD who do not receive services are at greater risk for behavioral and academic challenges, and ultimately delinquency and chemical dependency, than children with full FAS who do receive EI services (Streissguth et al., 2004).

Retrospectively, children with FASD are noted to have been irritable infants with difficulty sleeping and feeding (Eyler & Behnke, 1999) and were preschoolers described as mild-moderately inattentive and hyperactive with impulsivity and behavioral problems (Olson et al., 2007). Although these observations are clinically significant via longitudinal study, a fussy infant and active preschooler are not overt indicators of a significant disability. The developmental abnormalities associated with FASD are subtle in the first few years of life, and given the socioeconomic volatility of many families with FASD, may be overshadowed by more urgent environmental needs and issues.

When babies are born into unstable households that are plagued with chemical addiction and subsequent economic and environmental stress, there are negative ramifications. Many of these babies do not receive adequate postnatal medical care (Olson et al., 2007). Postnatal caregiving is very important for babies and their mothers to continue developing the bond that was formed prenatally, and is broken into three steps (Rossetti, 2001). First, babies make their needs known by crying or fussing. Then the mother attempts to meet the baby's needs, and finally the baby responds to that attempt, either by expressing pleasure or discontent. Learning the routine of a baby and his needs is time-consuming and tiring, but the process is critical for a strong mother–baby attachment (Rossetti, 2001).

In a situation where external factors take a mother's time and attention away from her baby, the disrupted attachment may lead to problems down the road. This is especially true for babies with FASD, who are biologically disadvantaged and have a decreased ability to cope with the chaos of their environments, and whose environments are more chaotic than their nonalcohol-exposed peers. The limited ability to cope lends itself to subsequent behavioral problems and even depression in children as young as preschool age (O'Connor & Paley, 2006). However, early recognition and EI services can capitalize on the plasticity of a baby or young child's brain and allow families the opportunity to advocate appropriately to facilitate improved language and coping skills for their children (Streissguth et al., 2004). Close examination of early skills such as an infant's ability to participate in elicited play can reveal clues about fetal alcohol exposure.

Molteno, Jacobson, Carter, and Jacobson (2010) completed a study that associated the quality of infants' elicited play with fetal alcohol exposure. Elicited play is when an infant attempts to imitate the mother (or other caregiver), and is considered the highest level of infant play (Belsky, Garduque, & Hrncir, 1984). Elicited play was negatively affected by living in a suboptimal home environment, how-

ever after controlling for the environmental factors within the study, the effects of prenatal alcohol exposure on elicited play persisted (Molteno et al., 2010). Elicited play is dependent on the quality of toys or other play materials provided for the child, as well as the mother's response to the infant's needs and attempts at imitation (Molteno et al., 2010). If the mother–baby attachment is limited and she does not provide the baby with appropriate feedback during play, the infant's reactions and attempts to imitate will decrease. Longitudinally, poor elicited play was associated with decreased verbal working memory in the children with FAS at 5 years old. Although FASD is rarely diagnosed in infants, Molteno et al. (2010) suggest the assessment of elicited play could become an integral part of the diagnostic process in an effort to diagnose during the EI years.

In the EI years, from birth to 3, the importance of a mother's connection with her child cannot be overstated. Ironically, the mother's drinking during pregnancy is precisely what causes the suboptimal bond when her baby is born with FASD. However, although the negative effects of prenatal alcohol exposure are abundant, identifying and emphasizing a child's strengths is important for both the child and the mother or caregivers (deBeer et al., 2010). Children with FASD are often outgoing and verbal, as well as active and energetic (deBeer et al., 2010). Although these attributes can ultimately lead to inappropriate social behavior, verbosity and hyperactivity, they can also be viewed as strengths and used to help the child and caregivers. When caregivers are knowledgeable about the effects of FASD and can appreciate the strengths of the child, they might feel more empowered to advocate for the child and to obtain additional services as directed by the EI team (Olson et al., 2007).

Speech and language intervention for children with full FAS should focus on parent education and direct interaction with the infant or toddler. Education regarding appropriate infant interaction and language development would focus on the importance of consistent caregiving and environmental safety, as well as reciprocal gaze, focusing on an object, looking around, early vocalizations, and playing with objects (Rosetti, 2001). As the infant grows into a toddler, the SLP will focus on eliciting expressive language, educating the parents on using simple, predictable language when interacting with the child, and teaching linguistic concepts like "in, on, under, through" to enhance receptive language skills.

Children with FASD who are labeled "at risk" benefit from different intervention. These children may not display overt developmental deficits, but are appropriate for preventative services tailored to needs that may arise, as well as maximizing appropriate environmental support and education regarding optimal caregiver/child interaction. For example, Olson et al. (2007) suggest that if a baby or young child presents with poor attachment to his mother, the EI team might work to examine the home setting and offer suggestions to modify and improve the child's surroundings. The caregivers would also be provided with education regarding typical developmental milestones to make them aware of what their baby should do in general timeframes.

Family and caregiver education is an important component of EI services regardless of a child's disability. However, the therapist working with children with FASD must be particularly sensitive to the social stigma and emotional burden associated with the disorder. FASD is preventable, and the effects can be long-lasting and devastating to an individual and family (Olson et al., 2007). Therapists should be trained to conduct an appropriate interview and be prepared for an array of responses from the interviewee, depending on whether that person is a biological parent and if alcohol use is still a part of the person's life. Feelings of guilt, shame, anger, and denial might be expressed. If the interviewee is still chemically dependent, the situation becomes more complicated. Persistent alcohol use might negatively impact parents' understanding of an FASD diagnosis and intervention plan (Olson et al., 2007).

Caregivers and living situations for children with FASD can vary greatly. Many children with FASD are placed in foster homes, which are often temporary. Inconsistent living situations make both the child's life and work of the therapist more complicated. However, a foster placement may outweigh a biological home plagued with addiction, in terms of improving cognition and behavior in children with FASD (Victor, Wozniak, & Chang, 2008). Beyond foster care, some children are adopted, and the adoptive parents may or may not appreciate the range of effects of FASD until the child ages (Olson et al., 2007). Families will require education and support as they try to provide the best home for a child who is difficult to raise. Children who are adopted by family members, called kinship adoptions, may continue to be subject to the influences of alcohol. So although a kinship adoption is ideal in terms of familial bond, the circumstances may be far less than ideal for the child in the presence of ongoing chemical addiction (Olson et al., 2007). The psychological factors associated with perpetual addiction, and guilt about the effects of such destructive behavior on the life of a child, are understandably intense. Therapists should be prepared to deal with these emotions both personally and professionally.

Working as a member of an EI team with children with FASD is a multifaceted job that requires specific training, clinical skills, and personal maturity, because of the complexity of each situation. Despite the challenges, the therapist has a unique opportunity to steer the lives of the one third of children with FASD in the right direction. By providing education and clinical services, children will gain skills and their caregivers will feel equipped to advocate for the children as they grow

out of EI and enter the school system. An important component of the EI team's work is to facilitate the transition into the schools, where the service delivery model is different (Clarren, 2004). See summary of items in Table 7–3.

School-Aged Intervention

The goal of service providers in the school system is inclusion of children with special needs into regular classroom settings when possible and appropriate (Kalberg & Buckley, 2007). In order for children with FASD to be successful in a regular education setting, specifically designed

Table 7–3. Summary of Info Presented and Cited in Chapter

Early Intervention	School-Aged Intervention
General:	**General:**
• Strong postnatal care provided in a safe environment	• Team approach includes students, caregivers, teachers, SLP, OT, PT, psychologist as appropriate
• Consistent caregiver attention to the baby's needs including nutrition, sleep, security	• Establish routines that are followed at home and at school to promote generalization of good behavior and reinforcement
• Establish attachment between caregiver and baby to foster trust and bond through routine	• Focus on caregiver education regarding pragmatic/behavioral effects of FASD
Speech-Language:	**Speech-Language:**
• Caregiver education regarding typical milestones	• Neuroconstructivist and/or domain-specific therapy
• Caregiver encourages baby's reciprocal gaze, visual focus on objects, early vocalizations, play with objects	• Emphasis on pragmatic training, may include social skills groups and self-regulation therapy
• Caregiver models expressive language by using simple, predictable language and reacts to baby's vocalizations	• Impose environment and task structure to activities
	• Executive function, language literacy and math skills are targeted as needed for each student

intervention is imperative. Jirikowic, Gelo, and Astley (2010) completed a summary of interventions recommended after diagnosis of FASD. Some of the services they suggested include medical, educational, developmental therapy (e.g., physical therapy, occupational therapy, speech-language pathology), mental health, social services, and safety-related intervention, among others. Research suggests a variety of successful intervention techniques, and the common conclusion is that the most effective plans involve both parents and children (Bertrand, 2009; Kalberg & Buckley, 2007). The scope of deficits associated with FASD is broad and impacts students and their families at home and in school, so including parents in the carryover of school-based strategies makes sense.

The behavioral challenges that present in infancy and during preschool years persist and become more complicated as a child with FASD gets older. Already frustrated parents become more desperate for effective techniques, and the strategies they use with nonalcohol-exposed children might not work well for children with FASD (Paley & O'Connor, 2009). When intervention focuses on educating parents about why their children misbehave, what to expect, and how to intervene, parents reported they felt less stressed, and their intervention plans for children with FASD became more effective (Bertrand, 2009; Clarren, 2004; Kalberg & Buckley, 2007; Paley & O'Connor, 2009; Schonfeld et al., 2006). Clarren (2004) suggested promoting regular interaction between parents and teachers, in addition to attending scheduled, structured team meetings.

Parents were directly involved in the test group of a social skills study for children with and without prenatal alcohol exposure (O'Connor et al., 2012). The children underwent specialized prag-matic training that addressed skills such as how to participate in conversations, sportsmanship, group dynamics, and bullying. Parents were trained to carry over their children's emerging social skills when they facilitated at-home play dates and helped their children to establish new friendships. Parents reported that selecting good friends was a challenge for their children with FASD. The children tended to gravitate toward people who were welcoming to them, and often those kids were not well-intentioned. The children with FASD did not have the judgment to appreciate they were being duped into manipulative relationships that often end with illegal behaviors (Watson, Hayes, Coons, & Radford-Paz, 2013).

Providing parents with specific strategies to help their children make good social judgments could lead to more healthy relationships and potentially deter children with FASD from illegal behaviors such as drug use, theft, and assault (Watson, Hayes, et al., 2013). Social skills groups were beneficial for children with prenatal alcohol exposure and their parents, as well as nonalcohol-exposed children with psychosocial dysfunction who were treated within the same groups (O'Connor et al., 2012). From a practical standpoint, parent involvement is a logical way to generalize change that begins in a therapy session. Less obvious, however, is how those changes occur neurologically.

Kodituwakku (2010) suggests considering the neuroconstructionist view of effective intervention for children with FASD. The neuroconstructivist hypothesis states that intervention should stimulate neural activity, which leads to neural plasticity, and subsequent changes in neural structures. This new neural circuitry would ideally facilitate greater generalization of intervention techniques (Kodituwakku, 2010). Neural pathways become stronger when used repeatedly, and therefore when interventions target broad areas of deficit like executive function and self-regulation (versus specific domains like math or phonics), the new pathways are reinforced constantly, because these skills are very commonly used (Kodituwakku, 2010).

Self-regulation and executive function skills are also targeted in research that suggests providing structure for children with FASD may help them to compensate for limitations in these skill areas (Kalberg & Buckley, 2007). Offering environmental and task structure can help a child to be more successful by eliminating extraneous distraction and facilitating understanding of the specific task at hand. Environmental structure includes reducing visual distractions like decorations on the walls, and auditory distractions like background hallway noise (Kalberg & Buckley, 2007). Establishing defined places within a classroom for specific work can also be helpful. For example, math is done at the math table, reading is done on the carpet, and current events are discussed by the map. When a classroom is structured in this fashion, a child knows when he is at the math table that he should only be working on math. Children with FASD benefit from the environmental support for behavioral and academic expectations (Kalberg & Buckley, 2007).

Environmental structure is important for the "big picture," and task structure provides extra support for the completion of specific tasks, both of which are helpful for children with FASD. One example of task support is the explicit explanation of directions for each assignment, because children with FASD have difficulty generalizing rules and processes from one task to another (Bertrand, 2009). For example, if a child with FASD writes a three-paragraph essay about his weekend plans on a Friday, he may not know to follow the same guidelines the following Friday, even though the assignment is recurring. The child must be told the expectations of the assignment each time it is presented. Directions should be presented clearly and thoroughly, and the child may benefit from seeing a model of the completed assignment or task. Visual structure could be added by using colors for specific steps of an assignment, or implementing a schedule for the task (Kalberg & Buckley, 2007).

While establishing the best structure for a child with FASD, teachers and therapists should be aware of the child's sensory processing. Many children with FASD have sensory processing differences that affect their ability to interact with the environment. Sensory processing differences can, in turn, lead to increased difficulty with learning and behavior, and deficits are specifically noted with executive function (Franklin, Deitz, Jirikowic, & Astley, 2008; Jirikowic, Olson, & Astley, 2012). Ideally, an occupational therapist (OT) would be on the interdisciplinary team, and would provide suggestions to the other team members regarding managing sensory differences in children with FASD. If an OT is not on the team and sensory differences are suspected, speaking with the other team members and referring out to an OT would most likely be appropriate.

Similarly, the team should be aware of potential motor deficits in children with FASD. Motor impairment could be fine motor, which might be manifested in difficulty writing or stacking blocks. Gross motor impairment would be evident if a child has difficulty walking, tends to fall, or has trouble with games and sports (Clarren, 2004). If impaired motor skills are suspected, the child with FASD should be referred to a physical therapist (PT) for assessment.

PTs, OTs, SLPs, and teachers should all be aware of the potential psychiatric and conditions of neglect associated with FASD. Studies related to the psychopathologies in children prenatally exposed to children were reviewed by O'Connor and Paley (2009) and included conditions such as depression, anxiety, attentional and social problems, mood disorders, suicide threats, binge drinking, drug dependence, and aggressive behavior. If a child with FASD demonstrates any symptoms of a psychiatric condition, a psychology referral is indicated. Similarly, if team members suspect the child might be a victim of neglect, a social work consultation should be pursued by members of the child's interdisciplinary team (Rogers-Adkinson & Stuart, 2007).

When teachers and therapists work together to develop assessment and treatment plans, children with FASD have a greater potential to succeed in school, at home, and out in the community. Additionally, implementation of consistent classroom and therapy routines provides children the opportunity to learn and practice appropriate behaviors repeatedly, which increases the chances for success (Paley & O'Connor, 2009). Utilizing these teaching strategies are ideal for instructing children with FASD. However, taking the time to explain each assignment in fine detail on every occasion it is assigned, providing multiple opportunities for practicing behaviors that typically developing children are able to generalize, and creating schedules for the day and specific tasks can be extremely consuming of teachers' time and attention (Paley & O'Connor, 2009). Therefore, a team approach is beneficial to best serve the children with and without FASD in a classroom. An aide

could help to reinforce behavioral strategies and an SLP could turn a classroom writing assignment into an activity targeting specific language goals. Including additional staff would provide appropriate support for the child with FASD without solely burdening the classroom teacher (Paley & O'Connor, 2009).

In addition to general intervention strategies, domain-specific research also reveals positive results and documents improvement of children with FASD within the areas of language literacy, math, safety, and social skills (Adnams et al., 2007; Bertrand, 2009; O'Connor et al., 2006; Paley & O'Connor, 2009). Children with FASD underwent specific intervention in these domains (within distinct studies) and all demonstrated improvement upon completion of the trials. However, their ability to generalize newly learned skills outside of the therapy session and the long-term efficacy of intervention varied, especially in the absence of follow-up longitudinal studies.

For example, Adnams et al. (2007) examined the effects of specific language-literacy training administered for 30 minutes twice weekly over a 9-month school year for third graders with FASD in South Africa. Their results were positive and the students did improve over that time in targeted skill areas such as phoneme identification, segmentation and blending, and manipulation of syllables and phonemes (Adnams et al., 2007). However, the students did not improve on normed "general scholastic" tests of reading and spelling (Adnams et al., 2007). One would assume that stronger preliteracy skills like phoneme identification, segmentation, and so forth would yield better reading and spelling test results, but this did not occur outside of the specific areas targeted during the study. The decreased ability to generalize knowledge and skills is not surprising, given the neurological basis of the deficits in children with FASD (O'Connor et al., 2006). Despite the practical and neurological challenges, generalization remains the ultimate goal of teachers and therapists working with children with FASD.

Reaching a consensus on the most effective intervention strategies for children and parents affected by FASD is challenging for several reasons. First, because of the broad range and varying degree of deficits experienced by children with FASD, a cognitive-behavioral phenotype for the disorder has not yet been developed (Adnams et al., 2007). Each child presents differently, and the areas of relative strength and deficits vary from one child to another. Additionally, identifying a large group of children with FASD to participate in well-designed, scientifically sound, intervention-based studies is challenging (Adnams et al., 2007; Davis, Gagnier, Moore, & Todorow, 2013). Additional research limitations include the social and environmental variables that often accompany FASD, which inhibit the inclusion of significant number of subjects within studies. Smaller sample sizes can decrease generalizability of results. However, despite the limitations of working with children and families with FASD, research does support the efficacy of intervention and documents improved outcomes for both children with FASD and their parents (Adnams et al., 2007; Bertrand, 2009; Kalberg & Buckley, 2007; Peadon, Rhys-Jones, Bower, & Elliott, 2009).

Caregiver Intervention

Parents and caregivers of children with FASD require support themselves as they live with the omnipresent effects of prenatal alcohol exposure. Watson, Coons, and Hayes (2013) conducted a study comparing the stress of parents of children with FASD to those with autism spectrum disorder (ASD). The Parenting Stress Index–Short Form was administered to parents in both groups, and results indicated that 95% of parents of children with FASD scored at or above the 90th percentile of overall parenting stress. In comparison, 53% of parents of children with ASD scored at or above the 90th percentile of overall parenting stress (Watson, Coons, et al., 2013). Therefore, although parents in both groups report substantial stress, those who have children with FASD are significantly more stressed.

Olson et al. (2009) compiled information about the demands that are placed on families of children with FASD and conducted surveys of parents' unmet needs. The survey results indicated that the greatest need is for parents to have the opportunity to speak with other parents of children with FASD. They also need a sense of hope, provision of respite care, explanation of the cognitive effects of FASD, and suggestions for behavior modification (Olson et al., 2009). Although physicians and therapists who specialize in FASD are equipped to meet some of these needs, the most urgent need is informal, community-based social support.

Olson et al. (2009) suggest several strategies to meet the needs of families of children with FASD. Primarily, access to social support is critical for parents. This support could be in a group setting, or one-on-one in person, by telephone or online. Also, having specific information about the effects of FASD and associated behavioral manifestations as a child ages would be helpful. The efficacy of caregiver intervention administered via information packets, in-person workshops, and

Web-based computer training was compared by Kable, Coles, Strickland, and Taddeo (2012). Parents of children with FASD were assigned to one of the three groups and data were collected based on parent satisfaction, knowledge of the material presented, and parent report of behavioral changes in their children with FASD. Parents were most satisfied with the workshop format, which supports the conclusions drawn by Olson et al. (2009). Both the Web-based and workshop groups improved in knowledge acquired; however, the workshop group reported the most behavioral changes in their children. The Web-based and workshop reported greater satisfaction than the information packet group in all three areas (Kable et al., 2012).

Regardless of the intervention modality, clinicians must consider the strengths and weaknesses of the family, their ability to learn and retain information and the severity of the child's FASD when deciding how to support parents and caregivers (Kable et al., 2012). Because parental support and carryover are critical elements in therapy for children with FASD, it is logical that the parents must feel prepared to take on that role (O'Connor et al., 2012). By improving family life and creating a more stable home environment, families affected by FASD can be better equipped to anticipate behavioral and cognitive differences, manage them as they arise, and feel supported and hopeful through the process.

Prevention

Although intervention strategies such as direct individual and group therapy for children with FASD and support for caregivers are effective, the best way to prevent the negative effects of prenatal alcohol exposure is to avoid exposure entirely. Because there is no safe threshold of alcohol consumption during pregnancy, the most effective prevention of FASD is maternal abstinence from drinking from conception to birth (Feldman et al., 2012). Several recent studies suggest strategies to eradicate maternal consumption of alcohol during pregnancy (Floyd, Weber, Denny, & O'Connor, 2009; Waterman, Pruett, & Caughey, 2013).

The first suggestion is to target medical personnel such as family practitioners and obstetricians/gynecologists. These health care professionals could potentially screen and educate women of reproductive age about the risks of alcohol consumption during pregnancy (Floyd et al., 2009; Waterman et al., 2013). Easy access to preconceptional and prenatal care would be beneficial for women to be educated about the risks of drinking during pregnancy prior to conception and throughout pregnancy. Screening women of reproductive age who drink alcohol could be done prior to medical appointments, or during initial intake, documented on a patient's electronic medical record, and updated routinely (Floyd et al., 2009; Waterman et al., 2013).

Public health awareness about the specific dangers of drinking alcohol during pregnancy is another important component of education. Improving awareness is a current work in progress through organizations such as NOFAS, The National Task Force on Fetal Alcohol Syndrome, the Substance Abuse and Mental Health Services Administration's FASD Center for Excellence, as well as medical groups like the American Academy of Pediatrics and the American College of Obstetricians and Gynecologists (Floyd et al., 2009). Effecting change through legislation and medical policy are formidable goals with potentially far-reaching outcomes.

In a more tangible sense, simple changes to the labels on alcohol containers could promote the dangers of fetal alcohol exposure at the very moment prior to alcohol consumption. The current labels have not changed since 1989. They are small in size and state, "According to the surgeon general, women should not drink alcoholic beverages during pregnancy because of the risk of birth defects." Waterman et al. (2013) suggest the labels might be more effective if they were larger in size, more prominently displayed on containers, provided specific information about the types of birth defects, and contained a picture of a child with FASD. Overall, a comprehensive prevention approach that targets health care providers and their patients, as well as the public at large, seems like a successful formula to reduce (and ideally eliminate) prenatal alcohol exposure and FASD.

Conclusion

Ideally, the comprehensive efforts of physicians, clinicians and legislators will ultimately eradicate prenatal exposure to alcohol and FASD. In the interim though, it is important to pursue research to better understand how alcohol exposure affects a developing fetuses, and how those prenatal changes lead to functional deficits as the baby grows, throughout childhood, and adulthood. Children with FASD and their families need specific education and treatment to identify their strengths and compensate for their weaknesses, which change as they get older. Care should be provided by a team of health care professionals trained in FASD intervention, as

well as community-based support from other families affected by FASD. Speech-language pathologists are valuable members of the interdisciplinary health care team, and can help to improve the functional communication of children with FASD at home, in school and in society.

Case Study 1: Jamie

Jamie's case study is presented as a think aloud, with case history information supplemented by the speech-language pathologist's thinking in italics.

Jamie is a 5-year-old female who was referred for a school-based speech-language assessment to establish her Individualized Education Plan (IEP) goals. She resides at home with her adoptive parents and one typically developing 10-year-old sister who was not adopted and was not exposed to alcohol in utero.

Jamie was placed in foster care with her current adoptive parents at 11 months old and was adopted 2 years later. Her birth mother admitted to alcohol use during pregnancy with Jamie, but details regarding quantity, frequency and type of alcohol are unknown. Jamie's birth mother is no longer involved in Jamie's life or care, and Jamie has since moved away from her birth family with her adoptive family.

Jamie is fortunate to have supportive and loving adoptive parents now. However, the circumstances of her first 11 months are largely unknown. Early bonding with her birth mother, adequate sleep and nourishment, an appropriate and nurturing environment, and a consistent routine are important for the development of newborns and infants. However, Jamie's exposure to consistent, quality care as a baby is unknown.

Jamie was a physically small baby who was difficult to soothe. She cried often and seemed inconsolable, which was stressful and challenging for her parents. They were aware of Jamie's birth mother's use of alcohol during pregnancy, but did not attribute Jamie's fussiness to FAS at that time. Jamie's speech and language were delayed, with deficits in both expressive and receptive language. Jamie spoke her first single word at 24 months and her parents reported she did not appear to understand their requests to select specific foods and toys. They attributed her speech and language delay to the transition into their family and the unknown circumstances of her first 11 months. Despite her delayed language, Jamie was physically affectionate and appeared to be forming a bond with her adoptive parents, which was very important to them.

As Jamie grew older, her language developed slowly. When she was 3 years old she was enrolled in a local preschool program. She was challenging to manage in the classroom because of difficulty following directions, inability to generalize the daily routine, and inattention. Jamie's parents reasoned with her teachers that her behaviors were a result of her background, and that she needed extra time and patience to adapt to the school environment.

Jamie was referred for speech-language and hearing evaluations after failing her respective screenings at school. Jamie's parents took her to the local university clinic for assessment, because her father is an employee of the university. A speech-language pathologist administered the Preschool Language Scale-Fifth Edition (PLS-5). Total administration time was about 45 minutes because Jamie reached the ceiling for both auditory comprehension and expressive communication rather quickly. Jamie was given a 5-minute play break after 20 minutes of testing due to her inattention. Directions were repeated whenever allowed per the administration manual, and Jamie required consistent redirection back to task throughout the assessment. She demonstrated impulsivity and got out of her seat repeatedly. Jamie answered questions quickly, often cutting off the clinician prior to the completion of the question or directions. She attempted to leave the room on one occasion, but was redirected back to her seat.

Jamie's auditory comprehension was relatively stronger than her expressive communication skills, however both fell within the third standard deviation below the mean. Areas of relative strength within expressive language included requesting objects, answering yes/no questions, and using noun/verb combinations. Receptively, areas of relative strength included identification of body parts, clothing, and understanding the verbs "eat, sleep, and drink" in context. She demonstrated difficulty with basic expressive language tasks such as using three-word combinations, using the present progressive tense, and naming described objects. Receptively, Jamie had difficulty understanding pronouns, spatial concepts, and quantitative concepts, as well as analogies.

The Articulation Screener component of the PLS-5 was also administered, and Jamie's score was "typical" for her age. Her speech was limited in content, but intelligible.

A full hearing evaluation revealed a mild bilateral sensorineural hearing loss and the audiologist anecdotally mentioned mild facial dysmorphology in her report, specifically questioning the presence of a short palpebral fissure. Copies of both the speech-language and audiology reports were sent to Jamie's parents and pediatrician. Neither the parents nor the pediatrician considered the audiologist's comments regarding facial dysmorphology.

Jamie was enrolled in weekly speech-language therapy at the university clinic for the next three years. She was likable and separated easily from her parents, but she was increasingly difficult for graduate student clinicians to manage because of her impulsive behavior and tangential language. Jamie's vocabulary was markedly limited and she was easily frustrated with age-appropriate tasks that were exceedingly difficult for her. For example, following three-step directions to make a simple craft and talking about the sequence afterward was challenging. She required consistent redirection to follow simple directions, use the materials appropriately, and complete the task. Additionally, although all therapy sessions concluded with a "recap" of the events of the session, Jamie was unable to generalize this pattern and consistently required a model to recall the first, next, and last activities. She got out of her seat repeatedly and tried to take toys off of high shelves as the clinicians redirected her back to the session.

Minimizing distractions and working with a schedule were two strategies that Jamie's SLP and audiologist suggested to improve her compliance in preschool. She was seated close to her teachers and they were instructed to face her when speaking with her. Background noise was also reduced by keeping the door to the hallway closed. Changes in the classroom routine were avoided as much as possible, including where in the room each activity occurred. For example, each morning began with circle time on the rug, followed by reviewing the calendar and weather by the window. By the end of the school year, Jamie required less redirection to progress through a typical day.

Jamie matriculated into public kindergarten after preschool. Her SLP corresponded with her kindergarten teacher shortly after the new school year began and provided strategies that were helpful to Jamie in preschool. Jamie had a difficult time transitioning into kindergarten, and she failed her speech-language screening. The school SLP is now ready to assess Jamie and, if appropriate, establish IEP goals and objectives to be implemented during the school year. The SLP reads Jamie's speech-language and audiology evaluation reports from the university clinic, and notices the audiologist's observation of facial dysmorphology.

The SLP worked with children with FAS previously and recognized the facial features in Jamie as well. After screening Jamie and reading the reports, she is suspicious of more than a receptive-expressive language disorder. The SLP is not qualified to diagnose FAS; however, she can mention her concerns to the team lead, her assistant principal. The SLP will read up on the speech and language characteristics of children with FAS and she can use the data to make more informed decisions about diagnostic and treatment plans.

Review Questions

1. What is the importance of Jamie's first 11 months in terms of speech and language development?

2. Why is the audiologist especially attuned to Jamie's facial dysmorphology?

3. Although the school SLP suspects Jamie might have FASD, she is not qualified to diagnose. What should she do next?

4. Who will be on Jamie's assessment team? Describe their respective roles.

5. After Jamie is diagnosed with FASD, her parents express their academic and social concerns to the school SLP. What information should she provide to Jamie's parents?

Case Study 2: Daniel

Daniel is a 16-year-old boy whose language and cognitive skills were recently reassessed to update his IEP goals. Daniel lives in a group home setting and attends a special education school. His classwork focuses on functional academic and life skills, preparing him to work within the community. Daniel was placed in foster care as an infant and resided with several families prior to his current group home. He was diagnosed with FAS when he was 6 years old, after a physician who treated other children with FASD recognized Daniel's facial dysmorphology, impulsivity and verbosity, and pursued a diagnostic assessment.

Daniel was diagnosed using the 4-Digit Diagnostic Code. He was small in stature, and was below the third percentile for both height and weight at the time of diagnosis (rank of 4 on growth deficiency scale). He presented with the characteristic facial phenotype for FAS, including a short palpebral fissure, thin upper lip, and smooth philtrum (rank of 4 on the facial phenotype scale). Daniel did not undergo brain imaging nor did he experience consistent neurological events such as seizures; however, he did display significant deficits across the areas of language, cognition, adaptation and achievements, and therefore he was given a rank of 3 on the brain damage scale. Daniel's birth mother did not change her preconception drinking habits when she became pregnant, and she consistently drank at least two drinks

multiple times per week throughout her pregnancy. She reported this information when she was approached during Daniel's evaluation process, though he was living in foster care at the time. Because Daniel's mother's consumption of alcohol during pregnancy was confirmed, Daniel was given a rank of 4 on the prenatal alcohol exposure scale. Daniels's 4-digit code "4434" placed him in Category A, "fetal alcohol syndrome (alcohol exposed)" (Astley, 2004, p. 49).

Subsequent to Daniel's diagnosis at age 6, he was placed with two foster families before moving to a group home when he was 10 years old. As Daniel grew older, his behavior, social skills and cognitive-linguistic deficits became increasingly difficult to manage. Daniel was impulsive and did not learn from his mistakes. He was caught stealing his classmates' and teachers' belongings on several occasions. Despite specific punishment and removal of privileges, he continued to be disrespectful to his peers and teachers, and he transferred from a regular education school where he received special education services, to a self-contained special education school. His transition to the new school and living situation was long and challenging. He continued to steal from his peers and his impulsive behavior and verbosity were disruptive in the group home and at school, but the teachers, therapists, nurses, and administrators collaborated to establish routines, schedules and support for Daniel.

His SLP administered the Comprehensive Assessment of Spoken Language (CASL) for objective reportable data for his IEP. The CASL was administered over three sessions to accommodate Daniel's attentional difficulties. Areas of relative strength included Antonym and Synonym subtests. Daniel demonstrated significantly more difficulty with language tasks that required higher level receptive and expressive skills, such as Syntax Construction, Paragraph Comprehension, and Pragmatic Judgment. Daniel also had difficulty with the Inferences, Ambiguous Language, and Meaning from Context subtests. The Grammaticality Judgment and Syntax Construction subtests were omitted in an effort to decrease frustration and because of previously established deficits in these areas. Daniel's scores across the Lexical/Semantic, Syntactic, Supralinguistic, and Pragmatic domains fell below the second standard deviation below the mean; he presented with significant, widespread language deficits. In general, Daniel's responses were impulsive and he asked for breaks repeatedly during the assessment sessions. He demonstrated decreased metacognitive awareness of his deficits and never asked for repetition of stimuli, even when his responses were consistently incorrect. Daniel was highly distractible and largely uncooperative during the assessment.

These behavioral observations and objective results of the CASL support the observations made in structured and unstructured naturalistic settings, including his classroom, off-campus work, and in his group home. His classroom teacher reports that Daniel does have instances of relatively improved behavior, typically when he is doing a functional activity of his choice. However, his behavior during the administration of the CASL was representative of his typical presentation most other times.

Generally, Daniel's language and actions are self-centered. He acts and speaks impulsively for immediate personal gratification, regardless of the circumstances. He interrupts during class and therapy sessions constantly by calling out what he would rather be doing at

that time, and getting up to walk around the room looking for different things to do. He requires consistent redirection to remain in his seat and to participate appropriately in class and therapy.

Daniel is currently in class with five other developmentally matched peers and they leave campus twice weekly to work at a local nursing home. At the nursing home, Daniel's responsibilities begin with greeting the receptionist by identifying himself and explaining where he will be reporting within the building. He is friendly and says hello and his name, but consistently requires cues to report his destination. Daniel reports to the dining room, where he stacks the chairs after the residents' breakfast, mops the floor, then arranges the tables and chairs for lunch. He places napkins, condiments and cutlery on each table. These jobs are the same each visit, and for the first several months Daniel required redirection throughout the morning to complete his tasks. His self-direction has improved over time and Daniel is now able to move through his morning jobs with minimal redirection, unless there is an unusual distraction. For example, one morning a therapist brought a resident to a table in the dining room for therapy and Daniel stopped what he was doing to talk with them. He chatted incessantly and the therapist and his SLP had to request that he leave the resident alone so that they could continue their session.

Once the dining room is set for lunch and the residents are ready to eat, Daniel and his peers from school report to a conference room where they eat lunch together with their teacher and SLP. During lunch, the students review their mornings in great detail, beginning with their conduct leaving school and on the bus, the appropriateness of their greetings, their interactions with one another and nursing home staff and residents, and completion of their assigned tasks. The teacher and SLP facilitate the conversation and provide cues for Daniel to compensate for his deficits in memory, self-awareness, and executive function. He is easily distracted by his peers and has difficulty recalling and critiquing his own behavior. The conversation follows the same structure during each visit, and at the end of lunch the students are allowed ten minutes of "free talking" during which time the teacher and SLP monitor the appropriateness of the students' conversation, but do not guide its content. After lunch, Daniel returns to the dining room and stacks the chairs, mops the floor and puts away the napkins, condiments and cutlery. Once he and his peers are finished, they report back to school together with the teacher and SLP on the bus.

Daniel prefers working at the nursing home to being at school. However, occasionally he loses the off-campus privilege because of poor behavior. Although he is small in stature, Daniel often uses physical violence and places himself and his peers in danger when he is frustrated. This is especially evident when he works on functional reading and auditory comprehension tasks that require sustained attention and receptive language skills. Daniel's teacher and therapists are deliberate in their choices of appropriate and applicable stimuli. For example, one task might be to find out the hours of Daniel's favorite restaurant by using Google and then answering questions and making choices from the menu. The SLP might role-play the waitress by asking about preferences for side orders and beverages.

These are functional and relevant tasks, because the students go on outings on the weekends to restaurants and arcades. But the tasks are difficult for Daniel because of his deficits in atten-tion, cognition, receptive language, and self-awareness. He is typically successful initially, but as the demands of the task become more complex, his accuracy decreases. He has to be reminded to pause and problem solve before answering, as he tends to reply to all questions at the same rate, regardless of their difficulty. When Daniel is corrected, he often gets angry. He has difficulty channeling and expressing his anger appropriately, in part because of a limited vocabulary, and he often resorts to violence.

Despite Daniel's propensity toward violence, he is a social student. He his highly verbal (though often verbose) and enjoys interacting with his peers, particularly the girls. Unfortunately his interactions are often impulsive and become inappropriate, so even casual interactions must be monitored and guided by the school staff. Because Daniel lives in a group home with other students from his school, his behavior and interactions are watched closely. He is currently on a certificate track, and will likely remain at the school and group home until he is 21 years old. Daniel's teachers and therapists think about his future when they consider his classes and therapy sessions, because their ultimate goal is to prepare him for a transition to a functional vocational position when he turns 21.

Review Questions

1. How might Daniel's memory, self-awareness, and executive functioning deficits impact his work at the nursing home?

2. What should the SLP assess in Daniel's re-evaluation?

3. Develop an age-appropriate lesson plan for a language/cognitive therapy

session for Daniel. What are some specific goals and objectives that could be targeted?

4. What type of accommodations should Daniel's teacher use in her classroom to facilitate his success?

5. Should Daniel be told about his FAS? Why or why not?

Case Study 3: Emily

Emily is 25 months old and is referred to the county Infants and Toddlers program for a speech-language pathology assessment because of delayed speech. She was born full-term weighing 3 lbs., 12 oz., and was 15 inches long. Emily's birth mother, Sarah, drank two to three drinks per night approximately two nights per week throughout her pregnancy, according to family report. Her pregnancy with Emily was unplanned and Emily's father was never involved in her life. Emily lived with Sarah until she was 6 months old.

Emily's infancy was generally difficult. She was irritable, rarely slept well, and was very fussy. Emily's behavior stressed and irritated Sarah, and she drank more frequently after Emily's birth than she did during her pregnancy. Sarah tried everything she could think of to soothe her daughter, including singing to her, swaddling, rubbing her back, changing her feeding schedule, more frequent diaper changes, and different brands of formula, bottles, and pacifiers. Nothing worked to improve Emily's sleep or make her happier when she was awake. Sarah felt like she was losing control of her baby and herself, and she looked forward to her drinks each evening to relieve her pain and anxiety.

Sarah's sister, Kate, lived in the same town and was married with a son who was 4 years old when Emily was born. Kate kept her son, Ben, away from Sarah because she believed Sarah was a bad influence, and she wanted her son to be sheltered from his aunt's bad habits. Kate predicted Sarah would get pregnant, and Kate kept her distance from her sister during the pregnancy. Kate knew about Sarah's persistent drinking from friends who saw Sarah out several nights per week throughout her pregnancy. Kate spoke to Sarah about stopping, but Sarah was not receptive to Kate's advice and became angry and belligerent when Kate brought up the topic of alcohol. As a result, Kate stayed away from Sarah because she could not stand to watch what her sister was doing to her unborn child.

Once Emily was born, Kate stopped by Sarah's house to see the baby regularly. Although Kate disapproved of Sarah's habits, she felt compelled to make sure her niece was doing as well as possible. Unfortunately, both Sarah and Emily seemed to be doing worse with every visit. Whereas Ben had settled into a routine by three months old, Emily had not, and her lack of sleep and irritability was taking its toll on Sarah. Kate described Emily's state as "jittery" and she had never seen her son behave in that way. Kate never saw Sarah enjoy those moments of attachment with Emily, like she remembered so fondly with Ben. Kate remembered gazing into Ben's eyes, playing peek-a-boo, and being thrilled when he grabbed at toys as an infant. Sarah's interactions with Emily always seemed functional, cold, and laden with frustration. Sarah eased her frustration through drinking, just like she had always done. She threatened to leave Emily and expressed her desire to move away from town and everything that caused her pain. As she was emotionally distancing herself from Emily, Kate was becoming closer to Emily.

When Emily was six months old, Kate and her husband adopted her, and Sarah moved to another state. Although Sarah was Emily's biological mother, Kate was now Emily's mother and was determined to provide love, care, and support to make up for Emily's first six months. Kate felt strongly that an adoption within the family (kinship adoption) would be the best for Emily because she would be surrounded by family her whole life, and that love was irreplaceable. She and her husband were planning to have another child, and instead they welcomed Emily into their home. Emily's transition into Kate's immediate family was a challenge for many reasons.

Emily's fussiness and irritability persisted. She still did not sleep well, and did not seem to enjoy playing with baby toys as much as Ben did when he was the same age. Ben was initially enamored by Emily, but he talked a lot about her frequent crying and although he had outgrown pacifiers, started sucking on Emily's when he was at home. Kate was concerned about Emily's behavior and Ben's regression, but attributed both to the newness of the situation and figured they would outgrow their respective phases as a family.

Gradually, Emily became better adjusted to their routine and was a bit less fussy, but her poor sleep patterns persisted. Kate spent a lot of time playing with Emily using Ben's old toys and books, but Emily tended to explore the toys briefly and then throw them. She seemed to enjoy when Kate sang to her, but she never attempted to sing along or participate in any way other than stopping what she was doing to attend to the

song briefly. Emily's first birthday came and went and she was still not speaking. The pediatrician recommended contacting Infants and Toddlers at 18 months if Emily was still not talking. Kate was busy caring for her ill mother, and finally called Infants and Toddlers when Emily was 23 months old.

The SLP from Infants and Toddlers came to assess Emily at 24 months and took a thorough history from Kate. She administered the Rossetti Infant-Toddler Language Scale and found that Emily's skills were generally grossly delayed, ranging from 0 to 3 months through 3 to 6 months. Emily's Interaction-Attachment was characterized by appropriate caregiver interaction; however, Emily's response was not complete within the 0 to 3 month range. For example, Emily did maintain brief eye contact during feeding, but did not smile purposefully in response to Kate. Emily's area of relative strength within Pragmatics was that she cried for attention (0–3 month skill), but did not respond to adult interaction or vary her cries for different reasons. In terms of Play, Emily momentarily looked at objects and played with a rattle briefly, but did not attempt to imitate any facial expressions. Language Comprehension and Expression were also impaired, with comprehension skills characterized by showing awareness of a speaker, moving in response to voice, and attending to the speaker's mouth or eyes. Expressive language was limited to crying for attention. Emily did not coo or vocalize sounds.

In addition to the Rossetti, the SLP observed Kate playing with Emily, as well as Emily playing independently. Kate was interactive and attempted to make good eye contact with Emily, used appropriate inflection, and initiated stimulating activities such as singing familiar songs with motions. Emily's responses were limited and characterized by brief attention to songs, toys, and books. She did not interact appropriately with toys, rather she tended to dump them from containers, mouth them, and then throw them. When Kate sang Itsy Bitsy Spider with accompanying gestures, Emily watched for a moment and then moved away. She did not attempt to imitate the gestures, sing along, or maintain attention during the song. Kate reported that she sings Itsy Bitsy Spider several times daily with Emily, so the song and gestures were familiar.

The SLP reviewed Emily's results with Kate, including objective information from the Rossetti and observations from Emily's play. The SLP was extremely complimentary of Kate and her efforts to stimulate Emily, maintain a sleep and feeding schedule, and provide a loving and nurturing environment for Emily. Kate got upset after the SLP explained Emily's deficits. She expressed her fatigue, frustration, and heartfelt concern about Emily's well-being.

Emily will be diagnosed with FASD following her 2-year-old checkup with her pediatrician, at which time Kate revealed Sarah's alcohol use during pregnancy and Emily's Infants and Toddlers assessment results. The pediatrician had not seen a baby with FASD in years, and in the absence of knowledge about Emily's prenatal exposure, had not considered FASD as a reason for her irritability and delayed language.

Review Questions

1. What are some pros and cons of a kinship adoption versus a traditional adoption?

2. What are some strategies the SLP might suggest to Kate to elicit language from Emily?

3. What other professionals should be on Emily's interdisciplinary EI team? What would each one be looking for in their assessments?

4. What information does Emily's play provide to her EI team?

5. What types of support would be beneficial for Kate and her husband as they face the myriad of challenges associated with raising a child with FASD?

References

Aase, J. M., Jones, K. L., & Clarren, S. K. (1995). Do we need the term "FAE"? *Pediatrics, 95*(3), 428–430.

Abel, E. L. (1999). Was the fetal alcohol syndrome recognized by the Greeks and Romans? *Alcohol and Alcoholism, 34*(6), 868–872.

Adnams, C. M., Sorour, P., Kalberg, W. O., Kodituwakku, P. W., Perold, M. D., Kotze, A., . . . May, P. A. (2007). Language and literary outcomes from a pilot intervention study for children with FASD in South Africa. *Alcohol, 41*(6), 403–414.

American Psychological Association. (2013). *Diagnostic and statistical manual of mental disorders* (5th ed.). Washington DC: Author.

Aragon, A. S., Kalberg, W. O., Buckley, D., Barela-Scott, L. M., Tabachnick, B. G., & May, P. A. (2008). Neuropsychological study of FASD in a sample of American Indian children: Processing simple versus complex information. *Alcoholism: Clinical and Experimental Research, 32*(12), 2136–2148. doi: 0.1111/j.1530-0277.2008.00802.x

Archibald, S. L., Fennema-Notestine, C., Gamst, A., Riley E. P., Mattson, S. N., & Jernigan, T. L. (2001). Brain dysmorphology in individuals with severe prenatal alcohol exposure. *Developmental Medicine and Child Neurology, 43*(3), 148–154.

Astley, S. J. (2004). *Diagnostic guide for fetal alcohol spectrum disorders: The 4-digit diagnostic code* (3rd ed.). Seattle, WA: University of Washington. Retrieved from http://depts.washington.edu/fasdpn/pdfs/guide04.pdf

Astley, S. J. (2011). Diagnosing Fetal Alcohol Spectrum Disorders (FASD). In S. A. Adubato & D. E. Cohen (Eds.), *Prenatal alcohol use and fetal alcohol spectrum disorders: Diagnosis, assessment and new directions in research and medical treatment*. Retrieved from http://depts.washington.edu/fasdpn/pdfs/astley-FASD-chapter2011.pdf

Astley, S. J., Aylward, E. H., Olson, H. C., Kerns, K., Brooks, A., Coggins, T. E., . . . Richards, T. (2009). Functional magnetic resonance imaging outcomes from a comprehensive magnetic resonance study of children with fetal alcohol spectrum disorders. *Journal of Neurodevelopmental Disorders, 1*, 61–80. doi:10.1007/s11689-009-9004-0

Astley, S. J., & Clarren, S. K. (1996). A case definition and photographic screening tool for the facial phenotype of fetal alcohol syndrome. *The Journal of Pediatrics, 129*(1), 33–41.

Astley, S. J., & Clarren, S. K. (2000). Diagnosing the full spectrum of fetal alcohol-exposed individuals: Introducing the 4-digit diagnostic code. *Alcohol and Alcoholism, 35*(4), 400–410.

Astley, S. J., Olson, H. C., Kerns, K., Brooks, A., Aylward, E. H., Coggins, T. E., . . . Richards, T. (2009). Neuropsychological and behavioral outcomes from a comprehensive magnetic resonance study of children with fetal alcohol spectrum disorders. *Canadian Journal of Clinical Pharmacology, 16*(1), 178–201.

Astley, S. J., Richards, T., Aylward, E. H., Olson, H. C., Kerns, K., Brooks, A., . . . Maravilla, K. (2009). Magnetic resonance spectroscopy outcomes from a comprehensive magnetic resonance study of children with fetal alcohol spectrum disorders. *Magnetic Resonance Imaging, 27*, 760–778. doi:10.1016/j.mri.2009.01.003

Becker, M., Warr-Leeper, G. A., & Leeper, H. A. (1990). Fetal alcohol syndrome: A description of oral motor, articulatory, short-term memory, grammatical, and semantic abilities. *Journal of Communication Disorders, 23*, 97–124.

Belsky, J., Garduque, L., & Hrncir, E. (1984). Assessing performance, competence, and executive capacity in infant play: Relations to home environment and security of attachment. *Developmental Psychology, 20*(3), 406–417.

Bertrand, J. (2009). Interventions for children with fetal alcohol spectrum disorders (FASDs): Overview of findings for five innovative research projects. *Research in Developmental Disabilities, 30*, 986–1006. doi:10.1016/j.ridd.2009.02.003

Bookstein, F. L., Streissguth, A. P., Sampson, P. D., Connor, P. D., & Barr, H. M. (2002). Corpus callosum shape and neuropsychological deficits in adult males with heavy fetal alcohol exposure. *Neuroimage, 15*(1), 233–251.

Chasnoff, I. J., Wells, A. M., Telford, E., Schmidt, C., & Messer, G. (2010). Neurodevelopmental functioning in children with FAS, pFAS, and ARND. *Journal of Developmental & Behavioral Pediatrics, 31*, 192–201.

Church, M. W., Eldis, R., Blakley, B. W., & Bawle, E. V. (1997). Hearing, language, speech vestibular, and dentofacial disorders in fetal alcohol syndrome. *Alcoholism: Clinical and Experimental Research, 21*(2), 227–237.

Church, M. W., Hotra, J. W., Holmes, P. A., Anumba, J. I., Jackson, D. A., & Adams, B. R. (2012). Auditory brainstem response (ABR) abnormalities across the lifespan of rats prenatally exposed to alcohol. *Alcoholism: Clinical and Experimental Research, 36*(1), 83–96. doi:10.1111/j.1530-0277.2011.01594.x

Clarren, S. G. B. (2004). *Teaching students with fetal alcohol spectrum disorder: Building strengths, creating hope*. Retrieved from http://education.alberta.ca/media/414102/fasd5.pdf

Clarren, S. K., & Smith, D. W. (1978). The fetal alcohol syndrome. *The Lamp, 35*, 4–7.

Coggins, T. E., Timler, G. R., & Olswang, L. B. (2007). A state of double jeopardy: Impact of prenatal alcohol exposure and adverse environments on the social communicative abilities of school-age children with fetal alcohol spectrum disorder. *Language, Speech, and Hearing Services in Schools, 38*, 117–127. doi:0161-1461/07/3802-0117

Cohen-Kerem, R., Bar-Oz, B., Nulman, I., Papaioannou, V. A., & Koren, G. (2007). Hearing in children with fetal alcohol spectrum disorder (FASD). *Canadian Journal of Clinical Pharmacology, 14*(3), e307–e312.

Coles, C. D., Platzman, K. A., Raskind-Hood, C. L., Brown, R. T., Falek, A., & Smith, I. E. (1997). A comparison of children affected by prenatal alcohol exposure and attention deficit, hyperactivity disorder. *Alcoholism: Clinical and Experimental Research, 21*(1), 150–161.

Cone-Wesson, B. (2005). Prenatal alcohol and cocaine exposure: Influences on cognition, speech, language, and hearing. *Journal of Communication Disorders, 38,* 279–302. doi:10.1016/j.jcomdis.2005.02.004

Crocker, N., Vaurio, L., Riley, E. P., & Mattson, S. N. (2011). Comparison of verbal learning and memory in children with heavy prenatal alcohol exposure or attention-deficit/hyperactivity disorder. *Alcoholism: Clinical and Experimental Research, 35*(6), 1114–1121. doi:10.0000/j.1530-0277.2011.01444.x

Davis, K. M., Gagnier, K. R., Moore, T. E., & Todorow, M. (2013). Cognitive aspects of fetal alcohol spectrum disorder. *WIREs Cognitive Science, 4,* 81–92. doi:10.1002-wcs.1202

de Beer, M., Kritzinger, A., & Zsilavecz, U. (2010). Young children with fetal alcohol spectrum disorder–communication profiles. *South African Journal of Communication Disorders, 57,* 33–52.

Disney, E. R., Iacono, W., McGue, M., Tully, E., & Legrand, L. (2008). Strengthening the case: Prenatal alcohol exposure is associated with increased risk for conduct disorder. *Pediatrics, 122,* e1225–e1230.

Dodge, N. C., Jacobson, J. L., Molteno, C. D., Meintjes, E. M., Bangalore, S., Diwadkar, V., . . Jacobson, S. W. (2009). Prenatal alcohol exposure and interhemispheric transfer of tactile information: Detroit and Cape Town findings. *Alcoholism: Clinical and Experimental Research, 33*(9), 1628–1637. doi:10.111/j.1530-0277.2009.00994.x

Eyler, F. D., & Behnke, M. (1999). Early development of infants exposed to drugs prenatally. *Clinics in Perinatology, 26*(1), 107–150.

Fast, D. K., Conry, J., & Loock, C. A. (1999). Identifying fetal alcohol syndrome among youth in the criminal justice system. *Developmental and Behavioral Pediatrics, 20*(5), 370–372.

Feldman, H. S., Jones, K. L., Lindsay, S., Slymen, D., Klonoff-Cohen, H., Kao, K., . . . Chambers, C. (2012). Prenatal alcohol exposure patterns and alcohol-related birth defects and growth deficiencies: A prospective study. *Alcoholism: Clinical and Experimental Research, 36*(4), 670–676. doi:10.1111/j.1530-0277.2011.01664.x

Floyd, R. L., Weber, M. K., Denny, C., & O'Connor, M. J. (2009). Prevention of fetal alcohol spectrum disorders. *Developmental Disabilities Research Reviews, 15,* 193–199. doi:10.1002/ddrr.75

Franklin, L., Deitz, J., Jirikowic, T., & Astley, S. (2008). Children with fetal alcohol spectrum disorders: Problem behaviors and sensory processing. *American Journal of Occupational Therapy, 62*(3), 265–273.

Goodlett, C. R., Horn, K. H., & Zhou F. C. (2005). Alcohol teratogenesis: Mechanisms of damage and strategies for intervention. *Experimental Biology and Medicine, 230,* 394–406. Retrieved from http://ebm.rsmjournals.com/content/230/6/394

Holland, B. A., Haas, D. K., Norman, D., Brant-Zawadzki, M., & Newton, T. H. (1986). MRI of normal brain maturation. *American Journal of Neuroradiology, 7*(2), 201–208.

Jirikowic, T., Gelo, J., & Astley, S. (2010). Children and youth with fetal alcohol spectrum disorders: Summary of intervention recommendations after clinical diagnosis. *Intellectual and Developmental Disabilities, 48*(5), 330–344. doi:10.1352/1934-9556-48.5.330

Jirikowic, T., Olson, H. C., & Astley, S. (2012). Parenting stress and sensory processing: Children with fetal alcohol spectrum disorders. *OTJR: Occupation, Participation and Health, 32*(4), 160–168. doi:10.3928.15394492-20120203-01

Jones, P. J., Leichter, J., & Lee, M. (1981). Placental blood flow in rats fed alcohol before and during gestation. *Life Sciences, 29*(11), 1153–1159.

Kable, J. A., Coles, C. D., Strickland, D., & Taddeo, E. (2012). Comparing the effectiveness of online versus in-person caregiver education and training for behavioral regulation in families of children with FASD. *International Journal of Mental Health Addiction, 10,* 791–803. doi:10.1007/s11469-012-9376-3

Kalberg, W. O., & Buckley, D. (2007). FASD: What types of intervention and rehabilitation are useful? *Neuroscience and Behavioral Reviews, 31,* 278–285. doi:10.1016/j.neubiorev.2006.06.014

Kodituwakku, P., Coriale, G., Fiorentino, D., Aragon, A. S., Kalberg, W. O., Buckley, D., . . . May, P. A. (2006). Neurobehavioral characteristics of children with fetal alcohol spectrum disorders in communities from Italy: Preliminary results. *Alcoholism: Clinical and Experimental Research, 30*(9), 1551–1561. doi:10.111/j.1530-0277.2006.00187.x

Kodituwakku, P. W. (2009). Neurocognitive profile in children with fetal alcohol spectrum disorders. *Developmental Disabilities Research Reviews, 15,* 218–224. doi:10.1002/ddrr.73

Kodituwakku, P. W. (2010). A neurodevelopmental framework for the development of interventions for children with fetal alcohol spectrum disorders. *Alcohol, 44,* 717–728. doi:10.1016/j.alcohol.2009.10.009

Kodituwakku, P. W., Adnams, C. M., Hay, A., Kitching, A. E., Burger, E., Kalberg, W. O., . . . May, P. A. (2006). Letter and category fluency in children with fetal alcohol syndrome from a community in South Africa. *Journal of Studies on Alcohol, 67*(4), 502–509.

Lebel, C., Roussotte, F., & Sowell, E. R. (2011). Imagine the impact of prenatal alcohol exposure on the structure of the developing human brain. *Neuropsychology Review, 21,* 102–118. doi:10.1007/s11065-011-9163-0

Lemoine, P., Harousseau, H., Borteyru, J. P., & Menuet, J. C. (2003). Children of alcoholic parents–observed anomalies: Discussion of 127 cases. *Therapeutic Drug Monitoring, 25*(2), 132–136.

Li, A., Ma, X., Peltier, S., Hu, X., Coles, C. D., & Lynch, M. E. (2008). Occipital-temporal reduction and sustained visual attention deficit in prenatal alcohol exposed adults. *Brain Imaging Behavior, 2*(1), 39–48.

Malisza, K. L., Buss, J. L., Bolster, R. B., deGervai, P. D., Woods-Frolich, L. Summers, R., . . . Longstaffe, S. (2012). Comparison of spatial working memory in children with prenatal alcohol exposure and those diagnosed with ADHD; A functional magnetic resonance study. *Journal of Neurodevelopmental Disorders, 4*(1), 12. Retrieved from http://www.jneurodevdisorders.com/content/4/1/12

May, P. A., & Gossage, J. P. (2011). Maternal risk factors for fetal alcohol spectrum disorders: Not as simple as it might seem. *Alcohol Research & Health, 34*(1), 15–26.

May, P. A., Gossage, J. P., Kalberg, W. O., Robinson, L. K., Buckley, D., Manning, M., . . . Hoyme, H. E. (2009). Prevalence and epidemiologic characteristics of FASD from various research methods with an emphasis on recent in-school studies. *Developmental Disabilities Research Reviews, 15,* 176–192. doi:10.1002/ddrr.68

May, P. A., Gossage, J. P., Marais, A. S., Adnams, C. M., Hoyme, H. E., Jones, K. L., . . . Vilgoen, D. L. (2007). The epidemiology of fetal alcohol syndrome and partial FAS in a South African community. *Drug and Alcohol Dependence, 88,* 259–271. doi:10.1016/j.drugalcdep.2006.11.007

Mirsky, A. F., Anthony, B. J., Duncan, C. C., Ahern, M. B., & Kellam, S. G. (1991). Analysis of the elements of attention: A neuropsychological approach. *Neuropsychology Review, 2,* 75–88.

Molteno, C. D., Jacobson, S. W., Carter, R. C., & Jacobson, J. L. (2010). Infant symbolic play as an early indicator of fetal alcohol-related deficit. *Infancy, 15*(6), 586–607. doi:10.1111/j.1532-7078.2010.00031.x

Mukherjee, A. B., & Hodgen, G. D. (1982). Maternal ethanol exposure induces transient impairment of umbilical circulation and fetal hypoxia in monkeys. *Science, 218*(4573), 700–702.

O'Connor, M. J., Frankel, F., Paley, B., Schonfeld, A. M., Carpenter, E., Laugeson, E. A., . . . Marquardt, R. (2006). A controlled social skills training for children with fetal alcohol spectrum disorders. *Journal of Consulting and Clinical Psychology, 74*(4), 639–648. doi:10.1037/0022-006X.74.639

O'Connor, M. J., Laugeson, E. A., Mogil, C., Lowe, E., Welch-Torres, K., Keil, V., . . . Paley, B. (2012). Translation of an evidence-based social skills intervention for children with prenatal alcohol exposure in a community mental health setting. *Alcoholism: Clinical and Experimental Research, 36*(1), 141–152. doi:10.1111/j.1530-0277.2011.01591.x

O'Connor, M. J., & Paley, B. (2006). The relationship of prenatal alcohol exposure and the postnatal environment to child depressive symptoms. *Journal of Pediatric Psychology, 31*(1), 50–64. doi:10.1093/jpedsy/jsj021

O'Connor, M. J., & Paley, B. (2009). Psychiatric conditions associated with prenatal alcohol exposure. *Developmental Disabilities Research Reviews 15*(3), 225–234. doi:10.1002/ddrr.74

Olson, H. C., Jirikowic, T., Kartin, D., & Astley, S. (2007). Responding to the challenge of early intervention for fetal alcohol spectrum disorders. *Infants and Young Children, 20*(2), 172–189.

Olson, H. C., Oti, R., Gelo, J., & Beck, S. (2009). "Family matters:" Fetal alcohol spectrum disorders and the family. *Developmental Disabilities Research Reviews, 15,* 235–249. doi:10.1002/ddrr.65

Olswang, L. B., Svensson, L., & Astley, S. (2010). Observation of classroom social communication: Do children with fetal alcohol spectrum disorders spend their time differently than their typically developing peers? *Journal of Speech, Language, and Hearing Research, 53,* 1687–1703. doi:10.1044/1092-4388(2010/09-0092)

Paley, B., & O'Connor, M. J. (2009). Intervention for individuals with fetal alcohol spectrum disorders: treatment approaches and case management. *Developmental Disabilities Research Reviews, 15,* 258–267. doi:10.1002/ddrr.67

Peadon, E., Rhys-Jones, B., Bower, C., & Elliot, E. J. (2009). Systematic review of interventions for children with fetal alcohol spectrum disorders. *BMC Pediatrics, 9*(35). doi:10.1186/1471-2431-9-35

Rasmussen, C., & Bisanz, J. (2009). Executive functioning in children with fetal alcohol spectrum disorders: Profiles and age-related differences. *Child Neuropsychology, 15,* 201–215. doi:10.1080/09297040802385400

Rich, S. (2012). Shifting diagnostic paradigms for improved treatment & surveillance of fetal alcohol spectrum disorder in the DSM-V. *Child & Adolescent Psychiatry Society of Greater Washington Newsletter,* (Fall-Winter), 4 & 7.

Riley, E. P., Infante, M. A., & Warren, K. R. (2011). Fetal alcohol spectrum disorders: An overview. *Neuropsychology Review, 21,* 73–80. doi:10.1007/s11065-011-9166-x

Rogers-Adkinson, D. L., & Stuart, S. K. (2007). Collaborative services: Children experiencing neglect and the side effects of prenatal alcohol exposure. *Language, Speech, and Hearing Services in School, 38,* 149–156. doi:0161-1461/07/3802-0149

Rossetti, L. M. (2001). *Communication intervention: Birth to three* (2nd ed.). Canada: Singular Thomson Learning.

Schonfeld, A. M., Mattson, S. N., & Riley, E. P. (2005). Moral maturity and delinquency after prenatal alcohol exposure. *Journal of Studies on Alcohol and Drugs, 66*(4), 545–554.

Schonfeld, A. M., Paley, B., Frankel, F., & O'Connor, M. J. (2006). Executive functioning predicts social skills following prenatal alcohol exposure. *Childhood Neuropsychology, 12,* 439–452. doi:10.1080/09297040600611338

Shor, S., Nulman, I., Kulaga, V., & Koren, G. (2009). Heavy in utero ethanol exposure is associated with the use of other drugs of abuse in a high-risk population. *Alcohol, 44*(7), 623–627. doi:10.1016/j.alcohol.2009.08.008

Sowell, E. R., Johnson, A., Kan, E., Lu, L. H., Darrell Van Horn, J., Toga, A.W., . . . Bookheimer, S. Y. (2008). Mapping white matter integrity and neurobehavioral correlates in children with fetal alcohol spectrum disorders. *The Journal of Neuroscience, 28(6),* 1313–1319. doi:10.1523/JNEUROSCI.5067-07.2008

Sowell, E. R., Lu, L. H., O'Hare, E. D., McCourt, S., Mattson, S. N., O'Connor, M. J., . . . Bookheimer, S. Y. (2007). Medial temporal and frontal lobe activation abnormalities during verbal learning in children with fetal alcohol spectrum disorders. *NeuroReport, 18,* 635–639.

Stephen, J. M., Kodituwakku, P., Kodituwakku, E. L., Romero, L., Peters, A. M., Sharadamma, N. M., . . . Coffman, B. A. (2012). Delays in auditory processing identified in preschool children with FASD. *Alcoholism: Clinical and Experimental Research, 36*(10), 1720–1727. doi:10.1111/j.1530-0277.2012.01769.x

Streissguth, A. P., Bookstein, F. L., Barr, H. M., Sampson, P. D., O'Malley, K., & Young, J. K. (2004). Risk factors for adverse life outcomes in fetal alcohol syndrome and fetal alcohol effects. *Journal of Developmental and Behavioral Pediatrics, 25*(4), 228–238.

Stuart, A. (n.d). *What is working memory and why does it matter?* Retrieved from http://www.ncld.org/types-learning-disabilities/executive-function-disorders/what-is-working-memory-why-does-matter

Thorne, J. C., & Coggins, T. (2008). A diagnostically promising technique for tallying nominal reference errors in narratives of school-aged children with fetal alcohol spectrum disorders (FASD). *International Journal of Language and Communication Disorders, 43*(5), 570–594. doi:10.1080/13682820701698960

Thorne, J. C., Coggins, T. E., Olson, H. C., & Astley, S. J. (2007). Exploring the utility of narrative analysis in diagnostic decision making: Picture-bound reference, elaboration, and fetal alcohol spectrum disorders. *Journal of Speech, Language, and Hearing Research, 50*(2), 459–474. doi:1092-4388/07/5002-0459

Timler, G. R., Olswang, L. B., & Coggins, T. E. (2005). "Do I know what I need to do?" A social communication intervention for children with complex clinical profiles. *Language, Speech, and Hearing Services in Schools, 36,* 73–85.

Victor, A., Wozniak, J. R., & Chang, P. N. (2008). Environmental correlates of cognition and behavior in children with fetal alcohol spectrum disorders. *Journal of Human Behavior in the Social Environment, 18*(3), 288–300. doi:10 .1080/10911350802427605

Ware, A. L., Crocker, N., O'Brien, J. W., Deweese, B. N., Roesch, S. C., Coles, C. D., . . . The Collaborative Initiative on Fetal Alcohol Spectrum Disorders (2012). Executive function predicts adaptive behavior in children with histories of heavy prenatal alcohol exposure and attention-deficit/hyperactivity disorder. *Alcoholism: Clinical and Experimental Research, 36*(8), 1431–1441. doi:10.1111/j.1530-0277.2011 .01718.x

Waterman, E. H., Pruett, D., & Caughey, A. B. (2013). Reducing fetal alcohol exposure in the United States. *Obstetrical and Gynecological Survey, 68*(5), 367–378.

Watson, S. L., Coons, K. D., & Hayes, S. A. (2013). Autism spectrum disorder and fetal alcohol spectrum disorder. Part I: A comparison of parenting stress. *Journal of Intellectual & Developmental Disabilities, 38*(2), 95–104. doi:10.3109 /13668250.2013.788136

Watson, S. L., Hayes, S. A., Coons, K. D., & Radford-Paz, E. (2013). Autism spectrum disorder and fetal alcohol spectrum disorder. Part II: A qualitative comparison of parenting stress. *Journal of Intellectual & Developmental Disabilities, 38*(2), 105–113. doi:10.3109/13668250.201 3.788137

Way, E. L., & Rojahn, J. (2012). Psycho-social characteristics of children with prenatal alcohol exposure, compared to children with Down syndrome and typical children. *Journal of Developmental and Physical Disabilities, 24,* 247–268. doi:10.1007/s10882-012-9269-1

Wozniak, J. R., Mueller, B. A., Muetzel, R. L., Bell, C. J., Hoecker, H. L., Nelson, M. L., . . . Lim, K. O. (2011). Inter-hemispheric functional connectivity disruption in children with prenatal alcohol exposure. *Alcoholism, Clinical and Experimental Research, 35*(5), 849–861. doi:10.1111/j.1530-0277.2010.0145.x.

Wozniak J. R., & Muetzel, R. L. (2011). What does the diffusion tensor imaging reveal about the brain and cognition in fetal alcohol spectrum disorders? *Neuropsychology Review, 21,* 133–147. doi:10/1007/s11065-011-9162-1

Wozniak. J. R., Muetzel, R. L., Mueller, B. A., McGee, C. L., Freerks, M. A., Ward, E. E., . . . Lim, K. O. (2009). Microstructural corpus callosum anomalies in children with prenatal alcohol exposure: An extension of previous diffusion tensor imaging findings. *Alcoholism, Clinical and Experimental Research, 33*(10), 1825–1835. doi:10.1111/j.1530-0277.2009.01021.x.

Wyper, K. R., & Rasmussen, C. R. (2011). Language impairments in children with fetal alcohol spectrum disorder. *Journal of Population Therapeutics and Clinical Pharmacology, 18*(2), e364–e376.

PART V

Emotional and Behavioral Disorders

CHAPTER 8

Communication Disorders Concomitant with Emotional and Behavioral Disorders

Marie R. Kerins

Chapter Objectives

Upon completing this chapter, the reader should be able to:

1. Paraphrase the federal definition of emotional disturbance and provide at least one reason why some professionals do not endorse the definition.
2. Name at least two psychiatric categories identified in DSM-5 that co-occur with speech and language disorders.
3. List several speech and language characteristics observed in clients identified with schizophrenia and depression.
4. Provide several descriptors associated with internalizing and externalizing behaviors.
5. List five other professionals likely to be on an interdisciplinary team and give their functions.
6. Describe a functional behavior assessment.
7. Describe an (a) early intervention strategy, (b) a school-age pragmatic intervention, and (c) an expressive arts intervention

Introduction

The speech-language pathologist (SLP) must understand the connection between speech and language development/disorders and psychiatric disorders. This is critical because of the high concomitance between speech and language disorders and emotional and behavioral disorders (Botting & Conti-Ramsden; 2008; Camarata, Hughes, & Ruhl, 1988; Lindsay & Dockrell, 2012; Loeber & Burke, 2011) indicating the likelihood of encountering a child or adolescent with co-occurring emotional or behavioral problems. This chapter describes many of these emotional and behavioral disorders. Some of the etiologies are known and others are only speculated. Language is intricately and intimately tied to socioemotional development, frequently making a differential diagnosis between a psychiatric disorder and a speech-language disorder difficult to discern. Over the past 30 years, researchers have demonstrated that a relationship between the two areas exists (Baker & Cantwell, 1987; Baltaxe & Simmons,

1988; Benner, Nelson, & Epstein, 2002; Botting & Conti-Ramsden; 2008; Camarata, Hughes, & Ruhl, 1988; Lindsay & Dockrell, 2012; Loeber & Burke, 2011), however a closer examination of the relationship between psychiatric disorders and speech and language disorders in the last dozen years has revealed more explicit information about the organic etiologies that affect communication in individuals identified with speech and language impairments. These recent advances are mostly evident in the research of individuals who are schizophrenic, or depressed, and those identified with an attention deficit disorder (e.g., ADHD) where brain imaging has revealed differences in brain structure and function (Castellanos, 2012; Liemburg et al., 2012; Price, 2010; Teicher, 2002). Other etiologies are less well understood and different theories are speculated. For example, although we know that early neural pathways in the immature cortex are dependent on experience (Perry, 2005) and some children lack the stimulation and experience to form secure attachments and to develop adequate language use (Pungello, Iruka, Dotterer, Mills-Koonce, & Reznick, 2009), children with insecure attachments are at risk for developing a host of behavioral issues that can be significant enough to become involved in the juvenile justice system (Snow, Powell, & Sanger, 2012). Further it is hypothesized that poor oral language skills can create an environment where the child is misunderstood or perceived as verbally disrespectful when the root of their problem may be language based and not behavioral (Barkley, 2000; Sibley, 2010; Tomblin, Zhang, Buckwalter, & Catts, 2000; Snow, Powell, & Sanger, 2012). Although etiology provides insight into the various disorders and theories

help to explain the relationship between behavior and language, further research is warranted.

Regardless of the theory, the speech-language pathologist (SLP) comes to recognize that the observed behaviors are real and must be considered a form of communication. The difficult part is disentangling the behaviors so the underlying problems can be treated. For this reason it is imperative that the SLP learn to function in an interdisciplinary environment distinguishing early on what other disciplines do and how speech and language is only a piece of a much larger puzzle. It is then that he or she can work collaboratively to peel off the layers of communication and behavior recognizing their dependency on one so an integrated treatment plan can be developed.

This chapter begins by reviewing definitions used in identifying children with emotional and behavioral problems. Then six commonly found psychiatric disorders in children and adolescents that occur with speech and language disorders are described in greater detail using the latest DSM-5 (American Psychological Association [APA], 2013) criteria. The DSM-5 is a classification system widely used by mental health professionals to diagnose disorders ranging from neurodevelopmental disorders such as intellectual disabilities, communication disorders, and attention-deficit disorder to depressive, anxiety, and trauma and stress-related disorders. The emotional and behavioral disorders often seen by the SLP that accompany speech and language disorders will be described according to general characteristics of the psychiatric disorder based on the DSM-5 criteria, speech-language characteristics often observed with the disorder, and other relevant details that may assist the

SLP in recognizing the psychiatric disorder. The latter part of the chapter provides an overview of assessment procedures that include collaborating with an interdisciplinary team, followed by interventions used with the populations identified in the chapter.

School-Age Population

School-age children with speech and language disabilities and/or emotional and behavioral disorders are most commonly served in the schools. Special education services are required by law if the child or adolescent qualifies for that service when the disability is determined to adversely affect the child's educational performance (IDEA §300.101(c)(1)). Other child and adolescent needs are met outside of the school by a private practitioner in an outpatient hospital setting or a clinical setting. Children served in the later environments elect to participate in those settings or their parents elect to have their children participate in those settings as either an adjunct to what they receive in the school or as a separate service. Regardless of setting, there is a strong concomitance between the two disorders and SLPs will likely encounter children and adolescents with emotional and behavioral issues on their caseload. A solid understanding of what constitutes an emotional disturbance in the schools will be helpful for SLP working with a pediatric population.

Children and adolescents are identified and provided services in the schools under the federal law that ensures an appropriate education to all children based on individual ability and need. This is commonly known as the Individuals with Disabilities Act (IDEA). President George W. Bush signed the reauthorized version of IDEA into law on December 3, 2004. Most provisions of the act became effective on July 1, 2005, with the final regulations published on August 14, 2006. This law covers special education services for children in the schools. There are two parts to the law, Part C for infants, toddlers, and their families and Part B for children and adolescents from 3 to 21. Part B is the primary focus for this chapter. For more details see ED.gov, the United States Department of Education's website (http://idea.ed.gov/).

Under the federal law 14 handicapping conditions are described. One of these conditions is referred to as emotional disturbance (ED). There is also a separate category to qualify the child for speech and/or language services (i.e., speech or language impairment). Familiarity with the law's content is important. The federal definition of ED is provided below and it should be noted that is has been modified slightly since 1997 eliminating under (2) the term autism.

IDEA defines emotional disturbance as

(1) A condition exhibiting one or more of the following characteristics over a long period of time and to a marked degree, which adversely affects educational performance:
   (a) An inability to learn which cannot be explained by intellectual, sensory, or health factors;
   (b) An inability to build or maintain satisfactory relationships with peers and teachers;
   (c) Inappropriate types of behavior or feelings under normal circumstances;

(d) A general pervasive mood of unhappiness or depression; or

(e) A tendency to develop physical symptoms or fears associated with personal or school problems

(2) The term includes children who are schizophrenic. The term does not include children who are socially maladjusted unless it is determined that they are seriously emotionally disturbed.

According to the Council for Exceptional Children, students who have emotional and behavioral disturbances exhibit significant behavioral excesses or deficits. The council also states that behavioral disorders have gained favor over emotional disturbance as a more accurate label leading to more objective decision-making and fewer negative connotations (see http://www.cec.sped.org). While the debate over the ED label persists, it is clear professionals still disagree over where to draw the line between youngsters who persistently act out with behavior that affects their educational performance versus those children and adolescents that have more classic symptoms of depression, anxiety, and thought disorders, which also impacts their educational performance.

Historically, the federal definition of emotional disturbance has been criticized for its lack of clarity and its exclusion of individuals who are socially maladjusted (Forness & Knitzer, 1992; Olympia et al., 2004; Webber & Sheuermann, 1997). Interestingly, in a review of the IDEA legislation, Skiba and Grizzle (1991) determined it was never the intent of Congress to deny services to students with emotional and behavioral disorders, but due to "poor legislation oversight and concern over opening the floodgates to juvenile delinquents" (Olympia et al., p. 836) the exclu-

sionary clause (i.e., socially maladjusted) remained through several iterations of the law. Although many have advocated for greater inclusion of individuals with behavioral disorders (see Duncan, Forness, & Hartsbough, 1995; Rosenblatt et al., 1998; Terrasi, Sennett, & Mackin, 1999; Webber & Scheuermann, 1997), the latest version of the law still maintains the language of excluding socially maladjusted youth. Regardless of the debate, the skilled educator will recognize that when the behavior of an individual is contextualized and interferes with learning or social development it becomes necessary to address and treat the issues of concern.

Gresham (2007) reported that as many as 20% of school-age children may have serious mental health issues, however only 1% to 2% of those children receive services under the IDEA label of emotional disturbance (ED). This under-representation of youngsters served under IDEA is alarming. What is also striking is that children and adolescents identified with an ED label may also incur language impairment. Hollo, Wehby, and Oliver's 2014 meta-analysis across 22 studies indicated the need for children identified as EBD to also be screened for language skills. They concluded from the studies that children identified as ED in kindergarten through eighth grade, as many as 4/5 of them had at least a mild language impairment. These numbers indicate that children's language needs may not be adequately served if one is not looking beyond the ED label. An SLP must be mindful of the ED/speech-language connection and be prepared to refer children with speech and language impairment to a mental health provider if warranted and likewise must serve to advocate and work collaboratively with mental health care providers to obtain appropriate speech and language services for youth identified with emotional and behavioral problems.

In summary, children served under the IDEA definition are children and adolescents with both emotional and behavioral disorders. Youth may also be served outside of the school setting, identified by a mental health care worker such as a psychiatrist or psychologist that use the DSM-5 classification system. Both IDEA and DSM-5 recognize a variety of disorders, however, categories of identification vary slightly; some of the DSM-5 diagnoses do not directly translate to services under IDEA. This is true especially for attention deficit disorder frequently observed by the SLP as a typical behavior disorder co-occurring with speech and language deficits. For the remainder of the chapter emotional and behavioral disorders (EBD) is the term used to describe youth with psychiatric disorders and the DSM-5 classification system will be utilized to organize the information. The EBD term will further be dichotomized by utilizing the categories of internalizing (emotional) and externalizing (behavioral) disorders, which are described below.

Methods of Categorization

Categorization of ideas, people, images, or words is an efficient method that allows one to retain and recall information (Seiler, Beall, & Mazer, 2014). Categorization of behavior also allows individuals to label the behavior and describe it. Unfortunately, when describing behavior or identifying a particular handicapping condition many individuals do not fit neatly into any one category. Achenbach (2001) and formerly, Achencbach and Edlebrock (1983), developed one checklist that is used demonstrat-ing this division between externalizing and internalizing behaviors. The Child Behavior Checklist (CBCL) maps 113 behaviors to eight different syndromes, which in turn can be clustered as either internalizing behaviors or externalizing behaviors. There are two forms of the CBCL, one for children and adolescents aged 4 to 18, and also a preschool version. On the CBCL, 4 to 18 form, there are also youth self-report and teacher report forms. The 113- and 100-item checklist, respectively, cluster behavioral into behavioral syndromes that are similar to the *Diagnostic and Statistical Manual of the American Psychiatric Association–Fourth Edition*. Because there is currently a newer version of the DSM, some renorming may be necessary to be consistent with the updated DSM-5. Lindsay and Dockrell (2012) consider externalizing behaviors consistent with the term behavior disorders and internalizing behaviors consistent with the term emotional disorders. These categories are briefly described.

Externalizing and Internalizing Behaviors

Externalizing behaviors describe the more overt actions children use. Externalizing behaviors are outward expressions that are obvious to anyone observing the individual. Adjectives used to describe this sort of behavior are: oppositional, impulsive, inattentive, aggressive, and combative. A child identified with Attention Deficit Hyperactivity Disorder (ADHD) is often viewed as having externalizing behaviors. The Child Behavior Checklist's broadband Externalizing scale scores is based on Delinquent Behavior and Aggressive Behavior scaled scores (Nelson, Benner, & Rogers-Adkinson, 2003).

Internalizing behaviors in contrast reflect one's internal state, and someone unknown to the child may not observe these signs as easily. Adjectives used to describe this disorder would include: withdrawn, unresponsive, anxious, or sad. The Child Behavior Checklist's broadband Internalizing scale is based on a sum derived from the Withdrawn, Somatic Complaints and Anxious/Depressed scale scores (Nelson et al., 2003). Externalizing behaviors and behavioral disorder are often considered synonymous, and similarly, internalizing behaviors and emotional disorders are considered synonymous. Recognizing that the lines between emotional disturbances and behavioral disorders are often blurred will give the SLP better insight into the child's behavior and will also be beneficial when developing a treatment plan. Children and adolescents can also be identified with both internalizing and externalizing behaviors. For example, a student identified with a conduct disorder (oppositional, impulsive) may also have a coexisting depression (sad, anxious). This merging of the two classification systems emphasizes the need for continued collaboration among the many educators and health care providers in developing a comprehensive treatment plan. The next section describes how externalizing and internalizing behaviors co occur with language disorders.

Concomitance of Emotional and Behavioral Disorders and Language

Speech-language disorders, learning deficits, and EBD frequently co-occur in children (Tomblin et al., 2000). The concomitance of these disorders has been the subject of much interest and study in the past several decades, resulting in two basic research strategies. The first involves identifying youth with emotional and behavioral problems in samples of individuals with known speech and/or language disorders. Youngsters identified with speech and language diagnoses demonstrated a high prevalence of EBD that ranged from 30% to 70% (Benner et al., 2002; Cohen, Lipsett, & Dip, 1991; Lindsay & Dockrell, 2012; Nelson, Benner, & Cheney, 2005). The second strategy identified children with emotional and behavioral disorders that have also been assessed with speech and language disorders (Gilmour, Hill, Place, & Skuse, 2004; Hollo, 2012; Mackie & Law, 2010). The language-learning connection is not a new one. It is a firmly established finding that children with language disorders are known to develop learning problems (Benner, Mattsion, Nelson, & Ralston, 2009; Catts, Adlof, Hogan, & Weismer, 2005; Justice et al., 2009; Tomblin et al., 2000). Data provided by the National Center for Educational Statistics indicated that for the 2011 to 2012 school year, the majority of students served under IDEA have learning disabilities (36%) followed by speech/language problems (21%). Many of the students identified with learning disabilities have problems with listening, speaking, reading, and writing; these are constructs within the scope of practice for the SLP (ASHA, 2010). Baker and Cantwell's landmark study in the 1980s, connecting emotional and behavioral disorders with speech and language disorders, provided researchers and clinicians with additional insight into the population they treat. Since the 1980s, researchers have continued to explore how language is connected to emotional and behavioral problems by attempting to identify which language disorders are associated with which emotional and/or behavioral disorder.

Benner, Nelson, and Epstein (2002) have looked more specifically at type of language impairment. Their findings indicated that children with pure receptive language deficits were at higher risk for antisocial behavior than children with speech only or speech and language deficits. This finding is consistent with Cohen, Davine, Horodezky, Lipsett, and Isaacson (1993) who supported that children with receptive language deficits were rated as the most delinquent and depressed by parents and the most aggressive by teachers, whereas children with expressive language deficits were rated more consistently with internalizing behaviors including being withdrawn and anxious. Children with expressive deficits may be reticent to reply and not confident in their ability to communicate their thoughts and feelings. Nelson, Benner, and Rodger-Adkinson's 2003 study found students in a K–12 environment with a comorbid EBD and language diagnosis more likely to have severe expressive language deficits rather than receptive deficits, and the expressive deficits increased in impact as children grew older, widening the expressive language gap. Most recently, a 2014 meta-analysis by Hollo, Wehby, and Oliver, showed participants generally had more difficulty with production than comprehension. Mean production scores were lower for expressive skills ($M = 75.9$) than receptive skills ($M = 82.2$). This new information indicates that expressive language skills are more impaired than receptive skills.

Although not all the researchers agree which area of language is more impaired in children with EBD, one area of consistency is the relationship between specific language impairment (SLI) and social relationships. It has been reported that between "27% and 30% of 8 to 12 year olds with SLI were rated by their teachers as having significant peer problems, this is approximately a three times greater prevalence than expected" (Lindsay & Dockrell, 2012, p. 446). Impaired social relationships are often the result of a pragmatic language deficit. Both Durkin and Conti-Ramsden (2007) and a later study by St. Clair, Pickles, Durkin, and Conti-Ramsden (2011) found that pragmatic language deficits and receptive language deficits were often a predictor of later behavioral difficulties. The correlations seem abundantly apparent between externalizing behaviors and language deficits, with the most recent meta analysis showing expressive language skills more of a factor than receptive language skills (Hollo et al., 2014).

Internalizing behaviors are less studied in terms of comorbity with language disorders. Hollo (2012) and Gresham (2007) pointed out that although 20% of school-age children may have serious mental health needs, only a few percent actually receive services under IDEA. Further, although the category of disability is labeled emotional disturbance it is those students with externalizing behavioral disorders who are more likely to receive special education services. This does not preclude children and adolescents with emotionally based disorders from receiving services but they are less well documented. Children diagnosed with anxiety disorders and/or depression had higher rates of absenteeism and lower academic achievement. In an article authored by DeSocio and Hootman (2004) they made a strong case for monitoring children's patterns of behavior that could indicate underlying emotional problems. Hart, Fujiki, Brinton, and Hart (2004) found no relationship between children's language and withdrawn behavior; however, a longitudinal study by Loeber and Burke (2011) demonstrated how aggressive patterns of behavior can shift, especially during adolescence, and develop into depression and/or anxiety. Loeber and Burke's study is one of the few studies that has tracked children over time and demonstrated the shift in diagnosis. Researchers continue to refine how to predict the nature and severity of disorders by observing the warning signs and symptoms that may signal more serious behavioral disorders. Better predictive abilities allow professionals to be proactive in their approaches to mitigating or lessening issues before they need specialized and intensive intervention. The work of early identification and prevention continues, and with a working knowledge of behaviors that may signal a communication problem. SLPs can join health care professionals to successfully intervene. Clearly there is need for further study to pursue developmental patterns that shift over time.

One psychiatric area of involvement the SLP may likely become involved in is the assessment and subsequent treatment of children who have been neglected and/or abused. These children may present as anxious or depressed due to circumstances and trauma. A closer look at their language abilities often reveals depressed language that is a result of biological changes to the brain (Atchison, 2007; Teicher, 2002) resulting in altered behavior and language function (Cicchetti & Lynch, 1995; Mills et al., 2010). These children need attention by a team of health care providers.

Interaction with children and adolescents manifesting emotional problems may also occur at the assessment stage due to abnormal speech patterns such as lack of prosody and slow rate of speech observed in individuals who are depressed, or the SLP may observe language processing problems and disorganized thinking typical in the early or prodromal stages of schizophrenia. To complicate matters, the literature also cites a group of individuals who typically have suffered some type of trauma that manifest speech problems that are psychogenic or have no organic basis for their expressed symptomatology. Etiologies of speech and language deficits especially those entwined with emotional and behavioral are varied and depend upon many factors making it impossible to draw generalizations. Regardless of the etiology, the SLP is often on the front line in helping either treat or diagnose individuals with concurrent speech-language and emotional disorders.

It is essential for the SLP to attend to signs and symptoms of both externalizing behaviors and internalizing behaviors to assist in an accurate diagnoses and treatment protocols. Keen observation will support other health professionals in a differential diagnosis. In the following section some of the major DSM-5 categories are discussed and speech and language characteristics observed with these diagnoses are highlighted.

Diagnostic and Statistical Classification System of Mental Disorders

Several clinically derived classification systems have been developed as noted previously. The system most widely used by the medical community is the American Psychiatric Association's *Diagnostic and Statistical Manual of Mental Disorders*

(DSM-5) (2013). The categories and sub-categories of the *Diagnostic and Statistical Manual of Mental Disorders* have become a standard reference for clinical practice in the mental health field and were mostly recently updated in May of 2013. The classification of disorders is congruent with the World Health Organization's International Classification System of Disease (ICD) (APA, 2013). In fact, the newest edition includes the coding systems for ICD- 9 as well as ICD-10, which will be required beginning October of 2014. One particularly helpful feature of the manual is the descriptive text that follows the criteria for each disorder. Another helpful feature is the common language it provides among professionals. These characteristics provide a basis on which to describe and compare children when communicating about them. This is especially important for aspiring professionals who have just mastered their own technical jargon within their chosen profession. This additional mastery of concepts and vocabulary improves the lines of communication between professionals and adds credibility to one's profession.

This chapter focuses primarily on categories deemed relevant for speech-language pathology including: (1) Disruptive, Impulse-Control, and Conduct Disorders, specifically Oppositional Defiant Disorder and Conduct Disorder, (2) Neurodevelopmental Disorders specifically Attention-Deficit/Hyperactivity Disorder, (3) Schizophrenia Spectrum and Other Psychotic Disorders specifically Schizophrenia, (4) Depressive Disorders specifically Disruptive Mood Dysregulation, and Depression, (5) Anxiety Disorders specifically Generalized Anxiety and Selective Mutism, (6) Trauma and Stressor Related Disorders specifically

Disinhibited Social Engagement Disorder and Post-traumatic Stress Disorder, and (7) Somatic Symptom and Related Disorders specifically Conversion Disorder. These categories are consistent with the new DSM-5 classifications. Prior to looking at each of the categories in more detail, some explanation of how emotional and behavioral disorders and speech-language disorders became a relevant area of study for the SLP is provided.

Disruptive, Impulse-Control, and Conduct Disorders

Based on the DSM-5 (2013) classification system, Oppositional Defiant Disorder and Conduct Disorder are two classifications that fall under this category and are the focus of the discussion that follows. Broadly defined and understood, disruptive behavior disorders are often synonymous with behavior disorders. The savvy SLP will recognize that individuals who are frequently characterized as having either oppositional defiant disorder or conduct disorder may have an underlying language-based learning disability. This finding is consistently revealed in the literature stating that anywhere from 30% to 80% of those identified with disruptive behavior disorders also had an identified language-based learning disability (Camarata et al., 1988; Cantwell & Baker, 1987; Cohen, Lipsett, & Dip, 1991; Lindsay & Dockrell, 2012; Loeber & Burke, 2011). The areas of difficulty often include expressive semantics, word retrieval, working memory, syntax and articulation, auditory comprehension, reading, writing, and spelling. All of these skills are necessary for successful completion of an academic program and will inevitably impact academic success.

Recent research has confirmed deficits in pragmatics or social use of language often were identified with a concomitant language disorder. Gilmour, Hill, Place, and Skuse (2004) identified two-thirds of their subjects with conduct disorders also were identified with pragmatic disorders. Their pragmatic deficits were similar in nature and degree to the children with autism who were also study participants. These findings appear to support the theoretical explanation put forth by Prizant and colleagues in 1990, who indicated that children with delayed and/or disordered language skills may have a difficult time establishing peer relationships, thus putting them even further behind their peers in the area of socio-emotional development. Individuals identified with Oppositional Defiant Disorder and Conduct Disorder are characteristically seen as having externalizing behaviors that may or may not develop into depression and anxiety. These two disorders are also overrepresented in correctional institutions and co-occur with individuals who have poor language and literacy skills.

Oppositional Defiant Disorder

The essential features of oppositional defiant disorder are the continuing pattern of anger and irritability, defiance, disobedience, or vindictive behavior with a first onset in childhood or adolescence (APA, 2013). The oppositional behavior is generally directed more toward figures the child knows well, which would include family and teachers. The noted behaviors are often part of a pattern of poor or problematic interaction with others and it is for this reason the SLP or interdisciplinary

team may consider language testing. Two commonly occurring conditions that coexist with oppositional defiant disorder are ADHD and conduct disorder (APA, 2013). First, conduct disorder is described followed by ADHD. Finally, fetal alcohol syndrome is another disorder that often co-occurs with both conduct disorder and ADHD, but is described separately in Chapter 7.

Conduct Disorder

The behaviors associated with conduct disorder are more severe in nature than oppositional defiant disorder. The individuals are typically male with displays of aggression and observations of poor peer relationships. The risk factors include lower than average verbal IQ and family history risk factors of rejection, neglect, and inconsistent child rearing practices and may include physical or sexual abuse.

Individuals with conduct disorder may have little empathy and show little concern for the feelings of others. Intentions of others are often misperceived; they feel threatened and often respond aggressively. These children and adolescents should be tested routinely for speech and language deficits. Self-esteem of these individuals could be low, or may appear inflated. Conduct disorder is differentiated from oppositional defiant disorder, which includes emotional dysregulation not identified with conduct disorder (APA, 2013). Speech and language characteristics for either of these diagnoses may or may not include receptive, expressive, or pragmatic language deficits. However, given the plethora of support for concomitance between children diagnosed with EBD and speech and language disorders, an evaluation should be considered.

Disruptive Behavior Disorders and the Juvenile Justice System

Externalizing behaviors or disruptive behavior disorders are problematic for the school-aged child but they also present a public health issue as many adolescents manifesting more severe externalizing behaviors such as oppositional defiant disorder and conduct disorder end up dropping out of school, developing an arrest record, and struggling with unemployment (Wagner & Newman, 2012). When considering all handicapping conditions, youth identified with EBD are the most highly represented category of youth with disabilities in the juvenile justice system (Gagnon & Richardson, 2008). The number identified with language deficits ranged from 50% impairment (Gagnon, Barber, Van Loan, & Leone, 2009) in one study, whereas Snow and Powell (2011) reported that out of a group of 100 juvenile offenders, two-thirds of this group was classified as having language impairment. In summary, the prevalence of those in the penal system with language impairment has ranged from 19% to 60% (Snow et al., 2012), depending on the sampling system and definitions used. A large and prominent study that followed the transition outcomes for youth with disabilities and tracked youths' progress post high school using several waves of student cohorts became known as the National Longitudinal Transition Study (NLTS). The NLTS demonstrated that, whereas adolescents' graduation rates improved between the 1990 and 2005 cohorts, arrest data increased from 36% for the 1990 cohort to 60.7% for the 2005 cohort (Wagner & Newman, 2012). Youth with EBD trail the general population in positive transition outcomes, and high rates of involvement in the criminal justice system are often cited as a probable trajectory for untreated youth. These data suggest more aggressive and earlier interventions. In addition, interdisciplinary training with collaborative efforts between SLPs, psychologists, counselors, social workers and other mental health providers will assist in mitigating negative outcomes because of increased knowledge between language processing, and social-emotional development.

There is concern among several advocacy groups that some youth are excluded from getting service in the schools because of the aforementioned social maladjustment clause written into the definition of what constitutes an emotional disturbance under IDEA. The Council for Children with Behavioral Disorders (CCBD) joined the National Juvenile Justice and Delinquency Prevention Coalition, and have advocated for at-risk and adjudicated youth to receive services (Jolivette & Nelson, 2010).

This bleak picture of high arrest rates and under identified language learning deficits depicts the incredible odds educators face when dealing with this very high-risk group. However, as mental health professionals become more knowledgeable about the possibility of language learning deficits co-occurring with EBD, more attention can be given to collaborative assessment and early intervention plans for children and adolescents that present with emotional and/or behavioral disorders. Advocacy groups such as CCBD and the National Juvenile Justice and Delinquency Prevention Coalition seek to address some of these issues by incorporating evidence-based education practices into the correctional institutions that have been successfully used in schools. Although this is encouraging, more advocacy and partnering is needed between all interested groups. Proactive approaches need to occur to avert later and more costly social issues such as incarceration.

Neurodevelopmental Disorder

Neurodevelopmental disorders as described and defined by the DSM-5 (APA, 2013) are a group of disorders that occur in early development and frequently co-occur with other neurodevelopmental disorders such as autism, intellectual impairment, or specific language impairment. In the following section the neurodevelopmental disorder of attention deficit/ hyperactivity disorder (ADHD) is addressed.

The essential features of ADHD include a "persistent pattern of inattention and/or hyperactivity-impulsivity that interferes with functioning or development, as characterized by inattention and/or hyperactivity and impulsivity" (APA, 2013, p. 59). According to the DSM-5 inattention may be characterized as wandering off task, difficulty with sustained attention, and being disorganized. Hyperactivity refers to excessive motor activity including not being able to sit still, or fidgeting; for adolescents and adults this may be described as restlessness. Finally, impulsivity refers to making a decision without considering the consequences, inability to delay gratification, or excessively interrupting (APA, 2013). ADHD is one of the most widely researched areas in childhood and adolescence. The disorder accounts for as many as 66% of referrals to child behavioral clinics, and roughly one child in every classroom is identified as hyperactive (Garfield et al., 2012).

Denckla (2012) reported that in children and adolescents between 5 and 17 years of age, the diagnosis rate rose from 7% to 9% in recent years. She further reported that ADHD persists into adolescence at a rate of 70% and into adulthood at 50%.

Studies have revealed decreased brain activity in the frontal lobe of persons identified with ADHD. The frontal lobe plays a key role in executive function and is involved in developing plans and organizing ideas. The frontal lobe is also involved in inhibiting behaviors necessary for attention (e.g., maintaining focus without being distracted by irrelevant stimuli in the environment). Cortex maturation is delayed in children with ADHD approximately three to five years as compared to typical peers. Children diagnosed with ADHD reach the peak of the thickening of their cortex in their teenage years rather than in their childhood years (Castellanos, 2012; National Institute of Mental Health, 2007). Ewen (2012) summarized common conclusions about ADHD that indicate that brain size is smaller with the cortex being thinner. Overall physical and functional maturation is delayed by two to five years. Finally, ADHD symptoms are related to cortical thickness and functional connectivity.

One of the problems with identifying ADHD is that the condition coexists with many other conditions and syndromes. In some cases, ADHD behaviors are involved in the condition; in other cases, ADHD characteristics are part of the condition. For this reason, it is important to understand comorbidity syndromes and medical and behavioral conditions that exist with ADHD. Flick (1998) describes the coexistence of ADHD associated with medical conditions and psychological conditions. The importance of recognizing these characteristics in diagnosing ADHD cannot be overstated. The fact that ADHD is one of the most common childhood disorders may be due to its coexistence with so many other syndromes as a primary or secondary characteristic. Many of the disorders that coexist with ADHD are described in this chapter. The most common comorbidities with ADHD include depression, anxiety, conduct disorder, and learning disabilities. Learning disabilities are referenced in a separate chapter in this text; this chapter explores three of the diagnoses, depression, conduct disorder, and anxiety that are frequently found to exist with ADHD.

ADHD Progression

Kratochvil (2012) reported that preschool children with ADHD are at greater risk for behavioral, academic, social, and family problems when compared to typical peers. They are also more likely to have been expelled or removed from preschool and daycare placements due to behaviors that are extremely disruptive. In addition, when entering school, these same children may already be delayed in understanding basic mathematical concepts, developing preliteracy skills, and in developing fine motor skills. The compounding difficulties of poor peer relationships and pragmatic deficits are additional risk factors in developing antisocial behaviors especially as children age up through elementary school. Barkley (2000) reported that 30% to 50% of children with ADHD between ages 7 and 10 are likely to develop symptoms of antisocial behavior and conduct disorder before they reach adolescence.

Whereas overactivity may subside by adolescence or adulthood, this characteristic is often replaced by a feeling of restlessness. Before the 1970s, many studies reported that children outgrow ADHD by adolescence. More recent research reveals the contrary. Barkley (2000) and Bussing, Zima, Mason, Porter, and Garvan (2011) reported that 70% to 80% of children clinically diagnosed with ADHD would continue to display these behaviors. Reportedly, 25% to 35% of this group may display antisocial behavior or conduct disorder; problems making and keeping friends due to deficits in social comprehension and decreased problem-solving skills are also evident (Sibley et al., 2010). Additionally, they may also have troubled relationships with parents, teacher, and school administrators (Barkley, Fisher, & Murphy, 2008). According to Kent et al. (2011), high school students with ADHD have a significantly lower GPA, a higher rate of course failure, a lower percentage of assignments completed and turned in, a higher rate of tardiness and absence, and an eight times greater chance of dropping out of school. These students are less likely to graduate and show decreased executive function and working memory skills (Galera, Melchior, Chastang, Bouvard, & Fombonne, 2009; Gau & Shang, 2010). Many adolescents display risk-taking behaviors experimenting with drugs and/or alcohol, and are more susceptible to peer pressure (Glass, Flory, Martin, & Hankin, 2011; Harty, Miller, Newcom, & Halperin, 2009). Those who go onto college may experience impairment in executive function as well as in academic, psychological, and social skills (DuPaul, Weyandt, O'Dell, & Varejao, 2009). According to DuPaul (2012), there is minimal data that exists on preparation for postsecondary education for adolescents with ADHD. Stimulant medication has been found to be anecdotally effective overall, but there are no controlled studies that exist. In addition, there are no studies on the effectiveness of the common types of accommodations that are given (extra time on tests, preferential seating).

Summary Findings for Oppositional Defiant Disorders, Conduct Disorder, and ADHD

The relationship between, speech and language problems, disruptive behavior disorders, conduct disorders, and ADHD has been demonstrated in the literature with the following conclusions:

1. Strong links between disruptive behavior disorders, ADHD, and language impairments have been documented. Although there is some conflict regarding which aspect of language is often most cited, studies have indicated that there are expressive deficits, receptive deficits, and overwhelming social deficits resulting in impaired social relationships. Because the externalizing behaviors tend to receive the most attention, underlying language deficits may be overlooked. Children with Conduct Disorder, Oppositional Defiant Disorder, and ADHD should be screened for language deficits.

2. The research cites the following weaknesses in language in related areas. Children with ADHD and oppositional defiant disorders are likely to manifest difficulties in receptive language including figurative language, and reading comprehension, expressive language such as formulating ideas and word retrieval. Syntax and semantics remain relatively intact (DaParma, Geffner, & Martin, 2011; Jacobson et al., 2011). Working memory deficits interfere with reten-

tion of material and learning to read. Impaired language leads to difficulties reading situations and expressing one's ideas and feelings fluently.

3. Research is beginning to track some of these children over time demonstrating the shifting patterns in behavior especially from childhood to adolescence. Longitudinal studies showed that youngsters with oppositional defiant disorders that have more affected domains tend to develop depressive symptoms whereas those that have more externalizing behaviors develop into conduct disordered categories (Loeber & Burke, 2011). Children with ADHD may likely carry symptoms into adolescence, but the hyperactivity may be replaced with a feeling of restlessness (APA, 2013; Denkla, 2012).

Schizophrenia Spectrum and Other Psychotic Disorders

Schizophrenia

Less common than disruptive behavior disorders and ADHD is psychosis in children and adolescents. The presenting speech and language features particular to psychosis have classically diagnosed the disorder and have aided psychiatrists in its diagnosis. Difficulties in producing a clear and coherent message are often a primary indicator of psychosis, and in clinical terms, this has been referred to as a formal thought disorder. In fact Baltaxe and Simmons (1995) have indicated that language dysfunction may be an early and significant neurodevelopmental indicator of schizophrenia in children and adolescents.

Features

The essential features of schizophrenia are defined by "abnormalities in one or more of the following five domains: delusions, hallucinations, disorganized thinking, grossly disorganized or abnormal motor behavior (including catatonia), and negative symptoms" (APA, 2013, p. 87). Delusions can take on many forms but simply put they are false beliefs held by an individual despite what the majority of individuals believe from a shared culture. Hallucinations are experiences that occur without an external stimulus with auditory hallucinations being the most frequent (APA, 2013). Disorganized thinking is probably one of the symptoms of most interest to the SLP because it is inferred from the individual's language and is characterized by language that jumps from topic to topic or responses to questions that appear unrelated or loosely related. More rarely, the language may be so severely disorganized it appears to be aphasic (APA, 2013). Disorganized behavior can "range from silliness to unpredictable agitation" (p. 88). The negative symptoms include restrictions in the range and intensity of emotional expression, in the productivity of thought and speech, and in the initiation of goal-directed behavior. A point of clarification is necessary for the student studying speech and language. *Speech*, within the discipline, is aimed at the phonological output of sound, whereas *language* is aimed at the content and use of sentences and narrative output. Throughout the DSM-5 the term *speech* is used when describing the disorganized thinking and should not be confused with the discipline-specific term of speech related to the phonological output of the sound structure of language.

Language Characteristics

Some argue that disorganized thinking is the single most important feature in schizophrenia that is mediated through language. The qualitative interpretation of language has become a principal means of assessing disorganized speech and in recent years with the advancement of technology, neuroimaging studies in schizophrenia patients have shown abnormalities in brain areas related to language processing (Price, 2010) with particular attention to the connectivity between brain regions. Whereas language deficits may be manifested during an assessment, a team approach is essential so all contributing factors can be weighed and the interactions between the factors explored for an accurate diagnosis. In several older but relevant studies the discourse of children with schizophrenia was assessed using many of the linguistic devices used by SLPs when analyzing narrative language samples.

Caplan (1996) analyzed the discourse of children with schizophrenia. He assessed their discourse using Halliday and Hasan's (1976) linguistic devices and compared their use of these devices that speakers employ to tie references made to people, objects, events, and ideas together. In Caplan's sample, 31 ten-year-old children with schizophrenia were matched with normally developing peers. The findings showed that the children with schizophrenia spoke less and did not provide the listener with enough links to previous utterances. Children with schizophrenia also provided the listener with fewer references to people, objects, or events mentioned in earlier utterances. In addition, the children appeared easily distracted by their immediate surroundings with little regard to the topic of conversation. Those children exhibiting loose associations confused the listener by using unclear and ambiguous references more than the children with no loose associations. These same findings were compared to other studies examining the language of adults with schizophrenia (Harvey, 1983; Rochester & Martin, 1979). Interestingly, the findings concluded that these youngsters did not have the "poverty of speech" found in the adult population with schizophrenia. Further, it was speculated that the onset of schizophrenia in middle childhood might also be associated with impaired maturation of social cognitive skills, including the development of logical thinking and topic maintenance. In conclusion, Caplan (1996) indicated that children with schizophrenia demonstrated deficits at the macrostructural and microstructural levels. The macrostructural deficits involved poor organization of topic maintenance and inadequate reasoning. The microstructural deficits involved impaired use of linguistic devices that link the contents of continuous speech and neighboring speech. Consequently, it was difficult to follow the line of thinking, which included whom subjects were talking about, what they were talking about, and how their topic was related to the topic of conversation. In another study by Baltaxe and Simmons (1995) analyzing the language skills of 47 children and adolescents ranging in age from 6;9 to 17;2, formal speech and language testing was administered. Of the 47, 83% demonstrated pragmatic deficits, 81% were observed to have disturbances of speech prosody, and 73% demonstrated auditory processing deficits, half of the subjects were impaired in receptive or expressive areas of language functioning. This study is further representation of the role the SLP may have in assessing individuals with schizophrenia.

Related Characteristics in Thought-Related Disorders

Individuals with thought disorders frequently exhibit emotional labiality. Affect may range from blunted and flat to euphoric and manic. Those who experience a flattened affect are frequently unable to experience pleasure. Anxiety, agitation, and confusion may be observed in these individuals. Exaggerated speech may also be characteristic of these individuals as they lose themselves in their delusions, rituals, and hallucinations.

Schizophrenia, a disorder of thinking, can often be diagnosed through a person's speech and writing. The SLP's contribution to the diagnosis of schizophrenia can be substantial because these are two modalities that are well within the domain of the SLP (see ASHA, 2010). France (1992) discusses four divisions when examining an individual's speech: stream, connection, possession, and content of thought.

- The stream of thought is how fast one thought follows another, which can be slowed down in depression or accelerated in a manic state.
- Disorders of connection involve a characteristic loosening of associations where two or more subjects can be woven together to combine thoughts, or where intruding stimuli become part of the thought process and adhere to the topic already initiated. Concrete thinking may be observed where the person with

schizophrenia cannot think in abstract terms.

- Disorders of possession include thought insertion, thought withdrawal, and thought broadcasting. Thought insertion is the belief that the thoughts one experiences come from someone else or somewhere else. Thought withdrawal, or the absence of thought, is the experience of one's thoughts being taken out of one's head. Thought broadcasting is an extension of thought withdrawal where thoughts travels outside the head only to have other people access them.
- Abnormalities of content of thought include delusions. Delusions are false beliefs, which may be either persecutory or paranoid, and reflect a distorted relationship between individuals and the world around them.

The more severe examples of psychosis are rare in the school setting. A clinician is more likely to see a child in the earlier stages of psychosis, or after the child has experienced some severe symptoms for which she or he is medicated. Continued monitoring of the child's speech and language functioning often provides helpful input for the consulting psychiatrist charged with the medical management of the child.

Individuals with schizophrenia are sometimes physically awkward and may display neurological "soft signs" such as left/right confusion or poor coordination. The psychotic features of schizophrenia typically develop between late adolescence and mid-thirties. So the SLP may see evidence of this in the older high school population.

Brain Studies to Support Language Impairment

Although schizophrenia is a severe, chronic, and heritable brain disorder it has been recently shown that there are functional and structural abnormalities evident in the language processing related areas of the brain. Brain studies have shown significantly weakened function of the left Broca's area with a right shifting pattern. This feature can be a potential biomarker of the disorder. Furthermore, in the high-risk and patient groups assessed there was a lack of communication between the hubs in the primary visual region and the phonological encoding, memory of visual word forms, and conceptual knowledge systems (Li, Xia, Bertisch, Branch, & DeLisi, 2012). Other areas of the brain that have been implicated include a reduced hippocampus, which has been linked to memory deficits often seen in schizophrenia (Hurlemann et al., 2008). It is unclear if the memory impairments cause the hippocampus to decrease in size or if a reduced hippocampus causes the memory impairments. Liemburg et al. (2012) observed increased functional connectivity between the attention and language networks of the brain. This increased connectivity was attributed to possibly suppressing unintended speech or excessive attention to internally generated speech. Connectivity was reduced between auditory and language networks, possibly contributing to language expression and comprehension difficulties. Finally, Wagner et al. (2006) demonstrated that the P300 amplitude used in hearing assessments was reduced in schizophrenics, revealing basal disturbances in information processing. As research continues to explore the brain of the schizophrenic with functional brain imaging, more objective measures will be identified in helping to proactively identify individuals at risk for schizophrenia and similarly, brain imaging could also be used to measure the effects of treatment.

Differential Diagnosis

Salokangas et al. (2013) has shown that mental health workers should be alert to adolescents identified with depression or anxiety due to the high prevalence of these disorders among this high-risk group for psychosis. In his European Prediction of Psychosis study, 245 patients were followed for clinical risk of psychosis, of those, 34% had depression and 39% had anxiety, certainly numbers that far exceed the prevalence in the normal population. As stated previously, the symptoms of psychosis are manifested in all aspects of communication. Speech and language characteristics prior to the onset of schizophrenia are helpful in diagnosing the illness. If this is not possible, awareness of what constitutes a formal thought disorder is useful; informal assessments such as oral or written narratives may provide additional insight for the interdisciplinary team.

Depressive Disorder

Depressive disorder, another category found in the DSM-5, includes disruptive mood dysregulation disorder and major depressive disorder, among others. Disruptive mood dysregulation and major depressive disorder will be the focus in this section. Although disruptive mood dysregulation is a new DSM-5 diagnosis it seems to fit with many of the externaliz-

ing behaviors evident in school-aged children. It serves as a logical bridge between the disruptive behavior disorders and the depressive disorders; the literature has consistently seen much overlap between the two disorders.

Disruptive Mood Dysregulation

Marked by chronic, severe irritability, disruptive mood dysregulation has two core manifestations. The first is frequent severe temper outbursts and chronic anger and irritability (APA, 2013). The onset is before the age of 10, and not assigned to a child who functions below a developmental age less than 6 years old. These children are at risk to develop depression or anxiety later in life. Because of the low frustration level in these children they typically have poor school performance and have difficulty developing and maintaining healthy relationships (APA, 2013). Many children may also meet the criteria of ADHD and carry a high risk for behavioral problems and mood problems. Although this is a new DSM-5 category it is very likely the SLP will cross paths with this population because of the marked impairment with relationships.

Depressive Disorder

Depressive disorder is characterized by depression, including the loss of the ability to enjoy life, feelings of sadness and grief, and possible suicidal ideation.

Family members may notice social withdrawal. Appetite may be reduced, whereas others with depression may experience increased appetite or cravings for specific foods. The most common sleep disturbance is insomnia. SLPs may notice the psychomotor changes that may involve agitation, including pacing or inability to sit still or conversely, slowed speech, and increased pauses before answering. "Speech is decreased in volume, inflection, amount of variety of content or muteness" (APA, 2013, p. 163).

France (1992) also reported that pitch changes may be evident, and resonance will sometimes be abnormally nasal or pharyngeal. In addition, many individuals report impaired ability to think, concentrate, or make decisions. They may appear easily distracted or complain of memory difficulties. The school-age child may show a drop in grades. Cognitive tests, such as IQ tests, may show lower verbal and performance scores. Research by Yingthawornsuk and Thanawattano (2010) has extracted the acoustic properties of the speech of depressed individuals including pitch contours, and formant changes. By using speech processors they have been able to differentiate depressed speech and also differentiate the tonal differences when one is suicidal. Although this data supports that there are changes in voice and speech when one is depressed it can also arm the SLP with objective data that can be shared with other health care providers when referring a client for additional services. Mundt, Vogel, Feltner, and Lenderking (2012) concurred with Yingthawornsu and Thanawattano's findings, who were also able to identify objective, noninvasive, physiologically based biomarkers from speech samples. Several acoustic properties identified in individuals with depression have included the duration and proportion of silences and vocalizations in voice samples, the mean and variability of the fundamental frequency (F_0), and the first and second formants (F_1 and F_2) produced by acoustic resonances of the vocal tract. These fea-

tures can certainly be helpful in lending objective data when assessing individuals suspected of clinical depression.

Nonverbal communication will also provide insight into how an individual feels. Restricted and flattened affect, reduced eye contact, and stooped or hunched posture may be apparent in an individual with depression (France, 1992). Poor nonverbal communication may be more evident in close relationships than in more superficial relationships, where the nonverbal interactions are not interpreted as abnormal (Segrin & Flora, 1998). Because SLPs are well versed in observing and interpreting nonverbal behaviors their observations may support a clinical diagnosis of depression.

Anxiety Disorders

Anxiety disorders consist of a subgroup of disorders that reflect abnormal and extreme responses to hypothetical and real stimuli. The triggers for the associated anxious feelings are either externally or internally generated. The focus of the anxiety often helps to differentiate the array of anxiety disorders. Generalized anxiety may be brought on by excessive worry. Selective-mutism is a less common anxiety disorder but one that an SLP may encounter. Generalized anxiety and selective-mutism will be discussed.

Generalized Anxiety Disorder

Excessive worries and concerns about real-life circumstances characterize generalized anxiety disorder. At least three additional symptoms that include restlessness, being easily fatigued, difficulty concentrating, irritability, muscle tension, and disturbed sleep must accompany the anxiety and worry, with only one of these symptoms required in children. Many individuals with generalized anxiety disorder also experience somatic symptoms such as nausea, diarrhea, and sweating. Disorders of autonomic hyperarousal, which include accelerated heart rate, shortness of breath, and dizziness, are less prominent in generalized anxiety disorders than in other anxiety disorders such as posttraumatic stress disorder. However, fidgety behavior and an inability to keep still may be apparent as a result of hypervigilance and the feeling that something is going to occur. The person is on constant alert and also may startle easily.

Anxiety disorders appear frequently in the general population and the disorder is often linked with depression. Twenge (2000) studied anxiety in young adults and has observed a substantial increase in the levels of anxiety since first tracking clients in the 1950s. With the increases in anxiety, professionals are beginning to look at symptoms in very young children. Although very young children cannot always articulate what is wrong with them, regressive behavior and mood changes may signal anxiety or depression in youngsters.

The causal connection remains unclear, but speech and language issues may often be overlooked when treating individuals with anxiety. The SLP may encounter this diagnosis with a range of speech and language problems including psychogenic disorders, autism spectrum disorder (Kreiser & White, 2014), ADHD, and others. A growing body of literature has shown that anxiety disorders frequently occur among the population of people with communication impairments, including those who are disfluent; this has been observed to be as high as 50% of this population (Iverach, Menzies, O'Brian, Packman, & Onslow, 2011).

Although this connection is not fully understood it does appear the SLP will encounter individuals with anxiety and depression, this will be seen in the upcoming sections on selective mutism, followed by trauma- and stress-related disorders, and finally conversion disorders. In the previous sections anxiety has also been shown to exist concurrently with ADHD.

Selective Mutism

Selective mutism (SM) is considered an anxiety disorder and is characterized by not talking in school or other community settings and impacts a child's development. Selective mutism is most commonly associated with social anxiety (Busse & Downey, 2011), and poorly developed language skills have also been implicated (Cohan et al., 2008; Klein, Armstrong, Shipon-Blum, 2013; Sharp, Sherman & Gross, 2007). Klein et al. found an underlying expressive language disability in 42% of their tested sample and even ventured to say that expressive language problems were a significant risk factor for the development of SM, including shorter narratives with fewer details according to McInnes, Fung, Manassis, Fiksenbaum, and Tannock (2004). Although the criteria is somewhat vague, Anstendig (1999) argued that children with language formulation problems, who also have a biological predisposition for behavioral inhibition and anxiety, are more likely to develop selective mutism. The child with selective mutism poses a unique challenge for the SLP and should be treated in conjunction with a licensed clinical social worker or school psychologist/counselor.

Trauma- and Stressor-Related Disorders

Two diagnoses that are worthy of mention under trauma- and stressor-related disorders are posttraumatic stress disorder (PTSD), which is triggered by exposure to an extremely traumatic event that may involve death, witnessing a violent crime, or physical or sexual abuse. Disinhibited Social Engagement Disorder that has an essential feature of "disinhibited social engagement" (APA, 2013 p. 269) can be observed in youth who have not formed secure attachments and/or who have been maltreated.

Posttraumatic stress disorder (PTSD) is the development of characteristics following exposure to one or more traumatic events (APA, 2013). The APA further defines features as those that involve intense fear, helplessness, and horror, and in children this response also includes disorganized or agitated behavior. Typically, the individual re-experiences the traumatic event repeatedly through dreams, or may avoid stimuli associated with the trauma. With young children under the age of 6, re-experiencing the symptoms through play that refers symbolically to the traumatic event may occur (APA, 2013). These symptoms begin three months after the trauma, although the PTSD diagnosis can occur years later. These events may include sexual and physical abuse, torture, terrorist attack, natural or man-made disasters, severe automobile accidents, or exposure to a medical incident such as waking up during surgery (APA, 2013). Events may be witnessed too. Impaired affect modulation, impulsive behavior, and impaired relationships with others are some of the symptoms that may occur, and may be overlooked as part of another disorder. In older children irritability or aggressive behavior may interfere with peer relationships (APA, 2013).

The SLP may have a child on his or her caseload that experienced traumatic and stressful events such as physical or sexual abuse and may manifest anxiety in more overt ways such as noncompliance and defiance of authority. Care must be taken to identify the root cause of the noncompliant behavior withholding judgments that the child is poorly behaved or in full control of their behavior. Sexual abuse is one of the most common causes of posttraumatic stress in children (Majcher & Pollack, 1996). When the abuse occurs before age 11 the event is three times more likely to result in PTSD (Davidson & Smith, 1990).

SLPs may be among the first to observe cognitive symptoms of stress that may include poor attention span, difficulty concentrating, difficulty in naming common objects, academic difficulties, lowered IQ, and poor communication skills (Richards & Bates, 1998). Affective symptoms may include panic and irritability, tension, constricted emotions, inability to express feelings, and avoidance of pleasurable activities (Richards & Bates, 1998). Functionally, impaired social interaction and educational difficulties may be evident. Regardless, it is important to consider why the child is performing the way he or she presents. This information may result in an altered form of intervention and indicate a referral to a school psychiatrist or psychologist.

Traumatized children experience biological brain changes as a result of repeated episodes of physical and emotional, abuse or neglect (Perry & Marcellus, 1997; Teicher, 2002). Treicher has described the impact of maltreatment on the function of the brain showing that the left hemisphere, largely responsible for language, is underdeveloped. Other observed behavior changes may include a constant state of hyperarousal, which are physical symptoms required for survival and activated through the release of stress hormones such as cortisol and adrenaline (Atchison, 2007). Although hyperarousal can be a necessary and adaptive condition in stressful situations, prolonged states of hyperarousal leads to hypervigilance. Hypervigilance is observed in some children who have been abused and neglected. It is marked by a tension or rigidity in behavior where one is continually surveying the environment for danger. Constant efforts to scan for danger leave little room for learning let alone establishing nurturing relationships.

Experience or lack of experience impacts brain development. Perry (2005) posited that the development of early neural pathways in the immature cortex is highly dependent on early experience, without the continual interactions the cortex does not develop the complex neural pathways important to learning. The early years in particular are critical for language and social-emotional development. Shared interactions that occur naturally in a healthy relationship such as turn-taking, eye-contact, and establishing joint attention are vital for language development and building a strong emotional attachment between infant and caregiver. Without these experiences a strong emotional attachment does not form and language behavior is altered. In some cases, the child fails to attach and fails to develop a meaningful repertoire of emotions. An unfamiliar term, alexithymia, is used to describe individuals who do not have the ability to recognize emotion in others and in extreme cases themselves. Although

the origins of the disorder may be difficult to determine, at least one of the sets of symptoms likely result from a childhood trauma such as abuse (Way, 2005). Factors that contribute to the development of emotions have their roots in early experiences with socialization (Espinosa, 2002); socio-emotional well-being continues to affect language and literacy development as the youngster develops. When this is disrupted through neglect and abuse, both social and language development are thwarted (Pungello, Iruka, Dotterer, Mills-Koonce, & Reznick, 2009).

A second trauma and stressor-related disorder related to childhood neglect is Disinhibited Social Engagement Disorder.

Disinhibited Social Engagement Disorder may be seen in children with a history of abuse and neglect "who lack attachments or whose attachments to their caregivers range from disturbed to insecure" (APA, 2013, p. 269). Social and interpersonal consequences, poor social and family relationships, and absenteeism from school may be observed. Although there has been limited research in the area comorbid conditions of cognitive and language delays may be present. In addition children may be diagnosed with ADHD and disinhibited social engagement disorder concurrently (APA, 2013).

Although these stress-related disorders may be less well connected with speech and language deficits they are nonetheless disorders the SLP may encounter particularly in settings that already have a high percentage of children identified with emotional and behavioral problems. Communication competence is central to mental health as it is the means one forges and maintains relationships. Substantial evidence links mother's mental status (i.e., depression) and parental responsiveness in general, with children's expressive and receptive language skills (Beeghly, 2006; Murray & Yingling, 2000; Pungello et al., 2009). This DSM-5 diagnosis fits squarely with the research related to maltreatment including abuse and neglect in the previous section. All trauma- and stress-related issues described in this section are viewed on a continuum with PTSD on one end and disinhibited social engagement disorder on another end of the continuum. It is important to note that although children may not attach adequately, there are language ramifications for both PTSD and attachment disorders that may not result in a DSM-5 label, but still impact the SLP.

Somatic Symptoms and Related Disorders

Conversion Disorder

With conversion disorders, the observed symptoms are not explained by neurological disease and this is detected in "clinical findings that show clear evidence of incompatibility of neurological disease" (APA, 2013, p. 319). Associated symptoms according to the DSM-5 manual (2013) include a history of somatic complaints often associated with some type of physiological or psychological trauma. For the speech-language pathologist conversion disorders are often seen in a subpopulation of clients with voice disorders (Baker, 2002), some individuals who stutter (Mahr & Leith, 1992), and it can also affect one's ability to swallow sufficiently (Koidou, Kollias, Sdravou, & Groulous, 2013). In the current literature the term conversion disorder goes by other names such as psychogenic disorders and functional disorders. As stated in Boone, McFarlane, Von Berg, and Zraick (2010), when describing

psychogenic voice disorders the voice problem is "typically resistant to change from various symptomatic voice therapy approaches" (p. 114). Boone et al. classifies the psychogenic voice disorders into four areas: falsetto, functional aphonia, functional dysphonia, and somatization or Briquet's dysphonia.

Falsetto

In essence, a falsetto voice is speaking in a high register voice, which is produced primarily by the adolescent or adult male who has already completed the physical maturational changes (Boone et al., 2010). It has also been identified in females. It is speculated that some young men have a difficult time transitioning into manhood and as a coping mechanism they maintain their prepubescent voices. The falsetto is diagnosed when the client is asked to cough uncovering a much lower and age-appropriate pitch. This demonstration of an incompatible symptom helps to support the diagnosis of a conversion or psychosomatic voice problem. A second technique to determine incompatibility is to apply pressure to the anterior thyroid cartilage requesting the client to produce a prolonged "ah" sound, which generally results in a lowered pitch.

Functional Aphonia

With this functional voice disorder, the client speaks in a whisper while maintaining normal prosody (Boone et al., 2010). To ensure there is no element of organic involvement a videoendoscopic exam is warranted to determine healthy vocal cords. Functional aphonia is seen in individuals with anxiety, stress, depression, and interpersonal conflict (Aronson, 1990). According to Boone and colleagues clients with functional aphonia communicate well and do not seem to avoid communication opportunities. They are quite effective in using their whisper and accompany this with adequate facial expressions and nonverbal communication strategies. Prognosis is considered very good.

Functional Dysphonia

Functional dysphonia appears to encompass a wide range of voice problems whereupon a physical examination does not reveal any physical or organic cause. The range is broad and Boone et al. (2010) describe some of the following as symptomatic of the diagnosis all which affect voice:

- Difficulties with phonation including breathiness or harshness
- Inappropriate pitch with voices too high or too low
- Excesses of mouth opening, head or jaw positioning affecting voice
- Excessive nasality

Similar to the other psychogenic voice problems, there is often a mix of emotional problems and voice usage problems.

Somatization Dysphonia (Briquet's Dysphonia)

More severe in nature than psychosomatic dysphonia, Briquet's dysphonia is characterized by more serious symptoms that may include "laryngeal pain, neck and shoulder stiffness, shortness of breath, fatigue, depression" (Boone et al., p. 120). Vocal characteristics include an elevated voice pitch and increased hoarseness with a greater prevalence in females than males (Verdolini, Rosen, & Branski, 2006).

All of the psychosomatic voice problems require a team approach, but particularly the latter due to the severity of symptoms.

Differential Diagnosis

A differential diagnosis between a speech and/or language disorder and a psychiatric disorder is not always discernible based upon the information observed. As a critical member of an interdisciplinary team, the SLP's job is to provide useful information that will contribute to the diagnosis and treatment of the individual. As a practitioner it is critical to have some background and awareness of the DSM classification system which is widely used in the diagnosis of psychiatric disorders.

Interprofessional Approach

Interdisciplinary education, team-based care has emerged as one of the recommendations from the ASHA's 2012 Health Care Summit. ASHA's Board of Directors has also identified interprofessional education (IPE) as a top priority. Some of the key elements for IPE include: (a) specific courses in graduate education, (b) opportunities for collaborative clinical education, and (c) collaborative practice in health care settings to maximize patients' functional outcomes (McNeilly, 2013). Although this is exciting news on the training front, practitioners have recognized for years the utility of interdisciplinary practice. Integrating IPE into health care professional programs minimizes losing valuable time learning about other disciplines "on-the-job" and allows professionals to immediately focus on their primary objective and that is the goal of increased quality of care for the client (McNeilly, 2013). Given this initiative, the sharing of information provided in this chapter is a step in the right direction by arming the SLP with knowledge of psychiatric conditions that often co-occur with speech and language deficits. Perhaps an additional challenge will be to share this information with psychiatrists, psychologists, and clinical social workers that provide treatment to individuals with emotional and behavioral problems.

Some of the more frequently co-occurring areas of overlap with speech and language deficits are seen between the neurodevelopmental disorder of ADHD, ODD, as well as between the disorders of depression and anxiety. One cannot nor should not be treating the child or adolescent in isolation and that is why a team approach presenting various perspectives is the most promising for improved quality of care.

Assessment

Language is central to human communication and development. The empirical research that is available supports a strong association between speech and language impairment and psychiatric disorder in childhood (Baker & Cantwell, 1987; Baltaxe & Simmons, 1988; Benner, Nelson, & Epstein, 2002; Botting & Conti-Ramsden; 2008; Camarata, Lindsay, & Burke, 2012; Loeber & Burke, 2011). Given this information, in any mental health setting or school setting specializing in care of students with emotional and behavioral disorders, a speech and language assessment should be part of the medical evaluation

of referred individuals. Likewise, SLPs evaluating youngsters with speech and language disorders must be aware of the issues and prevalence of psychiatric disorders that occur within this population.

Optimum circumstances encourage an interdisciplinary or interprofessional approach to assessment, including a psychologist, a psychiatrist, and an SLP, a clinical social worker, a general and/or special educator, parents/caregivers, and any other appropriate related service personnel, such as the occupational therapist or physical therapist.

Of obvious significance is the large role language and communication play in the team's diagnosis. An SLP has the unique training and expertise to be sensitive to this relationship and can be instrumental in interpreting findings. There has been a call for SLPs to continue to inform others about their unique role and educate those professionals that may not have the expertise to understand that youth with emotional and behavioral problems frequently have problems with receptive, expressive, and pragmatic language (McNeilly, 2013; Snow et al., 2012).

The Team

Psychiatrist

A psychiatric evaluation usually begins with the mental status examination, a tool most commonly used by psychiatrists. This examination presents a series of questions revolving around orientation of time, place, and person. In addition, keen observations of other characteristics are noted, such as hygiene, posture, affect, and general appearance. Characteristic behaviors are noted, and the quality of responses is judged. Psychiatrists regularly interpret the content of thought of their clients, questioning them about persistent thoughts, obsessions, hallucinations, or other occurrences that may help contribute to the diagnosis of one disorder over another. The information gleaned from this interview is used in conjunction with other observations and diagnostic information from other team members.

Occupational Therapist

The occupational therapist assesses the child both informally and formally. Observation in the child's classroom or another natural setting is important to assess how well sensory information is integrated for productive learning. The occupational therapist may look at motor planning, fine motor skills, visual motor skills, and ability to follow multistep directions. Formal assessment may involve tests such as the Beery-Buktenia Developmental Test of Visual Motor Integration (Beery, Buktenica, & Beery, 2010).

Social Worker

The social worker is a key individual in accessing important family information through face-to-face and phone interviews with family members. The social worker obtains information on developmental history, previous academic and behavioral history, and family dynamics. Additionally, the social worker will meet with the child, dialoguing to gain additional insights and to get the child's perspective on observed and reported difficulties she or he may have.

Nurse

In some settings the nurse may also play a role in the team assessment. Current health and general observations are made. School nurses are well positioned to interact daily with the child. The school health office is often a frequent stopping place for brief interactions and check-ins providing the nurse the opportunity to evaluate or monitor the situation. The nurse can provide information on medical issues related to the child's academic setting. Additional medical diagnosis such as diabetes or seizure disorders may need to be understood by the team and the nurse can provide this information. If medication is taken, the type and dosage is reported, as well as the child's compliance in taking the medication. For more complete information on the role of the school nurse in providing services for children with mental health needs see DeSocio and Hootman, 2004.

Special Educator

The special educator, or diagnostician, in charge of diagnostic testing is important for obtaining present levels of performance in major academic areas such as reading, math, and written language. One common instrument used is the Woodcock-Johnson III (Woodcock, McGrew, & Mather, 2007). Achievement tests yield standard scores, age scores, or grade scores that help in defining academic strengths and weaknesses, as well as identifying or supporting an existing learning disability. Specific reading batteries such as the Gray Oral Reading Test-5 (Wiederholt & Bryant, 2012) can provide useful information on the decoding and comprehension skills that may be impacting academic success.

Classroom Teacher

With the exception of the primary caregivers, the classroom teacher spends the most time with the child. Teachers are able to provide vital information on classroom performance, test results, and general observations of the child's behaviors. These may include reactions to situations and peers or recorded comments made by the child. Both formal assessment and informal curriculum based assessments can be used.

Psychologist

The psychologist provides information on cognitive functioning. Psychologists use a formal measure of intelligence such as the Wechsler Intelligence Scale for Children (WISC-IV) (Wechsler, 2003) that provides a global measure of intelligence using various subtests to cumulatively reflect a child's general intellectual ability. In addition to the IQ scores yielded from intelligence tests, other assessments are often completed. These tests may include projective tests, which are interpreted by the psychologist to gain insights into the child's personality.

Speech-Language Pathologist

The SLP figures prominently in the multidisciplinary team. Each team member uses language in his or her evaluation of the child. Oral responses from the child are interpreted by members of the team. Likewise, oral language is used to communicate information from the professional to the child. The levels of syntactic complexity and the length of utterances used by the professionals must be monitored or considered when weighing how well the child responded. SLPs are uniquely qualified to communicate what they observe in the language of youngsters to the health professionals and educators working with them (Cohen, Davine, & Meloche-Kelly,

1989; Giddan, Trautman, & Hurst, 1989). In addition to the assessment process, treatment plans used with children and families rely almost exclusively on verbal communication. The SLP must help professionals make informed decisions regarding appropriate language-based assessments matching the child's comprehension level to the therapy offered.

Formal Assessment. The SLP should screen the child's hearing or make a referral to the audiologist for a hearing assessment. Assessments of the child's receptive and expressive language should be made. Tools such as the Test of Language Development Primary: 4 (TOLD P: 4) (Hammill & Newcomer, 2008b) or TOLD Intermediate: 4 (Hammill & Newcomer, 2008a) or Clinical Evaluation of Language Fundamentals-5 (Semel, Wiig, & Secord, 2013) and the Comprehensive Assessment of Spoken Language (CASL) (Carrow-Woolfolk, 1999) are good starting points. However, in addition to traditional receptive and expressive measures, inclusion of pragmatic functioning, narrative analysis, and assessment of the child's ability to problem-solve is necessary to obtain a complete picture of language functioning. These formal test results are combined with informal findings completed through observation and conversation with individuals involved in the child's daily care.

Informal Assessment. Informal observations provide a measure of social validation to formal test results and provide qualitative data that are not always available in formal tests. Observations take place in settings where communication occurs naturally. If direct observations of the child's home environment are not possible, obtaining information from the child's primary caregivers helps to complete the communication picture. Participation by family members should be encouraged, as they are an integral part of diagnosis and intervention. There are checklists such as the Behavior Assessment System for Children–Second Edition (BASC-2) (Reynolds & Kamphaus, 2004) and Children's Communication Checklist–Second Edition (CCC-2), (Bishop, 2003) that are completed by various professionals as well as oral and written narratives that can be gathered and provide additional insight into language and behavioral functioning in multiple settings that can help create a more complete picture of the youngster.

Interdisciplinary Team— Considerations

After all formal and informal tests are performed it is necessary to review the information in a multidisciplinary meeting. These steps include:

- Convene with all the accumulated information
- Share information with an open mind until all perspectives are heard
- Come to a consensus on diagnosis
- Developing an appropriate treatment plan

Interventions

Interventions are divided primarily into two areas: those that deal with behavior and are used by a variety of educators and mental health care providers and interventions that are aimed at the social use

or pragmatics of language. Because of the interdisciplinary nature of working with children and adolescents with emotional and behavioral issues in tandem with speech and language deficits, interventions that are interdisciplinary in nature will also be emphasized. Each intervention presented does not necessarily have a strong evidence base to support it; however, it is felt that there is enough evidence or theory behind the intervention to present the intervention as promising and/or needing more research.

Early Intervention

Early language intervention has been consistently reported in the literature as a preventative method in the development or exacerbation of socio-emotional problems (Beitchman et al., 1996; Carson, Klee, Perry, Muskina, & Donaghy, 1998). One landmark study entitled The High/Scope Perry Preschool Project demonstrated the significant impact an early intervention could have on later development. Two groups of children were matched on significant variables then 58 children were assigned to an academic preschool program with weekly parental support and 65 were assigned to no program. The study tracked 3- to 4-year-old children from 1962 to 1991 and showed that those who were part of the preschool program were arrested less frequently, received less public assistance, earned more per month, and had a higher level of education (United States Department of Justice, 2000). The program is credited with promoting protective factors that reduce delinquency including early education, school readiness, and strengthening parenting skills. This is particularly significant even today as Snow and Powell (2011) reported on the oral language skills of 100 incarcerated young offenders with more than two-thirds of the group classified as language impaired. Prevention of the long-term effects of delinquency and incarceration is critical for a healthy society, which is a compelling reason for early intervention. This includes parent training, which has resulted in positive outcomes for children with behavioral problems and anxiety disorders (Delaney & Kaiser, 2001; Kendall et al., 1997; Webster-Stratton & Hammond, 1997). Teaching parents specific behavior management techniques with responsive interaction strategies is an ideal intervention and has resulted in both short-term and long-term changes in both reducing undesirable behaviors while improving language. Strategies used by Delaney and Kaiser can be seen in Table 8–1.

Certainly when dealing with very young children considered either at-risk for the development of speech and language problems or showing evidence of delay, early proactive approaches are imperative. When speech and language delays are misunderstood or masked by behavioral and emotional problems early intervention may be delayed. This chapter continually points out the striking occurrence of speech and language disorders among youth with emotional and behavioral problems. Therefore, SLPs must be continually evaluating the situation and intervening when necessary for preschool children demonstrating emotional and behavioral disorders.

Language of Feelings

Many youngsters, particularly those with pragmatic language deficits, cannot identify or articulate their feelings or the feelings of others. These skills develop in children as young as age 2. The language of feelings can be taught directly by the SLP either in individual therapy, group therapy, or a larger context (Giddan, Bade, Rickenberg, & Ryley, 1995; Giddan & Ross, 2001). It is important for children to understand the impact of their emotional outbursts on others. Addressing this issue and teaching alternative prosocial behaviors are encouraged (see positive behavior supports).

Preschoolers ages 3 to 5 can be taught the language of emotions in a purposeful manner by identifying facial features, vocal characteristics, and body postures associated with different emotions. The intervening professional should adapt lessons based on the different developmental levels when teaching the subtle nuances and shades of emotions. Cotreating with therapists skilled in expressive therapies (art, music, dance/movement) is also beneficial for generalization of these activities. This becomes more important for the child who has limited language and needs a nonverbal method of expression. Other more mainstream speech and language interventions can be found throughout this book in other chapters under treatment.

School-Age Intervention

The DSM-5 categories outlined in this chapter each feature a connection to communication. The Disruptive behavior disorders and neurodevelopmental disorder of ADHD share a strong concomitance with learning and language difficulties (Tomblin, et al., 2000). The emotional disorders of anxiety and depression feature speech and language characteristics that can be identified and used to solve a more complex diagnostic puzzle. The same patterns of anxiety and depression are also

Table 8–1. Intervention Goals, Rationales, and Measures of Parent Behavior

Goals of Intervention	Rationale	Measure
Balance turns	Creates a conversational framework for interaction	Discrepancy of turns (bases on number of parent verbal turns minus number of child verbal and nonverbal turns)
Give children an opportunity to respond	Encourages child-initiated utterances	Number of parents pause errors (i.e., two or more consecutive parent utterances without a 3-sec pause for child to respond)
Increase parent responsiveness to child verbal behavior	Meaningful, related responses encourage child communication and provide context-specific language models	% child verbalizations followed by semantically related parent verbalizations
Give simple, clear instructions	Children respond best if the instruction/command is at their language level and requests only one response	Number of total parent commands
Decrease frequency of instructions	Giving commands only for "important" behaviors will increase child compliance	% children's compliant and noncompliant behaviors to which parents responded appropriately
Increase positive responses following child compliance	Differentiates consequences for compliance and noncompliance; increases child compliance	% children's compliant and noncompliant behaviors to which parents responded appropriately
Increase corrective responses following child noncompliance	Differentiates a consequence for compliance and noncompliance; increases child compliance	Number of parent negative statements
Decrease parent negative verbal responses	Negative behavior by parent models negative behavior for the child and creates negative affect in the interaction	Number of parent praise statements
Increase parent praise	Children learn from positive consequences, and praise makes interactions more positive affectively	Number of expansions of child utterances at target level
Provide models of appropriate language	New language forms are learned through modeling	

Source: From The effects of teaching parents blended communication and behavior support strategy by Delaney, E. M., & Kaiser, A. P., *Behavioral Disorders*, Vol. 26, 2001, page 96. Copyright 2001 by The Council for Children with Behavioral Disorders. Reprinted with permission.

evident in children affected by abuse and neglect. Similarly, the increasing evidence of how the language centers of the brain are implicated in the diagnosis of schizophrenia make it likely that the SLP may play a role in diagnosing and individual in the early stages of schizophrenia. Baltaxe and Simmons were also able to clearly show the high prevalence rate of language disorders in children and adolescents with schizophrenia. Trauma-based disorders and somatic conversion disorders entail direct intervention by the SLP. Regardless of the diagnostic label, SLPs will have a role in either diagnosing or treating individuals with various emotional and behavioral difficulties. In the following section on intervention some of the more common interventions with these varied populations will be presented. It is important to emphasize that the treatments are not unique to populations with EBD, rather the treatment should be matched to fit the underlying speech or language weakness and these interventions may be found in other chapters in this book. Interventions in this chapter focus on (a) behavior, and (b) social communication, the core and essence of relationship building. Several nonevidence-based but promising interdisciplinary interventions will be shared and finally a table on pharmacological interventions is provided as a useful resource because so many individuals with a diagnosis of EBD are also treated with medication to deal with their symptoms.

Behavioral Intervention Plan

When IDEA was reauthorized in 1997 behavioral intervention plans (BIP) became a requirement and continue to be required under IDEA 2004. Behavioral interven-

tion plans are developed for individuals when the identified behavior is interfering with learning. Serving as the basis for the BIP is a functional behavioral assessment (FBA), which is typically initiated by the school psychologist who in turn works with a team of individuals involved with the child, although in more recent years a variety of practitioners and school personal are involved in conducting the FBAs (Gable, Park, & Scott, 2014). FBAs involve determining the nature of the behavior, the reason or motivation underlying the behavior, and under what conditions the behavior does and does not occur. Those conducting the FBA also try to identify what interests or motivates the student so the undesirable behavior can be replaced with more appropriate behaviors. In essence the team is attempting to identify a functional relationship between environmental events and the occurrence of a target behavior. Making this determination allows the educator to provide alternative behaviors that result in a more socially accepted response. Furthermore, an FBA serves as "one of the most important factors in determining the efficacy of an intervention" (Gable et al., 2014, p. 113).

An interview with the student may be part of the data collection to assist in collecting the information that precedes and influences the problem behavior. Direct observations can also be used to either formulate the hypothesis or more commonly confirm the hypothesis derived from the interview. Whereas teachers or psychologists often conduct these interviews and observations, many SLPs have added FBAs to their repertoire as suggested by the American Speech-Language-Hearing Association (ASHA, 2010) particularly as it relates to Augmentative and Alternative communication. SLPs are often quick to understand the connection between problem behavior and communication (Bopp, Brown, & Mirenda, 2004). An example of this may be the child observed hitting and sometimes eloping during academic tasks that involve written language. The team identifies this occurring when the child is frustrated during academic tasks and the identified function is to escape the task through negative behaviors. An alternative to the written task is developed that includes using a computer with word prediction software to assist with sentence creation. The maladaptive behaviors are replaced with more appropriate behaviors and the hitting and leaving the work area are reduced.

Positive Behavioral Interventions and Supports (PBIS)

Prevention is the best way to deal with problem behaviors. A clinician can address a problem behavior by identifying the antecedent that triggers the behavior. Planning for positive behavior supports by reinforcing positive behavior (replacement of the maladaptive behavior) increases the chances of the new behavior occurring again. PBIS is a three-tiered strategy implemented in schools to reduce behavior that disrupts learning (Wylene, 2013). The model is based on prevention that begins on a school-wide level and may include school rules that clearly define appropriate behavior. The second level is aimed at students who were not responsive to the school-wide program and may exhibit at-risk behaviors. The third level of prevention supports the at-risk students in a more intense and concentrated manner. Success of the PBIS has been measured by documenting the reduction of office discipline referrals (Flannery, Fenning, McGrath, Kato, & McIntosh, 2013) and improved social interactions (Hunter & Chopra, 2001). The goal of PBIS has been positive recognition of all students who are meeting behavioral expectations. PBIS is a proactive approach that attempts to create a positive school environment where students have clear expectations of what behaviors are acceptable. Unresponsive students may participate in a functional behavioral assessment to determine the cause of the behavior. Below are several positive behavior supports

- Prompting the student to review the classroom rules depicted by visual images before acting on an impulse, then rewarding his or her efforts through praise
- Charting behavior to show increases in making the right choices, which converts to earning a privilege or prize
- Rewarding the older student with extra computer time when he or she follows the behavioral plan specifically designed for him or her.

Cognitive Behavior Therapy

Cognitive Behavior Therapy (CBT) enjoys a strong evidence base and has been used with a variety of populations. CBT is a form of treatment that focuses on examining the relationships between thoughts, feelings, and behaviors. One population that SLPs frequently encounter is students with ADHD. In a document published by the National Institute for Health and Clinical Excellence (2009) CBT and social skills produced positive effects on ratings of conduct, and social skills in individuals with ADHD.

Because children and adolescents with speech and language deficits and emotional and behavioral difficulties benefit from interdisciplinary therapies care must be taken to match the treatment to the ability level, which sometimes requires adapting a more traditional CBT therapy approach. Sauter, Heyne, and Westenberg (2009) did an excellent job discussing how to adapt CBT strategies that combine both behavioral and cognitive theories based on the review of many research studies. Behavioral strategies emphasize principles such as positive reinforcement and extinction, whereas cognitive theory may involve self-monitoring of thoughts and feelings. Cognitive behavior therapy is used widely with youngsters who are anxious, depressed, and conduct disordered. It is also common to use CBT with clients who stutter. The CBT approach is language based and requires skills such as perspective-taking, reflection, adequate vocabulary, and language skills. It also requires the ability to understand the consequences of one's behavior with adequate skills in attention and memory (Sauter et al., 2009). Because of the reliance on language and executive function skills, which are often lacking in children with language disorders, adapting the CBT approach is useful. Please refer to Table 8–2 to see how some of these strategies can be adapted.

Table 8–2. Modifications to Cognitive-Based Therapy for Youth with Communication Impairments

Modification	Cognitive-Language Area Addressed
1. Employ the client's own vocabulary, using clear simplified language and task-oriented instructions (Ginsburg & Drake, 2002; Wilson & Sysko, 2006)	Language-impaired youth may not process complex sentences nor have the range of vocabulary to adequately express their thoughts and feelings
2. Use materials providing pictorial representations (Grave & Blissett, 2004); for example pictures of Stop, Think, Plan using a sentence strip and pictures	Visuals assist when a comprehension and memory problem exits
3. Provide visual analog scales for representing a wide range of emotions (Chorpita, 2007), shows gradation of emotions using a scale, for example, I feel annoyed, agitated, mad, furious, livid	Again the visuals aid in comprehension while assisting in depicting emotions as a range, helps nuance and differentiate emotion. This also works to develop vocabulary
4. Assist is self-monitoring by scaffolding and modeling for the client, continually moving them toward increased independence. Provide a model by "thinking out loud" what you would do in a given situation. View a video clip on bullying—"I get so mad I want to punch someone, this will only lead to trouble . . . "	Allows for reflection and perspective-taking; helps to establish a cause and effect relationship between actions and consequences

Executive Function Strategies

Students with language-based learning deficits that co-occur with ADHD, oppositional defiant disorder, and other emotional and behavioral disorders often manifest difficulties with executive function. Executive function skills are often compromised when the etiology of the disorder involves the frontal lobe. Struggles may be seen with initiating a task, planning, organizing, or recalling details. Structuring activities to mitigate these weaknesses often benefits the child or adolescent. Directly teaching self-regulation strategies has been useful in meeting the needs of individuals with emotional and behavioral problems (Kern, 1994) who demonstrate executive functions difficulties. Self-regulatory strategies include interventions that are student directed and include: (a) cognitive learning strategies, (b) strategies for independently learning how to use skills and when to use skills, and (c) self-monitoring strategies. They seem to be particularly useful for teaching generalization of material and can take many forms such as checklists, graphing progress, mnemonics, and goal setting. Perry, Albeg, and Tung (2012) completed a meta-analysis to determine the effectiveness of self-regulatory strategies by looking at single-subject design research for children and adolescents between 5 and 21 years old. The results of the analysis were consistent with previous findings stating that self-regulation was an effective means for improving academic performance. Although academic performance can be widely interpreted, self-regulatory strategies can be used for improving language skills.

Social Skills and Pragmatic Language Therapy

The lack of necessary social skills often serves as a deterrent in forming and maintaining adequate relationships for individuals with emotional and behavioral disorders. For younger children, social skills may involve greeting others, turn-taking skills in both play and conversation, and regulating emotions in a socially appropriate way. The child may exhibit avoidance of others or may not show a healthy skepticism when first meeting strangers. Older children may exhibit similar patterns of behavior with additional difficulties of taking another person's perspective, an inability to generate multiple solutions to problems, or an inability to work logically through a problem. Students have social skills deficits for many reasons. One reason may be lack of exposure to appropriate models, or a choice not to comply with social and cultural norms. Other individuals manifest a lack of awareness of the social expectations in a particular setting, due to primary language deficits. Although the reason for poor social skills may have a different origin, all of these children can benefit from social skills training. Typically, if the child demonstrates lack of social awareness due to primary language deficits he or she has a pragmatic language deficit.

Many programs are available to address pragmatic language skills such as role-playing and using scripts. Ciechalski and Schmidt (1995) were able to demonstrate that using role-playing along with performance feedback from guidance counselors positively affected the social interactions of students with disabilities. Most professionals agree that the key to generalizing the newly developed prosocial skills is adequate experience in several natural environments. Therapies involving the clinical social worker, the art therapist, or the special educator are natural ways to include pragmatic language skills in the child's intervention plan. Cotreatment is also a reciprocal process that allows different disciplines to learn from each other.

Cognitive and developmental levels must be considered when developing programs (see Sauter, Heyne, & Westenberg, 2009). The use of pictures and physical props may be necessary when instructing developmentally young children. Social skills stories developed by Carol Gray (1993) are a popular method for introducing some youngsters to appropriate social responses in various contexts and situations. Michele Garcia-Winner (http://www.socialthinking.com) has created a variety of materials for younger children and adolescents that help to develop a sense of others, or the ability to take someone else's perspective. Taking another's perspective is the lynchpin to developing social relationships and the lack of this skill can be the demise of developing and maintaining social relationships. The inability to take a person's perspective also influences academic skills such as inferencing and understanding a character's point of view in a story. Because of the interdisciplinary nature of addressing language skills, and emotional and behavioral disorders, working with mental health counselors becomes important particularly to assist the counselor in understanding the impact of the child or adolescent's language needs. When counselors rely on more traditional talk therapies, the success of the session may be impacted by the level of language used to interact with the client.

Social skills groups can be done in conjunction with a school counselor, psychologist, or social worker or by the SLP alone. For youngsters under the middle school age using parents as partners has been successful. In school settings the teachers should be included in the objectives and attempts should be made to generalize the skills to multiple settings including home and the classroom. The Social Communication Intervention Project (SCIP) has successfully used teachers as partners in improving social communication. Adams et al., (2012) conducted a randomized controlled study for 87 children between 5;11 and 10;8 who had been identified with pragmatic communication problems. Treatment goals incorporated areas of concern gleaned from both classroom teachers and parents. The SCIP treatment, was unique in that it supported language particularly comprehension monitoring and narrative structures which differs from many other treatments that directly target social language. While there was no significant difference found on standardized test measures there were significant differences between groups in overall conversation quality and parent-reported social communication, social behavior and language skills following the SCIP intervention. In a separate follow-up study that explored the parent and teachers perceptions following the treatment Baxendale, Lockton, Adams, and Gaile, (2013) found that parents and teachers alike described how the therapy had changed behavior and communication, including listening and attention while decreasing frustration and anxiety.

Social skills training has been shown to be effective with multiple populations including those individuals with social phobia (Sharfstein, Beidel, Finnell, Distler, & Cartner, 2011), child abuse victims (Moreno, Sanchez, Alonso, & Romero, 2012), ADHD (Corkum, Corbin, & Pike, 2011), and language impairment (Gerber, Brice, Capone, Fujiki, & Timler, 2012).

Components of the SCIP program (see Adams et al., 2012) include:

- Content guided by parent and teacher interviews
- Highly individualized based on unique profile

■ Support of language particularly comprehension monitoring and narrative structures

■ Language seen as a mediator in social communication intervention

■ Clear structure including: (a) language processing, (b) pragmatics, and (c) social understanding

More traditional language areas addressing receptive and expressive concerns can be found in other sections of this book (see Chapter 2 on Learning Disabilities).

In summary, social skills training is a viable intervention for improving social skills. A 2008 meta analysis supported social skills training particularly for improving the social competency of secondary students with emotional and behavioral disorders (see Cook et al., 2008 for complete review). One important question asked by the researchers in the review was if particular theoretical approaches appear to be more effective than others. Their findings were inconclusive but they did recognize that behavioral approaches were more effective than the social-cognitive approaches particularly for younger adolescents. Similarly those that included modeling and coaching yielded strong results (Cook et al., 2008). Also, of interest in this same meta analysis was the discussion of when to introduce social skills training in a child's development. The strongest effects were seen for adolescents, followed by preschool children and then elementary-aged children.

When children and adolescents lack the language skills needed to adequately express themselves supplementing talk therapy with expressive therapy often yields positive results.

Expressive Therapies

Other alternatives used to address both language deficits and emotional and behavioral problems have been in using expressive therapies including Dance-Movement and Music, Art, and Drama-Based approaches. Although these therapies do not share the same strong evidence base for improving language that other treatments demonstrate, they do show some promise for the SLP and merit further exploration. Most of these therapies can be used in an interdisciplinary manner, however, the SLP should have an understanding of these methods as he or she may want to integrate them into his or her own therapy techniques as these therapies typically have a reduced linguistic load.

Dance Movement Therapy/ Music Therapy

Using interdisciplinary approaches has been effective for many years. A 1987 study by Schmerling and Kerins revealed success with a child with selective mutism when combining dance and movement therapy with speech and language therapy. Music has also been used effectively with children with delayed speech development and social/pragmatic issues. Gross, Linden, and Ostermann (2010) effectively showed increased comprehension of sentences as well as improved phonological memory for nonwords and child-therapist relationship. SLPs reported that the children began communicating more frequently and started to socialize more (Gross et al., 2010) when listening to music. Music has been used for adults with aphasia as a method for stimulating speech and prosodic features for years. Implications for developing rhythmic prosodic abilities seem to be integral for language and social development; therefore music therapy may provide a supportive therapy for children with developmental speech delay without the lexical demands of language.

Art Therapy

McNamee (2004) presented an interesting case on using scribble drawings as a means of tying both verbal therapies with nonverbal therapies for a client with severe anxiety and depression. It was the nonverbal process driving the verbal process that facilitated therapy. Scribble drawings begin with a continuous line that eventually reveal shapes and images that the client can then identify, outline, and/or color. In McNamee'e example, the process of drawing was extremely beneficial and helped her client put words to a previously traumatic incident through the metaphor of drawing. In a similar vein, when therapists join together in an interdisciplinary fashion positive results can occur.

Drama-Based Therapy

One final expressive therapy that has gained ground in recent years has been drama-based therapy. Drama has been shown to be an excellent way of practicing body language, including facial expressions, by overacting different emotional states and role-playing scenarios. Drama activities have been promoted because they are interactive and address emotions, communication, cooperation, and imagination, and emphasize the reciprocity of interpersonal nonverbal cues (Goldstein & Winner, 2012; Lerner & Levine, 2007). Several studies (see Chung, Reavis, Mosconi, Drewry, Matthews, & Tasse, 2007;

Harper, Symon, & Frea, 2008) have used typically developing peers as models resulting in improved social responses from the impaired students. Guil, Semrud-Clikeman, Lerner, and Britton (2013) successfully piloted a creative drama program for youth with social difficulties, including ADHD, nonverbal learning disabilities, and autism entitled the Socialized Competence Intervention program, developed from creative drama activities. The program's goal is to improve social perception of nonverbal cues thereby improving social competence in natural settings. The program begins by focusing on the child's own emotional experience and then expanding that understanding to others. The results suggested generalized improvements in both positive interaction and decreased solitary play. The program seems best suited for preteenage children.

Although the therapies in the expressive arts have shown promise and anecdotally there have been improvements in both areas of language and social competence, the information has been largely anecdotal and does not have a strong evidence base at this time.

Another area that has been successfully used in conjunction with other therapies is pharmacological interventions. Although SLPs do not prescribe drugs many of their clients take medications. It is worth having some background knowledge on the various drug types and understands how the medications may impact speech and or language.

There are two very useful references for speech-language pathologists to assist in determining evidence-based practices in future years. The first resource, The Evidence-Based Compendium (http://www.asha.org/members/ebp/compendium/) includes systematic reviews tied to scientific evidence and guidelines in various areas. The American Speech-Language Hearing Association has attempted to develop clinical guidelines related to audiology and speech-language pathology. This resource is ongoing and is constantly being revised. A second resource for ASHA (and NSSHLA) members is the Beta site for ASHA's new practice portal. This is ASHA's attempt at placing clinical guidelines, practice documents, evidence maps, and client and patient handouts in one site. The SLP and audiologist should access the website periodically for updates and this can also be found on ASHA's website.

Pharmacological Interventions

Psychotropic medication is an important factor in the intervention of individuals with emotional and behavioral problems. Many of the above mentioned interventions are most effective when paired with the appropriate medications. However, a few studies have investigated the effects of medication in relation to the psychiatric diagnosis. A study by Hallfors, Fallon, and Watson (1998) showed that children who received a diagnosis of ADHD, schizophrenia, bipolar, or major depression were six times more likely to receive medication than other children in the study; children with conduct disorders were less likely to receive medication. Whereas this study did not address the effectiveness of the medications, it did show that children with conduct disorders were prescribed medication far less frequently than those with other disorders.

The developments in psychiatry have advanced from a psychoanalytical approach to one that is increasingly more grounded in medical-neurobiological findings. Scientists continue to make strides in discovering how medicine can be used to manage behaviors. A very brief overview of some of the common psychotropic medications is provided.

SLPs should be aware of the range of medications available to clients with psychiatric disorders as well as some of the side effects and the affect they may have on speech. A reference list is provided in Table 8–3 that details the DSM-5 diagnosis, typically prescribed medications and speech and/or language effects.

Interface Between School and Mental Health

Ideally, there should be meaningful communication between mental health facilities, private treatment professionals, and schools, but unfortunately this is not always the case. Communication between professionals that treat youth with emotional and behavioral disorders is essential. A problem exists when federal guidelines for eligibility for special education are not followed. The problem seems to be one of diagnosis and the subsequent eligibility for services. Children who are diagnosed in facilities outside of school may not be eligible for services unless communication between clinics and schools is consistent (McGinnis & Forness, 1988). The psychiatric diagnosis determined in the *Diagnostic and Statistical Manual-V* (APA, 2013) and eligibility for special education under the federal guidelines is not always easily transferable. Although many day treatment programs have their own staff psychiatrist who can communicate meaningfully with the day treatment staff, hospital and clinic professionals are not always versed in IDEA eligibility practices. Incorrect terminology between professionals and schools may result in a

Table 8–3. DSM-V Diagnosis, Speech, and Language Characteristics and Medication Side Effect

DSM-V Category	Speech/Language Characteristics	Common Medications	Side Effect of Medication
APA, 2013		Rappa and Viola, 2012	Vogel and Carter, 1995
Disruptive, Impulse Control, and Conduct Disorders *Oppositional Defiant, Conduct Disorder*	Phonological awareness issues/low reading; academic struggles; pragmatic issues	Same as ADHD and/or antidepressants	Dry mouth Pressured or rapid speech may be sign of overmedication with psychostimulants
Schizophrenia Spectrum and Other Psychotic Disorders *Schizophrenia*	Disorganized speech, (also may be diagnosed in writing sample) may not maintain topic, ambiguous references, loose associations (Caplan, 1996; Harvey, 1983)	Cloraril® Zyprexa® Risperdal® Ablify® Seoquel® Latuda®	Dysarthria for sedating drugs Neuroleptics may cause movement disorders affecting tongue or jaw Antipsychotic
Depression *Dysregulation Disorder, Major Depressive Disorder*	Slow speech, shortened responses, increased pause time, reduced pitch (nasal or pharyngeal quality) and decreased suprasegmentals Nonverbal communication: poor eye contact (France, 1992; Mundt et al., 2012)	MAOIs SSRIs SNRIs Remeron® Wellbutrin®	Dry mouth, slurred speech may indicate overmedication
Neurodevelopmental *ADHD*	Language formulation, word retrieval, working memory (Jacobson et al., 2011; DaParma et al., 2011)	Dexedrine® Ritalin® Concerta® Adderal®	Vocal tremor or rapid speech side effect of dextro-amphetamine
Anxiety Disorder *Selective Mutism, Generalized Anxiety*	Rapid naming, retrieval difficulty, poor expressive skills (Anstendig, 1999; Klein et al., 2013)	Tofranil® Nardil® Zoloft® Lexapro® Benzodiazepines	Impaired concentration and memory, dysarthric symptoms

psychiatric diagnosis without securing needed services for the child.

Eligibility is particularly problematic for those children and adolescents identified with the disruptive behavior disorders (opposition defiant disorder, conduct disorder, and ADHD) because of their identification with social maladjustment and the exclusion of socially maladjusted in under the federal definition of ED [EBD]. The play for services becomes a semantic game. Professionals must document accurately, thoroughly, and carefully to meet the definition under the IDEA. Ironically, the children with disruptive behavior disorders are among those most frequently identified in classrooms for youth with EBD (Mattison et al., 1986; Mattison, Morales, & Bauer, 1992). It is imperative that all professionals work toward a common language and understanding, so the child can be served comprehensively, at home, in the community, and at school.

As mental health issues continue to indicate an upward trend, services to treat those with emotional and behavioral disorders will continue to increase as well. SLPs need to feel confident of the vital role they play in the diagnosis and treatment of individuals with psychiatric disorders. Continued work and research continues to promote a greater level of confidence and understanding of the relationship between communication and socio-emotional development.

Case Study 1: Nine-Year-Old Psych-Educational Assessment

This case study is designed as a Think Aloud to facilitate understanding of how a clinician might think through a case. The clinician's thoughts are shown in italics.

Mason is a 9-year-old Caucasian male who is currently a third-grade student at a local parochial school. Mason's mother provided background information during the intake evaluation. Developmental milestones were within normal limits with the exception his speech and language development. Mason did not use words until 3½ years of age and then began speaking in sentences at 4 years old. He was diagnosed with apraxia of speech and received speech and language services through Infants and Toddlers program from the age of 18 months through 4 years old. Mason is not currently receiving services.

Mason has always performed well in school; however, recently there have been some concerns regarding Mason's difficulty following discussions in his higher-level reading group. His mother has also observed that he will forget assignments and textbooks from school. Furthermore, his mother has noted word-finding difficulty when conversing with friends and relatives.

Mason's mother reports that recently he has been struggling to control his anger when he is frustrated and has become more irritable in the past few months. He has been in several fights with peers at school and on occasion has verbally lashed out at his classroom teacher.

So far we have seen a classic pattern of phonological impairments impacting early language development then re-emerging during third grade when language and literacy demands increase. This classic pattern demonstrates the language-literacy connection and also demonstrates how an early speech and language delay can be predictive of later academic problems.

What is also typical is the relationship between academic struggles and behavior. Recall the divisions of externalizing and inter-

nalizing behaviors. Mason's academic struggles are causing him to lash out and become angry, which is classified as externalizing behaviors. Considering bringing in another mental health professional to assess the behaviors may be wise. In a school setting a functional behavioral assessment may be a good idea. Other professionals would be a licensed clinical social worker, or school counselor, or psychologist.

To assess Mason's cognitive ability, he was given the Weshsler Intelligence Scale for Children, Fifth Edition (WISC-V). Mason received a full-scale IQ of 100, which is in the average range of functioning. His verbal IQ of 95 was within the average range as was his performance IQ of 110. The psychologist also gave Mason the Wechsler Individual Achievement Test (WIAT-II), Third Edition to assess academic skills. In summary his WIAT-II profile suggests evenly developed and average to high average academic tasks in the areas of oral language, reading, writing, and mathematics.

Mason was assessed across multiple sessions; he was polite and socially engaged. During verbal tasks, Mason displayed concrete thinking, at times repeating the same answer instead of elaborating or rewording his response. He appeared distractible, fidgeting, and looking into the two-way mirror making faces at him.

The Verbal Comprehension index of the WISC-V showed some difficulties when defining words and concepts. He scored in the low average range with this subtest.

On the WIAT-III, Mason obtained an Oral Language composite of 90, with single-word receptive vocabulary weaker than his other skills in this area. His reading composite was also slightly depressed indicating his ability to read nonsense words (e.g., tashig) underdeveloped especially

when compared to his ability to read real words. Oral reading fluency was labored and reading comprehension was slightly delayed. Writing scores were evenly developed, but below average in his ability to spell words, write sentences, and express his thoughts in a cohesive essay.

Given the information on Mason's cognitive and achievement tests, a more fine-grained language analysis should be performed by the SLP. Word retrieval issues noted by his mother and below average oral language skills present some red flags. This is further corroborated by the depressed scores in reading nonsense words, which may indicate an underlying phonological issue. Finally, because written language is also an expressive language task, low spelling and sentence writing further support the need for a closer look at Mason's language. A referral should be made to the SLP.

If language testing supports the need for treatment and treatment is received, Mason's academic frustrations should subside. He will need continued support to access the general education curriculum and will need to be monitored by the school psychologist and counselor.

Review Questions

1. What were some of the classroom behaviors that Mason's mother reported? Were these externalizing or internalizing behaviors?

2. What were some red flags or signals in the psycho-educational report that indicate further testing by a SLP?

3. What other professionals should the SLP be collaborating with? Why?

4. What additional assessments should the SLP administer?

5. If Mason's language needs are not met, what could one expect about his behavior in and out of school?

Case Study 2:
13-Year-Old Male, EBD

Josh is a 13-year-old seventh grader enrolled in a program for individuals with emotional and behavioral disorders. Josh presents with a long history of involvement in the juvenile justice system, where he has been charged with theft and breaking and entering. Josh presently lives with his maternal grandmother. His mother is unable to care for him and his father is incarcerated. School records are incomplete, as Josh has relocated five times in his seven years of schooling. Records note consistently poor academic performance. A recent psychological test indicates a full-scale IQ of 67; however, the examiner felt test results were not valid because Josh "did not fully cooperate" during all tasks. A diagnostic assessment was recommended because of Josh's poor academic record, terse verbal output, and increasing aggression toward his grandmother and staff.

The school's special educator, psychiatrist, and SLP conducted assessments over a four-week period. Because of Josh's lack of trust in formal testing situations, much of the testing was completed informally. The special educator and SLP met daily with Josh to review his schedule, letting him know when he was in class and when he came to "speech." During speech diagnostic sessions Josh initially spent a good deal of time manipulating objects in the clinician's office such as Legos and three-dimensional puzzles. As he warmed up to the clinician he would respond to questions regarding likes, dislikes, and how he spent his time. When Josh was willing, the clinician would have him demonstrate some of his skills by reading words from standardized word lists and typing responses on a laptop. It was evident that Josh was functioning three to four years below grade level in some academic tasks. Josh was able to complete the Peabody Picture Vocabulary Test, which assesses one-word receptive vocabulary. He received a standard score of 85, demonstrating a low average performance in his understanding of words. Academically the special educator was able to assess classroom math and reading work. Josh was able to add, subtract, multiply, and divide two-digit numbers. He was able to use the calculator for multiplication and division tasks. Josh demonstrated the ability to read material at the fourth grade instructional level.

The psychiatrist met with Josh several times. He was unsuccessful in getting Josh to respond to him, deferring the psychiatric diagnosis of Josh at the time. The team met to discuss Josh's placement and educational plan. The team concurred that continued diagnostic assessment was needed to aid in a comprehensive picture of Josh's strengths and weaknesses. Continued support for a restrictive placement in a facility for emotionally and behaviorally disturbed children was necessary. The team agreed to continue to assess skills through informal assessments to supplement formal testing.

Several months later formal testing was completed indicating a language-based learning disability based on the Woodcock-Johnson Tests of Achievement, the Clinical Evaluation of Language Fundamental-IV, and the Comprehensive Test of Phonological Processes. Furthermore, Josh demonstrated difficulty with short-term auditory memory, word retrieval, and phonological production of multisyllabic words. These phonological core deficits contributed to a severe language-based learning disability affecting receptive and expressive language as well as academic skills, particularly reading. The following recommendations were made: (a) continued treatment in the day program for students with emotional and behavioral disorders; (b) enrollment in the Orton Gillingham Method of reading; (c) speech and language therapy targeting phonological awareness and strategies for word retrieval and memory; (d) special education help with math and written language; (e) weekly therapy with a licensed clinical social worker and an updated DSM diagnosis from the staff psychiatrist.

Review Questions

1. Why do you think the author chose to use the term *individual with emotional and behavioral disorder* as opposed to *individual with emotional disturbance?*

2. What language or label is used in the federal definition (IDEA) for children with psychiatric disorders?

3. How else could the SLP supplement the informal testing delineated in the case study? What risk factors would alert the SLP to the fact this student may have speech and language disabilities? Why? Why did the SLP choose to let the student play and manipulate "toys" before pushing him with formal assessments? What is the likelihood of a school-based SLP working with students with emotional and/or behavioral disorders?

4. Name three interventions used with this population. How are they the same or different as working with children with learning disabilities? ADHD?

Case Study 3: 15-Year-Old Male, Thought Disorder

Simon is a 15-year-old 10th grader recently receiving speech and language services in a regular public school setting. Simon was recently referred by the SLP for further testing because of increasing concerns over his "unusual behaviors and responses" observed in the classroom during push-in speech and language sessions. Past school history is positive for language-based learning disabilities in the areas of math and written language. Records also indicated speech and language therapy in the early elementary grades.

An interdisciplinary team that included the school psychologist, special educator, occupational therapist, SLP, and psychiatrist completed diagnostic testing. Assessments were completed both formally and informally while observing Simon during structured and unstructured times. Simon's parents were also interviewed to obtain a more complete family history and to discuss current concerns.

Results of the psychological assessment indicated a young man in the average range of intellectual functioning as demonstrated on the WISC-V. In fact, his ability to handle verbal abstractions and his fund of general knowledge was in the superior range of functioning. In contrast, performance areas including attention to detail, nonverbal reasoning, and ability to sequence items visually were comparatively low. Educational testing utilizing the Woodcock-Johnson Tests of Achievement, concurred with classroom observations and previous reports of below age level performance in the areas of math and written expression. Measures used by the occupational therapist (OT) assessed fine motor skills, sensory motor skill, and visual-perceptual skills. Simon demonstrated delays in letter formation, slow handwriting speed when copying, and poor cursive skills. Visual-perceptual skills were determined to be functional. Anecdotally, the OT noted inconsistent attention to tasks as well as tangential responses to questions. The psychiatrist reported behaviors consistent with a psychotic illness, including thought blocking, anxiety, and mental confusion.

Speech and language assessments completed the multidisciplinary testing. The Clinical Evaluation of Language Fundamentals-IV was administered to provide an overview of Simon's receptive and expressive language functioning. Simon demonstrated average skills perceiving semantic relationships between single words as well as the ability to interpret word relationships at the sentence level. However, Simon demonstrated a severe deficit in the ability to interpret, recall, and execute oral commands of increasing length and complexity. Expressively, Simon scored in the average range for all three subtests, indicating an average ability to understand and formulate original sentences using simple but appropriate syntax and morphology. Speech, voice, and fluency were assessed informally. Simon demonstrated adequate articulation skills but his prosody, rate, and inflection were flat and his rate of speech was judged to be slow.

The interdisciplinary team convened to review and discuss each discipline's finding. It was concluded that indeed Simon was presenting with symptoms consistent with a psychotic disorder that was affecting his performance across all academic and social settings. Although speech and language results showed evidence of a receptive language disorder it was the team's consensus that the receptive language problem was secondary to an emerging thought disorder. Because Simon showed a strong fund of general information and expressively showed average skills in sentence formulation, he was expected to be able to maintain himself in a structured classroom setting. The team recommended academic and psychiatric interventions including: (a) a small, self-contained setting; (b) goals addressing attention and organization; (c) indirect speech language services to provide comprehension strategies for the classroom teacher and suggestions for modifying written language assignments; (d) weekly sessions with the licensed clinical social worker; and (e) antipsychotic and antistimulant medications prescribed by and followed by the staff psychiatrist. Additionally, the SLP suggested that Simon participate in a weekly pragmatic language group to work on topic maintenance and appropriate responses, while improving his ability to take another person's perspective. The team agreed to meet about Simon on a quarterly basis to monitor his progress.

Review Questions

1. Why was an interdisciplinary team critical for this diagnosis?

2. What conclusion may have the SLP drawn if she had not worked as a collaborative team member?

3. What were some of the signs and symptoms generated formally and informally through assessment that helped lead to the diagnosis of a formal thought disorder?

4. What are some warning signs that may be seen in the early phases of schizophrenia?

5. Do you feel like the recommendation to place Simon in a Pragmatic Language group was appropriate? Why or why not?

References

Achenbach, T. M. (2001). *Manual for the Child Behavior Checklist/4-18 and 1991 Profile*. Burlington, VT: University of Vermont, Department of Psychiatry.

Adams, C., Lockton, E., Freed, J., Gaile, J., Earl, G., McBean, K., . . . Law, J. (2012). The social communication intervention project: A randomized controlled trial of the effectiveness of speech and language therapy for school-age children who have pragmatic and social communication problems with or without autism spectrum disorder. *International Journal of Language and Communication Disorders, 47*, 233–244.

American Psychiatric Association. (1980). *Diagnostic and statistical manual of mental disorders* (3rd ed.). Washington, DC: Author.

American Psychiatric Association. (2000). *Diagnostic and statistical manual of mental disorders* (4th ed.). Washington, DC: Author.

American Psychiatric Association. (2013). *Diagnostic and statistical manual of mental disorders* (5th ed.). Arlington, VA: Author.

American Speech-Language-Hearing Association. (2010). *Roles and responsibilities of speech-language pathologists in schools* [Professional issues statement]. Retrieved from http://www.asha.org/policy

Anstendig, K. (1999). Is selective mutism an anxiety disorder? Rethinking its DSM–IV classification. *Journal of Anxiety Disorders, 13*(4), 417–434. doi:10.1016/S0887-6185(99)99912-2

Aronson, A. E. (1990). *Clinical voice disorders. An interdisciplinary approach* (3rd ed.). New York, NY: Thieme-Stratton.

Atchison, B. (2007). Sensory modulation disorders among children with a history of trauma:

A frame of reference for speech-language pathologists. *Language Speech and Hearing Services in Schools, 38*, 109–116. doi:10.1044/0161-1461(2007/011)

Baker, J. (2002). Psychogenic voice disorders—heroes or hysterics? A brief overview with questions and discussion. *Logopedics Phoniatrics Vocology, 27*, 84–91. doi:10.1080/14015430 2760409310

Baker, L., & Cantwell, D. P. (1987). Factors with the development of psychiatric illness in children with early speech/language problems. *Journal of Autism and Developmental Disorders, 17*(4), 499–510. Retrieved from http://link.springer.com/journal/10803

Baltaxe, C., & Simmons, J. Q. (1988). Communication deficits in preschool children with psychiatric disorders. *Seminars in Speech and Language, 9*(1), 81–90. doi:10.1055/s-2008-1064453

Baltaxe, C., & Simmons, J. Q. (1995). Speech and language disorders in children and adolescents with schizophrenia. *Schizophrenia Bulletin, 21*(4), 677–692.

Barkley, R., Murphy, K., & Fischer, M. (2008). *ADHD in adults: What the science says.* New York, NY: Guilford Press.

Barkley, R. A. (2000). *Taking charge of ADHD: The complete authoritative guide for parents–revised edition.* New York, NY: Guilford Press.

Baxendale, J., Lockton, E., Adams, C., & Gaile, J. (2013). Parent and teacher perceptions of participation and outcomes in an intensive communication intervention for children with pragmatic language impairment. *International Journal of Language & Communication Disorders, 48*(1), 41–53. doi:10.1111/j. 1460-69 84.2012.00202.x

Beeghly, M. (2006). Translational research on early language development: Current challenges and future directions. *Development and Psychopathology, 18*, 737–757. doi:10.1017/S095 4579406060366

Beery, K. (1989). *Developmental Test of Visual-Motor Integration–3rd revision.* Cleveland, OH: Modern Curriculum Press.

Beery, K. E., Buktenica, N. A., & Beery, N. A. (2010). *Manual for the Beery-Buktenica Developmental Test of Visual-Motor Integration, Sixth Edition (VMI-6).* San Antonio, TX: Pearson Assessment.

Beitchman, J. H., Wilson, B., Brownlie, E. B., Walters, H., Inglis, A., & Lancee, W. (1996). Long-term consistency in speech/language profiles: II. Behavioral, emotional, and social outcomes. *Journal American Academy of Child and Adolescent Psychiatry, 35*(6), 815–970. doi:10.1097/00004583-199606000-00022

Benner, G., Mattison, R. E., Nelson, J. R., & Ralston, N. C. (2009). Types of language disorders in students classified as ED: Prevalence and association with learning disabilities and psychopathology. *Education and Treatment of Children, 32*(4), 631–653. Retrieved from http://digitalcommons.unl.edu/speechfacpub

Benner, G., Nelson, R., & Epstein, M. H. (2002). Language skills of children with EBD: A literature review. *Journal of Emotional and Behavioral Disorders, 10*(1), 43–59. doi:10.1177/106342660201000105

Bishop, D. (2003). *The Children's Communication Checklist–Second Edition (CCC-2).* London, UK: The Psychological Corporation.

Boone, D. R., McFarlane, S. C., Von Berg, S. L., & Zraick, R. I. (2010). *The voice and voice therapy* (8th ed.). Boston, MA: Allyn & Bacon.

Bopp, K. D., Brown, K. E., & Mirenda, P. (2004). Speech-language pathologist's roles in the delivery of positive behavior support of individuals with developmental disabilities. *American Journal of Speech-Language Pathology, 13*(1), 5–19. doi:1058-0360/04/1301- 0005

Botting, N., & Conti-Ramsden, G. (2008). The role of language, social cognition, and social skill in the functional outcomes of young adolescents with and without a history of SLI. *British Journal of Developmental Psychology, 26*(2), 281–300. doi:10.1348/026151007X235891

Burke, J. D., Hipwell, A. E., & Loeber, R. (2010). Dimensions of oppositional defiant disorder as predictors of depression and conduct disorder in preadolescent girls. *Journal of American Academy of Child and Adolescent Psychiatry, 49*(1), 484–492. doi:10.1097/00004583-201005000-00009

Busse, R. T., & Downey, J. (2011). Selective mutism: A three-tiered approach to prevention and intervention. *Contemporary School Psychology, 15*, 53–63.

Bussing, R., Zima, B. T., Mason, D. M., Porter, P. C., & Garvan, C. W. (2011). Receiving treatment for attention-deficit hyperactivity disorder: Do the perspectives of adolescents matter? *Journal of Adolescent Health, 49*(1), 7–14. doi:10.1016/j.jadohealth.2010.08.014

Camarata, S. M., Hughes, C. A., & Ruhl, K. L. (1988). Mild/moderate behaviorally disordered students: A population at risk for language disorders. *Language, Speech, and Hearing Services in Schools, 19*, 191–200. Retrieved from http://lshss.asha.org/

Cantwell, D. P., & Baker, L. (1987). Prevalence and type of psychiatric disorder and developmental disorders in three speech and language groups. *Journal of Communication Disorders, 20*(2), 151–160. Retrieved from http://www.journals.elsevier.com/journal-of-communication-disorders/

Caplan, R. (1996). Discourse deficits in childhood schizophrenia. In J. H. Beitchman, N. J. Cohen, M. M. Konstantareas, & R. Tannock (Eds.), *Language, learning, and behavior disorders* (pp. 156–177). New York, NY: Cambridge University Press.

Carrow-Woolfolk, E. (1999). *Comprehensive Assessment of Spoken Language (CASL).* Circle Pines, MN: American Guidance Services.

Carson, D. K., Klee, T., Perry, C. K., Muskina, G., & Donaghy, T. (1998). Comparisons of children with delayed and normal language at 24 months of age on measures of behavioral difficulties, social, and cognitive development. *Infant Mental Health Journal, 19*(1), 59–75. doi:10.1002/(SICI)1097-0355(199821)19:1<59::AID-IMHJ4>3.0.CO;2-V

Castellanos, F. (March, 2012). *What have we learned from neuroimaging. The spectrum of developmental disabilities XXXIV "ADHD: Too broad? Too narrow?"* Baltimore, MD: Johns Hopkins School of Medicine.

Catts, H. W., Adlof, S. M., Hogan, T. P., & Weismer, S. E. (2005). Are specific language impairment and dyslexia distinct disorders? *Journal of Speech, Language and Hearing Research, 48*(6), 1378–1396.

Cavendish, W. (2014). Academic attainment during commitment and postrelease education-related outcomes of juvenile justice-involved youth with and without disabilities. *Journal of Emotional and Behavioral Disorders, 22*(1), 41–52. doi:10.1177/1063426612470516

Chorpita, B. F. (2007). *Modular cognitive-behavioral therapy for childhood anxiety disorders.* New York, NY: Guilford.

Chung, K. M., Reavis, S., Mosconi, M., Drewry, J., Matthews, T., & Tasse, M. J. (2007). Peer-mediated social skills training program for young children with high-functioning autism. *Research in Developmental Disabilities, 28*(4), 423–436. doi:10.1016/j.ridd.2006.05.002

Cicchetti, D., & Lynch, M. (1995). Failures in the expectable environment and their impact on the individual development: The case of child maltreatment. In D. Cicchetti & D. J. Cohen (Eds.), *Developmental psychopathology: Vol. 2. Risk disorder and adaptation* (pp. 32–71). New York, NY: John Wiley & Sons.

Ciechalski, J. C., & Schmidt, M. W. (1995). The effects of social skills training on students with exceptionalities. *Elementary School Guidance and Counseling, 29*(3), 217–223. Retrieved from http://www.ebscohost.com/academic/academic-search-premier

Cohan, J. S., Chavira, D. A., Shipon-Blum, E., Hitchcok, C., Roesch, S. C., & Stein, M. B. (2008). Refining the classification of children with selective mutism: A latent profile analysis. *Journal of Clinical Child and Adolescent Psychiatry, 37*(4), 770–784. doi:10.1080/15374410802359759

Cohen, N. J., Davine, M., Horodezky, N., Lipsett, L., & Isaacson, L. (1993). Unsuspected language impairment in psychiatrically disturbed children: Prevalence and language and behavioral characteristics. *Journal of American Academy Child Adolescent Psychiatry, 32*(3), 595–603. doi:10.1097/00004583-199305000-00016

Cohen, N. J., Davine, M., & Meloche-Kelly, M. (1989). Prevalence of unsuspected language disorders in a child psychiatric population. *Journal of the American Academy of Child and Adolescent Psychiatry, 28*(1), 107–111. doi:10.1097/0004583-1989010000-00020

Cohen, N. J., Lipsett, L., & Dip, C. S. (1991). Recognized and unrecognized language impairment in psychologically disturbed children: Child symptomatology, maternal depression, & family dysfunction [Preliminary report]. *Canadian Journal of Behavioral Sciences, 23*(3), 376–389. doi:10.1037/h0079017

Cook, C. R., Gresham, F. M., Kern, L., Barreras, R. B., Thornton, S., & Crews, S. D. (2008). Social skills training for secondary students with emotional and/or behavioral disorders: A review and analysis of the meta analytic literature. *Journal of Emotional and Behavioral Disorders, 16*(3), 131–144. doi:10.1177/1063426608314541

Corkum, P., Corbin, N., & Pike, M. (2011). Evaluation of a school-based social skills program for children with attention-Deficit/Hyperactivity disorder. *Child and Family Behavior Therapy, 32*(2), 139. doi:10.1080/07317101003776472

Council for Children with Behavioral Disorders. (1987). *Position paper on identification of students with behavioral disorders.* Reston, VA: Author.

Council for Children with Behavioral Disorders. (1989). Best assessment practices for students with behavioral disorders: Accommodation to cultural diversity and individual differences. *Behavioral Disorders, 14,* 263–278.

Council for Exceptional Children. (1991). *Report of the CEC advocacy and governmental relations committee regarding the new proposed United States federal definition of serious emotional disturbance.* Reston, VA: Author.

DaParma, A., Geffner, D., & Martin, N. (2011). Prevalence and nature of language impairment in children with attention deficit/hyperactivity disorder. *Contemporary Issues in Communication Sciences and Disorders, 38,* 119–125. doi:1092-5171/11/3802-0119

Davidson, S., & Smith, R. (1990). Traumatic experiences in psychiatric outpatients. *Journal of Traumatic Stress Studies, 3*(3), 459–475. doi:10.1007/BF00974785

Delaney, E. M., & Kaiser, A. P. (2001). The effects of teaching parents blended communication and behavior support strategies. *Behavioral Disorders, 26*(2), 93. Retrieved from http://www.proquest.com/en-US

Denckla, M. (March, 2012). *ADHD after a quarter century.* Baltimore, MD: Johns Hopkins School of Medicine.

DeSocio, J., & Hootman, J. (2004). Children's mental health and school success. *The Journal of School Nursing, 20*(4), 189–196. doi:10.1177/10598405040200040201

Duncan, B. B., Forness, S. R., & Hartsough, C. (1995). Students identified as seriously emotionally disturbed in school-based day treatment: Cognitive, psychiatric, and special education characteristics. *Behavioral Disorders, 20*(4), 238–252. Retrieved from http://academia.edu/

DuPaul, G. (2012, March). *ADHD in high school and college. The spectrum of developmental disabilities XXXIV "ADHD: Too broad? Too narrow?"* Baltimore, MD: Johns Hopkins School of Medicine.

DuPaul, G., Weyandt, L., O'Dell, S., & Varejao, M. (2009). College students with ADHD:

Current status and future directions. *Journal of Attention Disorders, 13*(3), 234–250. doi:10 .1177/10807054709340650

Durkin, K., & Conti-Ramsden, G. (2007). Language, social behavior and the quality of friendships in adolescents with and without a history of specific language impairment. *Child Development, 78*(5), 1441–1457. doi:10.1111/ j.1467-8624.2007.01076.x

Espinosa, L. M. (2002). The connections between social-emotional development and early literacy. *The Kauffman Early Education Exchange, 1*(1), 30–32.

Ewen, J. (2012, March). *ADHD: Is it a matter of timing?* Baltimore, MD: Johns Hopkins School of Medicine.

Flannery, K. B., Fenning, P., McGrath Kato, M., & McIntosh, K. (2013). Effects of school-wide positive behavioral interventions and supports and fidelity implementation on problem behavior in high schools. *School Psychology Quarterly, 29*(2), 111–124. doi:10.1037/spq 0000039

Flick, G. L. (1998). Learning strategies and social skills training for students with ADHD. *Reaching Today's Youth, 2*(2), 37–40.

Forness, S. R., & Knitzer, J. (1992). A new proposed definition and terminology to replace "serious emotional disturbance" in Individuals with Disabilities Education Act. *School Psychology Review, 21*(1), 12–20. Retrieved from http://www.nasponline.org/

France, J. (1992). Depression. In R. Gravell & J. France (Eds.), *Speech and communication problems in psychiatry* (pp. 156–171). Clifton Park, NY: Delmar Learning.

Gable, R. A., Park, K. L., & Scott, T. M. (2014). Functional behavioral assessment and students at risk for or with emotional disabilities: Current issues and considerations. *Education and Treatment of Children, 37*(1), 111–135.

Gagnon, J., & Richards, C. (2008). *Making the right turn: A guide about improving transition outcomes of youth involved in the juvenile corrections system.* Washington, DC: National Collaborative on Workforce and Disability Youth, Institute for Educational Leadership.

Galera, C., Melchior, M., Chastang, J. F., Bouvard, M. P., & Fombonne, E. (2009). Childhood and adolescent hyperactivity-inattention symptoms and academic achievement 8 years later: The GAZEL youth study. *Psychological Medicine, 39*(11), 1895–1906.

Garfield, C., Dorsey, F., Zhu, S., Huskamp, H., Conti, R., Dusetzing, S., . . . Higashi, A. (2012). Trends in attention deficit hyperactivity disorder ambulatory diagnosis and medical treatment in the United States, 2000–2010. *Academic Pediatrics, 12*(2), 110–116. doi:10.1016/j .acap.2012.01.003

Gau, S., & Shang, C. (2010). Executive functions as endophenotypes in ADHD: Evidence from the Cambridge Neuropsychological Test Battery. *Journal of Child Psychology and Psychiatry, 51*(7), 838–849. doi:10.1111/j.1469-7610.2010.02215.x

Gerber, S., Brice, A., Capone, N., Fujiki, M., & Timpler, G. (2012). Language use in social interactions of school-age children with language impairments: An evidence-based systematic review of treatment. *Language Speech and Hearing Services in Schools, 43*, 235–249.

Giddan, J. J., Bade, K. M., Rickenberg, D., & Ryley, A. T. (1995). Teaching the language of feelings to students with severe emotional and behavioral handicaps. *Language, Speech, and Hearing in the Schools, 26*, 3–10. doi:0161-1461/95/2601-0003

Giddan, J. J., & Ross, G. J. (2001). *Childhood communication disorders in mental health settings.* Austin, TX: Pro-Ed.

Giddan, J. J., Trautman, R. C., & Hurst, J. B. (1989). The role of the speech and language clinician on a multidisciplinary team. *Child Psychiatry and Human Development, 19*(3), 180–185. Retrieved from http://link.springer.com/

Gilmour, J., Hill, B., Place, M., & Skuse, D. H. (2004). Social communication deficits in conduct disorder: A clinical and community survey. *Journal of Child Psychology and Psychiatry, 45*(5), 967–978. Retrieved from http://online library.wiley.com/

Ginsburg, D. S., & Drake, K. L. (2002). School-based treatment for anxious African-American adolescents: A controlled pilot study. *Journal of the American Academy of Child and Adolescent Psychiatry, 41*(7), 486–775. doi: 10.1097/00004583-200207000-00007

Glass, K., Flory, K., Martin, A., & Hankin, B. L. (2011). ADHD and comorbid conduct problems among adolescents: Associations with self-esteem and substance use. *Attention Deficit and Hyperactivity Disorders, 3*(1), 29–39. doi:10.1007/s12402-010-0042-y

Goldstein, T. R., & Winner, E. (2012). Enhancing empathy and theory of mind. *Journal of Cogni-*

tion and Development, 13(1), 19–37. doi:http://dx.doi.org/10.1080/15248372.2011.573514

Grave, J., & Blissett, J. (2004). Is cognitive behavior therapy developmentally appropriate for young children? A critical review of the evidence. *Clinical Psychology Review, 24*, 399–420. doi: 10.1016/j.cpr2004.03.002

Gray, C. A., & Garand, J. D. (1993). Social stories: Improving responses of students with autism with accurate social information. *Focus on Autistic Behavior, 8*(1), 1–10. doi:10.1177/108835769300800101

Gresham, F. M. (2007). Response to intervention and emotional and behavioral disorders: Best practices in assessment for intervention. *Assessment for Effective Intervention, 32*, 214–222. doi:10.1177/15345084070320040301

Gross, W., Linden, U., & Ostermann, T. (2010). Effects of music therapy in the treatment of children with delayed speech development–results of a pilot study. *BMC Complementary and Alternative Medicine, 10*, 39. doi:10.1186/1472-6882-10-39

Hallfors, D., Fallon, T., & Watson, K. (1998). An examination of psychotropic drug treatment for children with serious emotional disturbance. *Journal of Emotional and Behavioral Disorders, 6*(1), 56–72. doi:10.1177/106342669800600105

Halliday, M. A. K., & Hasan, R. (1976). *Cohesion in English*. London, UK: Longman Group.

Hammill, D. D., & Newcomer, P. L. (2008). *Test of Language Development-Intermediate Fourth Edition (TOLD I: 4)*. Austin, TX: Pro-Ed.

Hammill, D. D., & Newcomer, P. L. (2008). *Test of Language Development-Primary Fourth Edition (TOLD P: 4)*. Austin, TX: Pro-Ed.

Harper, C. B., Symon, J. B. G., & Frea, W. D. (2008). Recess is time-in: Using peers to improve social skills of children with autism. *Journal of Autism and Developmental Disorders, 38*(5), 815–826. doi:10.1007/s10803-007-0449-2

Hart, K. I., Fujiki, M., Brinton, B., & Hart, C. H. (2004). The relationship between social behavior and severity of language impairment. *Journal of Speech, Language, and Hearing Research, 47*(3), 647–662. doi:10.1044.1092-4388(2004/050)

Harty, S., Miller, C., Newcom, J., & Halperin, J. (2009). Adolescents with childhood ADHD and comorbid disruptive behavior disorders: Aggression, anger, and hostility. *Child*

Psychiatry Human Development, 40(1), 85–97. doi:10.1007/s10578-008-0110-0

Harvey, P. D. (1983). Speech competence in manic and schizophrenic psychoses: The association between clinically rated thought disorder and cohesion and reference performance. *Journal of Abnormal Psychology, 92*(3), 368–377. doi:10.1037/0021-843X.92.3.368

Hollo, A. (2012). Language and behavioral disorders in school-age children: Comorbidity and communication in the classroom. Perspectives on school-based issues. *Perspectives on School-Based Issues, 13*(4), 111–119. doi:10.1044/sbi13.4.111

Hollo, A., Wehby, J. H., & Oliver, R. M. (2014). Unidentified language deficits in children with emotional and behavioral disorders: A meta-analysis. *Exceptional Children, 80*(2), 169–186.

Hunter, L., & Chopro, V. (2001). The value of school based mental health programs. *Emotional and Behavioral Disorders in Youth, 1*, 57–58.

Hurlemann, R., Jessen, F., Wagner, M., Frommann, I., Ruhrmann, S., Brockhaus, A., . . . Maier, W. (2008). Interrelated neuropsychological and anatomical evidence of hippocampal pathology in the at-risk mental state. *Psychological Medicine, 38*(6), 843–851. doi:10.1017/S0033291708003279

Individuals With Disabilities Education Act of 1997, P. L. 105-17, 105th Cong., 1st Sess., H. R. 5. (1997).

Jacobson, L. A., Ryan, M., Martin, R. B., Ewen, J., Mostofsky, S. H., Denckla, M. B., & Mahone, E. M. (2011). Working memory influences processing speed and reading fluency in ADHD. *Child Neuropsychology, 17*(3), 209–224. doi:10.1080/09297049.2010.532204

Jolivette, K., & Nelson, C. M. (2010). Adapting positive behavioral interventions and supports for secure juvenile justice settings: Improving facility-wide behaviors. *Behavioral Disorders, 36*, 28–42.

Justice, L. M., Kaderavek, J. N., Fan, X., Sofka, A., & Hunt, A. (2009). Accelerating preschoolers' early literacy development through classroom-based teacher-child storybook reading and explicit print referencing. *Language, Speech, and Hearing Services in School, 40*(1), 67–85. doi:10.1044/0161-1461(2008/07-0098)

Kendall, P. C., Flannery-Schroeder, E., Panichelli-Mindel, S. M., Southan-Gerow, M., Henin, A., & Warman, M. (1997). Treatment of anxiety disorders in youths: A second randomized clinical trial. *Journal of Consulting and Clinical Psychology, 65*(3), 366–380. Retrieved from http://psycnet.apa.org/

Kent, K., Pelham, W., Molina, B., Sibley, M., Waschbusch, D., Yu, J., . . . Karch, K. (2011). The academic experience of male high school students with ADHD. *Journal of Abnormal Child Psychology, 39*(3), 451–462. doi:10.1007/s10802-010-9472-4

Kern, L., Dunlap, G., Childs, K. E., & Clarke, S. (1994). Use of a class wide self-management program to improve the behavior of students with emotional and behavioral disorders. *Education and Treatment of Children, 17,* 445–458.

Klein, E. R., Armstrong, S. L., & Shipon-Blum, E. (2013). Assessing spoken language competence in children with selective mutism: Using parents as test presenters. *Communication Disorders Quarterly, 34*(3), 184–195. doi:10.1177/1525740112455053

Koidou, I., Kollias, N., Sdravou, K., & Groulos, G. (2013). Dysphagia: A short review of the current state. *Educational Gerentology, 39*(11), 812–827. doi:10.1080/03601277.2013.766518

Kratochvil, C. (March, 2012). *Why preschoolers are special. The spectrum of developmental disabilities XXXIV "ADHD: Too broad? Too narrow?"* Baltimore, MD: Johns Hopkins School of Medicine.

Kreiser, N. L., & White, S. W. (2014). Assessment of social anxiety in children and adolescents with autism spectrum disorder. *Clinical Psychology: Science and Practice, 21*(1), 18–31. doi:10.1111/cpsp.12057

Lerner, M. D., & Levine, K. (2007). Spotlight method: An integrative approach to teaching social pragmatics using dramatic principles. *Journal of Developmental Process, 2*(2), 91–102. Retrieved from http://icdl.com/

Li, X., Xia, S., Bertisch, H., Branch, C., & DeLisi, L. (2012). Unique topology of language processing brain network: A systems-level biomarker of schizophrenia. *Schizophrenia Research, 141*(2–3), 128–136. doi:10.1016/j.schres.2012.07.026

Liemburg, E. J., Vercammen, A., Ter Horst, G., Curcic-Blake, B., Knegtering, H., & Aleman, A. (2012). Abnormal connectivity between attentional, language and auditory networks in schizophrenia. *Schizophrenia Research, 135*(1–3), 15–22. doi:http://dx.doi.org/10.1016/j.schres.2011.12.003

Lindsay, G., & Dockrell, J. (2012). Longitudinal patterns of behavioral, emotional, and social difficulties and self-concept in adolescents with a history of specific language impairment. *Language Speech and Hearing Services in Schools, 43,* 445–460. doi:10.1044/0161-1461(2012/11-0069

Loeber, R., & Burke, J. D. (2011). Developmental pathways in juvenile externalizing and internalizing problems. *Journal of Research on Adolescence (Blackwell Publishing Limited), 21*(1), 34–46. doi:10.1111/j.1532-7795.2010.00713.x

Mackie, L., & Law, J. (2010). Pragmatic language and the child with emotional/behavioural difficulties (EBD): A pilot study exploring the interaction between behaviour and communication disability. *International Journal of Language & Communication Disorders, 45*(4), 397–410. doi:10.3109/13682820903105137

Mahr, G., & Leith, W. (1992). Psychogenic stuttering of adult onset. *Journal of Speech and Hearing Research, 35*(2), 283–286. doi:10.1044/jshr.3502.283

Majcher, D., & Pollack, M. H. (1996). Childhood anxiety disorders. In L. Hechtman (Ed.), *Do they grow out of it? Long-term outcomes of childhood disorders* (pp. 139–169). Washington, DC: American Psychiatric Press.

Mattison, R. E., Humphrey, F. J., Kales, S. N., Handford, H. A., Finkenbinder, R. L., & Hernit, R. C. (1986). Psychiatric background and diagnoses of children evaluated for special class placement. *Journal of the American Academy of Child Psychiatry, 25*(4), 514–520. doi:10.1016/S0002-7138(10)60011-8

Mattison, R. E., Morales, J., & Bauer, M. A. (1992). Distinguishing characteristics of elementary schoolboys recommended for SED placement. *Behavioral Disorders, 17*(2), 107–114. Retrieved from http://www.eric.ed.gov/

McGinnis, E., & Forness, S. (1988). Psychiatric diagnosis: A further test of special education eligibility, hypothesis. *Monographs in Behavioral Disorder, 11,* 3–10.

McInnes, A., Fung, D., Manassis, K., Fiksenbaum, L., & Tannock, R. (2004). Narrative skills in children with selective mutism: An exploratory study. *American Journal of Speech-Language Pathology, 13*(4), 304–315. doi:1058-0360/04/130-0304

McNamee, C. M. (2004). Using both sides of the brain: Experiences that integrate art and talk therapy through scribble drawings. *Art Ther-*

apy *Journal of the American Art Therapy Association, 21*(3), 136–142. doi:10.1080/07421656.2004.10129495

McNeilly, L. (2013). Health care summit identified need for interprofessional education: Clinicians, researchers, and administrators agree: Changes in health care delivery and reimbursement models make interprofessional education and practice a must. *The ASHA Leader, 18.* doi:10.1044/leader.FTR4.18062013.np

Menzies, R. G., Onslow, M., Packman, A., & O'Brian, S. (2009). Cognitive behavior therapy for adults who stutter: A tutorial for speech-language pathologists. *Journal of Fluency Disorders, 34*(3), 187–200. doi:10.1016/j.jfludis.2009.09.002

Moreno Manso, J. M., García-Baamonde Sánchez, M. E., Blázquez Alonso, M., & Pozueco Romero, J. M. (2012). Pragmatic-communicative intervention strategies for victims of child abuse. *Children and Youth Services Review, 34*(9), 1729–1734. doi:10.1016/j.childyouth.2012.05.003

Mundt, J. C., Vogel, A. P., Feltner, D. E., & Lenderking, W. R. (2012). Vocal acoustic biomarkers of depression severity and response treatment. *Society of Biological Society, 72*(7), 580–587. doi:10.1016/j.biopsych.2012.03.015

Murray, A. D., & Yingling, J. L. (2000). Competence in language at 24 months: Relations with attachment security and home stimulation, *Journal of Genetic Psychology, 161*(2), 133–140. doi:10.1080/00221320009596700

National Center for Educational Statistics (n. d.). *Digest of educational statistics.* Retrieved from http://nces.ed.gov/programs/digest/d13/tables/dt13_204.30.asp

National Institute for Health and Clinical Excellence. (2009). *Attention deficit hyperactivity disorder: Diagnosis and management of ADHD in children, young people and adults* [Clinical guideline; no. 72]. London, UK: Author.

National Institute of Mental Health. (2007, November 12). *Brain matures a few years late in ADHD, but follows normal pattern.* Retrieved from http://www.nimh.nih.gov/science-news/2007/brain-matures-a -few-years-late-in adhd-but-follows-normal-patterns.html

Nelson, J. R., Benner, G. J., & Cheney, D. (2005). An investigation of the language skills of students with emotional disturbance served in public school settings. *Journal of Special Educa-*tion, *39*(2), 97–105. doi:10.1177/0022466905039002 0501

Nelson, J. R., Benner, G. J., & Rogers-Adkinson, D. L. (2003). An investigation of the characteristics of K–12 students with comorbid emotional disturbance and significant language deficits served in public school settings. *Behavioral Disorders, 29*(1) 25–33. Retrieved from http://academia. edu/

Olympia, D., Farley, M., Christiansen, E., Pettersson, H., Jensen, W., & Clark, E. (2004). Social maladjustment and students with behavioral and emotional disorder: Revisiting basic assumptions and assessment issues. *Psychology in the Schools, 41*(8), 835–847. doi:10.1002/pits. 20040

Perry, B. D., & Marcellus, J. E. (1997). The impact of abuse and neglect on the developing brain, *Colleagues for Children, 7,* 1–4.

Perry, V., Albeg, L., & Tung, C. (2012). Meta-analysis of single case design research on self-regulatory interventions for academic performance. *Journal of Behavioral Education, 21,* 217–229.

Price, P. J. (2010). The anatomy of language: A review of 100 fMRI studies published in 2009. *Annals of the N.Y. Academy of the Sciences, 1191*(1), 62–88. doi:10.111/j. 1749-6632.2010.05444.x

Prizant, B. M., Audet, L. R., Burke, G. M., Hummel, L. J., Maher, S. R., & Theadore, G. (1990). Communication disorders and emotional/behavioral disorders in children and adolescents. *Journal of Speech and Hearing Disorders, 55*(2), 179–192. Retrieved from http://jshd.asha.org/

Pungello, E. P., Iruka, I. U., Dotterer, A. M., Mills-Koonce, R., & Reznick, J. S. (2009). The effects of socioeconomic status, race, and parenting on language development in early childhood. *Developmental Psychology, 45*(2), 544–557.

Rappa, L., & Viola, J. *Condensed psychopharmacology 2013: A pocket reference for psychiatry and psychotrophic medications.* Ft. Lauderdale, FL: Rxpsych LLC.

Reynolds, C. R., & Kamphaus, R. W. (2004). *Behavior Assessment System for Children-Second Edition (BASC-2).* Circle Pines, MN: American Guidance Service.

Richards, T., & Bates, C. (1998). Helping children's post-traumatic stress. *Education Digest, 63*(8), 62–67. doi:10.1111/j.1746-1561.1997.tb01294.x

Rochester, S., & Martin, J. R. (1979). *Crazy talk: A study of the discourse of schizophrenic speakers.* New York, NY: Plenum Press.

Rosenblatt, J., Robertson, L., Bates, M., Wood, M., Furlong, M. J., & Sosna, T. (1998). Troubled or troubling? Characteristics of youth referred to a system of care without system-level referral constraints. *Journal of Emotional and Behavioral Disorders, 6*(1), 42–54. doi:10.1177/106342669800600104

Salokangas, R. K. R., Dingemans, P., Heinimaa, M., Svirskis, T., Luutonen, S., Hietala, J., . . . Klosterkötter, J. (2013). Prediction of psychosis in clinical high-risk patients by the schizotypal personality questionnaire. Results of the EPOS project. *European Psychiatry, 28*(8), 469–475. doi:10.1016/j.eurpsy.2013.01.001

Sauter, F. M., Heyne, D., & Westenberg, M. (2009). Cognitive behavior therapy for anxious adolescents: Developmental influences on treatment design and delivery. *Clinical Child and Family Psychology Review, 12*(4), 310–335. doi:10.1007/s10567-009-0058-z

Schmerling, J. D., & Kerins, M. R. (1987). Stimulating communication in a child with elective mutism: Collaborative interventions. *American Journal of Dance Therapy, 10*(1), 27–40. doi:10.1007/BF02251787

Segrin, C., & Flora, J. (1998). Depression and verbal behavior in conversations with friends and strangers. *Journal of Language and Social Psychology, 17*(4), 492–503. doi:10.1177/0261927X980174005

Seiler, W. J., Beall, M. L., & Mazer, J. P. (2014). *Communication making connections* (9th ed.). Upper Saddle River, NJ: Pearson.

Semel, E., Wiig, E. H., & Secord, W. A. (2013). *Clinical Evaluation of Language Fundamentals-Fifth Edition (CELF-5).* San Antonio, TX: Pearson.

Sharp, W. G., Sherman, C., & Gross, A. M. (2007). Selective mutism and anxiety: A review of the current conceptualization of the disorder. *Journal of Anxiety Disorders, 21*(4), 568–579. doi:10.1016/j.janxdis.2006.07.002

Skiba, R. J., & Grizzle, K. (1991). The social maladjustment exclusion: Issues in definition and assessment. *School Psychology Review, 20*(4), 580–598. Retrieved from http://ip-science.thomsonreuters.com/cgi-bin/jrnlst/jloptions.cgi?PC=SS

Snow, P. C., & Powell, M. B. (2011). Oral language competency in incarcerated young offenders: Links with offending severity. *International Journal of Speech-Language Pathology, 13*(6), 480–489. doi:10.3109/16549507.2011.578661

Snow, P. C., Powell, M. B., & Sanger, D. D. (2012). Oral language competence, young speakers, and the law. *Language Speech and Hearing Services in Schools, 43*(4), 496–506. doi:10.1044/0161-1461(2012/11-0065)

St. Clair, M. C., Pickles, A., Durkin, K., & Conti-Ramsden, G. (2011). A longitudinal study of behavioral, emotional, and social difficulties in individuals with a history of speech-language impairment. *Journal of Child Psychology and Psychiatry, 44*(2), 186–199. doi:10.1016/j.jcomdis.2010.09.004

Teicher, M. (2002). Scars that won't heal: The neurobiology of child abuse. *Scientific American, 286*(3), 68–77.

Terrasi, S., Sennett, K. H., & Mackin, T. O. (1999). Comparing learning styles for students with conduct and emotional problems. *Psychology in the Schools, 36*(2), 159–166. doi:10.1002/(SICI)1520-6807(199903)36:2<159::AID-PITS8>3.0.CO;2-O

Tomblin, J. B., Zhang, X., Buckwalter, P., & Catts, H. (2000). The association of reading disability, behavioral disorders, and language impairment among second grade children. *Journal of Child Psychology and Psychiatry, 41*(4), 473–482.

Twenge, J. M. (2000). The age of anxiety? Birth cohort change in anxiety and neuroticism. *Journal of Personality and Social Psychology, 79*(6), 1007–1011. doi:10.1037/0022-3514.79.6.1007

United States Department of Education, Office of Special Education. *Individuals with Disabilities Act (IDEA) database.* Retrieved May 22, 2013, from http://tadnet.public.tadnet.org/pages/712

United States Department of Justice. (2000). *The High/Scope Perry Preschool Project* [Juvenile Justice Bulletin]. Washington, DC: Office of Juvenile Justice.

Vogel, D., & Carter, J. E. (1995). *The effects of drugs on communication disorders.* San Diego, CA: Singular.

Wagner, M., Bechdolf, A., Ruhrmann, S., Klosterkoetter, J., Brinkmeyer, J., Woelwer, W., . . . Frommann, I. (2006). Wc5b auditory P300 is reduced in clinical ultra high risk subjects and may predict conversion to psychosis. *Schizophrenia Research, 86*, S12–S13. doi:10.1016/S0920-9964(06)70038-X

Wagner, M., & Newman, L. (2012). Longitudinal transition outcomes of youth with emotional disturbances. *Psychiatric Rehabilitation Journal,* *35*(3), 199–208. doi:10.2975/25.2.2012.199.208

Way, I., Yelsma, P., Van Meter, A., & Black-Pond, C. (2007). Understanding alexithymia and language skills in children: Implications for assessment and intervention. *Language, Speech and Hearing in Schools, 38,* 128–139. doi:0161-1461/07/3802-0128

Webber, J., & Scheuermann, B. (1997). A challenging future: Current barriers and recommended action for our field. *Behavioral Disorders, 22*(3), 167–178. Retrieved from http://www.eric.ed.gov/

Webster-Stratton, C., & Hammond, M. (1997). Treating children with early-onset conduct problems and a comparison of child and parent training interventions. *Journal of Consulting and Clinical Psychology, 65*(1), 93–109. doi:10.1037/0022-006X.65.1.93

Wechsler, D. (2003). *Wechsler Intelligence Scale for Children- Fourth Edition (WISC-4).* San Antonio, TX: Psychological Corporation.

Wiederholt, J. E., & Bryant, B. R. (2012). *Gray Oral Reading Test-Fifth Edition.* Austin, TX: Pro-Ed.

Wilcox, B. L., Turnbull, R., & Turnbull, A. P. (2000). Behavioral issues and IDEA: Positive behavioral interventions and supports and the functional behavioral assessment in the disciplinary context. *Exceptionality, 8*(3), 173–187. doi:10.1207/S15327035EX0803_4

Wilson, G. T., & Sysko, R. (2006). Cognitive-behavioural therapy for adolescents with bulimia nervosa. *European Eating Disorders Review, 14*(1), 8–16. doi: 10.1002/erv.668

Woodcock, R. W., McGrew, K. S., & Mather, K. (2007). *Woodcock-Johnson III Tests of Cognitive Abilities.* Itasca, IL: Riverside.

Yingthawornsuk, T., & Thanawattano, C. (2010). Comparative study of filter characteristics as statistical vocal correlates of clinical psychiatric state in human. *World Academy of Science, Engineering and Technology, 48,* 839–844. Retrieved from http://www.waset.org/

PART VI

Central Auditory Processing Disorders

CHAPTER 9

Central Auditory Processing Disorders

Donna L. Pitts

Chapter Objectives

Upon completing this chapter, the reader should be able to:

1. Identify and define terms relative to (central) auditory processing disorders [(C)APD]
2. Describe characteristics associated with [(C)APD]
3. Identify intervention strategies associated with specific (central) auditory processing deficits
4. Discuss the collaborative model between the speech-language pathologist and audiologist (and other related professionals) when addressing diagnostic and intervention needs of individuals with [(C)APD]

Introduction

(Central) Auditory Processing Disorder [(C)APD] is an umbrella term often used to describe a group of disorders that affect the way individuals perceive audi-

tory information. In easier terms, auditory processing is how one experiences sound after it leaves the peripheral mechanism, or "what you do with what you hear" (Katz, 1992), so a deficit may result in difficulty in listening. It is important, however, to realize that children with (C)APD may present with symptoms similar to children with hearing impairment; however, these children have normal peripheral hearing sensitivity. It can be assumed that some of these children's listening difficulties may be attributed to (C)APD. Essentially, this chapter refers to (C)APD as processes that occur in the Central Auditory Nervous System (CANS) in response to acoustic stimuli.

Terminology and Definitions Related to the Auditory System

The human auditory system is divided into two main parts. The *peripheral auditory system (mechanism)* refers to an anatomical subsystem of the auditory system consisting of the outer, middle, inner ear, and auditory nerve (CN VIII). The peripheral mechanism is responsible for detecting sound and changing the sound into electrical activity. The *central auditory nervous system* (CANS) refers to the anatomical subsystem consisting of a complex array of nuclei and neurological pathways that originates at the cochlear nucleus and terminates at Heschl's gyrus (cerebral cortex). It is critical to note that the CANS also includes structures in the right and left hemispheres as well as the corpus callosum (McLachlan & Wilson, 2010). The CANS interprets the sounds collected by the peripheral auditory system and interprets those sounds into meaning. *Hearing impairment* refers to a problem in the peripheral auditory system, which results in the inability to hear and differentiate sound. *Auditory processing disorder* is often used interchangeably with *central auditory processing disorder*. The "C" in (C)APD indicates that although APD generally occurs within the CANS, it is recognized that some auditory processing occurs prior to the CANS (ASHA, 2005; Campbell, 2011). Terminology necessary for understanding evaluative tasks of (C)APD is also necessary. *Monaural* refers to one ear stimulation whereas *binaural* refers to both ears being stimulated at the same time. *Dichotic* is similar to binaural in that both ears are stimulated at the same time, but with dichotic stimulation the ears. Finally, *ipsilateral* means on the same side and *contralateral* means on the opposite side.

Definition of (Central) Auditory Processing Disorders

Since it was first described by Mykelbust (1954) as the inability to "structure the auditory world (p. 8)," researchers have been trying to define what (C)APDs are and how they are diagnosed. Over the past several decades, there has been an increase in both professional and public awareness of (C)APD (ASHA, 1996, 2005). The Bruton Conference, which consisted of 14 senior research and clinical audiologists, met in separate groups and in a plenary session to attempt to arrive at a consensus regarding the problem of the diagnosis of auditory processing disorders in school-aged children (Jerger & Musiek, 2000). Additionally, these audiologists (known formally as the Working Group on Auditory Processing Disorders) came to a consensus that the disorder should be identified as an *auditory processing disorder* (APD) thus avoiding the assertion that an auditory processing disorder *must* occur in the central auditory pathway but rather that it is an interaction of disorders (ASHA, 2005). There are many working definitions of (C)APDs but it is broadly defined as a deficit processing information through the auditory modality and more specifically as an inability to process auditory information (ASHA, 2005; Bellis, Chermak, Weihing, & Musiek, 2012). The previously identified working group on (Central) Auditory Processing Disorders provides this definition of (C)APD:

> *(Central) auditory processing disorder* [(C)APD] refers to difficulties in the processing of auditory information in the central nervous system (CNS) as demonstrated by poor performance in one or more of the following skills: sound localization and lateralization; auditory discrimination; auditory pattern recognition; temporal aspects of audition, including temporal integration, temporal discrimination (e.g., temporal gap detection), temporal ordering, and temporal masking; auditory performance in competing acous-

tic signals (including dichotic listening); and auditory performance with degraded acoustic signals (p. 2).

It is crucial for one to understand what each of these processes means, and how a breakdown in one or more of them may lead to a diagnosis of (C)APD.

Sound localization and lateralization refers to the ability to know where a sound has occurred in space; localization is used to identify a source of sound, like a car horn or siren.

Auditory discrimination refers to the ability to distinguish one sound from another. The term is usually used for distinguishing speech sounds, such as phoneme /t/ from phoneme /d/ or /p/ from /b/.

Auditory pattern recognition refers to the ability to determine similarities and differences in patterns of sounds whether they are frequency, or intensity of time specific.

Temporal aspects of auditory processing refers to the ability to sequence sounds, integrate a sequence of sounds into words or other meaningful combinations, and perceive sounds as separate when they quickly follow one another.

Auditory performance with competing signals refers to the ability to perceive speech or other sounds when another signal is present. The other signal might be noise or another similar speech signal, and the competing signal might be soft or loud.

Auditory performance with degraded acoustic signals refers to the ability to perceive a signal in which some of the information is missing. A degraded signal might be one where parts of the sound spectrum have been filtered, or where the sound is compressed in time.

(C)APD and Comorbid Conditions

One dilemma that continually presents itself in the presence of (C)APD is the existence of disorders that share a cause/effect relationship with (C)APD. One such relationship is that of (C)APD and language/learning disabilities. There are varying opinions regarding (C)APD and deficits in language. Some professionals believe that (C)APD is another type of language disorder (Kamhi, 2010; Lovett, 2011; Sharma, Purdy, & Kelly, 2009; Vanni-asegaram, Cohen, & Rosen, 2010; Wallach, 2011). In a retrospective study of 150 children referred for diagnostic APD assessment, Wilson and Arnott (2013) found that the diagnosis of APD ranged from "7.3% to 96%" (p. 67) using criteria established by ASHA and respected researchers in the field of APD. Moreover, they argue that the use of (C)APD as a global label should either be abandoned, or, if a diagnosis is made it is qualified by a statement of criteria used to determine the diagnosis (Wilson & Arnott, 2013). Moore (2011) estimated that the diagnosis of APD could at best be 5%, whereas Campbell (2011) feels that prevalence is too difficult to establish because of a lack of a gold standard of diagnosis. Other research estimates have suggested a prevalence of 2% to 3% in the school-age population (Chermak & Musiek, 2001; Lovett, 2011). Finally, Bamiou, Musiek, and Luxon estimate that about

7% of children have (C)APD (2001). Others consider auditory processing deficits as a separate disorder that expresses deficits in language, attention, and learning. Research supports auditory processing skills to specific areas along the CANS (Campbell, 2011; Loo, Bamiou, & Rosen, 2013; Musiek et al., 2005). An abnormality anywhere along the CANS may cause a (C)APD thus triggering language and/or learning deficits.

Language Delay/Disorder

It is very difficult to separate language and listening skills during behavioral testing. One reason for this is that (C)APD and language disorders are heterogeneous, meaning that a diverse set of problems exists that make up the disorders (Cohen & Rosen, 2004; Medwetsky, 2011; Sharma, Purdy, & Rosen, 2009; Witton, 2010). Furthermore, not all (C)APDs lead to diagnoses of language disorders, and not all language disorders are due to (C)APD, though poor performance in one modality is likely to affect the other resulting in academic difficulties. Dawes and Bishop (2010) looked at comorbidity of APD, SLI, and dyslexia using a battery of tests that included an APD battery, language and literacy evaluation, and a nonverbal intelligence measure. They found a broad overlap between each disorder and felt that rather than focus on a specific diagnosis, the real benefit for children would be to begin an interdisciplinary remediation plan. Similarly, Kerins and Pitts (2005) found an overlap in diagnostic criteria for both APD and language impairment. Using a temporal processing measure (Gaps in Noise-GIN), Zaidan and Baran (2013) found that there was a statistically significant difference in the performance of chil-

dren with dyslexia and/or phonological processing disorder than children identified with normal reading skills. This led them to conclude that an auditory temporal processing deficit should be considered in children with dyslexia or phonological disorders (2013). Prior to that, Tallal (1975) reported poor temporal processing abilities in children who were poor readers so evidence of overlap has been reported for more than 4 decades. Additionally, on self-reported measures, Kreisman, John, Kreisman, Hall, and Crandell (2012) found psychosocial function could not be differentiated between individuals with (C)APD and those with language impairment. Witton (2010) feels strongly that (C)APD should be classified as a developmental disorder similar to other specific developmental disorders because most of the time, there is no obvious medical cause that pinpoints the disorder, and it is unlikely that one cause will ever be identified to determine its existence. There is endless debate on the association between auditory processing and its relationship with language. Some professionals even question if auditory processing disorder is its own disorder or simply a manifestation of a language disorder or delay (Kamhi, 2011; Wilson & Arnott, 2013). Because neuroscience has linked difficulties with auditory processing to specific areas in the central auditory nervous system it can be surmised that problems associated with auditory processing can and do cause complications in the development and processing of language, and, in fact, learning (Campbell, 2011; Moore, 2011; Musiek, 1983). Thus, the evidence supports that rather than focus on the etiology of one specific disorder, an interdisciplinary approach to treatment is essential. In fact, this should be considered before a differential diagnosis is even offered (Bellis, 2003).

Attention Deficit Hyperactivity Disorder

Research has indicated comorbidity of Attention Deficit Hyperactivity Disorder (ADHD) and (C)APD, which has raised the question as to whether the two are a separate diagnostic entity. A study by Riccio, Hynd, Cohen, Hall, and Molt (1994) found that most children diagnosed with ADHD had diagnostic criteria for (C)APD, but less than 50% of those diagnosed with (C)APD had the diagnostic criteria for ADHD (Lovett, 2011). Chermak, Tucker, and Seikel (2002), looking for overlapping behaviors between the two entities, polled audiologists and pediatricians and asked them to rank 58 behavioral symptoms as either (C)APD or ADHD. They found that pediatricians were more likely to rank symptoms of ADHD and audiologists' ranked symptoms for (C)APD. The symptoms of ADHD and (C)APD were comparatively exclusive for the identification of each, and, in fact, only two (inattention and distractibility) of 11 common characteristics of both disorders were found to be common to both. Without a doubt, evidence supports that there is no clear-cut diagnostic indicator to separate them and some estimate 25% to 45% of cases are actually comorbid existence of both. Lovett (2011) argues that (C)APD and ADHD are related disorders even if there is debate whether one can or does contribute to the other.

Characteristics Associated With Auditory Processing Disorder

Many features exist that can call into question the existence of an auditory processing deficit, and some of these features may overlap with other comorbid conditions such as: ADHD, language disorders, and learning disorders (Campbell, 2011; Lovett, 2011; Medwetsky, 2011; Miller, 2011; Wilson & Arnott, 2013; Witton, 2010). Because of this comorbity, it is often difficult to distinguish (C)APD from other similar disorders and to plan for adequate assessment. A child with (C)APD may demonstrate behavioral characteristics that cause concern. Generally, signs will be consistent with a hearing loss in the peripheral auditory system even though peripheral hearing sensitivity has been determined to be within normal limits. It is essential to note that behavioral characteristics do not make a diagnosis, so professionals in general look for a combination of the following characteristics to determine the need for (C)APD testing (AAA, 2010; ASHA, 2005). The list of behavioral characteristics below is not exhaustive but the presence of them can be considered as suspect of (C)APD (Jerger & Musiek, 2000).

- Difficulty comprehending speech in the presence of noise or in acoustic environments
- Decreased attention to auditory stimulus as compared to visual stimulus
- Inconsistent or inappropriate responses to auditory information
- Difficulty following and/or responding to rapid speech
- Difficulty comprehending/ following through multistep directions and/or tasks.
- Poor phonological and/or phonemic awareness skills
- Poor auditory discrimination skills
- Inconsistent responses to auditory stimuli
- Inconsistent auditory attention

Screening for APD

Screening tests and/or checklists for (C)APD may be used for the rudimentary identification of children considered at risk for (C)APD. Because there is no "gold standard" for screening, there is some controversy surrounding the use of them. AAA (2010) expressed concern that screening tools may not accurately identify individuals at risk for (C)APD and even called for more efficient screening tools.

Screening Tools

There are some widely accepted behavioral screening tools used to identify children who may have auditory processing disorders. These include the SCAN-3C (Keith, 2000) and the Differential Screening Test of Processing (Richard & Ferre, 2006). Screening subtests on the SCAN-C include Gap Detection, Auditory Figure Ground, and Competing Words Free recall. These subtests do not necessitate the use of a sound-treated audiometric booth and can be completed with a CD player and headphones in a quiet space, making it easier to utilize in school settings where audiometric equipment may not be standard. Nevertheless, once the screening protocol is complete, the results are then compared to norms and recommendations are made for further evaluation, if necessary.

Checklists

Other easily administered screening tools are checklists. Some of these checklists include Fisher's Auditory Problem checklist (Fisher, 1995); Children's Auditory Performance Scale (CHAPPS; Smoski,

Brunt, & Tannahill, 1998); and Screening Instrument for Targeting Educational Risk (SIFTER; Anderson, 1989). Checklists can be completed by teachers, speech and language pathologists, and/or other educational professionals. The checklists require observers in the classroom or other learning environment to judge students on:

- Attention span
- Listening comprehension
- Following multistep directions
- Phonics
- Immediate recall
- Responses to verbal stimuli
- Motivation for learning
- Distractibility

It is important to remember that checklists should only be used to identify students who may have the potential for (C)APD. In 2007, Wilson et al. found that these tests should only be used to highlight potential problems and those flagged for potential problems should be referred for an APD battery. Those identified should be referred for a complete (C) APD evaluation if selection criteria is met. A complete list of all checklists is found in Table 9–1.

Criteria for Testing

Although checklists may offer some insight into who should be referred for (C)APD evaluation, a set of criteria exist which, if not followed could confound the test results and/or influence the interpretation of the test results. Age is the primary consideration for testing in children. Most behavioral tasks are normed for children of at least 7 years of age (developmentally) (ASHA, 2005). Some tests have norms below that age but there are not

Table 9–1. Questionnaires and Checklists

Buffalo Model Questionnaire (BMQ)
Children's Auditory Performance Scale (CHAPS)
Children's Home Inventory for Listening Difficulties (CHILD)-Parent Version
Children's Home Inventory for Listening Difficulties (CHILD)-Self-reporting
Developmental Index of Audition and Listening (DIAL)
Fisher's Auditory Problems Checklist
Listening Inventory for Education (LIFE) Teacher Appraisal
Listening Inventory for Education (LIFE) Student Appraisal
Scale of Auditory Behaviors (SAB)
Screening Instrument for Targeting Education Risk (SIFTER) Preschool
Screening Instrument for Targeting Education Risk (SIFTER) Elementary
Screening Instrument for Targeting Education Risk (SIFTER) Secondary

enough of them to provide a comprehensive diagnostic battery. Another consideration for testing is cognitive status. Cognitive status (including mental age) of the individual should also be considered as the capacity to complete complex behavioral tasks may be compromised and make accurate interpretation challenging (AAA, 2010). Nonnative English speakers should have the expressive and receptive aptitude to complete the test battery because a language delay may render interpretation impossible (AAA, 2010). Finally, children considered for a (C)APD evaluation should have normal peripheral hearing status bilaterally.

APD Test Battery Determination

Behavioral Testing

There is no gold standard best practice test battery used for the diagnosis of (C)APD (Bellis, Billiet, & Ross, 2011; Jerger & Musiek, 2005). Most of the early empirical data on behavioral tests stems from studies on individuals for whom site of lesion was already established within the CANS (Fifer, Jerger, Berlin, Tobey, & Campbell, 1983; Katz, 1962; Musiek, 1983). These studies provide the foundation for the utilization of many of the behavioral tests used today. In addition, behavioral tests allow for the identification of specific auditory skill(s) weaknesses displayed by an individual. The use of a test battery to determine the presence of a (C)APD is of utmost importance as a battery will likely allow for identification of specific weaknesses or the lack thereof.

Electrophysiological Testing

More recently, the American Academy of Audiology (AAA) (2010) and ASHA (2005) have recommended the use of electrophysiological tests to assist in the diagnosis of (C)APD. Unlike behavioral tests, which require responses from the individual during the evaluation, electrophysiological measures require no response from the individual being tested. Information about the brain's response to sound is measured using electrodes and collected and evaluated against a set of standardized norms. Although electrophysiological testing may allow for testing of the sensory processing of information in the CANS, many clinicians do not have access to electrophysiological equipment, and even if equipment is present, the tests tend to be cost prohibitive to the patient.

Behavioral Tests

A behavioral test battery is one that should incorporate speech and nonspeech instruments that measure a variety of auditory mechanisms at different levels and areas of the CANS (ASHA, 2005). These include dichotic listening, temporal processing/patterning, monaural low redundancy, and binaural interaction and each are delineated below with rationale for the inclusion of each in the test battery.

Dichotic Listening

Dichotic listening tests require the simultaneous presentation of competing messages to each ear and provide information regarding interhemispheric transfer of auditory information. There are two tasks that can be measured with dichotic listening tests: *binaural integration and binaural separation.* Binaural integration requires the patient to repeat to the examiner what is heard in both ears, whereas binaural separation requires the patient to repeat what is heard in one ear while

ignoring what is presented to the opposite ear. A stimulus for dichotic listening tests ranges from digits, to phonemes, words or sentences. Because dichotic listening requires the transfer of information through the contralateral (crossed) pathways these tests provide important information about the development and function of the interactions between hemispheres and the corpus callosum (Jancke, 2002). A test battery for (C)APD should minimally include at least one test of dichotic listening, preferably two (one from binaural interaction and one from binaural separation). See Table 9–2 for a listing of all dichotic tests.

Temporal Processing/Patterning

Auditory signals can be distinguished by a few factors, including, but not limited to, temporal characteristics and spectral information (Robin, Tranel, & Demasio, 1990). Temporal (or time-based) processing of auditory signals is essential for the interpretation of speech and prosody, and complex auditory stimuli such as fundamental frequency and harmonic structure (Bellis, 2003; Johnson, Bellis, & Billiet, 2007; Robin et al., 1990). Additionally, temporal processing is essential for the perception of rapidly alternating speech sounds (Johnson, Bellis, & Billiet, 2007). Temporal behavioral tasks that are time based measure the ability to evaluate time differences in acoustic stimuli. These are frequently referred as to as gap detection tests. Gap detection tests require the patient to identify diminutive silent spaces (or gaps) between two consecutive auditory stimuli. Behavioral temporal sequencing (patterning) tasks require the patient to identify and discriminate sequential auditory events related to the

Table 9–2. Dichotic Listening Tests

Competing Environmental Sounds Test	Binaural Integration
Dichotic Consonant Vowel (CV) Test	Binaural Integration
Dichotic Digits	Binaural Integration
Dichotic Rhyme Test	Binaural Integration
Dichotic Sentence Identification Test	Binaural Integration
Multiple Auditory Processing Assessment (MAPA) Dichotic Digits	Binaural Integration
SCAN 3C Competing Words Subtest	Binaural Integration
Staggered Spondaic Word Test (SSW)	Binaural Integration
Competing Sentences Test (CST)	Binaural Separation
MAPA Competing Sentences Test	Binaural Separation
SCAN 3C Competing Sentences	Binaural Separation
Synthetic Sentence Identification with Contralateral Competing Message (SSI-CCM)	Binaural Separation

pattern of the signal over time (ASHA, 2005). In order for temporal sequencing to occur, there must be efficient interhemispheric communication, which makes these tests sensitive to issues associated with neuro-maturation and interhemispheric pathways dysfunction (Musiek, Pinhiero, & Wilson, 1980). There are two such types of tests of temporal sequencing: one involves frequency recognition and the second involves duration recognition. For the Frequency Pattern Test (FPT), two distinct frequencies are presented in different patterns and the patient is instructed to repeat the pattern given (high vs. low) (Musiek, 1994). For the Duration Pattern Test (DPT), the duration of the stimulus changes rather than the frequency. The patient is instructed to label the length of the signal (long vs. short). It is important to note that on both the FPT and DPT, acceptable responses can also be nonverbal (humming, pointing and/or gestur-

ing). A verbal response would require interhemispheric transfer of information whereas a nonverbal response would not. Patients who can provide a nonverbal response but not a verbal response lack intact interhemispheric interaction, making these tests sensitive to the detection of higher auditory processing problems (Musiek, Pinhiero, & Wilson, 1980). A test battery for (C)APD should include at least one test from each area (processing and patterning). Table 9–3 lists common tests for temporal processing/patterning.

Monaural Low Redundancy Tasks

Monaural low redundancy speech tasks measure the listener's performance on reduced redundancy of speech by changing the quality of the signal in various ways. This is referred to as auditory closure (and/or auditory discrimination) and

Table 9–3. Temporal Processing and Patterning Tests

Auditory Fusion Test-Revised	Temporal Resolution
Gaps in Noise Test	Temporal Resolution
MAPA Gap Detection (AFT-R)	Temporal Resolution
Random Gap Detection Test (RGDT)	Temporal Resolution
SCAN 3C Gap Detection	Temporal Resolution
Duration Pattern Test (DPT)	Temporal Ordering
MAPA Duration Patterns Binaural	Temporal Ordering
MAPA Pitch Pattern Test	Temporal Ordering
MAPA TAP Test	Temporal Ordering

in order to have auditory closure one must be familiar enough with speech and language to fill in what is missing when speech is not clear. The first such measure is Speech in Noise testing, or auditory figure-ground. This evaluates the ability to discriminate speech embedded in a noise signal such as multitalker babble usually presented monaurally. In the past, the ability to discriminate speech in the presence of competing noise was often thought of as the most prevalent characteristic of (C)APD; however, recent evidence suggests that speech in noise tests lack sensitivity in diagnosing APD (AAA, 2010; Iliadou & Bamiou, 2012; Moore, 2011). Children who have difficulty hearing and/or listening in noisy situations and have no known peripheral hearing loss are common in practice. Some researchers (Moore, 2011; Moore, Ferguson, Edmonson-Simers, & Ratib, 2010) suggest that poor listening skills are not associated with difficulty in auditory processing but are more related to children with poor attention skills or working memory deficits. Most evidence here indicates that there is little proof to support that diffi-

culty listening in noise has anything to do with auditory processing disorders. According to Iliadou and Bamiou (2012) when parents rated their children using checklists designed to assess auditory behaviors, there was no difference in the clinical groups (APD vs. non-APD) suggesting that listening in noise may not be a diagnostic characteristic of children with *only* (C)APD. Lagace, Jutras, Giguere, and Gagne (2011) suggest that hearing in noise is caused by a lack of myelination in the central nervous system, which is the cause of poorer listening in noise. In fact, Moore (2011) suggested that difficulty listening to speech in noise is more associated with poor attention or problems with working memory that may or may not specifically be related to audition. Nonetheless, this test is necessary for profiling a child's behavior in a noisy classroom situation. Other low redundancy tests alter the signal by filtering out frequency information, or maintain the quality of the signal but increase the rate at which they are presented. The test battery from this section should include minimally at least one that task that degrades the signal and one that measures performance with competing signals. Table 9–4 lists common tests for low redundancy.

Binaural Interaction (Fusion)

Binaural interaction, or fusion, tasks are indicative of how both ears work together in evaluating auditory input at the brainstem level. These tests are sensitive to time and intensity differences between ears that are primarily tasks of localization and lateralization (AAA, 2010). In one type of test, a patient would be required to attend to and repeat back nonsimultaneous or nonsequential information in a coherent pattern. In another, the patient may be presented with CVC words in which the consonants are presented to one ear and the vowel is presented to the opposite ear. Masking Level Difference (MLD) is another measure of binaural interaction fusion that compares speech threshold responses with masking noise presented in phase and out of phase with the test signal. An improvement in speech intelligibility usually occurs when the target (speech) is spatially separated (out of phase) from the masking and is referred to as a release of masking. When release of masking occurs, it is a good indication that lower brainstem function is intact. With the exception of the MLD, some

Table 9–4. Monaural Low Redundancy Speech (Children's Versions Only)

NU-6 Low-Pass Filtered	Auditory Closure
NU-6 Time Compressed	Auditory Closure
NU-6 Time Compressed + Reverberation	Auditory Closure
SCAN 3C Filtered Words Subtest	Auditory Closure
SCAN 3C Time Compressed Sentences	Auditory Closure
Time Compressed Monosyllabic Word Test	Auditory Closure
Time Compressed Sentence Test	Auditory Closure
Bamford-Kowal-Bench Speech in Noise (BKB-SIN)	Auditory Figure Ground
Discrimination of PB-K in Noise	Auditory Figure Ground
Listening in Spatialized Noise-Sentences (LISN)	Auditory Figure Ground
MAPA Monaural Selective Auditory Attention Test (SAAT)	Auditory Figure Ground
MAPA Speech in Noise for Children and Adults (SINCA)	Auditory Figure Ground
Pediatric Speech Intelligibility Test (PSI)	Auditory Figure Ground
SCAN 3-C Auditory Figure Ground Subtest	Auditory Figure Ground
Selective Auditory Attention Test (SAAT)	Auditory Figure Ground
Speech in Noise (SPIN)	Auditory Figure Ground
Synthetic Sentence Identification-Ipsilateral (SSI-ICM)	Auditory Figure Ground

evidence indicates that these tests are excellent at delineating conditions at the level of the brainstem but they lack sensitivity to (C)APD (Bellis, 2003). Nonetheless, both AAA (2010) and ASHA (2005) consider them to be a standard of the battery for (C)APD. Table 9–5 lists common tests for binaural interaction (fusion).

Other Behavioral Tests

The Phonemic Synthesis Test (PST) is not an audiological (C)APD test. It is a measure of short-term auditory memory, organizational skills, and phoneme decoding. This test requires the patient to discriminate individual speech sounds (phonemes) and synthesize them into words (Katz & Harman, 1981). During this test, individual phonemes are presented to the patient one at a time at about 1 per second and the patient has to say the word those phonemes produce. The test consists of 25 items and some test items include /s-u-p/ = soup and /d-r-e-s/ = dress.

Auditory attention is the ability to focus on specific sounds and then extract some meaning from the sounds. One specific test that is used for auditory attention is the Auditory Continuous Performance Test (ACPT; Keith, 1994). Generally, continuous performance tests require vigilance to a particular task. During the ACPT, the listener is required to raise his hand when one word (dog) is randomly presented in with many distractor words. No recent studies have looked at the overall effectiveness of this ability and previous results were mixed in that one showed a distinction between ADHD and (C)APD (Keith, 1994) and one did not (Riccio, Cohen, Hynd, & Keith, 1995). Moreover, Gomez and Condon (1999) found that auditory processing deficits were more in line with learning disabilities than ADHD. A list of other behavioral tests can be found in Table 9–6.

Electrophysiological Tests

Electrophysiological tests for (C)APD record the brainstem and associated pathways for the brain's response to acoustical stimuli. Some measures are good at evaluating malfunctions low in the brain (Auditory Brainstem Response or ABR) and some are good for assessing symptoms associated with deficits higher in the mid-brain and auditory cortex

Table 9–5. Binaural Interaction Tests

CVC Fusion Test
Intraural Intensity Difference Tonal Patterns (IID)
Masking Level Difference (MLD)
Rapidly Alternating Speech Perception (RASP)
Spondee Binaural Fusion

Table 9–6. Other Behavioral Tests

Auditory Continuous Performance Test (ACPT)
Auditory Processing Abilities Test (APAT)
Differential Screening Test for Processing
Functional Listening Evaluation (FLE)
Phonemic Synthesis Test (PST)
Test of Auditory Perceptual Skills (TAPS)

Note. Data for tables compiled from *Educational Audiology Handbook, Survey of Common Behavioral Audiological Tests of Auditory Processing*, Johnson and Seaton, 2012.

(middle latency responses, late auditory evoked responses, and P300 responses). Even so, electrophysiological test results are compared against a set of norms for determination of abnormalities. New research, which evaluates auditory brainstem (subcortical) responses to complex sounds (cABR), shows how sounds such as speech and music are behaviorally processed in the brain (Skoe & Kraus, 2010). cABR is used to denote that the electrophysiologic characteristics of the auditory brainstem response test are obtained using complex sounds rather than the typical tone bursts or clicks. This test, also known as Bio-Mark, is not yet commercially available but several studies show it can provide insight into how the brainstem processes acoustic information accurately and synchronously. Because this test is objective (electrophysiologic) and can be completed quickly it shows promise in understanding the neural aspect of auditory processing (Skoe & Kraus, 2010). Another study using Bio-Mark found a correlation between subcortical auditory function, and reading and phonological awareness abilities (Banai et al., 2009). Preliminary data show that Bio-Mark may be successful in understanding the differences between learning difficulties due to the temporal aspects of acoustic encoding versus learning difficulties due to other causes (Banai, 2009). Although the Bruton Conference and The Working Group strongly recommended the use of electrophysiological measures as part of a (C)APD battery because these tests have minimal cognitive demand and language influence (ASHA, 2005; Jerger & Musiek, 2000), Emanuel, Ficca, and Korczak (2011) conducted a survey of audiologists and found that very few of the respondents were using these tests in a (C)APD battery. Table 9–7 lists common electrophysiological tests.

Table 9–7. Electrophysiological Tests

Auditory Brainstem Response (ABR)
Middle Latency Response (MLR)
Mismatch Negativity (MMN)
P 300
cABR

Note. Data for table compiled from Clinical Practice Guidelines (AAA, 2010).

Diagnosis of (C)APD

The ASHA (2005) guidelines for (C)APD state that a diagnosis requires demonstration of a weakness of at least two standard deviations below normal in at least two of the following areas: auditory pattern recognition; temporal processing (including temporal integration, discrimination, ordering, and masking): auditory performance with degraded acoustic signals (monaural low redundancy); auditory performance with competing acoustic signals (including dichotic listening); auditory discrimination; and localization and/or lateralization (binaural interaction). Additionally, an individual may be diagnosed with (C)APD if there is a weakness of at least three standard deviations in any one of the above areas.

Ideally, a comparison of patterns of performance across all tests would assist in relating findings to behaviors that fall into profiles to determine if patterns of weakness are present throughout the testing, and that those weaknesses are categorized into models or profiles of (C)APD so that implementation of a modality-specific interdisciplinary auditory rehabilitation plan can be executed (ASHA, 2005). Two such models of (C)APD that are widely used are The Bellis/Ferre and The Buffalo

Model. These models are based upon the performance of the listener. It is important for professionals to remember that some individuals diagnosed with (C)APD may not fit neatly into one profile and, in fact, may display characteristics spread across several different profiles. Thus, clinicians should focus on intervention efforts that support the specific area(s) of weakness.

The Bellis/Ferre Model

These model subtypes were initially described by Ferre (1987) and expanded upon by Bellis and Ferre (2003) and Bellis (2003). The Bellis/Ferre Model has three primary types of (C)APD profiles and two secondary types of (C)APD profiles. The primary profiles are *Auditory Decoding Deficit, Integration Deficit,* and *Prosodic Deficit* and are likely indicative of a (C)APD. The secondary profiles are likely to be similar in the auditory manifestations of (C)APD but are caused by a related disorder and therefore are not be focused on in this chapter. An *Auditory Decoding Deficit* presents much like a child with peripheral hearing loss. Symptoms of this profile include difficulty with auditory discrimination and listening in noise. A child with this type of profile may exhibit difficulty with reading comprehension and spelling and often asks for repetition. Children who have *Auditory Decoding Deficit Profile* do poorly on monaural low redundancy tests of the (C)APD battery and may display a bilateral deficit on dichotic speech tests. The *Integration Deficit Profile* will display weaknesses in processing multisensory information (auditory and visual) and interhemispheric transfers of information. Typically the individual with this profile will have difficulty following multistep tasks and require more time to process information. On the (C)APD bat-

tery, this individual will display a left ear deficit on dichotic listening tasks. Additionally, on tests of Frequency and/or Duration patterns this individual may not be able to linguistically label tests (high vs. low; long vs. short) but will be able to hum or point to the pattern. The *Prosodic Deficit Profile* child has poor temporal processing skills and will have trouble understanding auditory messages because they cannot recognize rhythm, stress, and/or intonation. Some characteristics of this profile include misinterpreting messages, flat affect, poor pragmatic and/or social language skills, and possibly deficits in music appreciation or understanding. The reader is referred to Bellis (2003) for more complete information about this (C)APD model.

The Buffalo Model

The Buffalo Model (Katz, 1992) centers around performance on the Staggered Spondaic Word test (SSW), the Phonemic Synthesis test, and the Speech in Noise test. Additionally, test patterns and characteristics are noted on the SSW test that allows (C)APD to be diagnosed in four categories: *Decoding Deficit, Tolerance Fading Memory Deficit, Organization Deficit, and Integration Deficit.* The Buffalo Model also heavily favors collaboration between audiologists and speech-language pathologists and requires a speech and language evaluation in conjunction with the (C)APD evaluation. The *Decoding Deficit* is characterized by difficulty quickly and accurately processing what is heard. This results in children who have poor phonemic skills, difficulty following a conversation and/or directions and weak oral reading skills. Often, this child will not respond in a classroom situation. The *Tolerance Fading Memory* profile child will show difficulty understanding speech in adverse conditions (such as a noisy and active classroom) or have short-term auditory memory weakness, though in severe cases both characteristics may be present. The individual with the tolerance fading memory profile results in impulsive responses, poor reading comprehension, short attention span, distractibility, and hyperacusis. Children with this type of profile are often mislabeled as ADHD (Masters, Stecker, & Katz, 1998). The *Integration deficit* has two subtypes: *Type I* and *Type II. Integration Type I* has problems similar to a *Decoding Deficit* whereas *Integration Type II* has problems similar to *Tolerance Fading Memory Deficit.* The difference is that the weaknesses in the Integration subtypes are more significantly impaired than with either of the other two types (Katz, 1992). Individuals diagnosed with *an Integration Deficit* typically have been labeled with learning disabilities and occasionally are labeled as dyslexic because they have poor reading skills (Masters, Stecker, & Katz, 1998). Finally, the *Organization Deficit* is one in which individuals tend to be very disorganized both at home and at school. This deficit is not usually diagnosed as a single deficit but in conjunction with another deficit. The reader is referred to Masters, Stecker, and Katz (1998) for more information about this model of (C)APD

Management of (C)APD

Management of (C)APD should be interdisciplinary in nature. Specialists involved could include audiologists, speech-language pathologists (Ferre, 1997; Masters, Stecker, & Katz, 1998), psychologists (Medwetsky, 2009), social workers and/or and psychiatrists (Kreisman et al., 2012); classroom teachers, and learning disability special-

ists. The exact contribution of each team member should be based on the profile or characteristics displayed on the test battery. Regardless of profile, all children diagnosed with an (C)APD could benefit from intervention. Additionally, modality specificity should be indicated when beginning a management plan (Bellis & Ross, 2011; Cacace & MacFarland, 2005; Wallach, 2011; Witton, 2010). Treatment options typically focus on modifying the environment, teaching/using compensatory strategies, and/or remediating the auditory processing deficit (ASHA, 2005). Intervention and treatment are typically provided via a team approach with the audiologist being responsible for environmental changes and auditory training, the speech-language pathologist teaching compensatory strategies and assisting with the remediation of the deficit, and finally the classroom teacher and/ or learning disability specialist implementing and/ or utilizing the treatment plan. The treatment options will focus on the role and actions of the audiologist and speech-language pathologist and is typically based on whether the (C)APD is organic (caused by a specific disorder or lesion in the CANS) or functional (Moore, 2011).

Effective management should include the use of specific interventions to identify (C)APD weaknesses, and even though these may describe symptoms of a student with (C)APD, it does not always translate to the most appropriate intervention (Wallach, 2011). Wallach (2011) summarized the differences in remediation approaches between audiologists and speech-language pathologists, and insisted that the basic principle of intervention for (C)APD is about language. Nevertheless, intervention techniques and specific remediation strategies are based on the profiles outlined earlier in the chapter. Both *bottom-up* treatments and *top-down* treatments can and should be based on the efficacy of the specific problem as it relates to the identified deficit. Bottom-up treatment plans are stimulus driven and intended to improve the encoding of a signal through adaptive stimulation. Top-down treatment plans improve the ability to use metacognitive and metalinguistic strategies and enhance the listener's experiences and expectations to allow strategies to be used (Bellis, 2005).

Auditory Decoding Deficit

Keep in mind that a child with an auditory decoding deficit performs much like a child who has peripheral hearing impairment so most of the time they perform poorly in situations where there is reduced speech intelligibility. Therefore, environmental modifications that would enhance the signal-to-noise ratio may be the first line treatment. Enhancing the acoustic signal improves the overall quality of the signal. Environmental modifications are most likely to occur in the classroom and include:

- Use of an FM system or other assistive listening device
- Preferential classroom seating based on the location of the teacher, not necessarily the front of the classroom
- Reduction of extraneous noise sources if at all possible (i.e., keeping windows closed, not using fans; closed rather than open classrooms)
- Increased use of visual cues to provide auditory/visual association

Children with these types of deficits may also benefit from aural rehabilitation that uses both bottom-up activities that improve auditory perception and noise tolerance, and top-down activities that enhance the linguistic skills. Commercially available programs may also be utilized in the delivery of therapeutic materials. Some of the commercially available programs include Earobics® and Fast ForWord®.

Integration Deficit

With an integration deficit, the child has difficulty processing multimodal information such as visual and auditory, and interhemispheric sharing of information. For those diagnosed with this type of deficit the configuration of the signal (how it is structured) and the quantity of the signal should be the focus of remediation. Preteaching material, including the use of study guides, Spark notes, and note takers should be considered in the classroom. Dichotic listening training shows promise for the remediation of the comprised central auditory pathway. Introduced by Musiek, Chermak, and Weihing (2007), dichotic listening training involves using a decreasing signal on the unimpaired pathway while slowly increasing the signal of the impaired pathway. This allows the impaired pathway to get stronger over time. There are commercially available exercises (Differential Processing Training Program Acoustic Tasks), but this training can also be easily accomplished using recorded materials such as books or music.

Prosodic Deficit

Children with a prosodic deficit lack temporal processing skills and will have trouble understanding auditory messages because they cannot recognize rhythm, stress and/or intonation. Additionally, children with this type of deficit may lack pragmatics and interpreting nonverbal messages. Treatment for this type of deficit would include activities that improve pragmatic and nonverbal language and the use of patterning through rhythm and pattern recognition activities. Kraus and Chandrasekran (2010) evaluated the benefits of formal music training and found that music training sharpened one's sensitivity to the qualities of music and also increased the ability to detect emotional intonation in speech.

Conclusion

Despite the controversy, there is vast evidence to support the existence of a diagnosis of (C)APD. Further, a diagnosis cannot be made on the basis of one test, but rather should be made as a pattern of performances on a battery of tests. It is essential that collaboration between the audiologist, speech-language pathologist, and other appropriate professionals address these auditory deficits. Interdisciplinary efforts will ensure the most accurate diagnosis and remediation plan to address the needs of each individual child. Additionally, clinicians should periodically evaluate the effectiveness of the treatment.

Case Study 1: Stephen

The following case study shows the thinking of the audiologist throughout the assessment process. The commentary is noted in the italicized text.

Stephen, an 8-year, 2-months-old boy, was referred for an assessment to address

concerns noted by the classroom teacher and learning specialist at his school. He is finishing 2nd grade at a private Catholic school and is having difficulty with poor short-term memory as well as sound blending, which has led to difficulty with reading and spelling. A speech-language pathologist is currently seeing him twice a week for 30 minutes for articulation therapy. His parents, who reported that Stephen has a long-term history of middle ear effusion, which necessitated the surgical insertion of pressure equalization (PE) tubes on two separate occasions, accompanied Stephen to the evaluation. Reportedly, the second set of PE tubes is still in place. Mom reported that Stephen passed a hearing screening following the last set of PE tubes approximately 9 months ago. She also reported that Stephen's language milestones were delayed for first word (age 18 months; normal = 9–13 months), 2-word utterances (age 23 months; normal = 13–18 months), and sentences (age 4 years; normal = 2½–3 years).

Stephen is a very talkative child with multiple articulation errors, which makes it difficult to understand and follow the direction of his conversation. This could influence how certain parts of the evaluation may be scored, so in order to prevent articulation errors from interfering with the audiological evaluation, the Word Intelligibility by Picture Identification (WIPI) test will be used for word discrimination. Since parents reported PE tubes in place they should be visualized during otoscopy and tympanometry should yield flat tympanograms with high physical volume measures.

Cursory otoscopic inspection revealed unoccluded external auditory meati. Tympanic membranes (TM) were easily visualized and PE tubes were observed in each TM. Tympanometry results indicated flat Type B tympanograms, characterized by high physical volume in each ear. These results are consistent with patent PE tubes in each ear. Peripheral hearing sensitivity was evaluated using standard audiometric technique for octave band frequencies 250 Hz to 8000 Hz and indicated normal hearing sensitivity bilaterally. Picture spondee words were used to obtain Speech Reception Thresholds (SRT), and Word Intelligibility by Picture Index (WIPI) was used to determine word discrimination ability. SRTs were in good agreement with pure-tone averages and word discrimination was excellent in each ear.

Errors in articulation may unduly influence the results of the auditory processing evaluation so gestures and other nonverbal responses may be necessary for accurate scoring of the test results. A battery of tests for the evaluation will be based on specific issues with auditory processing but should also be sensitive to the multiple articulation errors noted on the speech and language evaluation. Tests that do not require spoken responses for every test item will be utilized as much as possible.

Stephen scored 2 to 3 standard deviations below normal on the SSW, slightly below one standard deviation below normal for in both ears for both the NU-6 Filtered Words Test and the NU-6 Time Compressed Words Test. The FPT test was well within normal limits in each ear as was Dichotic Digits.

Review Questions

1. Based on the selected test battery, which model of auditory processing should be used to determine the auditory processing profile?

2. Are there any additional tests that should have been completed?

3. Can a diagnosis of (C)APD be made based on the results of the test battery?

4. What recommendations would you make for Stephen?

Case Study 2: Adam

Adam is a 9-year, 11-month boy who will begin 4th grade next month. The psychologist at his school referred him for auditory processing evaluation based on classroom observations that included distractibility, irritability, and difficulty following multistep directions. A psycho-educational evaluation completed at the beginning of 2nd grade indicated a propensity toward Attention Deficit/Hyperactivity Disorder (ADHD). His full-scale IQ on the Wechsler Intelligence Scale for Children (WISC-IV) was 107 and there was no indication of a learning disability. He did demonstrate some scatter in areas related to continuous performance, which the examiner attributed to the possibility of ADHD. The examiner then provided checklists to Adam's classroom teacher and his parents and scores showed a tendency for ADHD, more so from the teacher than the parents.

His parents accompanied Adam to the evaluation, and indicated that although they felt he was overly active at times, they disagreed with the ADHD diagnosis. There were no complications at birth and Adam met all developmental milestones appropriately. His parents are concerned that Adam has begun to fall behind in his classes even though he has accommodations in place to address ADHD. They are hesitant to start Adam on medications for ADHD, but now wonder if that may ease his transition into 4th grade.

Adam presented as an active boy who easily engaged with the examiner. He had no difficulty following tasks or interacting with the examiner. He was inquisitive and even informed the examiner that he "remembered having his hearing tested at school when he was younger." Otoscopy indicated clear external meati and easily visualized tympanic membranes. Tympanometry results were consistent with normal middle ear function bilaterally. Peripheral hearing sensitivity was within normal limits for each ear. Adam was alert and attentive during all phases of testing. Results from test battery show very poor SPIN test results (32%/40%) and poor results on the NU-6 Time Compressed Words test. Furthermore, the ACPT was well within the normal limits of the test parameters.

Review Questions

1. Why do you think Adam had previously been diagnosed with ADHD?

2. What behaviors that Adam displayed prior to and during testing would assist with the findings of the evaluation?

3. Using the Buffalo Model as a guideline, which profile is most closely associated with Adam's profile?

4. What recommendations would you make for Adam?

Case Study 3: Emily

Emily is 13 years, 7 months and is a student in the 8th grade at Holy Angels Catholic School. She was referred for testing by her parents John and Susie who accompany her to the evaluation today. Developmental milestones were all reached at an appropriate age and dad noted that

Emily was "quite the chatterbox" even as a young toddler. Her parents report Emily is socially a little bit awkward. When she was in elementary school, it wasn't as apparent as it is now. They are concerned that her awkwardness will be even more apparent when she begins high school next year. Her parents also noted that schoolwork has been progressively and increasingly more difficult for Emily to complete and expressed concerned about the level of work she will have to complete in high school. Her report card went from As and Bs in elementary school to mostly Cs now. Both of her parents are musicians and love to play and listen to music but Emily does not share this appreciation. After forcing her to play piano for several years, they finally relented and let her stop because she was not getting better and hated to practice. Emily reported that she is a loner and does not have many friends. Lately, it seems to take forever for her to complete her schoolwork, which results in her bringing it home to finish. On top of this, she has homework to do and is often up late trying to complete her assignments. This results in late nights, early mornings, and grouchiness. She doesn't have friends because she doesn't have time for friends. She reports that her grades are OK but they used to be better and thinks her parents make too much of a deal about her grades. Emily had difficulty maintaining eye contact during the interview and seemed to have a flat affect.

Tympanometry results were indicative of normal middle ear function and no issues were noted during otoscopy. Peripheral hearing sensitivity was evaluated using standard audiometric technique for octave band frequencies 250 Hz to 8000 Hz, and indicated normal peripheral hearing sensitivity bilaterally. Quantitative results on the SSW were within normal limits; however, Emily displayed a large number of reversals of test material; she got the information correct, but in the wrong order. SPIN and Time Compressed Speech tests (given at the adult level of 60%) were normal for each ear. On the Frequency Pattern Test (FPT) and the Duration Pattern Test (DPT Emily scored more than 2 standard deviations below age-appropriate norms in each ear on both tests when using a verbal response mode. However, when Emily was reassessed for both FPT and DPT using a nonverbal response, her scores were within the normal limits in each ear.

Review Questions

1. What Bellis/Ferre Model deficit is Emily displaying based on test results?

2. What do you think the results of another monaural low redundancy test would be based on the findings?

3. Why were Emily's test results for FPT and DPT better for the nonverbal response mode?

4. What recommendations would you make for Emily?

References

American Academy of Audiology. (2010). *Guidelines for the diagnosis, treatment and management of children and adults with central auditory processing disorder.* Retrieved September 27, 2012, from http://www.audiology.org

American Speech-Language-Hearing Association. (1996). Central auditory processing: Current status of research and implications for clinical practice. *American Journal of Audiology, 5,* 2.

American Speech-Language-Hearing Association Working Group on Auditory Processing Disorders. (2005). *Central auditory processing.* Retrieved August 12, 2012, from http://www.asha.org/members/deskref-journals

Bamiou, D-E, Musiek, F. E., & Luxon, L. M. (2001). Aetiology and clinical presentations of auditory processing disorders—A review. *Archives of the Disordered Child, 85,* 361–365.

Banai, K., Hornickel, J. M., Skoe, E., Nicol, T., Zecker, S., & Kraus, N. (2009). Reading and subcortical auditory function. *Cerebral Cortex, 19,* 2699–2707. doi:10.1093/cercor/bhp024

Bellis, T. J. (2003). *Assessment and management of central auditory processing disorders in the educational setting: From science to practice.* San Diego, CA: Delmar Cengage Learning.

Bellis, T. J., Billiet, C., & Ross, J. (2011). The utility of visual analogs of central auditory tests in the differential diagnosis of (central) auditory processing disorder and attention deficit hyperactivity disorder. *Journal of the American Academy of Audiology, 22,* 501–514. doi:10.3766/jaaa.22.8.3

Campbell, N. (2011). Supporting children with auditory processing disorder. *British Journal of Nursing, 6,* 273–277.

Chermak, G. D., Tucker, E., & Seikel, J. (2002). Behavioral characteristics of auditory processing disorder and attention-deficit hyperactivity disorder: Predominantly inattentive type. *Journal of the American Academy of Audiology, 13*(6), 332–338.

Dawes, P., & Bishop, D. V. (2010). Psychometric profile of children with auditory processing disorder and children with dyslexia. *Archives of Disease in Childhood, 95,* 432–436. doi:10.11 36/adc.2009.170118

Emanuel, D. C., Ficca, K. N., & Korczak, P. (2011). Survey of the diagnosis and management of auditory processing disorder, *American Journal of Audiology, 20,* 48–60. doi:10.1044/10590889

Ferre, J. M. (1987). Pediatric central auditory processing disorder: Considerations for diagnosis, interpretation and remediation. *Journal of the Academy of Rehabilitative Audiology, 20,* 73–81.

Fey, M. E., Richard, G. J., Geffner, D., Kamhi, A. G., Medwetsky, L., Paul, D., . . . Schooling, T. (2011). Auditory processing disorder and auditory/language interventions: An evidence-based systematic review. *Language, Speech and Hearing Services in Schools, 42*(3), 246–264. doi:10.1044/0161-1461

Fifer, R. C., Jerger, J. F., Berlin, C. I., Tobey, E. A., & Campbell, J. C. (1983). Development of a dichotic sentence identification (DSI) test for use in hearing impaired adults. *Ear and Hearing, 4*(6), 300–306.

Fisher, L. I. (1980). *Fisher's Auditory Problems Checklist*. Cedar Rapids, IA: Grant Wood.

Gomez, R., & Condon, M. (1999). Central auditory processing ability in children with ADHD with and without learning disabilities. *Journal of Learning Disabilities, 32*(2), 150–158. doi:10.1177/002221949903200205

Iliadou, V., & Bamiou, D. E. (2012). Psychometric function of children with auditory processing Disorder (APD): Comparison with normal hearing and non-APD groups. *Journal of Speech, Language and Hearing Research, 55*(3), 791–799. doi:10.1044/1092-4388(2011/11-0035)

Jancke, L. (2002). Does "callosal delay" explain ear advantage in dichotic monitoring? *Laterality, 7,* 309–320.

Jerger, J., & Musiek, F. E. (2000). Report of the Consensus Conference on the Diagnosis of Central Auditory Processing Disorder in Children. *Journal of the American Academy of Audiology, 11,* 467–474.

Johnson, C. D., & Seaton, J. B. (2012). *Education audiology handbook* (2nd ed.). Clifton Park, NY: Delmar Cengage Learning.

Kamhi, A. G. (2010). What speech-language pathologists need to know about auditory processing disorder. *Language, Speech and Hearing Services in Schools, 42,* 265–272. doi:10.1044/0161-1461

Katz, J. (1962). The use of staggered spondaic words for assessing the integrity of the central auditory nervous system. *Journal of Auditory Research, 2,* 327–337.

Katz, J. (1992). Classification of auditory processing disorder. In J. Katz, N. Stecker, & D. Henderson (Eds.), *Central auditory processing: A transdisciplinary view*. St. Louis, MO: Mosby.

Katz, J., & Harmon, C. (1981). Phonemic synthesis: Diagnostic and training program. In R. Keith (Ed.), *Central auditory and language disorders in children*. Houston, TX: College Hill Press.

Keilmann, A., Läßig, A. K., & Nospes, S. (2013). Symptoms and diagnosis of auditory processing disorder. *HNO, 61*(8), 707–715. doi:10.1007/s00106-1=013-2732-1

Keith, R. W. (1994). *Auditory Continuous Performance Test*. Upper Saddle River, NJ: Pearson Products.

Keith, R. W. (2000). Development and standardization of the SCAN-C test for auditory processing disorders in children. *Journal of the American Academy of Audiology, 11*(8), 438–445.

Kerins, M. R., & Pitts, D. L. (2005). Auditory processing disorders in children: A interdisciplinary approach. *Perspectives on School-Based Issues, 6*(1), 20–24. doi:10.1044/sbi6.1.20

Kraus, N., & Chandrasekaran, B. (2010). Music training for the development of auditory skills. *Nature Reviews Neuroscience, 11,* 599–605. doi:10.1038/nrn2882

Kreisman, N. V., John, A. B., Kreisman, B. M., Hall, J. W., & Crandell, C. C. (2012). Psychosocial status of children with auditory processing disorder. *Journal of the American Academy of Audiology, 23*(3), 222–233. doi:10.3766/jaaa.23.3.8

Lagacé, J., Jutras, B., Giguère, C., & Gagné, J. P. (2011). Speech perception in noise: Exploring the effect of linguistic context in children with and without auditory processing disorder. *International Journal of Audiology, 50*(10), 385–395. doi:10.3109/14992027.2011.553204.

Lovett, B. J. (2011). Auditory processing disorder: School psychologist beware? *Psychology in the Schools, 48*(8), 855–867. doi:10.1002/pits.20595

Masters, M. G., Stecker, N. A., & Katz, J. (1998). *Central auditory processing disorders: Mostly management*. Boston, MA: Allyn & Bacon.

McLachlan, M. F., & Wilson, S. (2010). A central role of recognition in auditory perception: A neurobiological model. *Psychological Review, 117*(1), 175–196. doi:10.1037/a0018063

Medwetsky, L. (2011). Spoken language processing model: Bridging auditory and language processing to guide assessment and intervention. *Language, Speech and Hearing Services in Schools, 42,* 286–296. doi:10.1044/0161-1461

Miller, C. A. (2011). Auditory processing theories of language disorders: Past, present and future. *Language, Speech and Hearing Services in Schools, 42,* 309–319. doi:10.1044/0161-1461

Moore, D. R. (2011). The diagnosis and management of auditory processing disorder. *Language, Speech and Hearing Services in Schools, 42,* 303–308. doi:10.1044/0161-1461

Moore, D. R., Ferguson, M. A., Edmondson-Jones, A. M., Ratib, S., & Riley, A. (2010). Nature of auditory processing disorder in children. *Pediatrics, 126,* 382–390. doi:10.1542/peds.20092826

Moore, D. R., Roden, S., Bamoiou, D. E., Campbell, N. G., & Sirimanna, T. (2013). Evolving concepts of developmental auditory processing disorder (APD): A British Society of Audiology APD Special Interest Group "white paper." *International Journal of Audiology, 52*(1), 3–13. doi:10.3109/14992027.2012.723143.

Musiek, F. E. (1983). Assessment of central auditory dysfunction: Dichotic digits revisited. *Ear and Hearing, 4,* 316–322.

Musiek, F. E., Chermak, G., & Weihing, J. (2007). Auditory training. In F. E. Musiek & G. D. Chermak (Eds.), *Handbook of (central) auditory processing disorder: Comprehensive intervention* (Vol. 1, pp. 77–106). San Diego, CA: Plural.

Musiek, F. E., Pinheiro, M. L., & Wilson, D. (1980). Auditory pattern perception in "split-brain" patients. *Archives of Otolaryngology, 106,* 610–612.

Musiek, F. E., Shinn, J. B., Jersa, R., Bamiou, D., Baran, J. A., & Zaidan, E. (2005). GIN (Gaps in Noise) test performance in subjects with confirmed central auditory nervous system involvement. *Ear and Hearing, 26,* 608–618.

Mykelbust, H. R. (1954). *Auditory disorders in children: A manual for differential diagnosis.* New York, NY: Grune & Stratton.

Nickisch, A., & Massinger, C. (2009). Auditory processing in children with specific language impairments: Are there deficits in frequency discrimination, temporal auditory processing or general auditory processing? *Folia Phoniatrica et Logopaedica, 61*(6), 323–328. doi:10.1159/000252848

Pinheiro, M. L., & Musiek, F. E. (1985). Sequencing and temporal ordering in the auditory System. In M. L. Pinheiro & F. E. Musiek (Eds.), *Assessment of central auditory dysfunctions: Foundations and clinical correlates.* Baltimore, MD: Williams & Wilkins.

Riccio, C. A., Cohen, M. J., Hynd, J. W., & Keith, R. L. (1995). Validity of the auditory continuous performance test on differentiating central auditory processing disorders with and without ADHD. *Journal of Learning Disabilities, 29,* 561–566.

Riccio, C. A., Hynd, J. W., Cohen, M. J., Hall, J., & Molt, L. (1994). Comorbidity of central auditory processing disorder and attention-deficit hyperactivity disorder. *Journal of the American Academy of Child & Adolescent Psychiatry, 33*(6), 849–857. doi:10.1097/00004583-199407000-00011

Richard, G., & Ferre, J. (2006). *Differential Screening Test for Processing.* East Moline, IL: LinguiSystems.

Robin, D. A., Tranel, D., & Damasio, H. (1990). Auditory perception of temporal and spectral events in patients with focal left and right cerebral lesions. *Brain and Language, 39,* 539–555.

Sharma, M., Purdy, S. C., & Kelly, A. S. (2009). Comorbidity of auditory processing, language and reading disorders. *Journal of Speech, Language and Hearing Research, 52,* 706–722. doi:10.1044/1092-4388

Skoe, E., & Kraus, N. (2010). Auditory brainstem response to complex sound: A tutorial. *Ear and Hearing, 31*(3), 302–324. doi:10.1097/AUD.0b013e3181cdb272

Tallal, P. (1975). A different view of auditory processing factors in language disorders. *Journal of Speech and Hearing Disorders, 40,* 413–415.

Vanniasegaram, I., Cohen, M., & Rosen, S. (2004). Evaluation of selected auditory tests in school-age children suspected of auditory processing disorders. *Ear and Hearing, 25,* 586–597. doi:10.1097/01

Wallach, G. P. (2011). Peeling the onion of auditory processing disorder: A language/curricular based perspective. *Language, Speech and Hearing Services in Schools, 42,* 273–285. doi:10.1044/0161-1461

Wilson, W. J., & Arnott, W. (2013). Using different criteria to diagnose (C)APD: How big a difference does it make? *Journal of Speech, Language, and Hearing Research, 56*(1), 63–70. doi:10.1044/1092-4388

Wilson, W. J., Jackson, A., Pender, A., Rose, C., Wilson, J., Heine, C., . . . Khan, A. (2011). The CHAPS, SIFTER, and TAPS-R as predictors of (C)AP skills and (C)APD. *Journal of Speech, Language, and Hearing Research, 54*(1), 278–291. doi:10.1044/1092-4388

Witton, C. (2010). Childhood auditory processing disorder as a developmental disorder: The case for a multi-professional approach to diagnosis and management. *International Journal of Audiology, 49,* 83–87. doi:10.3109/14992020903289808

Zaidan, E., & Baran, J. A. (2013). Gaps in Noise (GIN) test results in children with and without reading disabilities and phonological processing deficits. *International Journal of Audiology, 52*(2), 113–123. doi:10.3109/149920207.2012.733421

Index

Note: Page numbers in **bold** reference non-text material.